A MEDICAL STUDY AND REVIEW
GUIDE FOR THE PANCE, PANRE
& MEDICAL EXAMINATIONS

2nd edition

PANCE PREP PEARLS

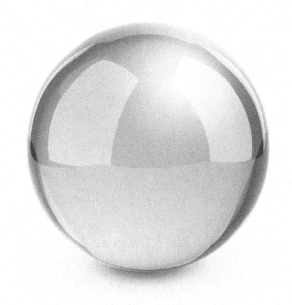

ISBN-13: 978-1542330299
ISBN-10: 1542330297
Library of Congress Control Number: 2017900426
CreateSpace Independent Publishing Platform, North Charleston, SC

Printed by CreateSpace, An Amazon.com Company

DEDICATION

I would like to thank the Cornell and Long Island University Physician Assistant Programs for giving me the platform to teach. Thanks to my foundation teachers Marion Masterson, Medea Valdez, Gerard Marciano. A very special thanks to Stacey Hughes (Words can't describe my gratitude to you), Sharon Verity and William Ameres for being my inspirational teachers as a student. To all those who contributed to making this profession great and to all my fellow educators who contribute to this field on so many levels.

Thanks to all of the owners of the photos. Your images helped to make this book a visual experience. Your contribution is invaluable. An extra special thanks to **Ian Baker**, the illustrator of most of the pictures in the book. You added a special touch to this project. Thanks Dr. Frank Gaillard and Jason Davis for your help during the process. Special thanks to **Kevin Young, Xiana Flowers & Kristen Risom** (the best illustrators I know!)

Special thanks to my parents Winifred & Robert Williams. Xiomara & Froylan Flowers (my second parents), Mercedes Avalon, Gilda Cain (the best nurse I know!) and my big brother Danilo Avalon.

To my gurus: Stacey Hughes, Tse-Hwa Yao, Ingrid Voigt, Dr. Antonio Dajer & Dr. Kenneth Rose.

Thanks to Isaak Yakubov (my Akim) for the Ultimate Mnemonic Comic Book and the amazing journey we have embarked on together. Thanks to Rachel Lehrer for allowing me to be a part of the FlipMed medical app project. I will make good on the promise I made to you.

To my amazing mentor John Bielinski Jr. Thank you for taking me under your wing and believing in me. I am forever grateful for all that you have done and I am looking forward to all of the things our synergy will have in store for us.

Pamela Bodley, the world's best manager. You are the real boss lady!

Last but not least a very special thank you to my PPP warriors. I enjoy our interactions on social media and at conferences. This book would not have been the success it is without the support of each and every one you! YOU ARE A WARRIOR.....WARRIORS WIN!

PREFACE

STUDENTS
This book is designed for use in both didactic and clinical education. It is formatted to make you a rockstar on clinical rotations! It is a **_review book_**, which means **it is not meant to replace textbook-based education** but as an additional study tool to enhance your knowledge base. Textbooks provide the foundation for understanding and learning medicine.

PRACTITIONERS
This book is purposed to increase your knowledge & retention of important clinical information and for use as a quick resource that is not time consuming.

THE STYLE OF PPP
Pance Prep Pearls is not written in the traditional style of a textbook but rather to feel like a collection of notes, drafts, charts, mnemonics and clinical pearls to make learning effective while entertaining. The use of bold and italics are to help you to organize the information and stress the importance of certain aspects of the disease states. The charts are designed for you to compare and contrast commonly grouped diseases and high-yield information. It is loaded with helpful algorithms to help you see the big picture on how to approach the disease.

I personally recommend that you use what I call the 5 P's of the **Patient-Centered Learning Model** as you study the different diseases:
1. **Pathophysiology:** imagine explaining the pathophysiology of a disease to your patient in 1 sentence (2 sentences maximum) in simple terms. Understanding the pathophysiology will often explain the clinical manifestations, physical examination findings, why certain tests are used and usually the treatment reverses the pathophysiology. This step is often skipped but is probably the most important (in terms of knowledge retention).
2. **Present** – based on the pathophysiology, how would this patient present? Know both the classic and the common findings and presentations (they aren't always the same).
3. **Pick it up**? – How would you diagnose the disease. Make sure to understand what is usually first line vs. gold standard (definitive diagnosis). Understand the indications and contraindications for each test.
4. **Palliate** – how do you treat (palliate) the disorder. Many people can list out the treatments but fail to remember first line treatments vs. alternative treatments. Make sure to understand the indications and contraindications of each treatment.
5. **Pharmacology** – understand the mechanism of action and understand why a medication is used for that disease. This helps to reinforce the pathophysiology as well as the presentation of the disease since the pharmacology often reverses the problem or treats the symptoms. A very important point is that if you see a medication that is used for different disorders, try to understand what connects the use of that drug to the different disorders.

TABLE OF CONTENTS

ABBREVIATIONS (SHORT-HAND) USED

Please note some are recognized medical abbreviations and many others are just abbreviations used to simplify layout of the material

±	May or May not	LAD	Lymphadenopathy
Δ	Changes	LDL	Low Density Lipoprotein
Ab/Ag	Antibody/Antigen	LLD	Left Lateral Decubitus
Abx	Antibiotics	LN	Lymph Nodes
AICD	Automated Implantable Cardioverter Defibrillator	LE/UE	Lower extremity/Upper Extremity
ALP	Alkaline Phosphatase	LES	Lower Esophageal Sphincter
Assoc	Associated	MC	Most Common
Asx	Asymptomatic	MOA	Mechanism of Action
b/c	Because	mos.	Months
Bx	Biopsy	Nml	Normal
C	With	NO	Nitric Oxide
Cx	Complication	NTG	Nitroglycerin
d	Days (d), weeks (wks), months (mos)	NSAID	Non Steroidal Antinflammatory Drugs
d/o	Disorder	N/V/D	Nausea/Vomiting/Diarrhea
DOC	Drug of choice	OCP	Oral Contraceptives
DOE	Dyspnea on exertion	PCI	Percutaneous Coronary Intervention
DM/DI	Diabetes Mellitus/Diabetes Insipidus	PG	Prostaglandins
Dx	Diagnosis	PE	Pulmonary Embolism or Physical Examination
Dz	Disease	PND	Paroxysmal Nocturnal Dyspnea
EGD	Endoscopy (Esophagogastroduodenoscopy)	PO/IM/IV	Oral/Intramuscular/Intravenous
ESLD	End Stage Liver Disease	PPM	Permanent Pacemaker
esp.	Especially	PUD	Peptic Ulcer disease
ETOH	Alcohol	Pt	Patient
EF	Ejection Fraction	r/o	Rule out
Ex.	Example	RUQ/LUQ	Right upper quadrant/Left Upper Quadrant
Fhx	Family history	Rxn	Reaction
GGT	Gamma-glutamyl transpeptidase	S	Without
h/a	Headache	S/E	Side effects
HCC	Hepatocellular carcinoma	SL	Sublingual
HCTZ	Hydrochlorothiazide	s/p	Status post (after)
HDL	High Density Lipoprotein	Sx	Symptoms
h/o	History of	TI	Therapeutic Index
HSN	Hypersensitivity	TWI	T-wave Inversion
HSV	Herpes simplex virus	Tx	Treatment
HTN	Hypertension	SBP/DBP	Systolic/Diastolic Blood pressure
Hx	History	US	Ultrasound
Ind	Indications	Us	Usually
Ind. Bili	Indirect Bili D. Bili = Direct Bilirubin	VZV	Varicella Zoster Virus
IP	Incubation Period	Wt	Weight
K, Na, Mg	Potassium (Kalium), Sodium (Natrium), Magnesium	w/u	Workup
L, R	Left, Right	XRT	Radiation Therapy

CHAPTER 1 – CARDIOVASCULAR DISORDERS

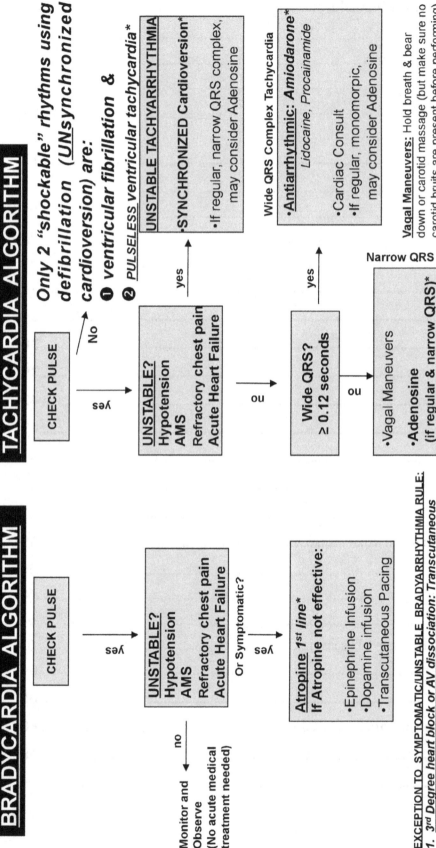

TACHYCARDIA ALGORITHM

Only 2 "shockable" rhythms using defibrillation (UNsynchronized cardioversion) are:
❶ ventricular fibrillation &
❷ PULSELESS ventricular tachycardia*

CHECK PULSE

No

yes

UNSTABLE?
Hypotension
AMS
Refractory chest pain
Acute Heart Failure

no

Wide QRS?
≥ 0.12 seconds

ou

yes

yes

Narrow QRS Complex

•Vagal Maneuvers
•Adenosine
(if regular & narrow QRS)*
•Beta Blocker or Calcium Channel Blocker

ou

UNSTABLE TACHYARRHYTHMIA

•SYNCHRONIZED Cardioversion*

•If regular, narrow QRS complex, may consider Adenosine

Wide QRS Complex Tachycardia

•Antiarrhythmic: *Amiodarone**
    Lidocaine, Procainamide

•Cardiac Consult
•If regular, monomorpic, may consider Adenosine

Vagal Maneuvers: Hold breath & bear down or carotid massage (but make sure no carotid bruits are present before performing)

3 IMPORTANT EXCEPTIONS TO STABLE TACHYARRHYTHMIA RULE:

1. ATRIAL FLUTTER: *Beta blocker or Calcium Channel Blocker 1st line** (skip adenosine).
2. ATRIAL FIBRILLATION: *Beta blocker or Calcium Channel Blocker 1st line** (skip adenosine even though A flutter is often regular with narrow QRS)
3. WOLFF-PARKINSON-WHITE (WPW): *Procainamide preferred** or Amiodarone
    Avoid use of AV nodal blockers (ABCD) in WPW
    ABCD = Adenosine, Beta blockers, Calcium channel blockers, Digoxin

BRADYCARDIA ALGORITHM

CHECK PULSE

yes

UNSTABLE?
Hypotension
AMS
Refractory chest pain
Acute Heart Failure

Or Symptomatic?

no

Monitor and Observe
(No acute medical treatment needed)

yes

Atropine 1st line*
If Atropine not effective:

•Epinephrine Infusion
•Dopamine infusion
•Transcutaneous Pacing

EXCEPTION TO SYMPTOMATIC/UNSTABLE BRADYARRHYTHMIA RULE:
1. 3rd Degree heart block or AV dissociation: *Transcutaneous pacing usually first line** followed by permanent pacemaker placement as definitive treatment.

β-Blockers:
Metoprolol, Esmolol, Propranolol

Calcium Channel Blockers
Non-dihydropyridines*
    Verapamil, Dilitiazem

ECG CHEAT SHEET

STEP 1: DETERMINE THE RHYTHM

Regular or Irregular?
   ☑ *Use Rhythm strip.* Check R-R intervals. If < 0.12 second difference, consider it a regular rhythm.

STEP 2: DETERMINE THE RATE

If *Regular* rhythm ⇨ 1500/# of small squares **OR** 300-150-100-75-60-50 method between an R-R interval.
If *Irregular* rhythm ⇨ count the number of R waves in a 6 second strip & multiply that number by 10.

STEP 3: DETERMINE THE QRS AXIS

	Normal	LAD	RAD
Lead I	+	+	-
aVF	+	-	+

If Left Axis Deviation (LAD) based on I and aVF ⇨ check lead II.
- *If QRS is predominantly positive in lead II ⇨ normal axis* ($0°$ to $-30°$)
- *If QRS is predominantly negative in lead II ⇨ LAD* ($< -30°$)

STEP 4: EVALUATE THE P WAVES/PR INTERVAL

(Look in Lead II and V_1 for P wave morphology)
   ☑ **Sinus?** If positive/upright in I, II, avF & negative in avR. *Each* P wave followed by QRS complex.
   ☑ **PR interval normal?** Normal PRI = 0.12 - .20 sec (or 3-5 boxes). Prolonged (> .20); shortened (< .12)
   ☑ **Atrial enlargement?**

LEFT ATRIAL ENLARGEMENT	RIGHT ATRIAL ENLARGEMENT
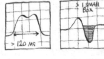 • *m-shaped P wave in Lead II* > .12 seconds (3 boxes) • Biphasic P in V1 with larger terminal component	• *tall P wave in Lead II* ≥3 mm • Biphasic P in V1 with larger initial component

STEP 5: EVALUATE THE QRS COMPLEX

   ☑ **Narrow v. Wide** (normal < .12 seconds). If QRS is narrow, skip looking for bundle branch blocks.
   ☑ **Bundle Branch Blocks?**

Left BBB	Right BBB
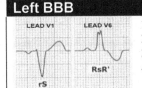 1. *Wide QRS > 0.12 seconds* 2. *Broad, slurred R in V5,6* 3. *Deep S wave in V1* 4. ST elevations V1-V3	1. *Wide QRS > 0.12 seconds* 2. *RsR' in V1,2* 3. *Wide S wave in V6*

   ☑ **Ventricular Hypertrophy**
      RIGHT VENTRICULAR HYPERTROPHY: look at V1: R>S in V1 or R >7mm in height in V1
      LEFT VENTRICULAR HYPERTROPHY:
         Sokolow-Lyon criteria: S in V1 + R in V5 (or V6) >35mm in men; >30mm in women.
         Cornell Criteria: R in aVL + S in V3 >28mm in men; >20mm in women.
   ☑ **Pathological Q waves?** Q wave >1 box (in depth or width).

STEP 6: EVALUATE ST SEGMENT

   ☑ ST depression or elevation >1 mm in depth/height?

STEP 7: EVALUATE T WAVES

   ☑ Any T wave inversions (TWI); T wave flattening? Is the QT interval prolonged?

AUTONOMIC NERVOUS SYSTEM CONTROL OF THE HEART

*1.*__SYMPATHETIC SYSTEM__: the hormones *epinephrine & norepinephrine* cause ❶increased excitability ❷ increased force of contraction ❸increased SA node discharge rate (↑ heart rate). *Epinephrine & Dobutamine are sympathomimetics* (they stimulate the sympathetic system).

*2.*__PARASYMPATHETIC SYSTEM__: the hormone *acetylcholine (regulated by the vagus nerve)* causes ❶decreased excitability ❷ decreased force of contraction ❸ decreased SA node discharge rate (↓heart rate). __CLINICAL CORRELATION:__ *"vagal stimulation" or "vagal maneuvers" slow down the heart rate.* Conversely, *anticholinergic drugs increase the heart rate.*

SUMMARY OF THE 12 LEADS AND THEIR RELATION TO THE HEART

Coronary Artery Anatomy   The leads and their relation to the coronary arteries

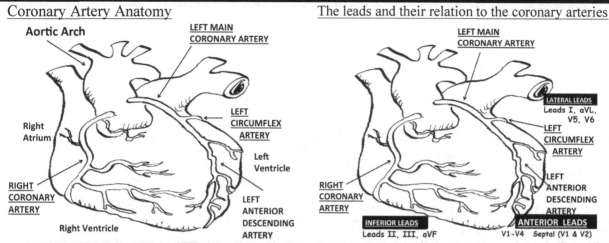

AREA OF INFARCTION	Q WAVES/ ST ELEVATIONS	ARTERY INVOLVED
ANTERIOR WALL	*V1 through V4*	*Left Anterior Descending (LAD)*
- SEPTAL	V1 & V2	Proximal LAD
LATERAL WALL	*I, aVL, V5, V6*	*Circumflex (CFX)*
ANTEROLATERAL	*I, aVL, V4 + V5 + V6*	Mid *LAD or CFX*
INFERIOR	*II, III, aVF*	*Right Coronary Artery (RCA)*
POSTERIOR WALL	*ST DEPRESSIONS V1-V2* (really the reciprocal changes since there are no "posterior" leads on a standard 12 lead ECG)	RCA, CFX

QRS AXIS DETERMINATION

Axis: the general direction of the impulses through the heart. It is the summation of all the vectors. Vectors move towards hypertrophy & away from infarction. *Normal QRS axis is -30° to +90°*

PERPENDICULAR	QUADRANT METHOD

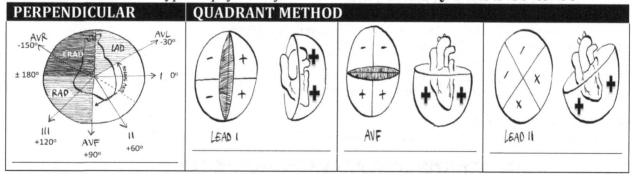

QUADRANT METHOD: *If LAD (based on I and aVF) ⇨ check lead II. If QRS is predominantly negative in lead II ⇨ LAD*

AXIS	Lead I	aVF	ETIOLOGIES OF LEFT & RIGHT AXIS DEVIATION
Normal	⊕	⊕	Normal
LAD	⊕	-ve	LBBB, LVH, inferior MI, elevated diaphragm, L anterior hemiblock, WPW
RAD	-ve	⊕	RVH, lateral MI, COPD, Left posterior hemiblock
ERAD	-ve	-ve	

LAD – vectors move towards hypertrophy (LVH) or away from infarction (inferior MI ± cause LAD).
RAD – vectors move towards hypertrophy (RVH) or away from infarction (lateral MI ± cause RAD).

SINUS RHYTHMS Impulses originate from the SA (sinoatrial) node in all sinus rhythms.

NORMAL SINUS RHYTHM (NSR)

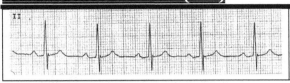

- Every P wave is followed by a QRS complex.
- P waves are positive/upright in leads I, II, aVF & negative in aVR.
- Rate 60-100 bpm.

SINUS TACHYCARDIA

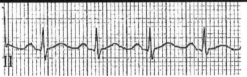

- Gradual onset & termination.

- Rarely >130 bpm.

- Same as normal sinus rhythm except *rate is >100 bpm.*
ETIOLOGIES
- **Physiologic:** exercise, emotional stress, young children/infants.

- **Pathologic:** fever, infection, hemorrhage, hypoglycemia, anxiety, pain, thyrotoxicosis, hypoxemia, hypovolemia, shock, sympathomimetics (ex. decongestants, cocaine).
- **MANAGEMENT:** *none usually. Treat the underlying cause.*

SINUS BRADYCARDIA

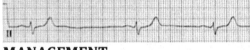

MANAGEMENT
- *Atropine 1st line treatment if symptomatic.**

- Epinephrine or transcutaneous pacing are options if no response to Atropine.

- Same as normal sinus rhythm except *rate is <60 bpm.*
ETIOLOGIES:
- **Physiologic:** well-conditioned athletes, vasovagal reaction, ↑intracranial pressure, nausea, vomiting.

- **Pathologic:** β-blocker, calcium channel blocker, Digoxin, carotid massage, SA node ischemia (inferior wall MI), gram-negative sepsis, hypothyroidism.
Because excess vagal stimulation is the most common cause of bradycardia, the anticholinergic Atropine is 1st line tx.*

SINUS ARRHYTHMIA

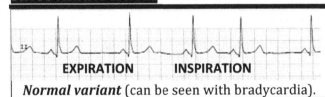

EXPIRATION   INSPIRATION

Normal variant (can be seen with bradycardia).

- Same as normal sinus rhythm except the *RHYTHM IS IRREGULAR:*
  - *heart rate increases during inspiration.*
  - heart rate decreases during expiration.

SICK SINUS SYNDROME (brady-tachy syndrome)

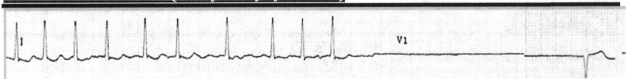

- Combination of *sinus arrest with alternating paroxysms of atrial tachyarrhythmias & bradyarrhythmias.* Commonly caused by sinoatrial node disease & corrective cardiac surgery.

MANAGEMENT: *± permanent pacemaker (PPM) if symptomatic* (dual chamber pacing usually preferred over ventricular pacing). If bradycardia alternating with ventricular tachycardia ⇨ *permanent pacemaker with automatic implantable cardioverter-defibrillator (AICD).*

ATRIOVENTRICULAR CONDUCTION BLOCKS

AV BLOCK: interruption of the normal impulse from the SA node to the AV node (AV node dysfunction).
- ***PR Interval (PRI) most helpful in determining the presence of AV conduction blocks.***

FIRST DEGREE AV BLOCK

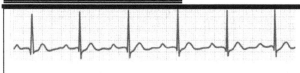

- **CONSTANT, PROLONGED PRI*** *(>0.20 seconds).*

- **QRS follows every P wave*** (all of the impulses are conducted from the atria to the ventricles).

MANAGEMENT: none, observation (may progress).

SECOND DEGREE AV BLOCK

- *2nd = not all of the atrial impulses are conducted to the ventricles.*
  This leads to some P waves that are not followed by QRS complexes ('dropped QRS').

MOBITZ I – WENCKEBACH

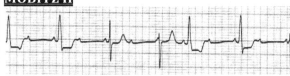

"Dropped QRS" Atrial impulse not Conducted to ventricle

P wave without QRS

MOBITZ I – WENCKEBACH
- **PROGRESSIVE PRI LENGTHENING*** ⇨ **dropped QRS.***
  Shortened R-R interval

MANAGEMENT
Symptomatic ⇨ **Atropine**, Epinephrine, ± pacemaker.
Asymptomatic ⇨ observation. ± Cardiac consult.

MOBITZ II

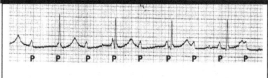

MOBITZ II: block commonly in the bundle of HIS.
- **CONSTANT/PROLONGED PRI*** ⇨ **dropped QRS.***

MANAGEMENT: *Atropine or temporary pacing.*
Progression to 3rd degree AV block common so
permanent pacemaker is the definitive treatment.

THIRD DEGREE AV BLOCK

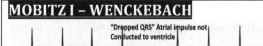

- **AV dissociation:*** *P waves NOT related to QRS.*
- **All P waves NOT followed by QRS** ⇨ ↓*cardiac output.*

MANAGEMENT
- Acute/symptomatic: *temporary pacing* ⇨ *PPM.*

- Definitive tx: *permanent pacemaker (PPM).**

ATRIAL DYSRHYTHMIAS

ATRIAL FLUTTER

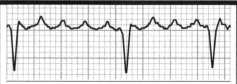

- ***Flutter ("saw tooth")* waves @***
  250-350 bpm *(no P waves)*
- The rate is usually REGULAR.

MANAGEMENT
- **STABLE:** *vagal, β-blocker or calcium channel blocker.*

- **UNSTABLE:** *direct current (synchronized) cardioversion.*

- **DEFINITIVE MANAGEMENT:** *radiofrequency ablation.**

Anticoagulation use is similar to atrial fibrillation.

ATRIAL FIBRILLATION (AF)

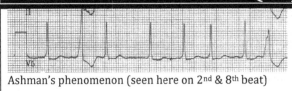

Ashman's phenomenon (seen here on 2nd & 8th beat)

- **IRREGULARLY IRREGULAR rhythm* with narrow QRS** usually.
- **No P waves** (characterized by the presence of *fibrillatory waves* @ 350-600 bpm).
- Ventricular rate is usually 80-140 bpm (rarely > 170).

- Atrial fibrillation is the most common chronic arrhythmia. Most patients are asymptomatic.

- The ineffective quivering of the atria **may cause thrombi** (clots) **to form, which can embolize** & cause ischemic strokes.
- ± Ashman's phenomenon: occasional aberrantly conducted beats (wide QRS) after short R-R cycles.

ETIOLOGIES:
Cardiac disease, ischemia, pulmonary disease, infection, cardiomyopathies, electrolyte imbalances, idiopathic, endocrine or neurologic disorders (ex. thyroid disorders), increasing age, genetics, hemodynamic stress, medications, drug or alcohol use.   Men > women;   Whites > blacks.

TYPES
- Paroxysmal: self-terminating within 7 days (usually <24 hours). ±Recurrent.
- Persistent: fails to self-terminate, lasts >7 days. Requires termination (medical or electrical).
- Permanent: persistent AF >1 year (refractory to cardioversion or cardioversion never tried).
- Lone: paroxysmal, persistent or permanent *without evidence of heart disease.*

MANAGEMENT
1. **STABLE:**
   RATE CONTROL: *usually preferred as initial management of symptomatic AF* over rhythm control.
   a. *β-blockers:* **Metoprolol, Esmolol. Cautious use in patients with reactive airway disease.** *
   b. *Calcium Channel blockers:* **Diltiazem**, Verapamil – (nondihydropyridines).
   c. **Digoxin** ± used in the elderly. **Digoxin is preferred for rate control in patients with hypotension or <u>congestive</u> heart failure.** Not generally used in active patients.

   RHYTHM CONTROL: may be used in *younger patients with lone A fib.*
   a. Direct current (synchronized) cardioversion (DCC): preferred over pharmacologic rhythm control. DCC can be done if ❶ AF present for <48 hours OR ❷ *after 3-4 weeks of anticoagulation & a transesophageal echocardiogram (TEE) shows no atrial thrombi.* Another option is to start IV heparin, cardiovert within 24h & anticoagulation for 4 weeks.
   b. Pharmacologic Rhythm control: Ibutilide, Flecainide, Sotalol, Amiodarone.
   c. Radiofrequency ablation ⇨ permanent pacemaker; catheter-based ablation or surgical 'MAZE" procedure.

2. **UNSTABLE:** ⇨ **direct current (synchronized) cardioversion** (DCC).

3. **Anticoagulation:** all patients with nonvalvular atrial fibrillation should undergo both:
   A. **Assessment of the risk of embolization.** The CHA2DS2-VASc or CHADS2 score mainly determines the risk.   The CHA2DS2-VASc score takes additional risk factors into consideration as well as assesses the risks differently and is now preferred by most. The use of anticoagulant therapy has been shown to reduce embolic risk by 70%.

   B. **Determination of the benefits vs. risks of anticoagulation.** Determine if the risk of embolization and stroke exceeds the potential risk of bleeding from anticoagulation. This is mainly determined by clinical judgment and a thorough discussion with the patient.

ANTICOAGULATION RISK STRATIFICATION IN NONVALVULAR ATRIAL FIBRILLATION

- **CHA_2DS_2-VASc score** (now recommended by most) or
- **$CHADS_2$ score**

CHA_2DS_2- VASc CRITERIA	POINTS	RECOMMENDED THERAPY
Congestive Heart Failure	1	**≥ 2 = Moderate to high risk:**
Hypertension	1	*chronic oral anticoagulation recommended.*
A₂ge ≥ 75y	2	
Diabetes Mellitus	1	1 = low risk:
S₂: Stroke, TIA, thrombus	2	Based on clinical judgment, consideration of risk to benefit assessment & discussion with patient. Anticoagulation may be recommended in some cases.
Vascular disease (prior MI, aortic plaque, peripheral arterial disease)	1	
Age 65 – 74y	1	0 = very low risk:
Sex (female)	1	*No anticoagulation needed.*
MAXIMUM SCORE	9	May be recommended in some (based on clinical judgment & consideration of risk to benefit ratio).

$CHADS_2$ CRITERIA	POINTS	RECOMMENDED THERAPY
Congestive Heart Failure	1	≥ 2 = High Risk: Warfarin
Hypertension	1	(maintain INR between 2-3)
Age ≥ 75y	1	
Diabetes Mellitus	1	1 = Moderate Risk: Warfarin or Aspirin
S₂: Stroke, TIA, thrombus	2	
MAXIMUM SCORE	6	0 = Low Risk: None or Aspirin

ANTICOAGULANT AGENTS:

1. **Non-vitamin K antagonist oral anticoagulants (NOAC):** *usually now preferred over warfarin in most cases* due to similar or lower rates of major bleeding as well as lower risk of ischemic stroke, convenience of not having to check the INR & less drug interactions.
   - **Dabigatran**: direct thrombin inhibitor (binds & inhibits thrombin).

   - **Rivaroxaban, Apixaban, Edoxaban**: factor Xa inhibitors (selectively binds to antithrombin III).

2. **Warfarin:**
   Indications: may be preferred in some of the following patients – some with severe chronic kidney disease, contraindications to the NOAC (ex. HIV patients on protease inhibitor-based therapy, on CP450-inducing antiepileptic medications such as carbamazepine, phenytoin etc), patients already on warfarin who prefer not to change, cost issues (Warfarin is less expensive). Warfarin usually bridged with heparin until warfarin is therapeutic.
   Monitoring: International Normalized Ratio *(INR) goal of 2-3.* Prothrombin Time (PT).

3. Dual antiplatelet therapy: (ex. Aspirin + Clopidogrel). Anticoagulant monotherapy is superior to dual antiplatelet therapy. Dual antiplatelet therapy may be reserved for patients who cannot be treated with anticoagulation (for reasons OTHER than bleeding risk).

LONG QT SYNDROME

ETIOLOGIES: congenital or acquired (ex. macrolides, TCAs, electrolyte abnormalities).
CLINICAL MANIFESTATIONS: recurrent syncope, ventricular arrhythmias & sudden cardiac death.

MANAGEMENT: Discontinue offending drugs & correct any electrolyte abnormalities.
AICD is the definitive management of congenital long QT or recurrent ventricular arrhythmias.

PAROXYSMAL SUPRAVENTRICULAR TACHYCARDIA (PSVT)

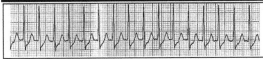

- Heart rate >100 bpm.
- **Rhythm** usually **regular with narrow QRS complexes.**
- P waves hard to discern due to the rapid rate.

- **"Paroxysmal"** = sudden onset & termination (*MC preceded by a premature atrial contraction*). **Supraventricular** = rhythm originates above the ventricles. SVT is an umbrella term when a more specific term cannot be applied to a tachyarrhythmia originating above the ventricles.

2 MAIN TYPES
❶ AV NODAL REENTRY TACHYCARDIA (AVNRT): **2 pathways** both **WITHIN** the **AV node** (slow & fast). *MC type.*

❷ AV RECIPROCATING TACHYCARDIA (AVRT): 1 pathway within the AV node & a **second accessory pathway** OUTSIDE the AV node ex. *Wolff-Parkinson-White (WPW)* & Lown-Ganong-Levine syndrome (LGL).

CONDUCTION PATTERNS
1. **Orthodromic (95%):** *impulse goes down the normal AV node pathway first* & returns via the accessory pathway in circles, perpetuating the rhythm ⇨ **narrow complex tachycardia.***

2. **Antidromic (5%):** *impulse goes down the accessory pathway first* & returns to the atria via the normal pathway ⇨ **WIDE complex tachycardia*** (mimics ventricular tachycardia).

MANAGEMENT OF SVT
1. **Stable (Narrow Complex):**
   - Vagal maneuvers (vagus nerve stimulation releases acetylcholine ⇨ ↓heart rate).
   - **ADENOSINE 1ST LINE MEDICAL TREATMENT FOR SVT*** (terminates 90% of narrow complex SVT).
     Note: the *use of Adenosine in patients with asthma/COPD may cause bronchospasm.*

   - **AV nodal blockers:** β-blockers or Calcium Channel Blockers.

2. **Stable (Wide Complex):**
   - **Antiarrhythmics:** *ex. Amiodarone. Procainamide if WPW is suspected.*

3. **Unstable** ⇨ *direct current (synchronized) cardioversion.**

4. **Definitive Management:** *radiofrequency ablation** (electrically destroys the abnormal pathway). Radiofrequency ablation ± indicated if patient experiences recurrent, symptomatic episodes.

WANDERING ATRIAL PACEMAKER (WAP) & MULTIFOCAL ATRIAL TACHYCARDIA (MAT)

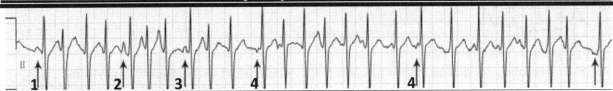

WANDERING ATRIAL PACEMAKER:
- Multiple ectopic atrial foci generate impulses that are conducted to the ventricles.
- **ECG: *heart rate <100 bpm & ≥3 P wave morphologies.****

MULTIFOCAL ATRIAL TACHYCARDIA:
- Same as wandering atrial pacemaker *except the heart rate is >100 bpm.*
- **ECG: *heart rate > 100 bpm & ≥3 P wave morphologies.****
- **MAT classically associated with severe COPD*** (chronic obstructive pulmonary disease).
Difficult to tx: Calcium channel blocker (ex. *Verapamil) or β-blocker* used if LV function is preserved.

WOLFF-PARKINSON-WHITE (WPW)

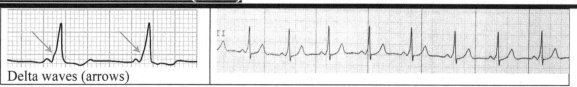

Delta waves (arrows)

- **WPW:** *accessory pathway (bundle of Kent) "pre-excites" the ventricles* ⇨ slurred, wide QRS. WPW is a type of AV reciprocating tachycardia (AVRT).

- Most patients are asymptomatic but they are prone to the development of tachyarrhythmias.

- **ECG:** ❶ _DELTA WAVE_* *(slurred QRS upstroke)* ❷ *wide QRS* *>0.12 seconds* & ❸ *Short PR interval.**

MANAGEMENT
1. <u>STABLE:</u>
   - Vagal maneuvers: ex. Valsalva, unilateral carotid massage (if no carotid bruits present).
   - *Antiarrhythmics: ex. Class IA:* _PROCAINAMIDE PREFERRED,_* Amiodarone, Flecainide, Ibutilide.

   - *Avoid the use of AV nodal blockers* (ABCD) *in WPW:** AV nodal blockade may cause preferential conduction through the fast (preexcitation) pathway ⇨ worsening of the tachyarrhythmia.
     ABCD = _Adenosine, Beta blockers, Calcium channel blockers, Digoxin_

2. <u>UNSTABLE:</u> *direct current (synchronized) cardioversion 1ˢᵗ line treatment.**

3. <u>DEFINITIVE MANAGEMENT:</u> *radiofrequency ablation** (electrically destroys the abnormal pathway). Radiofrequency ablation indicated if patients experience recurrent, symptomatic episodes.

LOWN-GANONG-LEVINE SYNDROME (LGL)

- Characterized by *short PR interval with a normal QRS complex.* Like WPW, LGL is an AVRT (leading to a short PR interval) but the accessory pathway (bundle of James) connects to the bundle of HIS, so the *QRS is narrow* in LGL (unlike the wide QRS seen in WPW).

AV JUNCTIONAL DYSRHYTHMIAS

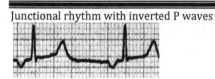
Junctional rhythm with inverted P waves

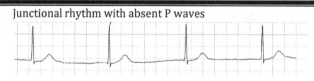
Junctional rhythm with absent P waves

- AV node/junction becomes the dominant pacemaker of the heart in AV junctional rhythms.

- **ETIOLOGIES:**   sinus disease, coronary artery disease, MC rhythm seen with Digitalis toxicity, myocarditis. May be seen in patients without structural heart disease.

- **ECG:** Regular rhythm. *P waves inverted (negative) if present* in leads where they are normally positive (I, II, aVF) *or are not seen.* Classically associated with a *narrow QRS* (± wide).
  Junctional Rhythm: heart rate is usually 40-60 bpm (reflecting the intrinsic rate of the AV junction).
  Accelerated Junctional: heart rate 60-100 bpm.
  Junctional Tachycardia: heart rate >100 bpm.

VENTRICULAR DYSRHYTHMIAS

> Ventricular dysrhythmias are frequently unpredictable, unstable & potentially lethal because stroke volume & coronary flow are compromised.
> Associated with *wide, bizarre QRS complexes.*

PREMATURE VENTRICULAR COMPLEXES (PVC)

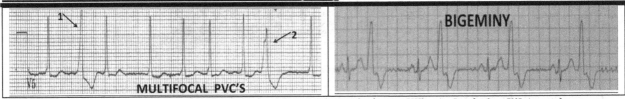

Unifocal (one morphology)   **Multifocal** (>1 morphology)   **Bigeminy** (every other beat is a PVC)   **Couplet** (two PVCs in a row)

- **PVC:** premature beat originating from the ventricle ⇨ *wide, bizarre QRS occurring earlier than expected.* With a PVC, *the T wave is in the opposite direction of the QRS* usually. Associated with a *compensatory pause =* overall rhythm is unchanged (AV node prevents retrograde conduction).
- **MANAGEMENT:** *no treatment usually needed.*   *Most ventricular arrhythmias occur after a PVC.*

VENTRICULAR TACHYCARDIA

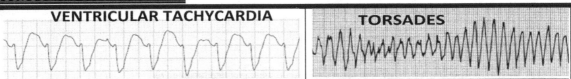

- **Ventricular tachycardia: ≥3 consecutive PVCs at a rate >100 bpm** (usually between 120-300 bpm). Must evaluate if the patient is *hemodynamically stable v. unstable* and if it is *sustained v. non-sustained.*
  - *Sustained is defined as having a duration of ≥30 seconds.*
    - **Ventricular Tachycardia: prolonged QT interval** a common predisposing condition.
    - **Torsades De Pointes:** MC due to **hypomagnesemia,** hypokalemia. V tach that "twists" around baseline.

MANAGEMENT:

Stable sustained VT	*Antiarrhythmics (Amiodarone,* Lidocaine, Procainamide).
Unstable VT with a pulse	*Synchronized cardioversion.*
VT (no pulse)	*- Defibrillation (unsynchronized cardioversion) + CPR (treat as Ventricular Fibrillation).*
Torsades de pointes	*IV Magnesium.** Correct electrolyte abnormalities.

VENTRICULAR FIBRILLATION

Coarse ventricular fibrillation   Fine ventricular fibrillation
MANAGEMENT: *unsynchronized cardioversion (defibrillation) + CPR*

PULSELESS ELECTRICAL ACTIVITY:

- *Organized rhythm seen on a monitor but patient has no palpable pulse* (electrical activity is not coupled with mechanical contraction).
MANAGEMENT: *CPR + epinephrine + checks for "shockable" rhythm every 2 minutes.*

ASYSTOLE (Ventricular standstill):

MANAGEMENT: Treated the same as PEA

CAUSES OF INCREASED JUGULAR PRESSURE

Increased JVP + crackles/rales in the lungs on pulmonary examination ⇨ congestive heart failure (CHF).
Increased JVP + normal pulmonary examination ⇨ pericardial (ex. tamponade or constrictive pericarditis).
Increased JVP + decreased breath sounds on pulmonary examination ⇨ tension pneumothorax.

CAUSES OF ST SEGMENT DEPRESSION

ST DEPRESSION: *usually indicates ischemia.**
- *Horizontal & downslope ST depressions are almost always pathological* & often indicate ischemia.

- *Upsloping may be benign.* An important exception is De Winter T waves = upsloping ST depressions with hyperacute T waves commonly seen with an acute occlusion of the proximal LAD, leading to infarction.

TYPES OF ST SEGMENT DEPRESSIONS
DOWNSLOPING	HORIZONTAL	UPSLOPING
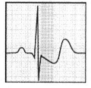	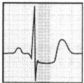	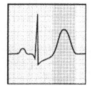

CAUSES OF ST SEGMENT ELEVATION

SHAPE OF ST ELEVATION

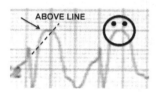

CONVEX ST ELEVATIONS "SAD FACE"
People who are vex become sad

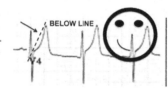

CONCAVE ST ELEVATIONS "HAPPY FACE"

CONVEX DOWN:	**CONCAVE UP:**
Most likely ischemic (ex. myocardial infarction)	*Usually benign* (*not always*) or reflects other causes of ST elevations ex. early repolarization abnormalities, pericarditis.

ETIOLOGIES OF ST ELEVATION ON ECG:
1. *Acute myocardial infarction*
2. Left ventricular hypertrophy (LVH)
3. Left bundle branch block (LBBB)
4. Acute pericarditis
5. Early repolarization abnormalities
6. Coronary vasospasm/Prinzmetal angina/cocaine
7. Brugada syndrome

EARLY REPOLARIZATION ABNORMALITIES

- ST elevation >2mm CONCAVE diffuse leads c̄ large T waves (esp precordial)
- Tall QRS voltage
- Fishhook (slurring/notching at J point)

Usually a normal variant.
May be seen in thin, healthy males; African-American males.

EARLY REPOLARIZATION ABNORMALITIES
- *Diffuse CONCAVE ST elevations* >2 mm with *large T waves* (especially precordial).
- *Tall QRS voltage.*
- Fishhook (slurring/notching) at the J point.

ACUTE PERICARDITIS

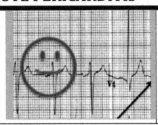

ACUTE PERICARDITIS
- *__Diffuse concave ST elevations in the precordial leads (V1 through V6).__**
- ***PR depressions in the same leads with the ST elevations.***
- <u>Lead aVR:</u> ST depression & PR elevation (opposite of what is seen in V1-V6).
- *No reciprocal changes.*
- T wave inversion will only occur AFTER ST elevations (acute MI may have T wave inversions simultaneously with ST elevations).

LVH with Left Ventricular STRAIN

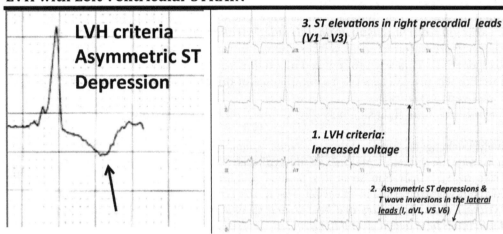

LVH criteria
Asymmetric ST
Depression

3. ST elevations in right precordial leads (V1 – V3)

1. LVH criteria:
Increased voltage

2. Asymmetric ST depressions & T wave inversions in the *lateral* leads (I, aVL, V5 V6)

Often seen in patients with left ventricular hypertrophy (LVH) who also suffer from ischemic disease. The coronary artery supply is "strained" trying to supply the excess hypertrophic cardiac muscle.

BRUGADA SYNDROME

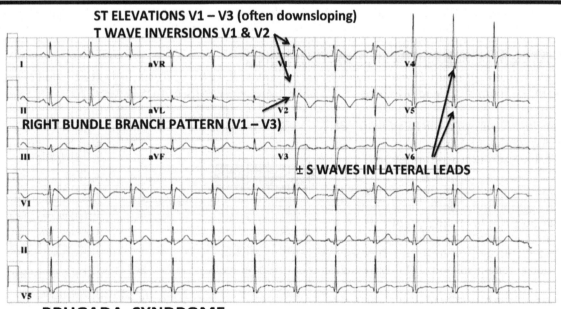

ST ELEVATIONS V1 – V3 (often downsloping)
T WAVE INVERSIONS V1 & V2

RIGHT BUNDLE BRANCH PATTERN (V1 – V3)

± S WAVES IN LATERAL LEADS

BRUGADA SYNDROME

BRUGADA SYNDROME ECG PATTERNS
- ***Right bundle branch block (RBB) pattern*** (often incomplete).
- ***ST elevation V₁-V₃ (often downsloping pattern).***
- T wave inversions *V₁ & V₂,* ***±S wave in lateral leads.***

- ***Genetic disorder*** associated with syncope, ***sudden cardiac death*** (from ***ventricular arrhythmias***).
- MC in ***Asian males.****

<u>**MANAGEMENT:**</u> AICD to prevent death from V fib.

19

CARDIOLOGY BASICS INTRO

BARORECEPTORS
1. Baroreceptors sense changes in arterial pressure (carotid artery stretching) & changes in the aortic arch.
   ***Clinical correlation: **Vagal maneuvers (ex carotid massage) decrease heart rate in tachyarrhythmias.**
   Vagal maneuvers increase carotid artery pressure ⇨ reflexive ↓ in heart rate (due to ↑vagal stimulation).

AUTOREGULATION
Process by which blood flow remains constant in an organ despite changing arterial pressures (perfusion) to the organ. **In the heart, the local vasodilators are nitric oxide, oxygen & adenosine.**

CARDIAC OUTPUT IN RELATION TO RESPIRATION
<u>CO = HR x SV.</u> Cardiac output (CO) on the left side is different than the cardiac output on the right. Normal physiologic variation = **during inspiration, left sided stroke volume decreases because:**
1. Negative intrathoracic pressure increases venous return to the right side of the heart (in order for blood to get oxygenated). This leads to reduced blood flow to the left side of the heart.
2. A decrease in the thoracic pressure increases compliance of the pulmonary vascular bed. This also reduces left-sided venous return.
3. Increased venous return on the right side may directly push on the septum towards the left side.

Left side CO is relatively unchanged *despite decreased stroke volume (SV) during inspiration because CO is maintained by compensatory ↑ in the heart rate (HR).* **This explains:**
a. PHYSIOLOGIC SPLITTING OF S_2: inspiration separates S_2 into A_2 followed by P_2. During inspiration, the decreased L-sided venous return results in an earlier A_2. ↑ R-side flow with inspiration results in later P_2.
b. MURMUR AUGMENTATION: **L-sided murmurs are best heard @ end expiration*** (maximum L-sided flow) whereas **R-sided murmurs best heard @ end inspiration*** (maximum R-sided flow).
c. SINUS ARRHYTHMIA: during inspiration, the compensatory ↑ in heart rate speeds up the rhythm. The rhythm slows during expiration. Normal variant.
d. PULSUS PARADOXUS: **>10 mmHg decline in SBP with inspiration.** Misnomer because in reality, it is an exaggeration of the normal physiologic drop in blood pressure. Normal cardiac auscultation BUT palpable peripheral pulses disappear with inspiration. Ex: *cardiac tamponade, tension pneumothorax.*
e. CAUTIOUS USE OF IV NITROGLYCERIN & MORPHINE IN R-SIDED & INFERIOR MI: because the right side is more dependent on preload & stroke volume to maintain cardiac output. Nitrogen & Morphine ↓'es preload.

RENIN-ANGIOTENSIN-ALDOSTERONE SYSTEM (RAAS):
Regulates blood pressure & water (fluid) balance. Activated with a decrease in systolic blood pressure.

If too much renin ⇨ ↑blood pressure	RENIN-ANGIOTENSIN-ALDOSTERONE SYSTEM (RAAS)
Hyperaldosteronism associated with ↑BP & hypokalemia (aldosterone enhances renal K^+ excretion & Na^+ retention) Some anti hypertensive drugs target RAAS: - **ACE Inhibitors:** block the effects of angiotensin II, leading to ↓BP. Because they inhibit aldosterone, hyperkalemia may occur (due to decreased aldosterone-mediated K^+ excretion). Because they potentiate other vasodilators (ex. bradykinin), patients may develop a cough or angioedema. - **Angiotensin II Receptor blockers (ARB):** block the receptor for AG II but don't cause angioedema & cough	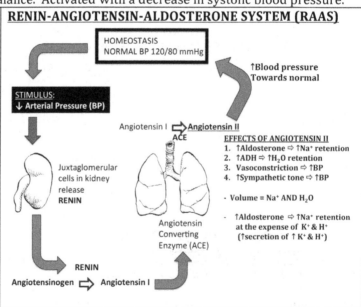

DIAGNOSTIC TESTS USED IN CARDIOLOGY

ELECTROCARDIOGRAM: evaluates rhythm disorders (*often initial test in evaluating cardiac disease*).

ANGIOGRAPHY: *gold standard* (definitive diagnosis) for coronary artery disease, peripheral arterial disease, renal artery stenosis & abdominal aortic aneurysms.

ECHOCARDIOGRAM: *most useful to diagnose heart failure*. May also be used in evaluating coronary artery disease (during stress testing).
> **TTE (Transthoracic Echocardiogram):** *primary noninvasive test for assessing cardiac anatomy & function.*
> **TEE (Transesophageal Echocardiogram):** *more invasive than TTE but provides better imaging of structures* - especially in patients with prosthetic valves, aortic disorders (ex aneurysms) & atrial abnormalities (ex. thrombi). TEE provides better visualization of posterior cardiac structures.

STRESS TESTING
- *Most useful noninvasive test in evaluating patients with suspected coronary artery disease.** Also used in patients with known cardiac disease to assess for progression. Usually done when the patient is stable & not having active symptoms or patients in whom acute MI has been ruled out.

❶**EXERCISE STRESS TESTING (ECG)**
  A. **Treadmill test:** ex. Bruce protocol: ⊕ if ST depressions, exercise-induced hypertension or hypotension, arrhythmias, symptoms or heart rate abnormalities occur during stress test.
  > **Ind:** initial test in most patients with normal resting ECG, low cost.
  > **Disadvantages:** doesn't localize ischemic regions, less sensitive if baseline ECG abnormalities present.
  > **CI:** unable to exercise, *baseline ECG abnormalities* (ex LBBB, WPW, baseline ST-T changes, pacing).
  B. **Radionuclide Myocardial Perfusion Imaging (MPI):** either Single Photon Emission Computed Tomography (SPECT using technetium or thallium) or Positive Emission Tomography (PET). *Benefits: localizes the regions of ischemia.*

❷**PHARMACOLOGIC STRESS TESTING:** *done in patients unable to exercise.*
  A.**Vasodilators with MPI:** *Adenosine or Dipyridamole. Vasodilators preferred with MPI.*
  > **MOA:** coronary vasodilators of normal (but not diseased) arteries.
  > **Ind:** preferred in patients with baseline ECG abnormalities (ex LBBB, ventricular pacing). *Localizes region of ischemia.*
  > **CI:** *bronchospastic disease* (ex. severe asthma & COPD because A2B receptor activation causes bronchospasm), 2nd/3rd degree heart block or sick sinus syndrome (Adenosine affects SA & AV node).
  > **Caution:** avoid vasoconstrictors 24 hours before test (ex Theophylline or caffeine).

  B. Dobutamine 2nd line

❸**STRESS ECHOCARDIOGRAPHY:** *localizes the regions of ischemia,* depicts wall motion abnormalities as well as visualizes the structure & function of the heart (assesses LV & valvular function).
  A. **Dobutamine:** sympathomimetic drug that stimulates β_1-mediated ↑HR/contractility. (positive inotrope/chronotrope) that ↑'es myocardial O_2 demand & provokes ischemia.
  > **Ind:** used in patients with contraindications to vasodilators or patients with recent vasoconstrictor use.
  > **CI:** sustained ventricular arrhythmias, significant LV outflow obstruction (ex. *severe aortic stenosis*), mod-severe hypertension, SBP >180 mmHg, aortic dissection or patients on β-blockers.

  B. Exercise stress echocardiography.

CHEST RADIOGRAPHS:
- Useful to assess signs of heart disease (ex. aortic dissection, CHF) or rule out other causes (ex. pulm, GI).

ULTRASOUND: used to assess arterial pulses or to evaluate AAA. Venous duplex for suspected DVTs.

CORONARY ARTERY DISEASE

- *INADEQUATE TISSUE PERFUSION/(ISCHEMIA)* due to imbalance between ↓*CORONARY BLOOD SUPPLY &* ↑*DEMAND.* *

ETIOLOGIES:
- *Atherosclerosis MC cause,* coronary artery vasospasm, aortic stenosis/aortic regurgitation, pulmonary hypertension, severe systemic hypertension, hypertrophic cardiomyopathy.

RISK FACTORS:
- *Diabetes Mellitus* (worst factor), *cigarette smoking* (most important modifiable risk factor), *hyperlipidemia (↑LDL, ↓HDL), hypertension, males, age* (>45y in men, > 55y in women), *family history* of coronary artery disease; Others risk factors include: obesity, hyperhomocysteinemia, ↑CRP.

PATHOPHYSIOLOGY OF ATHEROSCLEROSIS
A. **Formation of an atherosclerotic plaque:**
1. **Fatty streak formation:** *lipid deposition in the white blood cells* ⇨ smooth muscle proliferation. These "fatty streaks" are asymptomatic & can be seen as early as adolescence. Fatty streaks are the first step in the development of an atherosclerotic plaque.

2. Formation of an early Plaque: LDL enters the endothelium in the fatty streak ⇨ LDL is oxidized, attracting macrophages/smooth muscle cells to ingest harmful LDL (becoming foam cells). The foam cells attract more macrophages, fibroblasts & inflammatory cells.

3. Formation of a fibrous (mature) plaque: proliferating smooth muscle cells & connective tissue becomes incorporated into the mature plaque. *This "fibrous" cap results in narrowing of coronary arterial lumen.* *± calcification* (to stabilize plaque).

B. **Myocardial Ischemia:** the *narrowing of the arterial lumen reduces cardiac blood flow in conditions of increased demand (exercise, emotional stress)* ⇨ myocardial ischemia. *Usually ≥70% lumen reduction* is present when patients become *symptomatic.* Progressive compromise leads to collateral circulation in an attempt to perfuse the blood flow-deficient areas (long-term adaptation).

ANGINA PECTORIS

Angina Pectoris: *SUBSTERNAL CHEST PAIN* usually *brought on by exertion (due to ↓SUPPLY &* ↑*DEMAND).*

Class I: angina only with *unusually strenuous activity.* No limitations of activity.
Class II: angina with *more prolonged or rigorous activity.* Slight limitation of physical activity.
Class III: angina with usual daily activity. Marked limitation of physical activity.
Class IV: *angina at rest.* Often unable to carry out any physical activity.

CLINICAL MANIFESTATIONS
A. **HISTORY** *Clinical history is of utmost importance!*
1. **Chest Pain:** although there is significant clinical variation, patients usually complain of *substernal (chest pain/pressure/burning/tightness) poorly localized,* nonpleuritic, *exertional.* Radiation: *arm* (especially ulnar surfaces of the forearm & hand), *teeth, lower jaw,* back, epigastrium or shoulders; *usually short in duration (less than 30 minutes by definition but typically 1-5 minutes).* Levine's sign: clenched fist over chest.
         Pain relieved with: *rest or nitroglycerin (predictable pattern).*
         Pain precipitated by: *exertion/anxiety.*

2. **Associated symptoms:** dyspnea, nausea, diaphoresis (sweating), numbness, fatigue.

3. **Anginal equivalent:** *dyspnea, epigastric or shoulder pain instead of the classic chest pain.*

B. **PHYSICAL EXAM:** *often normal.* During attack, ± S_4 gallop, ± signs of left ventricular failure (S_3, pulmonary edema). You may see evidence of hyperlipidemia (xanthelasma).

DIAGNOSIS OF ISCHEMIC HEART DISEASE

Angina pectoris is primarily a historical diagnosis.
Workup: *ECG often initial test, stress testing usually after initial ECG. Angiography is gold standard.*

❶ ELECTROCARDIOGRAM (ECG):
1. *ST DEPRESSION:* *classic ECG finding** (especially horizontal or downsloping).
2. *The resting ECG is normal in 50%* of patients with stable angina.
3. ± T wave inversion/nonspp ST changes, poor R wave progression & T wave pseudonormalization.
4. The presence of left ventricular hypertrophy is associated with ↑adverse outcome.

❷ STRESS TESTING: *most useful noninvasive screening tool.**
- **STRESS ECG:** Bruce protocol: standard incremental increases in workload with monitoring of heart rate, blood pressure, ECG changes.
   Positive stress test = ST depressions, hypotension/hypertension, arrhythmias &/or symptoms.

- **MYOCARDIAL PERFUSION IMAGING STRESS** (exercise or pharmacologic) with thallium-201 or 99m-technetium sestamibi.
   Indications: *patients with baseline ECG abnormalities,** to *localize regions of ischemia.* Gives more information than a stress ECG.

   Pharmacologic agents: *Adenosine or Dipyridamole* (Persantine): coronary vasodilators of normal (but not diseased arteries). Used in *patients unable to tolerate exercise.*

   Contraindications: *asthmatics (± cause bronchospasm).*

- **STRESS ECHOCARDIOGRAM:** (exercise or pharmacologic): assesses left ventricular function, valvular disease, patients with pathologic Q waves. Can locate ischemia, *assess global & regional wall motion abnormalities & visualize heart structures.* Gives more information than a stress ECG.
   - *Dobutamine* (positive inotrope/ chronotrope) that ↑'es myocardial O_2 demand & provokes ischemia.

- CARDIAC MRI: performed with dobutamine infusion. Can assess perfusion & wall motion abnormalities. This may be used as an alternative to a stress test.

❸ CORONARY ANGIOGRAPHY: *definitive diagnosis/gold standard.** "Cath" outlines the coronary artery anatomy. Angiography also defines location & extent of coronary artery disease (CAD).
   Indications:
   1. Confirm/exclude CAD in patients with symptoms consistent with CAD.
   2. Confirm/exclude CAD in patients with negative noninvasive testing for CAD.
   3. Patients who may possibly need revascularization (PTCA or CABG).

REVASCULARIZATION TECHNIQUES FOR THE DEFINITIVE MANAGEMENT OF ANGINA

❶ PTCA (PERCUTANEOUS TRANSLUMINAL CORONARY ANGIOPLASTY):

Indications: *1 or 2 vessel disease <u>not</u> involving the left main coronary artery & in whom ventricular function is normal/near normal.* Should be a candidate for CABG. Restenosis occurs in 30% within 3 months after PTCA so restenosis can be reduced with stents.

Stents: provide safety net & *reduces restenosis* rates in about 30% of patients. Some stents have drug-eluting properties. The combination of Aspirin & Clopidogrel (Plavix) is effective in preventing coronary stent thrombosis.

❷ CABG (CORONARY ARTERY BYPASS GRAFT):

Indications: *left main coronary artery disease, symptomatic or critical stenotic* (>70%) *3-vessel disease* or decreased left ventricular *ejection fraction <40%.*

MEDICAL MANAGEMENT OF ANGINA

Angina is chest pain brought on by exertion (due to ↓SUPPLY & ↑DEMAND) so the pharmacologic treatment is effective by increasing supply while simultaneously reducing demand.

PHARMACOLOGIC MANAGEMENT OF STABLE (CHRONIC) ANGINA	
NITROGLYCERIN (Nitrates) Oral, spray, patch	❶**↑myocardial blood supply:** ↑O_2 & ↑collateral blood flow to ischemic myocardium, *reduces coronary vasospasm* & ↑'es coronary artery dilation. ❷**↓demand:** ↓cardiac work: *↓preload by venodilation.* ↓afterload. *Sublingual most effective.* Used when symptomatic or situations likely to induce angina. If no relief with 1st dose ⇨ give 2nd/3rd q5 minutes. No relief after 3rd dose, suspect ACS. Can be used prophylactically ~5 minutes before an activity likely to cause ischemia. **S/E:** headache, flushing, tolerance, hypotension, peripheral edema, *tachyphylaxis* after 24h (allow nitrate-free period for 8h). Deteriorates with moisture, light, air. **CI:** *SBP <90* mm Hg, *RV infarction, <u>use of Sildenafil & other PDE-5 inhibitors.</u>**
β – BLOCKERS **Cardioselective (β₁):** *Metoprolol, Atenolol* **Nonselective:** *Propranolol, Nadolol*	❶**↑myocardial blood supply:** *↑O_2 by prolonging coronary artery filling times* (coronary arteries fill during diastole). Beta blockers increase diastolic timing. ❷**↓Demand:** *reduces myocardial O_2 requirements during exercise/stress (negative chronotrope/inotrope).* *Good after myocardial infarction.* **Indications:** *1st line drug for chronic management** (reduces mortality, decreases symptoms & prevents ischemic occurrences).
CA CHANNEL BLOCKERS Nondihydropyridines: *Diltiazem* *Verapamil (long acting)*	❶**↑myocardial blood supply:** *prolongs diastolic filling times.* *Prevents/terminates ischemia induced by coronary vasospasm* by increasing coronary vasodilation. ❷**↓demand:** ↓'es contractility, ↓'es heart rate (AV node blocker) ↓'es afterload. **Indications:** used in patients unable to use beta blockers; *Prinzmetal angina.*
ASPIRIN	*Prevents platelet activation/aggregation* (by inhibiting cyclooxygenase ⇨ *↓thromboxane A_2* & inhibiting prostaglandins). Does not directly address the supply & demand problem but prevents progression from chronic stable angina to acute coronary syndrome (the first step in ACS is thrombosis after plaque rupture). Aspirin reduces the risk of thrombosis. Cautious use in patients with active peptic ulcer disease or ↑bleeding risk.

Reduction of risk factors: smoking cessation, control of hypertension/diabetes/cholesterol, diet & exercise.

Chronic (stable) angina: caused by *fixed plaque (coronary obstruction).* Usually relieved by rest/nitroglycerin.

CLASSIC OUTPATIENT REGIMEN: *daily aspirin, sublingual nitroglycerin as needed, daily beta blocker & statin.*

ACUTE CORONARY SYNDROME (ACS)

ACUTE CORONARY SYNDROME: symptoms of acute myocardial ischemia 2ry to _ACUTE PLAQUE RUPTURE_ _& varying degrees of CORONARY ARTERY THROMBOSIS (OCCLUSION)._

Includes: ❶ _Unstable angina_ (UA) ❷_Non ST elevation myocardial infarction_ (NSTEMI) &
        ❸ _ST elevation myocardial infarction_ (STEMI).

SPECTRUM OF ACUTE CORONARY SYNDROMES			
	UA	NSTEMI	STEMI
HISTORY	_Angina that is new in onset, crescendo, or at rest (usually >30 minutes). >90% occlusion can cause symptoms @ rest*_		
CORONARY THROMBOSIS	SUBTOTAL _occlusion_		TOTAL _occlusion_
ECG	ST DEPRESSIONS &/or T WAVE INVERSIONS		ST ELEVATIONS
CARDIAC ENZYMES	_Negative_	_Positive. Cell death seen in both NSTEM & STEMI_	

ETIOLOGIES

1. _Atherosclerosis: (MC cause of MI). Caused by plaque rupture_ ⇨ _acute coronary artery thrombosis_ with platelet adhesion/activation/aggregation along with fibrin formation. Vasculitis, embolism.
2. _Coronary artery vasospasm_ (2%): _cocaine-induced, variant (Prinzmetal) angina._

CLINICAL MANIFESTATIONS

1. **ANGINAL PAIN:** _retrosternal "pressure" (>30 minutes)_ NOT RELIEVED WITH REST/NITROGLYCERIN ±radiate to arms, neck, back, shoulders, epigastrium, lower jaw.   Levine's sign: clenched fist on chest. Frequency highest in AM. ± Dyspnea. _Pain at rest usually indicates >90% occlusion.*_

2. **SYMPATHETIC STIMULATION:** anxiety, diaphoresis, tachycardia/palpitations, N/V, dizziness.

3. SILENT MI: _~25% are atypical/silent: ex. **women, elderly, diabetics & obese** patients._ Atypical symptoms include: _abdominal pain, jaw pain or dyspnea_ without _chest pain._

4. **Physical Examination:** _usually normal._ ± _S4_ (especially with inferior), hyper or hypotension, _chest pain + bradycardia may be suggestive of an inferior wall MI.*_ ± New onset of regurgitant murmur.

DIAGNOSTIC STUDIES

A. **ECG (Electrocardiogram):**
   - **NSTEMI or UNSTABLE ANGINA:** ± ST depressions and/or T wave inversions. ECG ± be normal.
   - **STEMI:** _ST elevations ≥ 1mm in ≥ 2 anatomically contiguous leads._ ± _reciprocal changes_ in the _opposite leads. A **new left bundle branch block** is considered STEMI equivalent.*_

Hyperacute (peaked) T waves ⇨ ST elevations ⇨ Q waves ⇨ T wave inversions is natural STEMI progression.

			Pathologic Q wave:
Peaked T waves ⇨	_ST elevations_ ⇨	_Pathologic Q waves_	• Q wave ≥ 0.03 seconds & 0.1 mV deep. • Q wave depth @ least 25% of the associated R wave.

AREA OF INFARCTION	Q WAVES/ST ELEVATIONS	ARTERY INVOLVED
ANTERIOR WALL	_V1 through V4_	_Left Anterior Descending (LAD)_
- SEPTAL	V1 & V2	Proximal LAD
LATERAL WALL	_I, aVL, V5, V6_	_Circumflex (CFX)_
ANTEROLATERAL	_I, aVL, V4 + V5 + V6_	Mid _LAD or CFX_
INFERIOR	_II, III, aVF_	_Right Coronary Artery (RCA)_
POSTERIOR WALL	_ST DEPRESSIONS V1-V2_	RCA, CFX

B. **Cardiac Markers** Standard usually *3 sets every 8 hours. Troponin most sensitive & specific.*

	Appears	Peaks	Returns to baseline
CK/CK-MB	4-6 hours (h)	12-24 h	3-4 days
Troponin I & T	4-8 h	12-24 h	*7-10 days. Most sensitive & specific.** Also picks up smaller infarctions

^Troponin may be falsely elevated in patients with renal failure, advanced heart failure, acute PE, CVA.

MANAGEMENT OF UNSTABLE ANGINA (UA) or Non ST elevation MI (NSTEMI)

- **2 PART APPROACH:** ❶ *antithrombotic therapy* ❷ *adjunctive therapy & assess risk factors (TIMI score)*

1. ANTITHROMBOTIC TREATMENT IN UA or NSTEMI

ANTITHROMBOTIC TREATMENT IN UA or NSTEMI	
ANTI-PLATELET DRUGS	
Aspirin	*Prevents platelet activation/aggregation.* Inhibits COX ⇨ ↓thromboxane A_2
ADP INHIBITORS **Clopidogrel** (Plavix) Prasugrel Ticlopidine	**Ind:** *Good in patients with Aspirin allergy.* Give if conservative strategy or if PCI planned. 20% ↓in death/MI/stroke. **MOA:** *inhibits ADP-mediated platelet aggregation.* **Caution** *if CABG planned within 7d,* hepatic/renal impairment, bleeding.
GP IIb/IIIa Inhibitors • Eptifibatide (Integrilin) Tirofiban (Aggrastat) Abciximab (Reopro)	**MOA:** inhibits the final pathway for platelet aggregation. **Indication:** good for UA, NSTEMI, patients undergoing PCI. **CI:** internal bleeding within 30d; major trauma/surgery, thrombocytopenia.
ANTICOAGULANTS	
UNFRACTIONATED HEPARIN	**MOA:** *binds to & potentiates antithrombin III's ability to inactivate Factor Xa, inactivates thrombin (Factor IIa), inhibiting fibrin formation.* Prevents new clot formation (however, does not dissolve existing clots). **Ind:** *ACS patients with ECG changes or* ⊕ *cardiac markers* (↓ in death/MI).
LOW MOLECULAR WEIGHT HEPARIN *Enoxaparin* (Lovenox) *Dalteparin* (Fragmin)	**MOA:** *binds to & potentiates antithrombin III's ability to inactivate Factor Xa.* LMWH more specific to Factor Xa than UFH (LMWH less able to inhibit thrombin). **Ind:** *Same as UFH.* LMWH superior to UFH: longer ½ life (~12 hours) no need for IV infusion or PTT monitoring, ↓incidence of Heparin-induced thrombocytopenia, more reliable dosing. But long ½ life may be an issue if CABG planned. **S/E:** *thrombocytopenia* (obtain CBC prior to use). Obtain serum creatinine level (must be renally dosed if renal impairment to prevent complications).
Fondaparinux	Direct factor Xa inhibitor (binds to & enhances antithrombin). No direct effect on thrombin.

To form a clot, Factor Xa convers prothrombin (II) ⇨ thrombin (Factor IIa). Thrombin activates fibrinogen⇨ fibrin clot.

2. ADJUNCTIVE ANTI-ISCHEMIC THERAPY IN UA or NSTEMI

ADJUNCTIVE ANTI-ISCHEMIC THERAPY	
Drug	**Comment**
β-blockers *Metoprolol*	**MOA:** *lowers myocardial O_2 consumption; Antiarrhythmic effects* (titrated to pulse <70 bpm). S/E: fatigue, depression, erectile dysfunction, bronchospasm. **CI:** *severe bradycardia* (HR <50)*, hypotension* (SBP <90 mm Hg)*, decompensated CHF, 2nd/3rd heart block, cardiogenic shock, cocaine induced MI,* severe asthma/COPD.
Nitrates	decreases anginal symptoms but does not decrease mortality. Oral, sublingual, topical or IV.
Morphine	Relieves pain, ↓anxiety, *venodilation* ⇨ ↓preload.
Ca channel blockers Nondihydropyridines *Verapamil, Diltiazem* Dihydropyridines	Consider in patients who cannot tolerate β-blockers due to bronchospasm. *Calcium channel blockers drug of choice in vasospastic disorders - ex. Variant (Prinzmetal) angina or cocaine use.**

MANAGEMENT OF ST ELEVATION MI (STEMI)

- **3 part approach: ❶ *REPERFUSION therapy*** (most important) ❷ *antithrombotics* ❸ *adjunctive therapy*

❶ REPERFUSION THERAPY IN STEMI
MAINSTAY OF TREATMENT* – done **WITHIN 12 HOURS*** of symptom onset. Either ❶ PCI or ❷ thrombolytics

1. **PCI (Percutaneous Coronary Intervention):** *best within 3h of sx onset (esp c/n 90min)! PCI superior to thrombolytics.* Good especially for cardiogenic shock, large anterior MI, prior CABG and if thrombolytics are contraindicated.   *PCI = PTCA (Percutaneous Transluminal Coronary Angioplasty)*
   - *May need to do Coronary Artery Bypass Graft if >3-vessel disease, L main coronary artery, ↓left ventricle EF.*

2. **THROMBOLYTIC (FIBRINOLYTIC) THERAPY:**   Used if PCI is not an option/unable to get PCI early

THROMBOLYTIC (FIBRINOLYTIC) THERAPY	
Drug	**Comments**
Tissue Plasminogen Activators:	**MOA:** *dissolves clot by activating tissue plasminogen ⇨ plasmin.* Plasmin is a proteolytic enzyme that degrades fibrin.
• *Alteplase (rTPA)**	**Ind:** *STEMI (earlier patency of coronary artery, shorter half-life),** thrombotic strokes, pulmonary embolism. **S/E:** *higher rebleed risk.* Expensive.
• Reteplase (RPA)	↑ potency. Used in STEMI, pulmonary embolism.
• Tenecteplase (TNK)	Long ½ life. Used in STEMI.
Streptokinase	**MOA:** binds to plasminogen, activating it into plasmin. Derived from streptococcus. **Ind:** Less effective than TPA so only used in patients in whom PCI is contraindicated & patient has a high risk of intracerebral hemorrhage (*least chance of intracranial bleeding with streptokinase), cheap.* **S/E:** derived from streptococcus so usually only given once (tolerance develops).

Unlike <u>anti</u>thrombotic drugs that prevents new clots, thrombo<u>lytics</u> (fibrinolytics) dissolve existing clots.

❷ ANTITHROMBOTIC TREATMENT IN STEMI

ANTITHROMBOTIC TREATMENT IN STEMI	
Drug	**Comments**
Aspirin	*Lowers mortality by 20%. Chewed for faster absorption.*
Heparin (Unfractionated/LMWH)	**MOA:** inhibits thrombin by activating antithrombin III & inhibits factor Xa.
Glycoprotein IIb/IIIa Inhibitors	**MOA:** inhibits the final pathway of platelet aggregation. **Indications:** good for UA, NSTEMI, patients undergoing PCI.

❸ ADJUNCTIVE THERAPY IN STEMI

ADJUNCTIVE THERAPY	
Drug	**Comment**
β-blockers	15% ↓*in mortality (decreases wall tension, preventing complications of MI).* **MOA:** lowers myocardial O₂ consumption. Antiarrhythmic effects (titrated to pulse <70), *increases myocardial salvage in anatomic areas of infarct, prevents extension, reduces incidence of ventricular fibrillation.* Given within 12 hours of symptom onset. **S/E:** fatigue, depression, erectile dysfunction, bronchospasm. **CI:** *HR <50, SBP <100, decompensated CHF, 2nd/3rdº heart block, severe asthma/COPD, shock, cocaine-induced MI** (causes unopposed ↑alpha 1-mediated vasoconstriction).
*ACE Inhibitors**	• *slows the progression of CHF* during & after STEMI by ↓*ventricular remodeling,* (↓mortality) especially in patients with CHF, STEMI, LBBB, ejection fraction <40%. Given within the 1st 12-24h (after the patient is stable). **CI:** severe hypotension (SBP <100 mm Hg), renal failure. **S/E:** *angioedema & cough (due to ↑bradykinin – a potent vasodilator),* renal failure.
Nitrates	IV if continuing discomfort or STEMI complicated with HTN or pulm. edema. ~5% ↓mortality.
Morphine	Relieves pain, ↓anxiety, venodilation ⇨ ↓preload.

Additional: K+ & Mg+ repletion, **statin therapy,** monitor blood pressure & glucose & reduce risk factors.

Stable Plaque: thick fibrous cap, small amount of WBCs.

Unstable: thin fibrous cap, ↑WBCs. Unstable plaques have higher incidence of rupture.

MANAGEMENT OF ACUTE CORONARY SYNDROME OVERVIEW

- **AMI PROTOCOL:** *ECG within 10 minutes;*
  Door to thrombolytics within 30 minutes; Door to PCI within 90 minutes (± 30 minutes).*
- *"MONA regimen" – Morphine, Oxygen, Nitrates, Aspirin (Morphine if no pain relief with nitrates)*

STEMI:	ß blockers, NTG, Aspirin, Heparin, *ACEI, REPERFUSION (MOST IMPORTANT).**
UA or NSTEMI:	ß blockers, NTG, Aspirin, Heparin. NO emergent reperfusion!
COCAINE-INDUCED MI	ASA, NTG, heparin, anxiolytics *(avoid ß blockers because of vasospasm).*

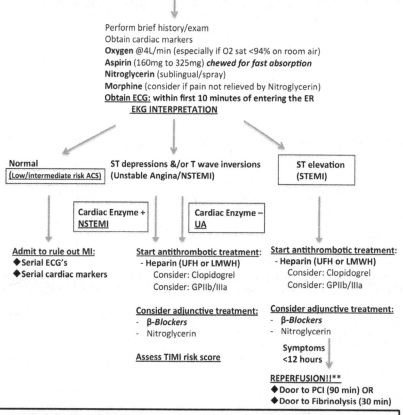

ACUTE CORONARY SYNDROMES

Symptoms associated with ischemia or infarction

Perform brief history/exam
Obtain cardiac markers
Oxygen @4L/min (especially if O2 sat <94% on room air)
Aspirin (160mg to 325mg) *chewed for fast absorption*
Nitroglycerin (sublingual/spray)
Morphine (consider if pain not relieved by Nitroglycerin)
Obtain ECG: within first 10 minutes of entering the ER
EKG INTERPRETATION

Normal
[Low/intermediate risk ACS]

ST depressions &/or T wave inversions
(Unstable Angina/NSTEMI)

ST elevation
(STEMI)

Cardiac Enzyme +
NSTEMI

Cardiac Enzyme –
UA

Admit to rule out MI:
◆Serial ECG's
◆Serial cardiac markers

Start antithrombotic treatment:
- Heparin (UFH or LMWH)
  Consider: Clopidogrel
  Consider: GPIIb/IIIa

Start antithrombotic treatment:
- Heparin (UFH or LMWH)
  Consider: Clopidogrel
  Consider: GPIIb/IIIa

Consider adjunctive treatment:
- β-Blockers
- Nitroglycerin

Assess TIMI risk score

Consider adjunctive treatment:
- β-Blockers
- Nitroglycerin

Symptoms <12 hours

REPERFUSION!!**
◆Door to PCI (90 min) OR
◆Door to Fibrinolysis (30 min)

> **EXCEPTIONS:**
> **1. Cocaine Induced MI:** O$_2$, ASA, *Benzodiazepines,* Heparin, CCB,NTG
>   **NO beta blockers!*** (causes unopposed alpha vasoconstriction)!
> **2. R ventricular (inferior wall) MI** – CAUTIOUS IV NITRATES & morphine use
>   (may cause unsafe drop in preload). *Give IV fluids for preload***
> **3. If Viagra or other erectile meds** – NO NITRATES (drops preload)

CONSERVATIVE MANAGEMENT

- Used in patients whose chest pain began >12 hours (<u>without</u> current/active chest pain) or low TIMI:
  - Aspirin (± *Clopidogrel* x 9 months), *statin, beta blocker, ACE Inhibitor. Nitroglycerin as needed.*

COMPLICATIONS OF MYOCARDIAL INFARCTION

- *Arrhythmias (ex. ventricular fibrillation), ventricular aneurysm/rupture,* cardiogenic shock,
  papillary muscle dysfunction, heart failure, left ventricular wall rupture.
- **Dressler syndrome:** *post-MI pericarditis* + fever + pulmonary infiltrates.

CORONARY VASOSPASM DISORDERS

❶ **VARIANT (PRINZMETAL) ANGINA:** *coronary spasm* ⇨ *TRANSIENT ST ELEVATIONS* usually without MI* (but MI can occur). Usually females, >50y, smokers, ±associated with vasospastic disorders (ex migraines, Raynaud's).

CLINICAL MANIFESTATIONS
CHEST PAIN USUALLY NONEXERTIONAL, OFTEN OCCURING AT REST.* Often occurs in the morning (may wake the patient up at night), occur with hyperventilation, emotional stress or cold weather.

DIAGNOSIS
- **ECG:** ± *TRANSIENT ST ELEVATIONS.**Angiography: vasospasm with IV Ergonovine administration.
- *Symptoms & ST elevations RESOLVE WITH CALCIUM CHANNEL BLOCKERS* or nitroglycerin.*

MANAGEMENT:
- *Calcium channel blockers (drug of choice),* nitrates as needed.* Both reduce spasms.
- In patients presenting with acute symptoms, Aspirin & Heparin may be given initially until atherosclerotic disease is ruled out.

❷ **COCAINE INDUCED MI:**
PATHOPHYSIOLOGY: *coronary artery vasospasm** due to cocaine's activation of the sympathetic nervous system & alpha-1 receptors ⇨ vasoconstriction of the coronary arteries. MI may occur if vasoconstriction is prolonged (due to decreased blood flow).

DIAGNOSIS:
- **ECG:** ± *TRANSIENT ST ELEVATIONS.** May induce myocardial infarction if prolonged constriction.

MANAGEMENT
- *Calcium channel blockers* & nitrates drugs of choice to reverse the vasospasm.*
- ± treated with Aspirin, Heparin & benzodiazepines until atherosclerotic disease is ruled out.
- *Avoid β-blockers in cocaine-induced MI** - ↑*risk of vasospasm (unopposed α-₁ constriction).**

TIMI AND RISK STRATIFICATION

TIMI risk score useful to assess the risk of death & ischemic events in patients with UA or NSTEMI to determine the benefit of invasive angiography to reduce mortality.

HISTORICAL		Score Interpretation:	
Age ≥65 y	1	% risk at 14 days of all-cause mortality, new or recurrent MI, or severe recurrent ischemia requiring urgent revascularization.	
≥ 3 CAD Risk Factors (FHx, HTN, ↑Chol, smoker, DM)	1		
Known CAD (stenosis ≥50%)	1	Score of 0-1 = 5% risk	
Aspirin use in past 7 days	1	Score of 2 = 8% risk	
PRESENTATION		Score of 3 = 13% risk	Score ≥ 3 = high risk
Recent (<24 h) severe angina	1	Score of 4 = 20% risk	
↑Cardiac markers	1	Score of 5 = 26% risk	
ST elevation 0.5 mm	1	Score of 6-7 = at least 41% risk	

THROMBOLYTIC CONTRAINDICATIONS IN ACS	
Absolute Contraindications:	Relative Contraindications:
• *Previous intracranial hemorrhage* • *Non-hemorrhagic stroke within 6 months or closed head/facial trauma within 3 months* • *Intracranial neoplasm, aneurysm, AVM* • *Active internal bleeding* • *Suspected aortic dissection*	• SBP >180 mm Hg on presentation • INR >2 or known bleeding diathesis • Trauma/major surgery within past 2 weeks • Recent internal bleed within 2 weeks • Prior streptokinase exposure, Pregnancy

HEART FAILURE (HF)

Heart failure: inability of the heart to pump sufficient blood to meet the metabolic demands of the body at normal filling pressures. *MC cause is coronary artery disease (CAD).* *

FORMS OF HEART FAILURE
These terms are not mutually exclusive: ex. left-sided systolic failure or left-sided diastolic failure etc.

1. **LEFT-SIDED vs. RIGHT-SIDED**
   - L-SIDED: *MC causes are coronary artery disease & hypertension.*
     Others include: valvular disease & cardiomyopathies.

   - R-SIDED: *MC cause of R-sided failure is L-sided failure.* *
     Pulmonary disease (COPD, pulmonary hypertension), mitral stenosis.

2. **SYSTOLIC vs. DIASTOLIC**
   - SYSTOLIC: *↓ ejection fraction, ± S_3 gallop. Systolic MC form of heart failure.*
     - **Etiologies:** *post myocardial infarction, dilated cardiomyopathy,* myocarditis.

   - DIASTOLIC: *normal/↑ejection fraction, ± S_4 gallop = forced atrial contraction into a stiff ventricle.* Associated with normal cardiac size.
     - **Etiologies:** *hypertension, left ventricular hypertrophy, elderly,* valvular heart disease, cardiomyopathies (hypertrophic, restrictive), constrictive pericarditis.

DIASTOLIC FAILURE		SYSTOLIC FAILURE
- *Normal/increased ejection fraction (EF)*	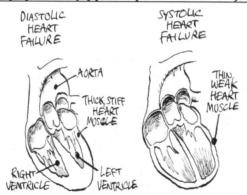	- *decreased ejection fraction (EF)*
- *thick* ventricular walls		- *thin* ventricular walls
- *small* LV chamber		- *dilated* LV chamber
- ⊕ S_4 on auscultation		- ⊕ S_3 on auscultation

3. **HIGH OUTPUT v. LOW OUTPUT**
   High output: the metabolic demands of the body exceeds normal cardiac function.
   – thyrotoxicosis, wet beriberi, severe anemia, AV shunting, Paget's disease of the bone.

   Low output: inherent problem of myocardial contraction, ischemia, chronic hypertension.

4. **ACUTE V. CHRONIC**
   Acute: *largely systolic* (ex. hypertensive crisis, acute MI, papillary muscle rupture).

   Chronic: typically seen in patients with dilated cardiomyopathy or valvular disease.

NEW YORK HEART ASSOCIATION FUNCTIONAL CLASS
Class I - No symptoms, no limitation during ordinary physical activity.
Class II – Mild symptoms (dyspnea &/or angina), slight limitation during ordinary activity.
Class III – Symptoms cause marked limitation in activity (even with minimal exertion) comfortable only at rest.
Class IV – Symptoms even while at rest, severe limitations & inability to carry out physical activity.

PATHOPHYSIOLOGY OF HEART FAILURE

Initial insult leads to ↑*afterload,* ↑*preload* &/or ↓*contractility.* The injured heart tries makes short-term compensations that, over time, promote cardiovascular deterioration. Compensations include:

❶ Sympathetic nervous system activation

❷ Myocyte hypertrophy/remodeling

❸ RAAS activation: *fluid overload, **ventricular remodeling**/hypertrophy* ⇨ CHF

CLINICAL MANIFESTATIONS

LEFT-SIDED FAILURE: ↑*pulmonary venous pressure* from FLUID BACKING UP INTO THE LUNGS:*

1. **Dyspnea MC symptom.*** Initially exertional ⇨*orthopnea* (dyspnea when the patient is supine – ↑'ed venous return & cardiac work) & *paroxysmal nocturnal dyspnea* (same reasons) ⇨ dyspnea @ rest (seen in advanced disease).

2. **Pulmonary congestion/edema:** **rales** (fluid in alveoli), **rhonchi, chronic nonproductive cough** (commonly missed) especially with **pink frothy sputum** *(surfactant)*, wheezing "cardiac asthma" due to airway edema. **CHF MC cause of transudative pleural effusions,*** nocturia.

3. **Physical exam***: hypertension*, rapid/shallow breathing (tachypnea), **Cheyne-Stokes breathing** (deeper faster breathing with gradual decrease & periods of apnea), cyanosis.
   - **S_3** (especially systolic failure), **S_4** (especially diastolic failure). Lateral displaced PMI.

4. **Increased adrenergic activation:** dusky, pale skin; diaphoresis, sinus tachycardia, cool extremities (due to poor perfusion & peripheral arterial vasoconstriction), fatigue, AMS.

RIGHT-SIDED FAILURE: ↑*systemic venous pressure* ⇨ signs of SYSTEMIC FLUID RETENTION:*

1. **Peripheral edema:*** ex. pitting edema in the legs. May develop cyanosis.

2. **Jugular Venous Distention (JVD):** ↑jugular venous pressure.

3. **GI/hepatic congestion:** anorexia, nausea/vomiting (due to edema of the GI tract), hepatosplenomegaly, RUQ tenderness, hepatojugular reflex (↑JVP with liver palpation).

DIAGNOSIS OF HEART FAILURE

1. **ECHOCARDIOGRAM** *most useful test to diagnose HF.** Measures ventricular function & ejection fraction (EF). **Ejection Fraction most important determinant of prognosis.*** Normal EF = 55-60%. EF <35% = ↑mortality ⇨ cardioverter defibrillator placement to reduce mortality.

   - **Systolic Failure: *decreased EF, thin ventricular walls, dilated LV chamber, ⊕ S_3***

   - **Diastolic Failure: *normal/↑EF, thick ventricular walls, small LV chamber, ⊕ S_4***

2. **CXR:** *especially useful in congestive heart failure.* Cephalization of flow ⇨ Kerley B lines ⇨ butterfly pattern ⇨ **cardiomegaly** infiltrates, **pleural effusions** ⇨ **pulmonary edema.**

3. ↑ **B-type natriuretic peptide (BNP) may identify CHF as the cause for dyspnea in ER.** Indicates severity & prognosis. Ventricles release **B-type natriuretic peptides during volume overload** (congestive heart failure) in attempt to reverse the process (causing ↓renin-angiotensin-aldosterone activation, ↓total body fluid volume, ↑sodium excretion).
   - BNP >100 = CHF is likely. **N-terminal pro-BNP may also be used.** Order cardiac enzymes to r/o MI.

LONG TERM MANAGEMENT OF HEART FAILURE

Initial management: *ACEI (& diuretic for symptoms). ACEI > beta blockers best 2 drugs for ↓mortality.**

	DRUG/INTERVENTION	COMMENTS
VASODILATORS (↓ AFTERLOAD)	Diet/exercise	Na restriction <2g/d; fluid restriction <2L/d, exercise smoking cessation
	ACE INHIBITORS* *Captopril* (Capoten) *Enalapril* (Vasotec) *Ramipril* (Altace) *Benazepril* (Lotensin) *Lisinopril* *Quinapril* *Trandolapril*	**MOA:** ↓preload/afterload, ↓aldosterone production (↓synthesis of AG II). Potentiates ***vasodilators*** (bradykinin, prostaglandins, nitric oxide). ↑'es exercise tolerance. **INDICATIONS:** *1ST LINE TREATMENT OF HF:** ↓mortality (post MI), ↓rehospitalization, *reverses the pathology by ↓'ing renin/sympathetic activation, ↓ventricular remodeling.* **S/E:** *1st dose hypotension, renal insufficiency* (esp if Cr >3, CrCl <30, dilation of efferent arteriole), **hyperkalemia**; *Cough & angioedema (due to ↑bradykinin).** **CI:** *hypotension, pregnancy* (teratogenic).
	ANGIOTENSIN II RECEPTOR BLOCKERS (ARB)*	**IND:** *patients unable to tolerate ACEI. Blocks effects of angiotensin II* (not its production, so there is no increase in bradykinin ⇨ no cough/angioedema). • *Losartan* (Cozaar); *Valsartan* (Diovan), *Candesartan, Irbesartan* (Avapro)
	BETA-BLOCKERS* *Carvedilol* nonselective *(β₁,₂,α₁)* *Metoprolol & Bisoprolol* (cardioselective: β₁ only)	*35% ↓mortality (↑EF & reduces ventricular size). Added after ACEI** or ARB. **S/E:** Carvedilol ± cause dizziness, hypotension (2ʳʸ to α₁ -receptor blockade); EF ↓'es transiently then increases so *stop or reduce βB dose during decompensated CHF.**
	HYDRALAZINE + NITRATES* *COMBINED*	Consider if not able to tolerate ACEI or βB; not as good as ACEI. Vasodilators that ↓'es mortality. **Good for African-Americans.** Hydralazine safe in pregnancy.* **MOA:** NTG ↓*preload* (venous- relaxation) & afterload; *Hydralazine ↓'es afterload* **S/E:** *dizziness, headache, tachyphylaxis (8 hour nitrate-free period to prevent it).**
↓PRELOAD	**DIURETICS** **LOOP DIURETICS** *Furosemide* (Lasix) *Bumetanide* *Torsemide*	*Most effective treatment for symptoms* for mild-moderate CHF.* **Ind:** CHF, hypertension, severe edema, mild renal disease. **MOA:** inhibits water transport across Loop of Henle ⇨ ↑excretion of H₂0, Cl⁻, Na⁺, K⁺. **S/E:** volume depletion, **hypOkalemia/calcemia/**natremia, **hyperglycemia**, **hyperuricemia**, sulfa allergies, hypochloremic metabolic alkalosis.
	POTASSIUM SPARING DIURETICS* *Spironolactone* *Eplerenone*	**MOA:** aldosterone antagonist. *Spironolactone associated with ↓mortality* - added in severe CHF (Class III & IV heart failure). **S/E:** hyperkalemia. *Gynecomastia with Spironolactone.* **CI:** renal failure, hyponatremia.
	Hydrochlorothiazides **Metolazone**	**S/E:** *hypOnatremia/*kalemia; metabolic alkalosis, **hyperuricemia, hyperglycemia.** Thiazide-like diuretic. **IND:** refractory edema, commonly used in combo with loop.
POSITIVE INOTROPES	**SYMPATHOMIMETICS** *(Positive Inotropes)* **DIGOXIN**	*Used SHORT TERM in severe acute CHF. Digoxin is the only one that is used long-term.* **IND:** *HF + A fib,* ↓hospitalization/symptoms but *NO MORTALITY BENEFIT WITH DIGOXIN.** **MOA:** ⊕ *inotropic agent* – prolongs intracellular calcium/contraction via Na⁺/K⁺ pump inhibition; **negative chronotrope** (↓HR); **negative dromotrope** (↓conduction speed). **S/E:** *narrow TI – arrhythmias, CNS (seizures, dizziness), GI* (anorexia, N/V/D); **visual: (double/blurred vision green/yellow, halos around lights), gynecomastia.** **Digoxin Toxicity:** digitalis effect on ECG: downsloping sagging ST segment, junctional rhythms. *Hypokalemia worsens toxicity.** Mgmt: *Digoxin Immune Fab (antidote).*
	Dobutamine	↑contractility (β₁ agonist), produces peripheral vasodilation.
	Dopamine	High doses acts as β/α agonist. @ low doses acts as a diuretic by ↑renal blood flow.

Nesiritide | **MOA:** *synthetic BNP (↓'es RAAS activity, ↑'es Na⁺ excretion).* Only used in ER or inpatient settings.

MEDS THAT ↓MORTALITY: *ACEI, ARB, β-blockers, Nitrates + Hydralazine, Spironolactone.*

Calcium channel blockers not generally used in systolic HF* (exceptions: angina with HF or normal EF).

HF OUTPATIENT REGIMEN *ACE + diuretic initially ⇨ add β–blockers;** ±Hydralazine + NTG, Digoxin.

➢ *Implantable Cardioverter Defibrillator in patients with EF <35% (because they tolerate arrhythmias poorly).*

NOVEL MEDICATIONS FOR SYSTOLIC HEART FAILURE

1. Ivabradine: selective sinus node inhibitor (slows the sinus rate). Associated with ↓hospitalization & ↓mortality. Used in symptomatic chronic stable heart failure with LVEF ≤35%, in sinus rhythm with a resting pulse of ≥70 bpm & already maxed out on the beta-blocker dose or are unable to take beta-blockers.

2. Sacubitril-Valsartan (Entresto):
   MOA: Sacubitril is an angiotensin receptor neprilysin inhibitor ⇨ increased levels of natriuretic peptides. Valsartan is an angiotensin II receptor blocker.
   Ind: reduces mortality & ↓hospitalization for chronic heart failure (Class II-IV) with reduced EF.

CONGESTIVE (DECOMPENSATED) HEART FAILURE (CHF)

CHF: acute decompensated heart failure with worsening of baseline symptoms, pulmonary congestion (worsening of dyspnea, rales, pink frothy sputum etc.); CXR findings of congestion & sympathetic activation.

CXR FINDINGS IN CONGESTIVE HEART FAILURE

Cephalization of flow ⇨ Kerley B lines ⇨ batwing appearance ⇨ pulmonary edema.

Cephalization: ↑vascular flow to the apices as a result of increased pulmonary venous pressure. Occurs with pulmonary capillary wedge pressures of 12-18mm Hg (normal PCWP is 6 – 12 mm Hg).

Kerley B Lines (PCWP 18-25 mmHg)
Short linear markings @ lung periphery

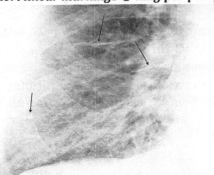

Butterfly (Batwing) Pattern (PCWP >25mmHg)

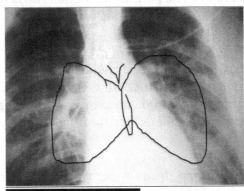

CONGESTIVE HEART FAILURE SIGNS

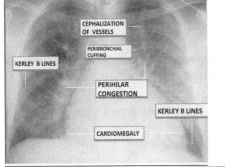

PULMONARY EDEMA

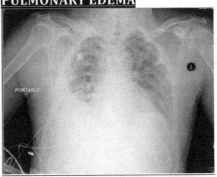

MANAGEMENT OF ACUTE PULMONARY EDEMA/CONGESTIVE HEART FAILURE

"LMNOP": Lasix, Morphine, Nitrates (venodilators), Oxygen, Position (place upright to ↓venous return). Lasix (Furosemide) removes fluids (relieves symptoms). Morphine reduces preload, reducing heart strain (limited use in CHF). Nitrates reduce preload & afterload. May need inotropic support if severe.

DIASTOLIC HEART FAILURE

MANAGEMENT: heart rate control, blood pressure control & relief of ischemia (β-blockers, ACE inhibitors & calcium channel blockers). Diuretics for volume overload.

PERICARDIAL DISEASES

ACUTE PERICARDITIS

ACUTE PERICARDITIS: *acute fibrinous inflammation of the pericardium.* May cause an effusion.
<u>Serous:</u> noninfectious (ex. RA, SLE); If fibrin adhesion occurs⇨ fibrinous or serofibrinous (ex. post MI).

ETIOLOGIES
1. *2 MC causes are idiopathic (probably viral-related) & <u>viral</u> (especially the Enteroviruses-Coxsackie & Echovirus).** Neoplastic, Dressler syndrome (post-MI pericarditis), autoimmune, systemic, uremia, bacterial, radiation therapy, drugs: ex. Procainamide, INH, Hydralazine.

CLINICAL MANIFESTATIONS
1. CHEST PAIN: *Pleuritic (sharp & worse with inspiration), Persistent & Postural (worse when supine & relieved by sitting/leaning forward).* ± Radiate to trapezius, back, neck, shoulder, arm, epigastric area. ± Dyspnea & odynophagia. *Fever usually present.*

2. PERICARDIAL FRICTION RUB: *best heard at end expiration while upright & leaning forward.* 3 components. The pericardial friction rub is notoriously variable (can be transient).

DIAGNOSTIC STUDIES
A. ECG: *diffuse ST elevations in precordial leads* (concave up in V1 through V6) & associated PR depressions.** (aVR ⇨ atrial injury associated with PR elevation & ST depression) ⇨ T wave inversions ⇨ resolution. 30% ±have ⊕ cardiac enzymes because of concurrent myocarditis.
B. Echocardiogram: *used to assess for complications of acute pericarditis (effusion or tamponade).* Isolated pericarditis ⇨ normal echo. Effusions are common; Tamponade is rare.

MANAGEMENT
1. *Anti-inflammatory drugs - aspirin or NSAIDs** x7-14 days. (sx usually subside within 24h). *Colchicine is 2nd line management.*
2. *± Corticosteroids if symptoms > 48h & refractory* to 1st line meds. *Dressler: Aspirin or Colchicine.**

PERICARDIAL EFFUSION

- **Pericardial Effusion:** *increased fluid in the pericardial space.*

ETIOLOGIES
Pericarditis, malignancy, infection, radiation therapy, dialysis/uremia, collagen vascular disease, etc.

PHYSICAL EXAMINATION
1. *Distant (muffled) heart sounds** (because fluid interferes with sound conduction).

DIAGNOSTIC STUDIES
A. ELECTROCARDIOGRAM:
1. *Low voltage QRS complex:** suggests a large effusion* or tamponade.
2. *Electric alternans:* cyclic beat to beat shift in QRS amplitude (heart swinging in fluid).
B. ECHOCARDIOGRAM: ↑*pericardial fluid. Used to assess for tamponade physiology.*
C. CXR: *cardiomegaly.*

MANAGEMENT OF PERICARDIAL EFFUSION
1. Observation if small & no evidence of tamponade. *Treat the underlying cause.*
2. ± Pericardiocentesis if tamponade or large effusion. Pericardial window drainage if recurrent.

ACUTE PERICARDITIS

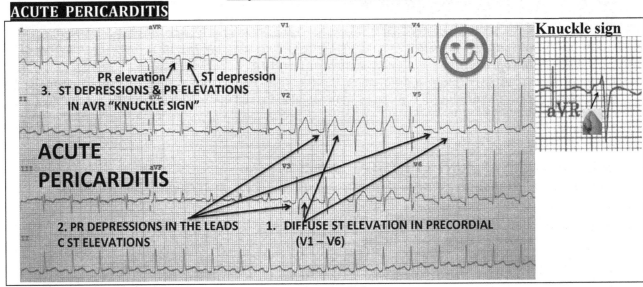

Knuckle sign

PR elevation / ST depression
3. ST DEPRESSIONS & PR ELEVATIONS
   IN AVR "KNUCKLE SIGN"

ACUTE
PERICARDITIS

2. PR DEPRESSIONS IN THE LEADS
   C ST ELEVATIONS

1. DIFFUSE ST ELEVATION IN PRECORDIAL
   (V1 – V6)

- **_Diffuse ST segment elevation (concave upwards)._**
- **_PR segment depressions_** in the leads with ST elevations.

- <u>Lead aVR</u>: PR elevation with ST depression (knuckle sign) reflects atrial injury.

NORMAL ECG EVOLUTION IN ACUTE PERICARDITIS

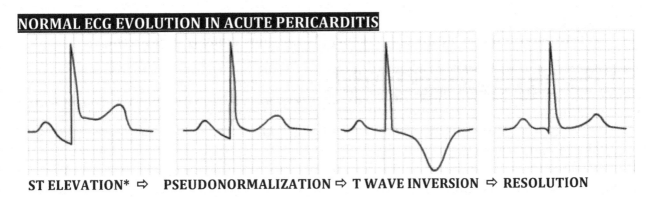

ST ELEVATION* ⇨ PSEUDONORMALIZATION ⇨ T WAVE INVERSION ⇨ RESOLUTION

ELECTRIC ALTERNANS

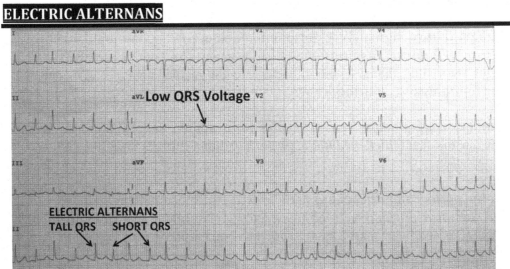

Low QRS Voltage

ELECTRIC ALTERNANS
TALL QRS   SHORT QRS

Sinus tachycardia with electric alternans. Notice the shift in amplitude of QRS complexes with the taller waves alternating with shorter waves & low QRS voltage.

PERICARDIAL TAMPONADE

- **Tamponade:** *pericardial EFFUSION CAUSING SIGNIFICANT PRESSURE ON THE HEART* ⇨ *restriction of cardiac ventricular filling* ⇨ *decreased cardiac output.**
- The time of pericardial effusion development is of critical importance. Small, rapidly developing effusions of a few hundred cc's can cause tamponade. In chronic diseases (ex malignancy), the pericardium can stretch to accommodate up to 1L of pericardial fluid without causing hemodynamic compromise.

CLINICAL MANIFESTATIONS & PHYSICAL EXAMINATION
1. BECK'S TRIAD:* ❶ *distant (muffled) heart sounds* ❷↑*JVP** ❸ *systemic HYPOtension.*

2. *Pulsus paradoxus:* *exaggerated >10 mmHg decrease in systolic blood pressure with inspiration* ⇨↓pulses with inspiration. Increased filling of the right side of the heart during inspiration decreases left sided ventricular filling, leading to pulsus paradoxus.
3. Dyspnea, fatigue, peripheral edema, shock: hypotension, reflex tachycardia, cool extremities.

DIAGNOSTIC STUDIES
1. **Echocardiogram:** presence of effusion + *__diastolic collapse of cardiac chambers__** (due the pericardial fluid pressure being greater than the chamber pressure ⇨ collapse).

MANAGEMENT
1. *Pericardiocentesis (immediate).** ± Pericardial window drainage if recurrent.

CONSTRICTIVE PERICARDITIS

- **Constrictive pericarditis:** *THICKENED, FIBROTIC, CALCIFIED PERICARDIUM* (from chronic pericarditis & inflammation) *that __restricts ventricular diastolic filling__* ⇨↑venous pressures, ↓stroke volume (decreased cardiac output).

CLINICAL MANIFESTATIONS
1. *Dyspnea MC symptom,** fatigue, orthopnea.

2. **Right-sided heart failure signs:** ↑JVD, peripheral edema, N/V, hepatojugular reflux. *Kussmaul's sign*:* ↑*JVD during inspiration.* ± also be seen in restrictive cardiomyopathy. Impaired right ventricular filling ⇨ blood backs into the jugular veins ⇨ ↑JVD (jugular venous distention/pressure) with inspiration.

3. PERICARDIAL KNOCK:* *high-pitched 3rd heart sound* due to *sudden cessation of ventricular filling* in early diastole from *thickened inelastic pericardium.* Often Sounds like S_3.

DIAGNOSTIC STUDIES
1. **Echocardiography:** *pericardial thickening.** (CT or MRI ± be more sensitive).
2. CXR: *pericardial calcification** may be seen (especially on lateral views), clear lung fields. Normal/slightly increased heart size. "Square root sign" on cardiac catheterization.

Differential dx: *constrictive pericarditis often confused with restrictive cardiomyopathy.*

MANAGEMENT
Pericardiectomy: definitive treatment.* Diuretics may be used for symptomatic control.

PERICARDIAL DISEASES

	ACUTE PERICARDITIS	PERICARDIAL EFFUSION	PERICARDIAL TAMPONADE	CONSTRICTIVE PERICARDITIS
DEFINITION	*Inflammation of the pericardium.*	↑ fluid in pericardial space.	*Pericardial effusion ⇨ pressure on the heart* ⇨ *limits ventricular diastolic filling & ↓cardiac output.*	*Fibrotic, calcified pericardium limits ventricular diastolic filling*
ETIOLOGIES	• 2 most common causes are idiopathic (probably postviral) & viral (*esp Enteroviruses: Coxsackievirus & Echoviruses*). • Neoplastic, autoimmune (SLE, RA) • Inflammatory, vascular etc. • *Dressler's syndrome: post MI*	Same as acute pericarditis.	Same as pericarditis. May be traumatic.	Same as pericarditis Chronic inflammation
CLINICAL MANIFESTATIONS	5 P's of pericarditis: • Chest Pain - Pleuritic (sharp pain worse with inspiration)* - Postural (pain worse supine, relieved with sitting forward).* - Persistent chest Pain • Pericardial Friction Rub	• *Distant (muffled) heart sounds.* • ± sx of pericarditis.	• BECK'S TRIAD* ❶ *Distant heart sounds (effusion)* ❷ ↑JVP (jugular venous pressure) ❸ *Systemic HYPOtension* • *Pulsus paradoxus* – drop >10mmHg of systolic BP with inspiration (pulses disappear with inspiration). - *Kussmaul's sign:* ↑JVP c̄ inspiration.	• *Dyspnea MC sx* • *R-SIDED FAILURE SX*: - Peripheral edema - ↑JVP - Hepatic congestion, N/V • *PERICARDIAL KNOCK* 3rd heart* sound from sudden cessation of ventricular filling. • *Pulsus paradoxus* • *Kussmaul's sign*
DIAGNOSIS	• ECG: - *Diffuse ST elevations* (concave up) in precordial leads with PR depressions in same leads* ⇨ T wave inversions ⇨ resolution. - aVR: ST depression & PR elevation. • ECHOCARDIOGRAM: - Normal (± pericardial effusion). Used mainly to r/o tamponade.	• ECG: - *Low voltage QRS complex* - Electric Alternans • ECHOCARDIOGRAM: - ↑*pericardial fluid.* - No hemodynamic compromise.	• ECG: - *Low voltage QRS complexes* - Electric Alternans • ECHOCARDIOGRAM: - ↑*pericardial fluid + diastolic collapse of cardiac chambers* hemodynamic compromise.*	• ECHOCARDIOGRAM: - *PERICARDIAL THICKENING* & calcification*
MANAGEMENT	• *ASPIRIN OR NSAIDs tx of choice* • *Colchicine 2nd line* • *Steroids if refractory (sx > 48h)* • *Dressler's syndrome:* *Aspirin or Colchicine*	• *Treat underlying cause* • *Pericardial window if recurrent*	• *PERICARDIOCENTESIS*	• *PERICARDIECTOMY*

MYOCARDITIS

- **MYOCARDITIS:** *inflammation of the heart muscle.*
  Complications of heart failure more common in children.

- *MC due to viral infection* *(or postviral immune-mediated cardiac damage).*

ETIOLOGIES OF MYOCARDITIS	
INFECTIOUS	*Viral:* ENTEROVIRUSES (ESP. COXSACKIE B) MC CAUSE,* adenovirus; Parvovirus B19, Human herpesvirus 6, Epstein-Barr virus (HHV-4), HIV, Varicella zoster. *Bacterial:* Rickettsial *(Lyme disease, Rocky Mountain spotted fever, Q fever),* other, Chagas disease – rare in US but seen in South/Central America. Diphtheria. Fungal: actinomycosis, coccidioidomycosis, histoplasmosis, candidiasis. Parasitic: trichinosis, toxoplasmosis.
TOXIC	Scorpion envenomation, diphtheria toxins.
AUTOIMMUNE	*Systemic lupus erythematosus, Rheumatic fever,* Rheumatoid arthritis, Kawasaki syndrome, Ulcerative colitis.
SYSTEMIC	Uremia (develops in $^1/_3$ especially if on hemodialysis), Hypothyroidism.
MEDICATIONS	*Clozapine,** Methyldopa, antibiotics (Tetracycline, Amphotericin-B, penicillin), Isoniazid, Cyclophosphamide, Acetazolamide, Indomethacin, Phenytoin, sulfonamides.

PATHOPHYSIOLOGY
➤ Myocellular damage ⇨ myocardial necrosis & dysfunction ⇨ ± *heart failure (due to systolic dysfunction, cardiac enlargement & myocardial fibrosis).*

CLINICAL MANIFESTATIONS
1. *Viral prodrome:* (fever, myalgias, malaise) for several days ⇨ HEART FAILURE SYMPTOMS.*

2. *Heart failure:* dyspnea @ rest, exercise intolerance, syncope, tachypnea, tachycardia, hepatomegaly. *Impaired systolic function (S_3, ±S_4).* Severe: hypotension, poor pulses & perfusion, altered mental status. GI symptoms: *ex. megacolon.*
3. *± concurrent pericarditis:* fever & chest pain, pericardial friction rub, pericardial effusion.

DIAGNOSTIC STUDIES
1. **CXR:** *cardiomegaly classic* (dilated cardiomyopathy),* ±normal.
2. **ECG:** nonspp: *sinus tachycardia MC,* ± show atrial/junction/ventricular arrhythmias. ±normal ECG. ± show pericarditis (precordial ST elevations + PR depressions), pericardial effusion (alternans).

3. **Cardiac Enzymes:** ⊕ *CK-MB & Troponin (reflecting myocardial necrosis due to the disease process – not usually due to occlusion).* ⊕ Cardiac enzymes help to distinguish myocarditis from chronic dilated cardiomyopathy.

4. **Echocardiography:** *ventricular dysfunction,* ± pericardial effusion or mitral regurgitation. Echocardiogram most useful to assess cardiac function.
5. **Other:** ↑*ESR.* Workup may include: CBC, viral cultures & titers.

6. **Endomyocardial biopsy:** *gold standard in diagnosing myocarditis.* Commonly shows infiltration of lymphocytes with myocardial tissue necrosis.* Done in patients with new onset of heart failure unrelated to structural disease. Helps with the diagnosis & prognosis.

MANAGEMENT
1. *Supportive mainstay of treatment, standard systolic heart failure tx:* diuretics, afterload reducing agents (ex ACEI), inotropic drugs if severe (Dopamine, Dobutamine, Milrinone).
2. Beta blockers generally not used in the management of pediatric patients.
3. Intravenous immune globulin (IVIG) may be helpful in some patients.

DILATED CARDIOMYOPATHY (DCMP)   95% of cardiomyopathies

- *Systolic dysfunction* ⇨ *ventricular dilation* ⇨ *dilated, weak heart.** MC 20-60y. *MC in men.*

ETIOLOGIES
IDIOPATHIC: *(50%)*. Postviral probably MC cause of idiopathic.
VIRAL MYOCARDITIS: *Enteroviruses MC* (ex Coxsackie B, echovirus), PB19,* HIV. Lyme dz, *Chagas dz*
TOXIC: *alcohol abuse** (7-8 drinks/day x 5y), *cocaine, anthracyclines (Doxorubicin),** radiation tx.
Other: *pregnancy,* infiltrative, autoimmune, metabolic (ex. hyperthyroid/hypothyroid disorders).

CLINICAL MANIFESTATIONS
1. *Heart failure: systolic heart failure sx:* ⊕ *S₃;* fatigue, signs of left & right-sided CHF, lateral displaced PMI, ± mitral or tricuspid regurgitation (annular dilation, displaced papillary muscle).
2. *Embolic events* (~10%); *Arrhythmias;* Chest pain on exertion.

DIAGNOSTIC STUDIES
1. ECHOCARDIOGRAM: ❶ *left ventricular dilation* (thin ventricular walls), large ventricular chambers,* ❷ ↓*ejection fraction (EF),** ❸ regional or global *left ventricular hypokinesis.*
2. CXR: *cardiomegaly*, pulmonary edema, pleural effusion. ECG: sinus tachycardia or arrhythmias.

MANAGEMENT OF DILATED CARDIOMYOPATHY
1. *Standard heart failure tx:* ACEI, diuretics, beta blockers (if not in decompensated CHF), Digoxin, Na⁺ restriction; Implantable Defibrillator (AICD) if EF <30-35%; Cardiac transplant.

DIFFERENTIAL DIAGNOSIS
- Dilated heart failure due to cardiac disease: ischemia, valvular disease, hypertension. These are the MC causes of decreased EF & LV dilation (however not true DCMP as they are cardiac causes).
- **Takotsubo Cardiomyopathy:** APICAL LEFT VENTRICULAR BALLOONING* following an event that causes a catecholamine surge (ex. emotional stress *"broken heart syndrome"*, surgery), especially postmenopausal. ECG: ST elevations, ⊕ cardiac enzymes (but no thrombosis on catheterization).

RESTRICTIVE CARDIOMYOPATHY (RCMP)   1%

- *Impaired diastolic function with relatively preserved contractility.* *Ventricular rigidity impedes ventricular filling* (↓*compliance).* The stiff ventricle only fills with great effort.

ETIOLOGIES
1. *Infiltrative disease:* AMYLOIDOSIS MC CAUSE,* sarcoidosis, idiopathic myocardial fibrosis, hemochromatosis, metastatic disease, scleroderma, chemotherapy, radiation therapy.

CLINICAL MANIFESTATIONS
1. *Right-sided failure sx more common** than *left-sided,* poorly tolerated tachyarrhythmias.

PHYSICAL EXAM
1. *Kussmaul's sign (JVP increases with inspiration):* Stiff, inelastic RV ⇨ impaired filling of RV causes increased blood flow to back up in the venous system; Signs of heart failure, ± S₃.

DIAGNOSTIC STUDIES
CXR: normal ventricular chamber size, enlarged atria, may have pulmonary congestion.
ECG: low voltage, ± arrhythmias. *Echo ± show bright (speckled) myocardium in amyloidosis.*
Echocardiogram: ❶ *Ventricles nondilated with normal wall thickness* (± slightly thick). ❷*MARKED DILATION OF BOTH ATRIA.** *Diastolic dysfunction.* Systolic dysfunction ± seen if advanced.

MANAGEMENT
1. *No specific treatment.* Treat underlying disorder (ex. chelation for hemochromatosis, steroids for sarcoidosis etc.). Treatment is basically symptomatic (ex. *gentle* diuresis, vasodilators).

HYPERTROPHIC CARDIOMYOPATHY (HCMP) 4% (IDIOPATHIC HYPERTROPHIC SUBAORTIC STENOSIS)

> ➤ Inherited <u>genetic</u> disorder of inappropriate LV and/or RV hypertrophy (especially septal).

PATHOPHYSIOLOGY

- **SUBAORTIC OUTFLOW OBSTRUCTION** narrowed LV outflow tract 2ry to: ❶ *hypertrophied septum* + ❷ *systolic anterior motion (SAM)* of the mitral valve & papillary muscle displacement. *↑SAM seen with:*
   a. *↑contractility:* ex. Digoxin, beta agonists, exercise.
   b. *↓LV volume:* ex. decreased venous return, dehydration, Valsalva maneuver.

- **DIASTOLIC DYSFUNCTION:** stiff ventricular chamber ⇨ *impaired ventricular relaxation/filling* (because thickened walls lead to a smaller left ventricular volume & ↓ left ventricular filling).

CLINICAL MANIFESTATIONS
Often asymptomatic, first symptom may be sudden cardiac death.
   1. *Dyspnea most common initial complaint** (90%). Fatigue.

   2. *Angina pectoris (chest pain)* 75%. Usually in the setting of a normal angiogram.

   3. <u>Syncope:</u> includes pre syncope & dizziness (due to inadequate cardiac output on exertion).
   4. *Arrhythmias* A fib; VT/VF (palpitations, syncope, sudden cardiac death).

   5. *Sudden cardiac death:* especially in adolescent/preadolescent children *(especially during times of extreme exertion).* Usually due to *ventricular fibrillation.**

PHYSICAL EXAM
   1. *Harsh systolic crescendo-decrescendo murmur:** best heard @ LLSB *(sounds similar to AS).*
      - ↓ *murmur intensity:* handgrip; *increased venous return (ex squatting, lying supine)* because *↑LV volume preserves outflow* (↑fluid pushes septum out of the way & ↓'es SAM of mitral valve).

      - *↑murmur intensity with decreased venous return** (ex: Valsalva & standing).
      - Usually *no carotid radiation.** May have *loud S₄,* mitral regurgitation, S₃ or *pulsus bisferiens.*

DIAGNOSTIC STUDIES
   1. **ECHOCARDIOGRAM:** *asymmetrical wall thickness (esp septal)** ≥15mm, *systolic anterior motion of mitral valve*; small LV chamber size, dynamic outflow obstruction, ± mitral regurgitation.

   2. <u>ECG:</u> *LVH,* atrial enlargement, anterolateral & inferior pseudo q waves. <u>CXR:</u> cardiomegaly.

MANAGEMENT
   - Focus on early detection, medical management, surgical and/or *ICD placement.**
   - *Counseling to avoid dehydration & extreme exertion/exercise very important!**
      1. **Medical**: *BETA BLOCKERS 1ST LINE MEDICAL TX,** CCB (Verapamil), Disopyramide. All 3 are negative inotropes that ↑ ventricular diastolic filling time. *Cautious use of Digoxin, nitrates & diuretics** (Digoxin ↑'es contractility; Nitrates & diuretics ↓'es left ventricular volume)

      2. **Surgical (Myomectomy):** resection of the hypertrophied septum. Myomectomy usually performed in patients with severe, refractory symptoms despite medical management.

      3. **Alcohol Septal Ablation:** (alternative to surgical management with good outcomes). Medical "myomectomy". Ethanol destroys the extra myocardial tissue.

Secondary HCM: due to longstanding hypertension, aortic stenosis (however not true HCM).

CARDIOMYOPATHIES

Cardiomyopathy: disease of the heart muscle (myocardial tissue) with cardiac dysfunction NOT due to other heart diseases*

	DILATED CARDIOMYOPATHY (95%)	RESTRICTIVE CARDIOMYOPATHY (1%)	HYPERTROPHIC CARDIOMYOPATHY (4%)
DEFINITION	• *SYSTOLIC DYSFUNCTION* ⇨ *ventricular dilation* ⇨ *"dilated, weak heart** • MC present 20-60y. • MC in men	• *DIASTOLIC DYSFUNCTION** with relatively preserved contractility • Ventricular rigidity impedes ventricular filling (↓ ventricular compliance)	• *DIASTOLIC DYSFUNCTION** due to *impaired ventricular relaxation/filling* • *SUBAORTIC OUTFLOW OBSTRUCTION**: - *hypertrophied septum* PLUS - systolic anterior motion (SAM) of mitral valve & SAM is increased with: ❶ ↑contractility (exertion) & ❷ ↓LV volume (ex. ↓decreased venous return, dehydration).
ETIOLOGIES	• *Idiopathic MC cause,** autoimmune • *Viral myocarditis** (ex. enteroviruses) • *Toxic: ETOH*, cocaine, pregnancy • XRT, *doxorubicin*, daunorubicin	•Infiltrative diseases - *Amyloidosis MC cause** - Sarcoidosis, Hemochromatosis - Scleroderma, metastatic disease; Idiopathic	• Inherited genetic disorder of inappropriate *left and/or right ventricular hypertrophy (especially septal).*
CLINICAL MANIFESTATIONS	•*SYSTOLIC HEART FAILURE SX* - Both L & R-sided •Embolic phenomena, arrhythmias •*Viral Myocarditis: viral prodrome a few weeks* ⇨ signs of heart failure or chest pain, ⊕ cardiac enzymes, nonspp ST-T changes	•*RIGHT-SIDED FAILURE SX* more common than left-sided* •Poorly tolerated tachyarrhythmias	•Often asymptomatic •*Dyspnea* 90%. *Most common initial complaint**. •*Angina pectoris. Syncope* •*Arrhythmias* AF; VT/VF (palpitations, syncope). •*Sudden cardiac death*: esp in adolescent/preadolescent children (especially exertion) due to *Vent. Fibrillation**
PHYSICAL	•L-sided heart failure - Pulmonary congestion: *rales, tachycardia,* cough, pleural effusion •R heart failure - Peripheral edema, ↑JVP, hepatic congestion	•*Kussmaul's sign:* ↑JVP with inspiration •R-sided heart failure Peripheral edema, ↑JVP, hepatic congestion	•*Harsh systolic cres-decrec murmur @LLSB* sounds like AS* - ↓*murmur intensity:* ↑*venous return* (ex squatting, supine); handgrip (increases afterload) - ↑*murmur: ↓venous return* (Valsalva & standing) & exertion (because ↓LV volume & ↑contractility will ↓CO), amyl nitrate • Usually *no carotid radiation*.* Normal pulse, *Loud S₄*. ± MR
DIAGNOSIS	•ECHOCARDIOGRAM: - ❶ *left ventricular dilation: thin walls* - ❷ ↓*ejection fraction (EF)* - ❸ *Regional or global LV hypokinesis.* •CXR: - *Cardiomegaly*, pulmonary edema, pleural effusion	•ECHOCARDIOGRAM: - Ventricles nondilated with normal wall thickness. - *MARKED DILATION OF BOTH ATRIA** - *Diastolic dysfunction* with normal or near normal systolic function.*	•*ECHOCARDIOGRAM:* - *Asymmetric wall thickness (esp septal)*,* SAM mitral v. •*ECG:* - *Left ventricular hypertrophy**
MANAGEMENT	*Standard systolic heart failure treatment**: -*ACEI, diuretics,* digoxin, beta blockers, sodium restriction -Implantable defibrillator (AICD) if EF <35%	•*No specific treatment* Treat underlying cause	Avoid exertion, Implantable Defibrillator to prevent VF. •*Medical: BETA BLOCKERS**, Verapamil, Disopyramide. •*Cautious use of digoxin, nitrates & diuretics** (digoxin ↑'es contractility while nitrates & diuretics ↓volume) •*Surgical*: Myomectomy, ETOH ablation

RHEUMATIC FEVER

- *Acute autoimmune inflammatory multi-systemic illness* mainly affecting ***children 5-15y.****

PATHOPHYSIOLOGY: *symptomatic or asymptomatic* **infection with GABHS Group A β-Hemolytic Streptococcus*** *(aka **Strep pyogenes**)* stimulates antibody production to host tissues & damages organs directly. The infection usually precedes the onset of rheumatic fever by 2-6 weeks.

COMPLICATIONS: *rheumatic valvular disease: mitral* (75-80%)*, aortic* (30%); tricuspid & pulmonic (5%).

DIAGNOSIS

JONES CRITERIA FOR RHEUMATIC FEVER	(2 Major OR 1 major + 2 minor)
MAJOR CRITERIA	**MINOR CRITERIA**
1. **J**oint *(migratory polyarthritis)* 2. **O**h my heart *(active carditis)* 3. **N**odules (subcutaneous) 4. **E**rythema marginatum 5. **S**ydenham's chorea	**CLINICAL** Fever (≥101.3° F/≥ 38.5° C) Arthralgia (joint pain) **LABORATORY** ↑acute phase reactants (↑ESR, CRP, leukocytosis) ECG: prolonged PR interval
PLUS ***Supporting evidence of a recent group A streptococcal infection*** ex. positive throat culture or rapid antigen detection test &/or elevated/increasing streptococcal antibody titers (ASO)	

MAJOR CRITERIA

1. **POLYARTHRITIS:** (75%) *2 or more joints affected* (simultaneous more diagnostic) *or migratory (lower ⇨ upper joints). Medium/large joints MC affected* (knees, hips, wrists, elbows, shoulders). *Heat, redness, swelling, severe joint tenderness must be present.* Joint pain (athralgia) without other symptoms doesn't classify as major. Usually lasts 3-4 weeks.

2. **ACTIVE CARDITIS:** (40-60%) can affect valves (especially mitral & aortic), myocardium (myocarditis) &/or pericardium (pericarditis). *Carditis confers great morbidity & mortality.*

3. **SYDENHAM'S CHOREA** (<10%) "Saint Vitus dance" may occur 1- 8 months after initial infection. Manifestations include sudden involuntary, jerky, non-rhythmic, purposeless movements especially involving the head/arms. Usually resolves spontaneously. MC in females.

4. **ERYTHEMA MARGINATUM:** often accompanies carditis. Macular, erythematous, non-pruritic annular rash with rounded, sharply demarcated borders (may have central clearing). MC seen primarily on the trunk & extremities (not the face). Crops last hours-days before disappearing.

5. **SUBCUTANEOUS NODULES:** *rare.* Seen over joints (extensor surfaces), scalp & spinal column.

Other findings not associated with Jones criteria: abdominal pain, facial tics/grimaces, epistaxis.

MANAGEMENT

1. **Anti-inflammatory:** *Aspirin* (2-6 weeks with taper); ± Corticosteroids in severe cases & carditis.

2. ***Penicillin G antibiotic of choice (or Erythromycin if PCN-allergic)*** both in acute phase & after acute episode. Prevention is the most important therapeutic course. Therefore all patients (even if presenting with acute rheumatic fever) should be treated with antibiotics.

VALVULAR DISEASE INTRO

- 4 valves ensure blood flow in one direction.
- Atrioventricular (AV) valves = mitral (L); tricuspid (R) Semilunar valves = aortic (L), pulmonary (R)

HEART SOUNDS

SYSTOLE	S_1: _**AV valve closure**_ (**S_1 marks beginning of systole**) S_1 (First heart sound) comprised of mitral (M_1) followed by tricuspid (T_1) valve closure. _S_1 normally loudest @ the apex_ c diaphragm. Palpation of carotid impulse helps to identify S_1 (S_1 is lower pitched and of longer duration than S_2). Exercise increases the force of velocity of ventricular contraction & thus S_1 intensity.
	S_2: _**Semilunar valve closure**_ (**S_2 marks the end of systole**). Second heart sound. Composed of aortic (A_2) followed by pulmonic (P_2) closure. _**S_2 best heard at base**_ (aortic & pulmonic areas). **Physiologic split of S_2:** inspiration separates S_2 into A_2 followed by P_2. **Fixed split of S_2:** doesn't vary with inspiration. Seen with L to R shunt (ASD, VSD) or delayed P_2 closure **(Pulmonary HTN, mitral regurgitation)**. **Paradoxical split of S_2:** Maximally on expiration & P_2 followed by A_2. Delayed in AV valve closure (prolonged LV emptying, LBBB, **severe aortic stenosis**).
	**Ejection click: mitral valve prolapse** (chordae tendinae abruptly pulls the mitral valve tight).
DIASTOLE	S_3: _**rapid "passive" ventricular filling.**_ Occurs in early diastole when blood enters into right ventricle. Commonly heard in children, adolescents and in some young adults. Physiologic S_3 usually disappears when the patient sits or stands or if the heart rate is low. **When heard over age 30y**, it is called a **"protodiastolic gallop" sound** and is a pathologic: ex **left ventricular systolic failure.*** Mimicked by the sound " **lub de bub**".
	S_4: _**atrial contraction**_ into the ventricles. A physiologic S_4 may be heard in infants, small children, and adults over 50y. It is usually heard only @ apex. Pathologically associated with **decreased compliance of left ventricle (atria contracting into stiff ventricle). Seen with hypertension, left ventricular hypertrophy & aortic stenosis.** Mimicked by the sound **"belup dub"**.
	Opening snap: _**opening of stenotic mitral valve (MS).**_ OS best heard @ apex

- **Murmurs:** abnormal blood flow backwards (regurgitation) through a valve that should be closed or abnormal forward flow through a (stenotic) valve that should be open.

QUALITY OF THE MURMUR

- **HARSH/RUMBLE SOUNDS = think STENOSIS***: AS, MS:** abnormal forward flow of blood through (stenotic) valve that should be open. Stenotic lesions lead to pressure overload. Regurgitation leads to volume overload.

- **BLOWING sound – think REGURGITATION***: AR, MR:** abnormal backflow of blood (regurgitation) through an incompletely closed valve. Regurgitation leads to volume overload.

TIMING

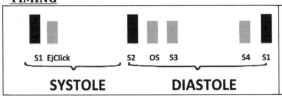

- _Systolic (AS, MR)_

- _Diastolic (AR, MS)_   ****remember "ARMS rest"****
  <u>A</u>ortic <u>R</u>egurgitation & <u>M</u>itral <u>S</u>tenosis heard during diastole (rest).

LOCATION OF INTENSITY _Bell: <u>low-pitched sounds</u> (think "Below") Diaphragm: high pitched_

"<u>A</u>pple <u>P</u>ies <u>T</u>astes <u>M</u>mmmm"	
<u>A</u>ortic: R 2nd ICS (R upper sternal border) <u>P</u>ulmonary: L 2nd ICS (L upper sternal border) <u>T</u>ricuspid: L 4th ICS (L lower sternal border) [Erbs @ 3rd ICS] <u>M</u>itral: 5th ICS (Midclavicular line) apex	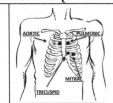

RADIATION

• Carotid (AS)	• No radiation (MS)
• L upper sternal border (AR)	• Axilla (MR)

MURMUR ACCENTUATION MANEUVERS

POSITION
- **AORTIC**: *SITTING UP & LEANING FORWARD ACCENTUATES AORTIC MURMURS (AS, AR).*
- **MITRAL:** *LYING ON LEFT SIDE ACCENTUATES MITRAL MURMURS (MS, MR).*

INCREASED VENOUS RETURN
- *↑venous return INCREASES ALL MURMURS/opening Snap* (left & right side)
  - squatting, leg raise, lying down
- ***exceptions: ↓ murmur of hypertrophic cardiomyopathy & delayed ejection click (decreased prolapse/shorter murmur duration) of MVP*****

DECREASED VENOUS RETURN
- *↓venous return (Valsalva/standing) DECREASES ALL MURMURS/Opening Snap* (left & right side).
- ***exceptions: ↑murmur of hypertrophic cardiomyopathy & earlier ejection click (increased prolapse & longer murmur duration) of MVP*****

INSPIRATION
- Inspiration ↑'es venous return on right side:
  ↑ALL murmurs/opening snap on the R side (↓ejection click R side)
    - ***Right-sided murmurs best heard with inspiration.***

- Inspiration ↓'es venous return on left side:
  ↓ALL murmurs/opening snap on the L side (earlier ejection click on the L side)

EXPIRATION
- Expiration ↑'es venous return on left side:
  ↑ALL murmurs/opening snap on the L side (delayed ejection click on the L side)
    - ***Left-sided murmurs best heard after maximal expiration.***

- Expiration ↓'es venous return on right side:
  ↓ALL murmurs/opening snap on the R side (earlier ejection click R side).

HANDGRIP
- *↑'es afterload* (by compressing the arteries of the upper extremity) leading to ↓LV emptying (decreased forward flow & *increased backward flow*).
    - AS, MVP, hypertrophic cardiomyopathy murmurs ↓ with handgrip (note that *handgrip & amyl nitrate are the only maneuvers that affect hypertrophic cardiomyopathy & AS in the same direction – because both maneuvers affect AFTERLOAD & FORWARD FLOW*). Because handgrip increases afterload, the increased afterload prevents blood from being ejected from the ventricles, lessening the blood flowing through the stenotic aortic valve and less blood ejected in hypertrophic cardiomyopathy, thus lessening both murmurs.
    - *AR, MR,↑'es with handgrip* (due to ↑backward flow); MS ↑'es due to ↑afterload.

AMYL NITRATE
- *↓'es afterload* (direct arteriolar vasodilator) leading to ↑LV emptying (increases forward flow & decreases backward flow of blood).
    - AS, MVP, hypertrophic cardiomyopathy murmur ↑ with amyl nitrate
    - *AR, MR ↓'es with amyl nitrate*
      This is why afterload reducers like ACEI are used in the management of AR, MR.

AORTIC STENOSIS (AS)

- **AORTIC STENOSIS:** *obstruction of left ventricular outflow of blood* across the aortic valve.
- MC valvular disease. Patients usually become symptomatic when AoV <1 cm^2 (Normal area 3-4 cm^2).

ETIOLOGIES
1. **Degenerative heart disease:** *calcifications* (ex atherosclerotic/wear & tear) *common in patients >70y.*
2. **Congenital heart disease:** (ex. *bicuspid Aov*) common in patients *<70y.*
3. *Rheumatic heart disease:* AS usually accompanied by AR or mitral disease (but may be isolated).

PATHOPHYSIOLOGY
- Stenosis ⇨ LV outflow obstruction (fixed CO) ⇨ ↑afterload (pressure overload) ⇨ LVH ⇨ LV failure.

CLINICAL MANIFESTATIONS
- Once symptomatic, lifespan is <u>dramatically</u> shortened if valve replacement not performed.
- Dyspnea is the most common symptom if patients become symptomatic.
  To **remember symptoms, think "Aortic Stenosis Complications":** Angina, **Syncope, CHF**
1. **Angina:** (5y mean survival). ↑O$_2$ demand (LVH coupled with exertion) + ↓O$_2$ supply (2^{ry} to fixed cardiac output) ⇨ subendocardial ischemia; ± associated coronary artery disease present.
2. **Syncope (exertional):** (3y survival). Exertional peripheral vasodilation in the setting of fixed CO ⇨ insufficient cerebral perfusion during exercise/exertion.
3. **Congestive Heart Failure:** (2y survival) *worst prognosis!* Dyspnea & pulmonary edema.

PHYSICAL EXAMINATION
1. *SYSTOLIC "EJECTION" CRESCENDO-DECRESCENDO MURMUR @ RUSB THAT RADIATES TO CAROTID (NECK).*
   - ↓*murmur intensity:* ↓*venous return:* (ex. *Valsalva, standing*); inspiration; *handgrip.* ↓S$_2$.

   - ↑*murmur with* ↑*venous return (ex. squatting, leg raise)*; expiration; *sitting & leaning forward*
   - **Signs of severity:** *late peaking murmur*, pulsus parvus et tardus, paradoxically split S$_2$, Signs of left ventricular hypertrophy: LV heave & loud S$_4$ (due to contraction into stiff ventricle).
2. *PULSUS PARVUS ET TARDUS: small, delayed, carotid pulse. NARROWED PULSE PRESSURE,** hypertension.

DIAGNOSTIC STUDIES
1. **Echocardiogram:** ❶small aortic orifice during systole, ❷ LVH, ❸ thickened/calcified Aov.
2. ECG: *left ventricular hypertrophy,** ± strain; Nonspp: LAE, LBB, ± A fib, ischemic changes.
3. CXR: nonspecific (poststenotic aortic dilation, AoV calcification, ± pulmonary congestion).
4. Cardiac catheterization: definitive diagnosis. Useful in symptomatic patients prior to surgery.

MANAGEMENT
A. **Surgical therapy:** *aortic valve replacement <u>only</u> effective treatment (treatment of choice)!**
   1. **AoV replacement (AVR):** *symptomatic AS,* asymptomatic severe AS (↓EF or area <0.6cm^2).
      -mechanical: prolonged durability but thrombogenic (ex. stroke), bleeding. Must be placed on long-term anticoagulant therapy.
      - bioprosthetic: less durable but minimally thrombogenic (usually used in patients that that are not candidates for anticoagulant). Heterograft (porcine valve); pericardial.
   2. Percutaneous aortic valvuloplasty (PAV): results in 50% ↑AoV area, but 50% restenosis @ 6-12 months so used as a bridge to AVR, if not a surgical candidate or in pediatric patients.
   3. Intraortic balloon pump: used for temporary stabilization as a bridge to valve replacement.

B. **Medical therapy:** *no medical treatment truly effective!*
   - No exercise restrictions in patients with mild AS.
   - *severe AS:* because patients are dependent on preload to maintain CO ⇨ *avoid physical exertion/venodilators* (ex. nitrates)/*negative inotropes* (Ca^{+2} channel blockers, β-blockers).

45

AORTIC REGURGITATION (AR) or AORTIC INSUFFICIENCY (AI)

ETIOLOGIES
1. **Valve disease:** *rheumatic heart disease* (mixed AS/AR); *Endocarditis,* Bicuspid AoV.
2. **Aortic root disease/dilation:** hypertension, Marfan syndrome, syphilis, rheumatoid arthritis, systemic lupus erythematosus, aortic dissection, ankylosing spondylitis.

PATHOPHYSIOLOGY
• Incomplete AoV closure during diastole ⇨ regurgitation of blood from Ao to LV (in addition to the normal antegrade flow from LA to LV) ⇨ LV volume overload ⇨ LV dilation ⇨ CHF.

CLINICAL MANIFESTATIONS
Acute: (ex. acute MI, aortic dissection, endocarditis) ⇨ pulmonary edema, ± hypotension.
Chronic: clinically silent while LV dilates ⇨ LV decompensation ⇨ *CHF.*

PHYSICAL EXAMINATION
1. *DIASTOLIC, DECRESCENDO, BLOWING MURMUR MAXIMAL @ LUSB** (high-pitched).
   - ↑*murmur intensity:* ↑**venous return (ex. *squatting); sitting forward; handgrip, expiration.* Severity of AR proportional to the duration of murmur** (except in acute/late disease); displaced PMI, ± thrill. May radiate along the left sternal border.

   - ↓intensity: ↓venous return *(Valsalva, standing),* inspiration, **amyl nitrate.**
   - ± *Austin Flint murmur* (mid-late diastolic rumble at the apex 2ry to retrograde regurgitant jet competing with antegrade flow from left atrium into the ventricle).
2. *BOUNDING PULSES:** 2ry to ↑stroke volume (↑SV).*
3. *WIDE PULSE PRESSURE.** Laterally & inferior displaced point of maximum impulse (PMI).

Classic Signs of WIDENED PULSE PRESSURE in AR/AI (seen ONLY with chronic AR/AI)	
SIGN	DESCRIPTION
Water Hammer pulse	*Swift upstroke & rapid fall of radial pulse accentuated with wrist elevation.*
Corrigan's pulse	Similar to water hammer pulse but referring specifically to the carotid artery.
Hill's sign	Popliteal artery systolic pressure > brachial artery by 60mmHg *(most sensitive).*
Duroziez's sign	Gradual pressure over femoral artery ⇨ systolic and diastolic bruits.
Traube's sound (pistol shot)	Double sound heard @ femoral artery c̄ partial compression of femoral artery.
De Musset's sign	*Head-bobbing* with each heartbeat (low sensitivity).
Müller's sign	Visible systolic pulsations of the uvula.
Quincke's pulses	Visible *fingernail bed pulsations* with light compression of fingernail bed.

4. **Pulsus Bisferiens:** double pulse carotid upstroke. *Seen with combined AR + AS or severe AR.*

DIAGNOSTIC STUDIES
1. **Echocardiogram:** regurgitant jet seen with Doppler flow. Catheterization definitive diagnosis.
2. ECG: Nonspecific: (± LVH, LAD). CXR: nonspecific: ± cardiomegaly (due to LV dilation).

MANAGEMENT
Variable progression. CHF associated with a 2-year mean survival rate.
A. **Medical therapy:** *afterload reduction* with vasodilators (ACEI, ARBs, Nifedipine, Hydralazine) because afterload reduction *improves ventricular performance by increasing forward flow* (↓LEDV, improve ejection fraction, ↓ LV mass, degree of LVH).

B. **Surgical therapy:** *Definitive management.* Indicated in acute or symptomatic AR; asymptomatic AR with LV decompensation: ejection fraction (EF) <55%. Although 55% is a normal EF, these patients need a hyperdynamic ventricle to maintain adequate cardiac output.

MITRAL STENOSIS (MS)

ETIOLOGIES
1. **_Rheumatic heart disease (RHD): MC cause by far*_** *(almost always caused by rheumatic heart disease)* leading to a "fish mouth valve." MC in 3rd/4th decade.
2. Congenital, left atrial myxoma, thrombus, valvulitis (SLE, amyloid, carcinoid).

PATHOPHYSIOLOGY
Obstruction of flow from LA to LV 2ry to narrowed mitral orifice ⇨ blood backs up into the left atrium.
   ↑L-atrial pressure/volume overload ⇨ pulmonary congestion ⇨ **_pulmonary HTN_** ⇨ CHF.

CLINICAL MANIFESTATIONS
Slow progression until symptoms occur (then progression becomes rapid).
1. **_Pulmonary symptoms:_ dyspnea** (MC sx), pulmonary edema, **hemoptysis,** cough, frequent bronchitis, **pulmonary HTN** (if rheumatic in origin, symptoms usually begins in 20s – 30s).
2. **_Atrial fibrillation:_** secondary to atrial enlargement ⇨ thromboembolic events (ex. CVA).
3. Right-sided heart failure: due to prolonged pulmonary hypertension.
4. **_Mitral facies = ruddy (flushed) cheeks_ with facial pallor** (chronic hypoxia).
5. Signs of left atrial enlargement: dysphagia (esophageal compression), Ortner's syndrome: recurrent laryngeal nerve palsy due to compression by the dilated left atrium ⇨ hoarseness.

PHYSICAL EXAMINATION
1. **_Prominent (loud) S_1_** (due to delayed forceful closure of mitral valve). ± split S_2 prior to the OS.

2. **_OPENING SNAP* (OS):_** high-pitched early diastolic sound of the opening of stenotic valve. Valve area proportional to S_2-OS interval (tighter valve ⇨ shorter the interval).
   Severity of MS: a) shorter S_2-OS interval & b) prolonged diastolic murmur.

3. **_EARLY-MID DIASTOLIC RUMBLE @ APEX (LOW-PITCHED) ESP IN LLD POSITION*_** (± preceded by OS).
   - ↓ **murmur intensity:** ↓**venom return** *(Valsalva, standing); inspiration.*
   - ↑**murmur intensity:** ↑**venous return** *(lying supine, squatting); expiration, **exercise, left lateral decubitus position placement.***

DIAGNOSTIC STUDIES
1. **Echocardiogram:** narrowed mitral valve (↑LA pressure, ±pulmonary HTN).
   LV function is usually normal. Cardiac catheterization.
2. ECG: **_left atrial enlargement* (LAE/P mitrale)_**; ± **_A fib*_** or RVH (pulmonary HTN).
3. CXR: nonspp. LAE (straightening of L heart border, left mainstem bronchus elevation).

MANAGEMENT
A. **Surgical Management:**
   1. **_Percutaneous balloon valvuloplasty/valvotomy: best treatment in younger patients_** and in patients with noncalcified valves.
   2. Open mitral valvotomy: if percutaneous valvotomy is unsuccessful or not possible.
   3. **Mitral valve repair or replacement: symptomatic MS,** pulmonary HTN. Mechanical better than porcine (porcine not as suitable in replacement). Replacement may be needed if unable to perform valvotomy.

B. Medical Management: does not alter the natural history nor delay the need for surgery.
   - Loop diuretics & Na^+ restriction (if congestion), β blockers; Digoxin (if A fib).

MITRAL REGURGITATION

ETIOLOGIES
1. **Leaflet abnormalities:** *mitral valve prolapse MC cause,** *rheumatic heart disease, endocarditis,* valvulitis, annulus dilation (any cause of LV dilation), Marfan syndrome.
2. **Papillary muscle dysfunction:** *ischemia/infarction,* displacement 2^{ry} to cardiomyopathy.
3. Ruptured chordae tendinae: collagen vascular disease, dilated cardiomyopathy.

PATHOPHYSIOLOGY
- *Retrograde blood flows from the LV into the LA* (but the refluxed blood in the LA returns to the LV during diastole) ⇨ ***LV volume overload*** ❶*LA dilation* as the blood flows into the pulmonary circulation ⇨ ↑LA/pulmonary pressures ❷↓cardiac output (due to diminished effective forward flow).

CLINICAL MANIFESTATIONS
1. **Acute:** *pulmonary edema* (rapid volume overload on LA), hypotension. **Dyspnea,** fatigue.
2. **Chronic:** *A fib,* progressive dyspnea on exertion, fatigue, CHF, pulmonary HTN, hemoptysis.

PHYSICAL EXAMINATION
1. *BLOWING, HOLOSYSTOLIC (PANSYSTOLIC) MURMUR @ APEX** with *RADIATION TO AXILLA* (high-pitched).
   - ↓ **murmur intensity:** ↓*venous return (Valsalva, standing); inspiration; amyl nitrate.*
   - ↑**murmur intensity:** ↑*venous return (squatting, supine); inspiration, handgrip, left lateral decubitus position placement.*
2. *Widely split S_2* (↓LV ejection time results in early A_2, pulmonary HTN results in delayed P_2).
3. Laterally displaced PMI, ±thrill, ± S_3 gallop (LV dysfunction), ± decreased S_1 if severe.

DIAGNOSTIC STUDIES
1. **Echocardiogram:** regurgitant jet, *hyperdynamic LV.* Ejection fraction <60% = LV impairment.
2. ECG: *nonspecific:* left atrial enlargement (P mitrale), LVH, ± atrial fibrillation.
3. CXR: *nonspecific:* cardiomegaly (dilated LA/LV), ± pulmonary congestion.

MANAGEMENT
A. **Surgical:**
   1. ***repair preferred over replacement.**** Acute or symptomatic MR; asymptomatic MR with *LV decompensation/dilation* (EF <55-60%). Balloon pump for stabilization/bridge to surgery.
B. **Medical:** indicated in a nonoperative symptomatic patient. ***Vasodilators to ↓afterload*** (*ACEI,* hydralazine/nitrates); ↓***preload*** (↓amount of MR – diuretics); Digoxin (A fib or need for ⊕ inotropy).

MITRAL VALVE PROLAPSE (MVP)

ETIOLOGIES: myxomatous degeneration of the mitral valve apparatus, associated with connective tissue diseases (ex Marfan's, Ehlers-Danlos, osteogenesis imperfecta). *MC in young women* (15-35y).

CLINICAL MANIFESTATIONS: *most are asymptomatic!* ❶*Autonomic dysfunction:* anxiety, atypical chest pain, panic attacks, palpitations (arrhythmias), syncope, dizziness, fatigue. ❷*symptoms associated with MR progression:* fatigue, dyspnea, PND, CHF. ❸ stroke, endocarditis.

PHYSICAL EXAM: ± *narrow AP diameter, low body weight, hypotension, scoliosis, pectus excavatum.*
- *MID-LATE SYSTOLIC EJECTION CLICK** best heard @ the apex ± mid-late systolic murmur.
   - *Any maneuver, which makes the LV smaller (Valsalva, standing), results in earlier click* & longer murmur duration (2ry to *increased prolapse*). Squatting decreases & delays click onset.

DIAGNOSIS: echocardiogram shows posterior bulging leaflets (with tissue redundancy).
MANAGEMENT: *reassurance only (good prognosis). Beta blockers ONLY if autonomic dysfunction.*

PULMONIC STENOSIS (PS)

- Pulmonic stenosis: right ventricular outflow obstruction of blood across the pulmonic valve.
- **_Almost always congenital_** & a **_disease of the young_** (ex. congenital rubella syndrome).

PHYSICAL EXAMINATION
1. _HARSH MIDSYSTOLIC EJECTION CRESC-DECRESCENDO MURMUR (MAXIMAL @ LUSB) RADIATES TO NECK._*
   - **_Murmur increases with inspiration._** The longer the murmur duration = ↑stenosis.
   - Signs of R-sided heart failure.
   - **_Systolic ejection click_** (often "buried" in S1) may precede the murmur (click increases with expiration); Wide, split S_2 (delayed P_2), ± S_4.

MANAGEMENT: balloon valvuloplasty is the preferred treatment.

PULMONIC REGURGITATION (PR)

Etiologies: pulmonary hypertension, tetralogy of Fallot, endocarditis, rheumatic heart disease.
Pathophysiology: retrograde blood flow from pulmonary artery into RV ⇨ R-sided volume overload.
Clinical manifestations: most clinically insignificant. If symptomatic ⇨ R-sided failure symptoms.

PHYSICAL EXAMINATION
Graham Steell murmur: **_brief decrescendo early diastolic murmur @ LUSB_** (2nd L ICS) **_with full inspiration._** Severe pulmonary HTN ↑'es the velocity of the regurgitation.
   - ↑**(augmented) murmur:**↑**_venous return (squatting, supine, inspiration)._**
   - ↓ (diminished) murmur: ↓ _venous return (Valsalva, standing, expiration)._
Management: no treatment needed in most (most well tolerated). **_Almost always congenital._**

TRICUSPID STENOSIS (TS)

- blood backs up into the right atrium ⇨ ↑ right atrial enlargement ⇨ right-sided heart failure.*
PHYSICAL EXAMINATION
1. _MID-DIASTOLIC MURMUR @ LEFT LOWER STERNAL (XYPHOID BORDER)* (4TH ICS)._ Low frequency
   - ↑ **_intensity_**: ↑_venous return: (squatting, laying down, leg raising, **inspiration**)._
2. Opening snap (OS): usually occurs later than the opening snap of mitral stenosis.

Medical Management: decrease right atrial volume overload with diuretics & Na^+ restriction.
Surgical Management: commisurotomy or replacement if right heart failure or ↓cardiac output.

TRICUSPID REGURGITATION

PHYSICAL EXAMINATION
1. _HOLOSYSTOLIC BLOWING HIGH-PITCHED MURMUR @ SUBXYPHOID AREA (L MID STERNAL BORDER)._*
   Little to no murmur radiation. ↑murmur intensity: ↑venous return: (ex. squatting, inspiration).
2. **_Carvallo's sign:_*** **_increased murmur intensity with inspiration_** (due to increased right sided blood flow during inspiration). Helps to distinguish TR from MR. ±Pulsatile liver.

MANAGEMENT
Medical: diuretics (for volume overload & congestion). If LV dysfunction - standard HF therapy.
Surgical: suggested for patients with severe TR despite medical therapy. Repair >replacement.

	AORTIC STENOSIS (AS)	MITRAL STENOSIS (MS)	AORTIC REGURGITATION	MITRAL REGURGITATION	MITRAL VALVE PROLAPSE
PATHO PHYSIOLOGY	• LV outflow obstruction ⇨ fixed CO*. ↑afterload ⇨ LVH*	• Obstruction of flow from LA to LV ⇨ ↑L-atrial enlargement & ↑LA pressure ⇨ pulm HTN	• Backflow from Aorta to LV ⇨ LV volume overload*	• Backflow from LV into LA ⇨ LV volume overload* ⇨ ↓CO	• Myxomatous degeneration of mitral valve (floppy, redundant valve)
ETIOLOGIES	• Degeneration (>70y)* • Congenital (<70y)* • Rheumatic disease	• Rheumatic Heart disease (RHD) MC cause by far*	• Rheumatic disease, HTN • Endocarditis, Marfan • Syphilis • Ankylosing spondylitis	• MVP MC cause* • Rheumatic, Endocarditis • Ischemia (ruptured papillary muscle/chordae tendinae post MI)	• MC in young women • Connective tissue disease (ex Marfan, Ehrlos Danlos)
CLINICAL	• Angina (5y survival s AVR) • Syncope (3y s AVR) • CHF (2y s AVR)	• R-SIDED heart failure* • Pulmonary HTN - Hemoptysis • ATRIAL FIBRILLATION* • Mitral Facies* (flushed cheeks)	• L-SIDED heart failure*	• Acute: pulmonary edema, dyspnea • Chronic: A fib, CHF. May have Pulmonary HTN (not as often as MS)	• Most asymptomatic • ❶Autonomic dysfunction: chest pain, panic attacks; arrhythmias causing palpitations, syncope, dizziness, fatigue • ❷ Sx associated with MR progression: fatigue, dyspnea, CHF. • ❸ Stroke, endocarditis, PVC's
MURMUR	• SYSTOLIC "EJECTION" CRESCENDO-DECRESCENDO @ RUSB* • Later peaking murmur = ↑severity	• DIASTOLIC RUMBLE @ APEX (LOW) IN LLD* May be preceded by OPENING SNAP* • Shorter S₂-OS duration = ↑severity	• DIASTOLIC DECRESCENDO BLOWING @ LUSB. ↑'es with handgrip* with amyl nitrate ↓ • ±Austin Flint Murmur: mid-late diastolic rumble @ apex	• BLOWING HOLOSYSTOLIC MURMUR @ APEX ↑'es with handgrip, LLD* ↓'es with amyl nitrate	• MID TO LATE SYSTOLIC EJECTION CLICK* @ apex. ↓venous return (Valsalva, standing, inspiration) ⇨ earlier click (↑prolapse) & longer murmur duration • ±mid-late systolic murmur (MR)
RADIATION	• CAROTID ARTERIES*	• NO RADIATION	• Along L-sternal border	• AXILLA*	
PULSE	• PULSUS PARVUS ET TARDUS* (weak, delayed pulse) • Narrow pulse pressure*	• Usually reduced intensity (due to decreased cardiac output)	• BOUNDING PULSES* (↑SV) • WIDE pulse pressure* • Pulse Bisferiens (if combined AS +AR)*	May have a brisk upstroke (due to hyperdynamic ventricle from ↑preload & ↓afterload)	
PHYSICAL EXAM	• LV heave due to LV hypertrophy	• Left atrial enlargement	• Hill- popliteal mmHg >brachial pressure • DeMussets- Head bobbing • Quincke pulses – nail bed pulsations • Water hammer pulse • Pistol shot over fem art.		• Narrow AP diameter • Low Body weight (thin) • Hypotension • Scoliosis, Pectus Excavatum
HEART SOUNDS	• Paradoxically split S₂ (If severe) • S₄ if LVH	• Prominent S₁ ="closing snap" ± diminish with ↑severity • OPENING SNAP* (OS)		• Widely split S₂ • ± S₃, decreased S₁	
MANAGEMENT	Aortic valve replacement (AVR) once sxatic* Severe AS is preload dependent ⇨ avoid exertion, venodilators & negative inotropes (CCB, B-blockers)	Valvotomy in young patients if rheumatic dz is cause, sxatic & valve orifice < 1.0 cm²; Repair preferred over replacement	Meds: Vasodilators (↓afterload increases forward flow); Surgery: acute or sxatic AR or ↓LV <55% (need hyperdynamic ventricle to maintain CO)	Meds: vasodilators;↓Afterload increases forward flow (ACEI); Surgery: valve repair preferred vs. valve replacement* (Acute/sxatic or ↓LV <55%)	- Reassurance good prognosis in asymptomatic patients or mild sx* - Beta blockers for autonomic dysfunction*
MURMUR MANEUVERS	↓venous return (Valsalva/standing) DECREASES ALL MURMURS EXCEPT: ❶ ↑'es the murmur of hypertrophic cardiomyopathy* & ❷ causes earlier click of MVP ↑venous return (lying supine, squatting, leg raise) INCREASES ALL MURMURS EXCEPT: ❶ ↓ murmur in hypertrophic cardiomyopathy* & ❷ later click of MVP Inspiration ↑'es all R-sided murmurs, Expiration ↑'es all L-sided murmurs. AORTIC (AR,AS): ↑'es if sitting forward; MITRAL (MR,MS): ↑'es with left lateral decubitus				

HYPERTENSION

DEFINITION & DIAGNOSIS OF HYPERTENSION (HTN)

JNC 8 CLASSIFICATION		
Category	Systolic (mmHg)	Diastolic (mmHg)
Normal	<120	<80
Pre-HTN	120-139	80-89
Stage 1 HTN	140-159	90-99
Stage 2 HTN	≥160	≥100

- ***Elevated BP ≥ 2 readings on ≥ 2 different visits.***
- ***Systolic ≥ 140*** mmHg ***&/or diastolic ≥ 90*** mmHg.

Isolated systolic shows greater risk for cardiovascular disease than isolated diastolic in patients >50y.

ETIOLOGIES

1. **PRIMARY (ESSENTIAL):** *(95%) hypertension due to idiopathic etiology.* Onset 25-55 yrs; ⊕ Fhx.

2. **SECONDARY:** (5%). *HTN due to an underlying, identifiable & often correctable cause.* **Suspect secondary hypertension if blood pressure is refractory to antihypertensives or severely elevated.**
   - *Renal: renovascular MC cause of 2ry** (4%).* ***Renal artery stenosis:***
     Fibromuscular dysplasia MC cause in young patients, atherosclerosis in the elderly.
   - Endocrine: (0.5%): 1ry hyperaldosteronism, pheochromocytoma, Cushing's syndrome.
   - Coarctation of aorta (↑BP upper>lower); sleep apnea, ETOH, oral contraceptives, COX-2 inhibitors.

PATHOGENESIS OF HYPERTENSION

- Increased sympathetic activity.
- Increased angiotensin II activity.
- Increased mineralocorticoid activity (sodium & water retention).

COMPLICATIONS OF HYPERTENSION

Cardiovascular: coronary artery disease, heart failure, myocardial infarction, left ventricular hypertrophy, aortic dissection, aortic aneurysm, peripheral vascular disease.
Neurologic: TIA, stroke (CVA), ruptured aneurysms, encephalopathy.
Nephropathy: renal stenosis & sclerosis. *HTN 2nd MC cause of end stage renal disease in the US.**
Optic: retinal hemorrhage, blindness, retinopathy.

CLINICAL MANIFESTATIONS: examination may help to reveal possible causes or complications.
Goals: ❶ identify CV risk factors ❷ reveal 2° causes of hypertension ❸ assess for end organ damage.

1. **Funduscopic exam:** *papilledema signifies an advanced stage of malignant hypertension. More prognostic than an isolated BP measurement.*

GRADES OF RETINOPATHY
I. arterial narrowing	III. I-II + hemorrhages & soft exudates (accelerated)
II. A-V nicking	*IV. I-III + papilledema (malignant HTN)**

2. skin: uremic appearance (CRF); striae (Cushing's disease); neck: carotid bruits, jugular vein exam.
3. cardiopulmonary: check for loud component of S2, presence of an S4.
4. abdomen: pheochromocytoma, polycystic kidney disease, bruits over the renal artery (stenosis); dilation of the aorta or truncal obesity.
5. arterial pulses: decreased or absent femoral pulses (peripheral vascular disease); blood pressure greater in the upper extremities > lower suggests aortic coarctation; Edema (CHF, nephrosis).

MANAGEMENT GOALS OF HYPERTENSION

- ***Goal <140/90 mmHg in general population, diabetics or chronic renal disease.** <150/90 if >60y.*
- Treatment results in 50% ↓ of heart failure; 40% ↓of strokes, 20-25% ↓of myocardial infarctions.
- Lifestyle modifications: (each ↓SBP ~5mmHg)
  - Weight loss: achieve BMI 18.5-24.9. Smoking cessation, sodium restriction: ≤2.4 g/day.
  - Dash Diet: ↑ fruits & vegetables with ↓saturated/total fats & low sodium.
  - Exercise: ≥30 minutes of exercise/day for most of the week.
  - Limited alcohol consumption: ≤2 drinks/d in men; ≤1 drink/d in women (& patients with low BMI).

PHARMACOLOGIC MANAGEMENT OF HYPERTENSION

DRUG/INTERVENTION	COMMENTS
DIURETICS *Hydrochlorothiazides* *Chlorthalidone* Metolazone	↓ blood volume/blood pressure by increased Na+/H2O excretion. **Ind:** *treatment of choice as initial therapy in uncomplicated HTN* *Cardioprotective;* Low cost and very effective. **MOA:** affect BP by reducing blood volume, prevent **kidney Na+/water reabsorption at the distal diluting tubule.** Lowers urinary Ca+ excretion. **S/E:** hyponatremia, hypokalemia, <u>hypercalcemia</u> mild ↑ in cholesterol, <u>**hyperuricemia & hyperglycemia**</u>, so **caution** in patients **with gout, DM.**
Loop diuretics *Furosemide, Bumetanide*	**Ind:** HTN, CHF, hypercalcemia, severe edema, mild renal disease. **MOA:** *inhibits water transport across the <u>loop of Henle</u>* ⇨ ↑excretion of water, Na+, Cl+ K+. *Strongest class of diuretics.* **S/E:** *volume depletion, hypokalemia*/natremia/calcemia, hyperuricemia, **hyperglycemia,** hypochloremic **metabolic alkalosis. Ototoxicity.** **CI:** *sulfa allergy.*
Potassium sparing diuretics *Spironolactone* *Amiloride* *Eplerenone*	**MOA:** *inhibits aldosterone-mediated Na+/H2O absorption* (spares potassium). Weak diuretic, most useful in combination with loops to minimize K+ loss. **S/E:** *hyperkalemia. Gynecomastia with Spironolactone.* **CI:** renal failure, hyponatremia.
ACE INHIBITORS *Captopril* (Capoten) *Enalapril* (Vasotec) *Ramipril* (Altace) *Benazepril* (Lotensin)	**MOA:** *cardioprotective, synergistic effect when used with thiazides;* ↓preload/afterload, (↓ synthesis of AG II/aldosterone production), potentiates other vasodilators (bradykinin, prostaglandin, nitric oxide); ↑exercise tolerance, *renoprotective.* **Indications:** *HTN (especially if history of DM, nephropathy, CHF, post MI).* **S/E:** *1st dose hypotension,* azotemia/renal insufficiency (esp if Cr >3, CrCl <30), *hyperkalemia, <u>cough & angioedema (due to ↑bradykinin)</u>, hyperuricemia.* **CI:** pregnancy.
ANGIOTENSIN II RECEPTOR BLOCKERS (ARB)	**Ind:** *consider in patients not able to tolerate beta blockers/ACEI.* Blocks the effects of angiotensin II (not its production). *CI in pregnancy.* • *Losartan* (Cozaar); *Valsartan* (Diovan), *Irbesartan* (Avapro), *Candesartan*
CALCIUM CHANNEL BLOCKERS *Dihydropyridines* Nifedipine (Procardia XL) Amlodipine (Norvasc) *Non-dihydropyridines* Verapamil (Calan/covera) Diltiazem (Cardizem CD)	❶ **Dihydropyridines:** *potent vasodilators (little or no effect on cardiac contractility or conduction)* neutral or increased vascular permeability. *Dihydropyridines often used to treat HTN.* ❷ **Non-dihydropyridines:** *affect cardiac contractility & conduction,* potent vasodilators. *Non-dihydropyridines used in HTN with concomitant A fib.* **Ind:** HTN, Angina, Raynaud's phenomenon **S/E:** vasodilation: *headache, dizziness, lightheadedness, flushing, peripheral edema.* **Verapamil:** *constipation,* cautious use if on beta blocker therapy. **CI:** *CHF (especially nondihydropyridines), 2nd/3rd heart block.*
β – BLOCKERS **Cardioselective (β₁):** *Atenolol, Metoprolol, Esmolol* **Nonselective (β₁, β₂):** *Propranolol* Both α & β₁,₂: *Labetalol, Carvedilol*	**Ind:** HTN (especially if history of MI, tachycardia); angina (stable & unstable), acute MI, heart failure, pheochromocytoma, migraines, essential tremor. **Beta blockers NOT used as 1st line monotherapy.** **MOA:** catecholamine inhibitor. **Blocks "adrenergic" renin release.** **S/E:** *fatigue, depression, impotence; masks sympathetic symptoms of hypoglycemia (so use with caution in diabetics).* **CI:** *2nd/3rd heart block, decompensated heart failure; Nonselective agents CI asthma/COPD and may worsen peripheral vascular disease/Raynaud's phenomenon, hypotension or pulse <50 bpm.*
α₁ BLOCKERS *Prazosin (Minipress)* *Terazosin (Hytrin)* *Doxazosin (Cardura)*	**Ind:** antihypertensive, also ↑'es HDL & ↓'es LDL, improves insulin sensitivity. *Good for a hypertensive with benign prostatic hypertrophy (BPH).* **S/E:** *1st dose syncope,* dizziness, headache, weakness. *Not used as 1st line.*

DIURETICS · **VASODILATORS**

MANAGEMENT OF UNCOMPLICATED HYPERTENSION (NO OTHER COMORBIDITIES)

Choosing initial medication in **uncomplicated HTN in non-African American patients:** any 1 of the 4 drugs from the following classes may be used:

1. *Thiazide-type diuretics**   3. Angiotensin Receptor Blockers
2. ACE inhibitors   4. Calcium Channel Blockers

MANAGEMENT OF HYPERTENSION WITH THE FOLLOWING COMORBIDITIES

Choosing an antihypertensive medication largely depends on treating other comorbid diseases:

Disease	Optimum therapy
Atrial Fibrillation (rate control)	β-blockers or Calcium channel blockers (non dihydropyridines: Verapamil, Cardizem)
Angina	β-blockers, Calcium channel blockers
Post Myocardial Infarction	β-blockers, ACE Inhibitors
Systolic Heart Failure	ACEI, ARB, β blockers, diuretics
Diabetes mellitus/Chronic kidney disease	*ACEI,** ARB
Isolated systolic HTN in elderly	Diuretics, (± Calcium channel blockers)
Osteoporosis, **No other comorbidities**	Thiazides*
BPH	α_1 *blockers*
African-Americans (nondiabetic)	*Thiazides, Calcium channel blockers*
Young, Caucasian males	Thiazides ⇨ ACE inhibitors, ARB ⇨ β-blockers
Gout	Calcium channel blockers Losartan is the only ARB that doesn't cause hyperuricemia (so it can be safely used).

ACUTE COMPLICATIONS OF HYPERTENSION

- Includes hypertensive urgency & emergency.
  PATHOPHYSIOLOGY:
  - The triggering event of hypertensive urgency/emergency is an **abrupt rise in BP** associated with **increased systemic vascular resistance.** Sustained dangerous blood pressure elevations lead to **endothelial cell deterioration** (the increased pressure causes capillary leakage with exudation of fibrinogen & proteins, leading to swelling and fibrinoid necrosis of the vessel wall).

HYPERTENSIVE URGENCY

↑BP + NO apparent acute end organ damage.
  MANAGEMENT
  ↓BP (mean arterial pressure) by 25% over <u>24-48 hours</u> *using ORAL agents.**
  Goal of management is blood pressure reduction to ≤160/≤100 mmHg. Mean arterial pressure should not be lowered by more than 25% over the first several hours.

ORAL DRUGS USED FOR HYPERTENSIVE URGENCIES		
Drug	**Mechanism of Action**	**Adverse Effects**
Clonidine	*Centrally acting α-2 adrenergic agonist (short-term use only)*	Headache, tachycardia, nausea, vomiting, sedation, fatigue dry mouth, *rebound hypertension* if discontinued abruptly - (mimics pheochromocytoma).*
Captopril	ACE Inhibitor	Angioedema, acute kidney injury.
Furosemide	Loop diuretic	Electrolyte abnormalities, alkalosis.
Labetalol	α 1 β 1 β 2 blocker	CI in severe asthma/COPD, AV heart block, <u>congestive</u> heart failure.
Nicardipine	Calcium channel blocker	Reflex tachycardia, headache, nausea, flushing

HYPERTENSIVE EMERGENCY

↑BP + *ACUTE END ORGAN DAMAGE**

Usually systolic blood pressure ≥ 180 and/or *diastolic blood pressure ≥120* (no specific threshold #).
Note: JNC 8 did not define hypertensive emergency parameters. BP ≥180/120 as per JNC7 guidelines.
2015 ACOG guidelines defines HTN in pregnancy as acute onset of BP 160/110 persisting >15 minutes.

Neurological damage: encephalopathy, hemorrhagic or ischemic stroke, seizure.
Perform a neurological exam (may need CT scan to rule out stroke).

Cardiac damage: acute coronary syndrome, aortic dissection, acute heart failure/pulmonary edema.
ECG, CXR (to rule out dissection, look for pulmonary edema), CK-MB/Troponin.

Renal damage: acute kidney injury; proteinuria, hematuria (glomerulonephritis).
Order UA ⇨ if proteinuria and/or hematuria ⇨ may need chemistries to look for ↑BUN/creatinine.

Retinal damage:
*Malignant HTN/Grade IV retinopathy (papilledema).** May present with blurred vision.

MANAGEMENT

Decrease blood pressure (mean arterial pressure) by no more than 25% within the first hour & an
additional 5-15% *over the next 23* hours **using IV agents.** 2 important exceptions:
1. **Acute phase of an ischemic stroke**. In general, blood pressure is not lowered in ischemic
   stroke unless it is ≥185/110 mmHg in patients who are candidates for thrombolytics or
   ≥220/120 in patients who are not candidates for thrombolytics.
2. **Acute aortic dissection**: BP often rapidly reduced to SBP of 100-120 mmHg within 20 minutes.

EMERGENCY	FIRST LINE	NOTES
NEUROLOGIC **HTN ENCEPHALOPATHY**	*Nicardipine or Clevidipine* *Labetalol,* Fenoldopam Sodium Nitroprusside	Must r/o stroke. *HTN encephalopathy often presents with confusion, headache, nausea & vomiting.** Symptoms improve with lowering of the blood pressure. Nitroprusside, Nitroglycerin & Hydralazine may increase intracranial pressure.
HEMORRHAGIC STROKE	Nicardipine or Labetalol	Benefits vs. risks of lowering blood pressure must be weighed in hemorrhagic strokes.
ISCHEMIC STROKE	Nicardipine or Labetalol	*Avoid cerebral hypoperfusion if ischemic.* Reduce blood pressure ONLY if BP is: ≥220/120 (not a thrombolytic candidate). ≥185/110 (if a thrombolytic candidate).
CARDIOVASCULAR **AORTIC DISSECTION**	**β-blocker**: *Esmolol, Labetalol* Sodium Nitroprusside (± add to beta blocker) Nicardipine, Clevidipine	Decreases shearing forces. Beta blocker tx target: systolic BP 100-120mmHg & pulse <60 bpm achieved within 20 minutes.
ACUTE CORONARY SYNDROME	*Nitroglycerin* *Beta blockers* (ex. Esmolol, Metoprolol) Nitroprusside	*Nitroglycerin not used if suspected right ventricular infarction or phosphodiesterase - 5 inhibitor use within 24-48h (ex. Sildenafil).*
ACUTE HEART FAILURE	*Nitroglycerin, Furosemide* Sodium Nitroprusside	Avoid Hydralazine & Beta blockers in CHF. Only if no evidence of cardiac ischemia.
RENAL	Fenoldopam	

HYPERLIPIDEMIA

ETIOLOGIES
1. Hypercholesterolemia: hypothyroidism, pregnancy, kidney failure.
2. Hypertriglyceridemia: Diabetes Mellitus, ETOH, obesity, steroids, estrogen.

CLINICAL MANIFESTATIONS OF HYPERLIPIDEMIA
1. Most patients are asymptomatic. Hypertriglyceridemia may cause pancreatitis.
2. May develop Xanthomas (ex. Achilles tendon) or Xanthelasma (lipid plaques on the eyelids).

GOALS
- Weight reduction, increased exercise.
- Dietary restriction of cholesterol & carbohydrates, decreased trans fatty acids.
- Goal of lipid-lowering agents: plaque stabilization, reversal of endothelial dysfunction, thrombogenicity reduction & atherosclerosis regression.

SCREENING FOR HYPERLIPIDEMIA
Based on risks: sex, age, cardiac risk factors such as smoking, hypertension, family history of coronary heart disease (first-degree male relative with CHD before age 55; first-degree female relative with CHD before age 65).

1. <u>American College of Cardiology/American Heart Association:</u> (2013): in adults between the ages 20 to 79 who are free of cardiovascular disease (CVD) it is "reasonable" to assess risk factors every 4 – 6 years to calculate their 10-year CVD risk.

There is considerable controversy regarding the optimal age for initiating screening.
- <u>Higher risk</u> = >1 risk factor (hypertension, smoking, family hx) or 1 severe risk factor. initiate screening at age 20 to 25 for males; 30 - 35 for females.

- <u>Lower risk:</u> initiate screening at age 35 for males; 45 for females.

LIPID GUIDELINES FOR THE INITIATION OF STATIN THERAPY
Determined by a 10-year and lifetime risk calculator instead of strict numbers only. The risk factors include: gender, age, race, smoking, blood pressure, blood cholesterol levels & diabetes mellitus. It recommends treatment in the following patients:

1. Patients with type 1 or 2 Diabetes Mellitus between the ages 40-75 years of age.

2. Patients without cardiovascular disease ages 40-75 years of age & ≥7.5% risk for having a heart attack or stroke within 10 years.

3. People ≥21 years of age with LDL levels ≥190 mg/dL.

4. Any patient with any form of clinical atherosclerotic cardiovascular disease.

BENEFIT OF LIPID LOWERING MEDICATIONS
- ***Best meds to lower elevated LDL*** ⇨ ***Statins,**** *Bile acid sequestrants.*
- ***Best meds to lower elevated triglycerides*** ⇨ ***Fibrates,**** *Niacin.*
- ***Best meds to increase HDL*** ⇨ ***Niacin,**** *Fibrates.*
- Type II DM ⇨ Fibrates, Statins
     *(Niacin may cause hyperglycemia so use in caution in patients with diabetes mellitus)**

Omega 3 fatty acids used for hypertriglyceridemia. Salmon, flaxseed, canola oil, soybean oil, nuts

GOALS: LDL <100 mg/dL is optimal, total cholesterol <200 mg/dL, HDL >60 mg/dL.

LIPID LOWERING AGENTS

	HDL	LDL	TG	INDICATIONS & MOA	SIDE EFFECTS & CONTRAINDICATIONS
NIACIN (NICOTINIC ACID) - Vitamin B$_3$	↑*	↓	↓*	• *BEST drug to increase HDL*.* • 2nd best drug to reduce triglycerides. • *Has been shown to decrease cardiovascular complications.* • **MOA:** *Increases HDL* (delays HDL clearance), reduces plasma fibrinogen levels. ↓*hepatic production of LDL* & its precursor VLDL.	• *Flushing, headache, warm sensation & pruritus 80%* (prostaglandin – mediated).* • *Aspirin or ibuprofen prior to dosing may decrease flushing* • S/E: *hyperuricemia:* may precipitate *gout,* *hyperglycemia.* • **CI:** peptic ulcer disease, hyperglycemia, hepatotoxicity, paresthesias, nausea (may last minutes to hours), vomiting, diarrhea, dry skin.
HMGcoA REDUCTASE INHIBITORS - Atorvastatin - Rosuvastatin - Lovastatin - Simvastatin - Pravastatin	↑	↓*	↓	• **BEST DRUG TO DECREASE LDL.*** • **MOA:** *inhibits the rate-limiting step in hepatic cholesterol synthesis (HMGcoA reductase inhibitor):* ↑'es *LDL receptors* (removes LDL from the blood). Reduces triglycerides. • *Shown to decrease cardiovascular complications*	• *Myositis*/myalgias/rhabdomyolysis* (especially when used with fibrates, niacin). • *Hepatitis** (1%): ↑LFTs (usually within the 1st 3 months). • Gastrointestinal symptoms, headache, proteinuria. • Much higher incidence of S/E if used with tetracyclines & antibiotics • Atorvastatin & Rosuvastatin strongest in the class. Fewer drug reactions with Pravastatin & Rosuvastatin. • Statins best given at bedtime (when cholesterol synthesis is maximal).
FIBRATES - Gemfibrozil - Fenofibrate	↑	↓	↓*	• **BEST DRUG TO DECREASE TRIGLYCERIDES.*** • **MOA:** *inhibits peripheral lipolysis & reduces hepatic triglyceride production* (by decreasing hepatic extraction of fatty acids). ↑HDL synthesis.	• ↑LFTs, *myositis & myalgias especially with concomitant statin use* (due to CYP3A4-related reduction in statin metabolism). • ↑*bile lithogenicity (gallstones).* • **CI:** hepatobiliary disease or severe renal disease.
BILE ACID SEQUESTRANTS - Cholestyramine - Colestipol - Colesevelam	↑	↓*	↑*	• **MOA:** *binds bile acids in intestine blocking enterohepatic reabsorption of bile acids,* reducing cholesterol pool, lowering intrahepatic cholesterol. The liver has to make new bile acids, so it ↑ its LDL receptors thereby *removing LDL from the blood.* • Mild- mod ↑es in HDL (via intestinal formation of HDL). • *Bile acid sequestrants are most useful in combining with a statin or niacin to aggressively lower LDL* cholesterol levels. • *Only meds safe in pregnancy!* (not systemically absorbed & excreted in feces). • *Bile acid sequestrants used for pruritus associated with biliary obstruction.*	• **GI side effects:** nausea, vomiting, bloating, crampy abdominal pain, ↑**LFTs.** • *Causes increased triglycerides** (so best used in patients with ↑LDL and normal triglyceride levels). Osteoporosis with long-term use. • May impair the absorption of Digoxin, Warfarin, fat-soluble vitamins (so give those meds 1 hour before or 4 hours after bile acid sequestrants).
EZETIMIBE (Zetia)		↓		• **MOA:** *inhibits intestinal cholesterol absorption* (lowers LDL). May be used with statins.	• S/E: ↑LFTs especially with statin use.

INFECTIVE ENDOCARDITIS

- Infection of the endothelium/valves 2ry to colonization (ex. during transient/persistent bacteremia).
- *Mitral valve MC valve involved** (*M>A>T>P). **Exception is IVDA (Tricuspid valve MC in IV drug users.)**

TYPES OF ENDOCARDITIS

❶ **ACUTE BACTERIAL ENDOCARDITIS (ABE):** infection of *normal valves* with a virulent organism (ex *S. aureus).*

❷ **SUBACUTE BACTERIAL ENDOCARDITIS (SBE):** indolent infection of *abnormal valves* with less virulent organism (ex *S. viridans).*

❸ **ENDOCARDITIS IN IV DRUG USERS:** ex. *MRSA,** Pseudomonas, Candida.

❹ **PROSTHETIC VALVE ENDOCARDITIS (PVE):** *early (within 60 days): Staphylococcus epidermis MC.**
    Late (after 60 days) resembles native valve endocarditis.

MICROBIOLOGY

- *STREP VIRIDANS - MC organism in SUBACUTE bacterial endocarditis* - *oral flora* source of infection.

- *STAPH AUREUS - MC in ACUTE bacterial endocarditis & IVDA (especially MRSA),** patients with HIV.

- *Enterococci - MC in men 50y with history of GI/GU procedures.** Others: fungi, yeasts, gram negative rods.

- **HACEK organisms: H**aemophilus, **A**ctinobacillus, **C**ardiobacterium, **E**ikenella, **K**lingella. HACEK = gram-negative organisms that are associated with the development of large vegetations & are often hard to culture.

CLINICAL MANIFESTATIONS

1. *Fever (80-90% - including fever on unknown origin),* anorexia, weight loss, fatigue. *ECG conduction abnormalities.*
2. Peripheral Manifestations:
   - *JANEWAY LESIONS - painless erythematous macules on the palms & soles* (emboli/immune).
   - *ROTH SPOTS:* retinal hemorrhages with pale centers. *Petechiae* (conjunctiva, palate).
   - *OSLER'S NODES: tender nodules on the pads of the digits*.
   - *Splinter hemorrhages* of proximal nail bed, clubbing, hepatosplenomegaly. *Septic emboli:* (ex CNS, kidneys, spleen)

DIAGNOSTIC STUDIES

1. **Blood cultures:** (before antibiotic initiation). *3 sets at least 1 hour apart* if the patient is stable.
2. **ECG:** at regular intervals to assess for new conduction abnormalities (*prone to arrhythmias).*
3. **Echocardiogram:** obtain TTE first; consider TEE if TTE is nondiagnostic or increased suspicion. *Transesophageal echocardiogram (TEE) much more sensitive than TTE** (>90% v 50% in NVE) (82%v 36% in PVE).
4. **Labs: *CBC: leukocytosis, anemia* (normochromic, normocytic); ↑*ESR/Rheumatoid Factor.*

MODIFIED DUKE CRITERIA	
MAJOR	**MINOR**

• **SUSTAINED BACTEREMIA** *2 ⊕ blood cultures* by organism known to cause endocarditis.
 	
• **ENDOCARDIAL INVOLVEMENT**: documented by either:
  - ⊕ *echocardiogram*: (vegetation, abscess, valve perforation, prosthetic dehiscence)
 	
- clearly established *new valvular regurgitation* (aortic or mitral regurgitation)
	• *Predisposing condition*
	  abnormal valves, IVDA, indwelling catheters, etc.
	• *Fever* (>38° C /100.4°F).
	• *Vascular & embolic phenomena:* Janeway lesions, septic arterial or pulmonary emboli, ICH.
	• *Immunologic phenomena:* Osler's nodes, Roth spots,
	  - ⊕ Rheumatoid factor
	  - Acute glomerulonephritis
	• ⊕ Blood culture not meeting major criteria.
	• ⊕ echocardiogram not meeting major criteria (ex. worsening of existing murmur).

Clinical criteria for infective endocarditis: 2 major OR 1 major + 3 minor OR 5 minor (80% accuracy)	

INDICATIONS FOR SURGERY

- Refractory CHF; persistent or refractory infection, invasive infection, prosthetic valve, recurrent systemic emboli, fungal infections.

MANAGEMENT OF INFECTIVE ENDOCARDITIS: suggested Empiric therapy:

ACUTE (NATIVE VALVE)	- *Nafcillin + Gentamicin x 4- 6 weeks* OR - *Vancomycin (if suspected MRSA or PCN allergic) + Gentamicin*
SUBACUTE (NATIVE VALVE)	- *Penicillin or Ampicillin + Gentamicin.* *Vancomycin in IVDA.* - Ceftriaxone or Vancomycin plus Gentamicin.
PROSTHETIC VALVE	- *Vancomycin + Gentamicin + Rifampin* (for Staph aureus)
FUNGAL	- *Amphotericin B (treat 6-8 weeks).* - Patients often need surgical intervention for fungal cases

Penicillin & Vancomycin have great gram-positive coverage. Gentamicin has great gram-negative coverage.

- In acute endocarditis, antibiotics are started promptly after culture data is obtained.
- In subacute endocarditis, if the patient is hemodynamically stable, antibiotics may be delayed in order to properly obtain blood culture data, especially if prior treatment with antibiotics.
- Adjust the antibiotic regimen based on organism, culture & sensitivities. Fever may persist up to 1 week after appropriate antibiotic therapy has been initiated.
- *Duration of therapy usually 4-6 weeks* (with aminoglycosides used only for the first 2 weeks).

ENDOCARDITIS PROPHYLAXIS INDICATIONS	
Cardiac conditions	1. *Prosthetic (artificial) heart valves.* 2. *Heart repairs using prosthetic material (not including stents).* 3. *Prior history of endocarditis.* 4. *Congenital heart disease.* 5. Cardiac valvulopathy in a transplanted heart.
Procedures	1. *Dental:* involving manipulation of gums, roots of the teeth, oral mucosa perforation. 2. *Respiratory:* surgery on respiratory mucosa, rigid bronchoscopy. 3. *Procedures involving infected skin/musculoskeletal tissues* *(including abscess incision & drainage).*
Regimens	AMOXICILLIN* 2g 30-60 minutes before the procedures listed above. CLINDAMYCIN 600mg if penicillin allergic.* Macrolides or Cephalexin are other options.

**NOTE prophylaxis is no longer routinely recommended for gastrointestinal or genitourinary procedures.
**NOTE prophylaxis no longer routinely recommended for most types of valvular heart disease (including mitral valve prolapse, bicuspid aortic valve, acquired mitral or aortic valve disease, hypertrophic cardiomyopathy).
Good oral hygiene recommended to reduce temporary episodes of bacteremia.

NONBACTERIAL VERRUCOUS ENDOCARDITIS (LIBMAN-SACKS ENDOCARDITIS):
Small, warty, sterile vegetations on both sides of the leaflets that can be a source of embolization. Seen especially with systemic lupus erythematosus (SLE).
MANAGEMENT: manage the SLE. May need anticoagulation.

PERIPHERAL ARTERIAL DISEASE

• Atherosclerotic disease of the lower extremities (and vessels outside of the heart & brain).

CLINICAL MANIFESTATIONS

1. **INTERMITTENT CLAUDICATION:** *MC presentation. Reproducible pain/discomfort in the **lower extremity brought on by exercise/walking & relieved with rest.*** Symptoms occur distal to lesion.

VESSEL INVOLVED	AREA OF CLAUDICATION	PERCENTAGE
AORTIC BIFURCATION/COMMON ILIAC	*Buttock, hip, groin.*	25-30%
	Leriche's syndrome: triad: ❶ *claudication (buttock, thigh pain)* ❷ *impotence &* ❸ *decreased femoral pulses.*	
FEMORAL ARTERY OR BRANCHES	*Thigh, upper calf*	*80 -90%*
POPLITEAL ARTERY	*Lower calf,* ankle and foot	
TIBIAL AND PERONEAL ARTERIES	Foot	40-50%

2. **Resting leg pain:** limb-threatening ischemia. Rest pain = advanced disease.
   Typically occurs while lying in bed at night. Pain usually lessened with foot dependency.
3. **Acute arterial embolism:** *usually caused by sudden occlusion: 6 P's (paresthesias, pain, pallor, pulselessness, paralysis, poikilothermia). Livedo reticularis (mottling of the skin).*
4. **Gangrene:** when arterial perfusion is so poor that *spontaneous necrosis occurs.* The tissue goes from purplish/blue ⇨ black. Gangrene is a complication of acute/chronic arterial occlusion.
   - wet gangrene: *ulcers* ⇨ malodorous, copious, purulent, infected, blackened regions.
   - dry gangrene: mummification of the digits.

PHYSICAL EXAM

1. **Pulses:** *decreased/absent pulses; ± bruits* (>50% occlusion). *↓capillary refill.*
2. **Skin:** *atrophic skin changes:* muscle atrophy; thin/shiny skin, hair loss, thickened nails, cool limbs. Usually no edema. May develop painful, black areas of necrosis at points of trauma, toes.
3. **Color:** *pale on elevation, dusky red with dependency (dependent rubor),* cyanosis. If ulcers are present, they usually involve the toes or points of trauma (ex. *LATERAL malleolar ulcers*).

DIAGNOSIS

1. **Ankle-brachial index (ABI):** *simple, quick, noninvasive most useful screening tool for chronic.*
   - ⊕ *PAD if ABI <0.90* (0.50 is severe). Rest pain if < 0.4. Normal ABI 1-1.2.
   - >1.2 ⇨ possible noncompressible (calcified) vessels – may lead to a false reading.
   - ABI of at least 0.85 needed to heal ulcers in diabetics (0.6-0.8 needed in nondiabetics).

2. **Arteriography:** *gold standard* because it shows length, location & degree of occlusion.
   Clinically usually only performed if revascularization is planned.
3. Duplex B mode ultrasound: noninvasive. Used for visualizing stenosis.
4. **Hand Held Doppler:** may be used to help assess distal blood flow & pulses. Often used in the ER.

MANAGEMENT

A. **Platelet inhibitors:** ❶ *Cilostazol mainstay of tx. Helpful for intermittent claudication* [*vasodilator & ADP inhibitor,* ↑RBC flexibility (phosphodiesterase-3 inhibition)]. ❷ *Aspirin* ❸ *Clopidogrel (Plavix):* ADP inhibitor. Pentoxifylline: ↓'es blood viscosity & ↑RBC flexibility, ↑microcirculation.

B. **Revascularization:** ❶ PTA (percutaneous transluminal *angioplasty*); ❷ Bypass grafts *fem-pop bypass* (autogenous in situ saphenous vein bypass grafts). ❸ Endarterectomy.

C. **Supportive:** foot care, *exercise:* fixed distance walking to the point of claudication, resting and continuing until symptoms occurs (do this for 1h/day); ↓risk factors (HTN, DM, lipid levels).

D. Acute Arterial Occlusion: Heparin for acute embolism; Thombolytics if thrombus; Embolectomy.

E. Amputation: if severe or gangrene occurs.

ABDOMINAL AORTIC ANEURYSM (AAA)

Focal dilation of the aortic diameter @ least 1-1.5x diameter measured @ level of the renal arteries.
- **>3.0 cm generally considered aneurismal. MC occurs INFRARENALLY.**

RISK FACTORS FOR AAA DEVELOPMENT
- **ATHEROSCLEROSIS MC RISK FACTOR.** **Age >60y** (increases dramatically after age 60y).
- **Smoking: major risk factor** - promotes rate of aneurysm formation, growth and rupture.
- *Males* (5x MC in men); *Caucasians:*African-Americans (2:1).
- Hyperlipidemia, connective tissue disorder (ex. Marfan's syndrome), Syphilis. Hypertension.

PATHOPHYSIOLOGY OF AAA
- Although inciting event is unknown, there is *proteolytic degeneration of aortic wall,* connective tissue, inflammation and an immune response.
- Laplace's law: wall tension = (pressure x radius)/tensile force dictates that as the aorta dilates ⇨ the force on the aortic wall increases ⇨ further dilation *(larger aneurysms expand more quickly).* Average rate 0.25 to 0.5 cm/year. All expanding aneurysms will eventually rupture.

CLINICAL MANIFESTATIONS
1. **Asymptomatic AAA:**
   - *Most asymptomatic* until they rupture. Often *incidental finding* on US, CT or MRI when doing workup for other problems or on physical exam *(palpable, expanding, pulsatile abdominal mass).*

2. **Acute leakage/rupture:**
   - **Classic presentation**: *older male (>60y) with* ❶ *severe back or abdominal pain who presents with* ❷*syncope or hypotension &* ❸ ⊕ *tender, pulsatile abdominal mass* (may be obscured by obesity); May complain of unilateral groin/hip pain. ±*Flank ecchymosis.* Femoral pulsations usually normal. Acute may be rapidly fatal. *>5 cm* ⇨↑*rupture risk.*
3. Chronic-contained rupture: uncommon. Rupture may be tamponaded by surrounding retroperitoneum.
4. Aortoenteric fistula: presents as acute GI bleed *in patients who underwent prior aortic grafting.*

DIAGNOSIS OF AAA
1. **ABDOMINAL ULTRASOUND:** *initial imaging study of choice in suspected AAA* to determine aneurysm presence, size & extent. Also used to monitor for progression in size (expansion).* Bedside ultrasound often done in ER to r/o AAA in patients presenting with nonspecific abdominal pain > 60y.

2. **CT SCAN:** *test of choice for thoracic aneurysms* & for further evaluation of patients with known AAA* (clearly defines the anatomy of the aneurysm for planning surgery).

3. **Angiography:** *gold standard.** Often used before surgical intervention.
4. **MRI/MRA:** increased use in lieu of angiography.
5. Abdominal radiograph: may show calcified aorta in 65% of patients with aneurysmal disease.

MANAGEMENT OF AAA
Surgical Repair definitive management. Endovascular stent graft or open repair.

≥5.5 cm OR > 0.5 cm expansion in 6 months	*IMMEDIATE SURGICAL REPAIR (even if asymptomatic), symptomatic patients or patients with acute rupture.*
>4.5 cm	Vascular surgeon referral.
4 – 4.5 cm	Monitor by ultrasound every 6 months.
3 - 4 cm	Monitor by ultrasound every year.

- **β-blockers: reduces shearing forces,** ↓'es expansion & rupture risk. ↓ risk factors

AORTIC DISSECTION

- **AORTIC DISSECTION:** *tear in the innermost layer of aorta (intima)* due to cystic medial necrosis.
- **65% ascending,** 20% descending, 10% aortic arch. MC site is ascending: near the aortic arch or left subclavian. *Ascending = high mortality.**

PATHOPHYSIOLOGY

- **Intimal wall tear*** ⇨ propagation of tear: blood under high systemic pressure flows into the media at the point of the tear. This tear causes a false lumen (channel). The blood may propagate proximal or distal to the tear (sometimes both).
- Another type is an intramural hematoma (bleeding into the media).

RISK FACTORS

1. **HYPERTENSION*** (80%): **most important predisposing factor.**
2. **Age: MC 50-60y** (patients with history of Marfan may present in 20-30y); Men 2 times MC.
3. Vasculitis (rare), trauma, family history of aortic dissection, Turner's syndrome.
4. Collagen disorders: (ex. Marfan's syndrome, Ehlers-Danlos). Cocaine use.

CLINICAL MANIFESTATIONS

1. **Chest Pain** (96%): **sudden onset of** SEVERE, TEARING (RIPPING, KNIFE-LIKE)* **chest/upper back pain*** accompanied with nausea, vomiting, diaphoresis. Symptoms depend on the location:
   - ascending aorta ⇨ anterior chest pain (especially Type A).
   - aortic arch ⇨ neck/jaw pain.
   - descending aorta ⇨ interscapular pain (especially with Type B).

2. **Decreased peripheral pulses** (50%): radial, carotid or femoral.
   VARIATION IN PULSE (>20 MMHG DIFFERENCE BETWEEN THE RIGHT & LEFT ARM).*

3. **Hypertension**: MC in distal/Type B: ascending (70:36). May be hypotensive.
4. Ascending dissections: **acute new-onset aortic regurgitation** (diastolic decrescendo murmur if the dissection involves the aorta & aortic valve); acute MI, cardiac tamponade.
5. Descending dissections: back pain, HTN (60%), hypotension/shock (3%), spine ischemia.
6. Neurological deficits: including stroke, hemiplegia & syncope.

DIAGNOSIS

1. **CT scan with contrast: CT 3-D is rapidly becoming the test of choice** (especially in the ER). CT, MRI & Transesophageal echocardiogram are the MC used first-line imaging modalities.

2. **MRI Angiography: gold standard.** Best if hemodynamically stable but is time-consuming.
3. **TEE (Transesophageal echocardiography):** accurate & portable. *May be used to initially evaluate patients especially if hemodynamically unstable.*

4. **CXR:** WIDENING OF THE MEDIASTINUM CLASSIC* (60-90%). 10% may have normal CXR so it cannot be used to rule out dissection (especially if distal dissection is suspected).

MANAGEMENT

1. **SURGICAL MANAGEMENT:** done in ACUTE PROXIMAL* (Stanford A/ DeBakey I and II) or **acute distal** (Type III) **with complications** (vital organ involvement, impending rupture, etc).

2. **MEDICAL MANAGEMENT:** done in DESCENDING IF NO COMPLICATIONS (Stanford B/Debakey III).
   - **Esmolol, Labetalol 1st line** - target: SBP 100-120mmHg & pulse <60 bpm achieved in 20 minutes.
   - **Sodium nitroprusside added if needed**; ± Nicardipine.

ACUTE ABDOMINAL AORTIC ANEURYSM

ABDOMINAL AORTIC ANEURYSMS (AAA)

DIAGNOSIS

ABDOMINAL ULTRASOUND

- Determine aneurysm presence, size & extent. Also used to monitor for progression in size (expansion).

ABDOMINAL AORTIC ANEURYSMS (AAA)

Patient with h/o prior AAA (Abdominal aorta shows graft from old rupture - black arrow) with acute new AAA c extravasation of the contrast dye (white arrow)

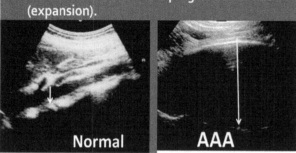

Normal / AAA

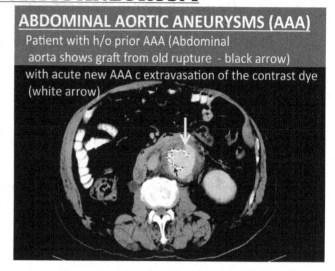

AORTIC DISSECTION

DIAGNOSIS OF AORTIC DISSECTION

Chest X Ray:
- Widening of mediastinum*, 10% normal

NORMAL / AORTIC DISSECTION

AORTIC DISSECTION

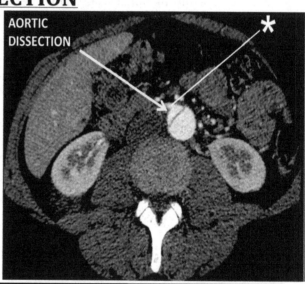

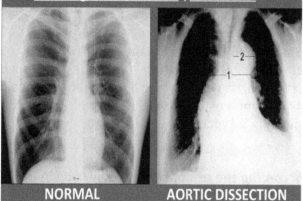

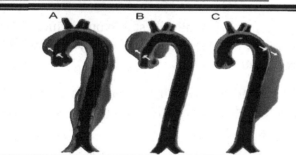

Type	DeBakey I	DeBakey II	DeBakey III
	Stanford A		Stanford B
	Proximal		Distal

AORTIC DISSECTION CLASSES

DeBakey

Type I – Originates in ascending aorta, propagates at least to the aortic arch and often beyond it distally.

Type II – Originates in and is confined to the ascending aorta.

Type III – Originates in descending aorta, rarely extends proximally but will extend distally.

Stanford

A – Involves ascending aorta and/or aortic arch, & possibly descending aorta.

B – Involves the descending aorta (distal to left subclavian artery origin), without involvement of the ascending aorta or aortic arch.

THROMBOANGIITIS OBLITERANS (BUERGER's DISEASE)

- **_Nonatherosclerotic inflammatory disease of small & medium arteries & veins._**
  - Characterized by segmental vascular inflammation & vasoocclusive phenomena.

- **_Strongly associated with tobacco*_** (smoking, chewing etc).
  - **_MC in young men 20-45y._** MC in India, Asia & the Middle East.

- **_Suspect in young smokers/tobacco users with distal extremity ischemia/ischemic ulcers or gangrene of the digits._**

PATHOPHYSIOLOGY
- Immunologic disorder ⇨ vasodysfunction & _microthrombi_ (hypersensitivity to tobacco). Affects both arteries & veins.

CLINICAL MANIFESTATIONS
- **Triad of ❶ _superficial migratory thrombophlebitis_ ❷ _claudication_ & ❸ _Raynaud's phenomenon._**
  1. SUPERFICIAL MIGRATORY THROMBOPHLEBITIS: large, erythematous tender superficial veins causing nodules that follow the venous distribution.

  2. DISTAL EXTREMITY ISCHEMIA: **_CLAUDICATION & finger/toe ischemia MC presentation._** Paresthesias of the hands/feet. **_Ischemic ulcers or gangrene_** seen on exam. Usually involves the distal vessels but may progress to proximal vessel involvement. 80% involve 3-4 limbs.
     - _Think thromboangiitis obliterans in the differential in a young patient with foot claudication._

  3. RAYNAUD'S PHENOMENON: 40%. Involves the hand & fingers. **_Reversible vasospasm-induced tri-color_** (❶ pallor-white ❷ cyanosis-blue ❸ reperfusion hyperemia-red) _changes of fingers, toes, ears, nose, tongue that worsen with cold exposure, smoking or emotional stress._ May develop numbness, tingling & pain. May be asymptomatic.

DIAGNOSIS
1. **Aortography:** _nonatherosclerotic, segmental_ **occlusive lesions of small/medium vessels** with **_corkscrew collaterals_** (collateralization around areas of occlusion - not specific for Buerger's). **_Gold standard diagnosis.*_**

2. **Abnormal Allen test:** Allen test assesses the patency of the radial and ulnar arteries. Decreased patency & delayed reperfusion are seen in patients with thromboangiitis obliterans.

3. <u>Labs:</u> usually normal but often ordered to rule out other diseases (ex. vasculitis).

MANAGEMENT
1. **_Tobacco cessation:_** **_only definitive management of Buerger's disease._**

2. <u>Wound care:</u> debridement, moist dressings, negative pressure wound therapy. Amputation if gangrene occurs or to avoid the spread of infection in severe ischemic cases.

3. **_Calcium channel blockers for Raynaud's phenomenon:*_**
   - _Dihydropyridines: ex. Nifedipine, Nicardipine, Amlodipine_

4. <u>Iloprost:</u> prostaglandin analog that may be helpful in patients with critical limb ischemia while patient is in the process of smoking cessation. Prostaglandins keep blood vessels patent.

PERIPHERAL VENOUS DISEASE

1. **SUPERFICIAL VENOUS SYSTEM:** *greater/lesser saphenous veins.* Not well supported.
2. **DEEP VENOUS SYSTEM:** accompanies major arteries. Carries 90% of venous return & well supported. *Includes the femoral, iliac, popliteal, posterior tibial & "superficial" femoral.*
3. **PERFORATING VEINS:** communicate between the deep & superficial systems.

THROMBOPHLEBITIS: inflammation/swelling of a vein caused by a blood clot. 2 main types: superficial thrombophlebitis and deep vein thrombosis (deep, larger veins).

VIRCHOW'S TRIAD: patients with thrombi may have a combination of factors:
❶ *Intimal damage:* ex. trauma, infection, inflammation.
❷ *Stasis:* ex. immobilization or prolonged sitting >4 hours.
❸ *Hypercoagulability:* ex. *Factor V Leiden mutation*, Protein C or S Deficiency, antithrombin III deficiencies, oral contraception use, malignancy, pregnancy.

SUPERFICIAL THROMBOPHLEBITIS

- **INFLAMMATION &/OR THROMBUS OF A SUPERFICIAL VEIN.** Usually a benign, self-limited disease.
- *MC associated with IV catheterization, trauma, pregnancy & varicose veins.* May be infectious (septic).

- **TROUSSEAU'S SIGN OF MALIGNANCY (TROUSSEAU SYNDROME):** *migratory thrombophlebitis associated with malignancy* ex. pancreatic cancer. May also be seen with vasculitic disorders.

PATHOPHYSIOLOGY
Inflammatory reaction leads to formation of a thrombus of a superficial vein under the skin.

CLINICAL MANIFESTATIONS:
1. **Local phlebitis:** *tenderness, pain, induration, edema, erythema along the course of the superficial vein ±palpable cord* (thrombosed superficial vein). Fever (if septic).

DIAGNOSIS
1. **Venous duplex ultrasound:** *noncompressible vein* with clot, vein wall thickening. Clinical dx.

WORKUP
Most patients don't need a workup unless an underlying cause is suspected:
1. Hypercoagulability workup: *Factor V Leiden (MC cause),* prothrombin gene mutations, Protein C and S, antiphospholipid antibodies, lupus anticoagulant, factor VII, homocysteine.
2. Migratory phlebitis: malignancy workup: carcinoembryonic antigen (CEA), prostate specific antigen (PSA), colonoscopy, CT scan, mammography (as indicated based on suspicion).

MANAGEMENT OF THROMBOPHLEBITIS
1. *Supportive management mainstay of treatment:** extremity elevation, warm compresses,* normal daily activity, *NSAIDs, elastic support compression stockings.* Bed rest if severe.

2. Aseptic: NSAIDs. May consider Heparin & Warfarin if the clot is near the saphenofemoral junction.

3. Septic: IV Antibiotics: penicillin + aminoglycoside. Suspect septic if high fever or if purulent.

4. Vein ligation/excision (phlebectomy): if extensive varicose veins, septic phlebitis or persistent symptoms despite supportive measures.

DEEP VENOUS THROMBOSIS

- *Most important consequence is pulmonary embolism (50%):* both are manifestations of a single entity. ***Most DVTs originate in the calf.****
- RISK FACTORS: Virchow's triad: ❶*venous stasis:* car rides/plane flight >4 hours, prolonged bed rest, immobilization ❷*endothelial damage:* lower leg injury ❸*hypercoagulability:* malignancy, pregnancy, OCPs.

CLINICAL MANIFESTATIONS

1. *UNILATERAL SWELLING/EDEMA OF LOWER EXTREMITY:* *>3cm most specific sx/sign of DVT.* Swelling due to forced retrograde flow of blood. Warm skin. Surface veins become more visible.
2. *Calf pain/tenderness 50%.* Tenderness on palpation often present. **Homan's sign:** calf pain with dorsiflexion with a flexed knee (not reliable). **Phlebitis:** warmth, erythema, palpable cord.
3. Rare, massive DVT of proximal vein: cerulea alba: milky white pallor with occlusion of the deep venous system ⇨ cerulea dolens: cyanosis & swelling of limb with sudden pain due to the progression of compression of the deep + superficial veins of the lower limb.

DIAGNOSTIC STUDIES

1. VENOUS DUPLEX ULTRASOUND: *FIRST LINE IMAGING TEST (NONINVASIVE).** Thrombus will show *noncompressible echogenicity* & altered flow. MRI: similar to ultrasound.

2. D-DIMER: fibrin degradation products (highly sensitive but not specific). ❶*A negative D-dimer can rule out DVT in a LOW risk patient** (Wells DVT score <1) *not to confirm dx.* ❷ Used in probable or high-risk patient with negative venous US to determine if serial US needed. All patients with positive D-dimer & all patients with moderate-high risk of DVT (Wells score >2) require US.
   False positives: pregnancy, liver disease, inflammation, malignancy, trauma, hospitalized patients.*

3. VENOGRAPHY: *gold standard.** Filling defect or nonfilling of the deep veins is diagnostic of DVT.
4. Plethysmography: not as reliable or sensitive as duplex. Size of leg doesn't increase if ⊕DVT.

MANAGEMENT OF DVT

Main goal is preventing pulmonary emboli (PE).

1. **Anticoagulation therapy:** *Heparin (LMWH or unfractionated)* ⇨ *Warfarin.* Consider lifelong anticoagulation in patients with Protein C/S or antithrombin III deficiencies, Factor V Leiden.
   - UNFRACTIONATED HEPARIN Ind: prevents further emboli rather than treat existing one. Usually the first episode doesn't kill, subsequent PEs are more deadly. Titrate to *PTT 1.5-2.5 x normal value.*
     MOA: *potentiates antithrombin III,* inhibits thrombin & other coagulation factors.
     S/E: *protamine sulfate antidote for heparin toxicity.* Heparin–induced thrombocytopenia.
   - LOW MOLECULAR WEIGHT HEPARIN: Enoxaparin. No need to monitor PTT. SQ injection that lasts 12 hours so patient can be discharged home. Safe in pregnancy. **CI:** thrombocytopenia, renal failure if Cr >2.0.
   - WARFARIN (COUMADIN): MOA: *inhibits vitamin K-dependent coagulation factors of EXTRINSIC pathway: 2, 7, 9 & 10. Inhibits protein C & S. Coumadin should be overlapped with heparin for at least 5 days* AND until INR >2.0 -3.0 @ least 24h. *Vitamin K is the antidote for toxicity. Avoid cruciferous vegetables with* ↑*Vit K* (Spinach, Kale, Brussel sprouts, Greens), green tea, cranberry juice, ETOH.

RISK FACTORS VENOUS THROMBOEMBOLISM (VTE)	RECOMMENDED DURATION OF THERAPY
1st event with reversible or time-limiting RF for VTE	*at least 3 months** (Risk factors: trauma, surgery, OCPs etc).
1st episode of IDIOPATHIC DVT (no malignancy) - Proximal DVT or PE - Distal DVT	Long-term anticoagulation 3 months if severely symptomatic distal DVT No tx & surveillance (ultrasound) if asymptomatic distal DVT
Pregnancy	LMWH preferred as initial & long-term therapy.
Malignancy	LMWH as initial & long-term therapy. Warfarin or direct oral anticoagulants are alternatives to LMWH in these patients.

2. **IVC filter:** *in patients with contraindications to or who failed anticoagulation treatment.**

2016 ACCP guidelines: novel oral anticoagulants (Apixaban, Dabigatran, Edoxaban, Rivaroxaban) are preferred over Warfarin therapy in the management of DVT/PE (if no cancer is present).

APPROACH IN SUSPECTED DVT

If ultrasound is negative, repeat US within 1 week if intermediate or high clinical probability.

WELL'S CRITERIA FOR DVT

Clinical feature	Points	
Active cancer (including treatment within 6 months, or palliation)	1	
Paralysis, paresis, or immobilization of lower extremity	1	
Bedridden for more than 3 days because of surgery (within 4 weeks)	1	
Localized tenderness along distribution of deep veins	1	
Swelling of entire leg	1	
Unilateral calf swelling of greater than 3 cm (below tibial tuberosity)	1	
Unilateral pitting edema	1	
Collateral superficial veins	1	
Alternative diagnosis as likely or more likely than DVT	-2	
Total points		

LOW MOLECULAR WEIGHT HEPARIN (LMWH)

- **MOA:** *potentiates antithrombin III* - works more on factor Xa than thrombin (Factor IIa).

- *SQ injection. Compliant, low-risk patients can be discharged home during bridging therapy.*

- *Duration of Action ~12 hours.*

- *No need to monitor PTT* (weight based – more predictable dosing).

- *Protamine Sulfate is the antidote* (not as effective as it is for UFH).

- *Lower risk of HIT* (higher anti Xa-IIa ratio means less potential binding with platelets).

- **CI:** *Renal failure* (Cr >2.0) because LMWH excreted by kidneys, *Thrombocytopenia.*

UNFRACTIONATED HEPARIN (UFH)

- **MOA:** *potentiates antithrombin III, inhibits thrombin & other coagulation factors.*

- Continuous IV drip – requires hospitalization for bridging therapy.

- *Duration of Action: 1h p IV drip is discontinued.*

- *Must monitor PTT 1.5-2.5x normal value.*

- *Protamine Sulfate is the antidote.*

- *Heparin Induced Thrombocytopenia* – Heparin acts as a hapten (stimulates the immune response when attached to platelet factor 4). This complex activates platelets, causing simultaneous thrombocytopenia & thrombosis. **Management:** other anticoagulants: ex: Argatroban or Bivalirudin. DO NOT use Warfarin (may develop necrosis)

Peripheral VENOUS disease

- **Leg pain:**
  Worse c leg dependency, standing/prolonged sitting.

  IMPROVES with walking, elevation of leg.*

- *Cyanotic leg with dependency.**

- **Leg ulcers:**
  Esp @ MEDIAL malleolus,* uneven ulcer margins

- **Skin Findings:**
  Stasis dermatitis: eczematous rash, thickening of skin BROWNISH PIGMENTATION.

  Pulses & temperature usually normal.

  Prominent edema common.

Peripheral ARTERIAL disease

- **Leg pain:**
  Better with leg dependency, rest.

  WORSE with walking, elevation of leg, cold.

- *Redness leg with dependency - DEPENDENT RUBOR* & cyanotic leg with elevation.*

- **Leg ulcers:**
  Esp @ LATERAL malleolus,* clean margins

- **Skin Findings:**
  Atrophic skin changes: thin shiny skin, loss of hair, muscle atrophy, pallor, thick nails. Livedo reticularis (mottled appearance).

  ↓pulses & temperature usually cool.

  Minimal to no edema.

VARICOSE VEINS

- **Varicose veins:** dilated, tortuous superficial veins 2^{ry} to defective valve structure & function of the superficial veins (especially the superficial saphenous veins).
- Intrinsic weakness of the vein wall & ↑intraluminal pressure leads to reversal of venous flow.
- *Seen especially with ↑**estrogen: OCPs, pregnancy;** ↑stress on legs: **prolonged standing, obesity.***

PATHOPHYSIOLOGY
- Muscle contractions compress the deep veins (pumping action produces ↑transient deep venous pressures). This pressure gets transferred to the superficial venous system.
- *Exposure to high pressures causes the superficial veins to dilate because superficial veins lack support & are thin-walled.* The deep veins can withstand higher pressures because they are supported well.

CLINICAL MANIFESTATIONS
1. Often asymptomatic but may be a cosmetic issue for some patients. ***Dilated, tortuous veins.***
2. Dull ache or pressure sensation ***worsened with prolonged standing & relieved with elevation.***
3. ***Venous stasis ulcers:*** severe varicosities resulting in skin ulcerations. ± Mild ankle edema.
4. Visual inspection of the leg in the dependent position usually confirms the presence of varicosities.

MANAGEMENT:
1. ***Conservative: leg elevation, elastic compression stockings,*** avoid prolonged standing & girdles.
2. Sclerotherapy, radiofrequency or laser ablation & ambulatory phlebectomy commonly used.

CHRONIC VENOUS INSUFFICIENCY

- Vascular incompetency of either the deep and/or superficial veins.
ETIOLOGIES: *MC occurs after superficial thrombophlebitis, after DVT or trauma to the affected leg.*

CLINICAL MANIFESTATIONS
1. **Leg pain:** burning, aching, throbbing, cramping, muscle fatigue, "heavy leg".
   - *Pain/color worse with: prolonged standing/sitting, foot dependency.*
   - *Pain/color improves with: leg elevation* & walking.*
2. Leg edema: ↑leg circumference, pitting edema, varicosities, erythema. *Pulses/temperature normal.*
3. ***Stasis dermatitis:*** eczematous rash, itching, scaling, weeping erosions with crusting ± cellulitis.

4. ***BROWNISH HYPERPIGMENTATION:**** hemosiderin deposition in the skin from damaged vessels.

5. ***Venous stasis ulcers*** with uneven margins may occur, especially at the ***MEDIAL malleolus.****
6. Atrophie blanche: atrophic, hypopigmented areas with telangiectasias & punctate red dots.

DIAGNOSTIC STUDIES:
1. **Trendelenburg test:** tests perforator function & saphenofemoral vein competency. Elevate one leg @ 90^0 (empties it of venous blood) ⇨ occlude great saphenous vein at the upper thigh. After patient stands for 20 seconds, ***slow filling at the ankle suggests perforator competency.***
2. **Ultrasound:** especially if procedures are planned.

MANAGEMENT
1. ***Compression mainstay of treatment: periods of leg elevation, elastic compression stockings,*** avoid prolonged periods of standing or sitting. Patient should exercise regularly.
2. **Ulcer management:** wet to dry dressings, Unna boot, edema control.
   Severe ⇨ skin grafting, hyperbaric oxygen.
3. Venous valve transplant.

POSTURAL (ORTHOSTATIC) HYPOTENSION

• Marked reduction of blood pressure from supine to upright position (ex. supine to standing).

PATHOPHYSIOLOGY

❶ Impaired autonomic reflexes &/or ❷ reduced intravascular volume:

Medications: antihypertensives (ex. alpha-1 blockers, ACE inhibitors); vasodilators, diuretics, narcotics, antipsychotic medications, antidepressants, alcohol consumption.

Neurologic: diabetic autonomic neuropathy, Parkinson disease, polyneuropathies, Guillain-Barré syndrome.

CLINICAL MANIFESTATIONS

1. Dizziness, weakness, lightheadedness, visual, syncope with changes in position.
2. Syncope (may be recurrent), change in mental status (due to hypoperfusion).
3. ± Weak pulse, cool extremities, tachycardia, hypotension & tachypnea.

DIAGNOSIS

Within 2-5 minutes of quiet standing (after a 5-minute period of being supine) there is EITHER a:
  • ***fall in the systolic blood pressure ≥20 mmHg*** and/or
  • fall of the diastolic blood pressure ≥10 mmHg with changes in position.

> The pulse rate normally rises on standing. The absence of an increase in heart rate as compensation for the fall in blood pressure is associated with autonomic dysfunction. If secondary to hypovolemia, it may be accompanied with an ***increase of pulse rate >15 beats per minute.***

WORKUP: includes: basic metabolic panel, CBC and ECG to look for other causes.

MANAGEMENT

Treat underlying disease, remove offending medications, if possible and support blood pressure.

1. Nonpharmacologic: remove offending medications whenever possible, increase salt & fluid intake, gradual exercise, elastic stockings. Usage of caffeine. Maintain the head of the bed elevated, gradual changes in position. Usually tried before pharmacologic treatment.

2. Pharmacologic: Fludrocortisone. Midodrine may be added on if additional therapy is needed or if unable to take fludrocortisone. Midodrine is a vasopressor/antihypotensive agent.

ATRIAL MYXOMA

• Most common primary cardiac tumor in adults (rare). Usually pedunculated (± sessile).
• 90% occur in atria (often arises from the interatrial septum near the fossa ovalis).
• Often seen on echocardiogram.

CLINICAL MANIFESTATIONS

• nonspecific flu-like symptoms, fever & palpitations. May develop syncope if it causes a "ball-valve" obstruction of the mitral valve orifice. May embolize, causing metastatic disease.

PHYSICAL EXAMINATION

• low-pitched diastolic murmur that changes character with changing body positions.

CIRCULATORY SHOCK

- *Inadequate organ perfusion & tissue oxygenation* to meet the body's oxygenation requirements. *Often associated with hypotension (but not always).* *Shock is determined by* **EITHER:**
  1. **Low cardiac output**   **OR**
  2. **Low systemic vascular resistance** *(SVR). SVR = the resistance to blood flow through the circulatory system (determined by peripheral blood vessels). Peripheral vasoconstriction increases SVR. Vasodilation decreases SVR.

4 MAIN TYPES OF SHOCK	
1. HYPOVOLEMIC	*loss of blood or fluid volume* (ex. hemorrhage).
2. CARDIOGENIC	*primary myocardial dysfunction* ⇨ reduced cardiac output (ex. MI).
3. OBSTRUCTIVE	*extrinsic or intrinsic obstruction to circulation* (ex. pericardial tamponade).
4. DISTRIBUTIVE	*maldistribution of blood flow* from essential organs to nonessential organs (ex. septic or neurogenic shock).

PATHOPHYSIOLOGY OF SHOCK
1. **Inadequate tissue perfusion:** inability to meet the body's metabolic oxygen requirements ⇨ metabolic acidosis & organ dysfunction.
2. **Autonomic nervous system activation:** in an attempt to improve systemic O_2 delivery.
   - Sympathetic nervous system activation: causes vasoconstriction (↑SVR) & ↑contractility (to ↑CO). ↑Norepinephrine, dopamine & cortisol release. The ↑SVR helps to maintain cerebral & cardiac perfusion by causing vasoconstriction of splanchnic, musculoskeletal & renal blood flow.
   - RAAS activation: water & sodium retention (↓urine output to minimize renal water & salt loss). Also causes vasoconstriction to help maintain cardiac output.
3. **Systemic effects of shock:**
   - ATP depletion ⇨ ion pump dysfunction leading to cellular dysfunction, cell swelling & death.
   - *Metabolic acidosis*: due to lack of oxygen ⇨ *cells resort to anaerobic metabolism, producing lactic acid* as a byproduct. Order lactate levels as part of workup.
   - Multiorgan Dysfunction Syndrome (MODS): physiologic consequences of shock on organ systems. Includes lung, kidney, heart & brain dysfunction as well as DIC (disseminated intravascular coagulation).
   - Multisystemic Organ Failure (MSOF): organ failure if the conditions persist.

CLINICAL MANIFESTATIONS OF SHOCK
1. Generally acutely ill, altered mental status, decreased peripheral pulses, tachycardia, skin usually cool and mottled (may be warm and flushed in distributive shock), systolic blood pressure <110 mmHg (some patients in shock may be normotensive initially).
2. Laboratory tests: include CBC, BMP (Chem-7), lactate, coagulation studies, cultures (to look for potential infectious sources), ABG and other studies depending on the likely etiology.

GENERAL MANAGEMENT OF SHOCK ABCDE's
1. **A**irway: may need intubation.
2. **B**reathing: mechanical ventilation & sedation decreases the work of breathing (reducing the oxygen demand associated with tachypnea).
3. **C**irculation: isotonic crystalloids (Normal Saline, Lactated Ringer's). Often given multiple liters & titrated to central venous pressure (CVP) of 8-12mmHg OR urine output of 0.5ml/kg/hr (30ml/hr) OR an improved heart rate.
4. **D**elivery of Oxygen: monitor lactate levels.
5. **E**ndpoint of Resuscitation: urine output (UOP): 0.5ml/kg/hr, CVP 8-12mmHg, mean arterial pressure (MAP) 65-90mmHg, central venous oxygen concentration >70%.

HYPOVOLEMIC SHOCK

- **LOSS OF BLOOD OR FLUID VOLUME*** due to hemorrhage or fluid loss.

ETIOLOGIES

- **_Hemorrhagic:_** ex. GI bleed, AAA rupture, massive hemoptysis, trauma, ectopic pregnancy, postpartum hemorrhage.

- **_Non-blood fluid loss:_** GI: vomiting, bowel obstruction, pancreatitis; severe burns, diabetic ketoacidosis (causes osmotic diuresis in response to hyperglycemia).

PATHOPHYSIOLOGY

Loss of blood or fluid volume ⇨ ↑heart rate, vasoconstriction (↑SVR), hypotension, ↓CO.
  Body's response to hypovolemia:
  - <u>rapid</u>: peripheral vasoconstriction, ↑cardiac activity.

  - <u>sustained</u>: arterial vasoconstriction, Na⁺/water retention, ↑cortisol.

CLINICAL MANIFESTATIONS

Loss of volume ⇨ ↑heart rate (tachycardia), hypotension, ↓CO (oliguria or anuria), vasoconstriction (↑SVR) ⇨ **_pale cool dry skin/extremities, slow capillary refill >2 seconds, ↓skin turgor, dry mucous membranes,_** AMS.

Usually does not cause profound respiratory distress.

CLASSES OF HEMORRHAGIC SHOCK		
I	< 15% blood loss	Pulse usually normal, systolic blood pressure (SBP) usually normal.
II	15 – 30% blood loss	**_Tachycardia_** (pulse >100). SBP usually >100mmHg.
III	30 – 40% blood loss	Tachycardia, **_decreased systolic blood pressure_** (<100mmHg), confusion, decreased urine output.
IV	>40% blood loss	Tachycardia, decreased SBP, **_lethargy, no urine output._**

DIAGNOSIS

<u>Hallmark:</u>
  _Vasoconstriction (↑SVR), hypotension, ↓CO & decreased pulmonary capillary pressure._*

- <u>CBC</u>: ↑Hgb/Hct = dehydration (hemoconcentration). ↓Hgb/Hct is late sign in hemorrhagic shock.

- Decreased CVP (central venous pressure)/PCWP (pulmonary capillary wedge pressure).

MANAGEMENT

1. ABCDE's, Insert 2 large bore IV lines or a central line.
2. **_Volume resuscitation: crystalloids (Normal Saline or Lactated Ringer's)_** _often given 3-4 liters to_ restore blood volume. Monitor urine output to assess success of resuscitation.
3. Control the source of hemorrhage to prevent further sequelae. ± Packed RBC blood transfusion if severe hemorrhage: (O-negative or cross-matched).
4. Prevention of hypothermia, treat any coagulopathies.

CARDIOGENIC SHOCK

- **PRIMARY CARDIAC/MYOCARDIAL DYSFUNCTION*** ⇨ inadequate tissue perfusion ⇨ ↓CO (cardiac output) with ↑systemic vascular resistance (SVR).   Often systolic in nature.
- Cardiogenic often produces increased respiratory effort/distress whereas hypovolemic does not.

ETIOLOGIES:
Cardiac disease: myocardial infarction, myocarditis, valve dysfunction, congenital heart disease, cardiomyopathy, arrhythmias.

PATHOPHYSIOLOGY
↓CO & evidence of tissue hypoxia in the presence of adequate intravascular volume. Sustained hypotension in the presence of ↑*pulmonary capillary wedge pressure* (>15mmHg).
Vasoconstriction (↑SVR), hypotension ↓CO & ↑ pulmonary capillary wedge pressure.*

MANAGEMENT
1. Oxygen, isotonic fluids (*avoid aggressive IV fluid treatment - use smaller amounts of fluid*).
   NOTE CARDIOGENIC SHOCK IS THE ONLY SHOCK IN WHICH LARGE AMOUNTS OF FLUIDS AREN'T GIVEN.
2. *Inotropic support:* drugs to increase myocardial contractility & cardiac output:
   - Dobutamine (positive inotrope), Epinephrine (positive inotrope & vasoconstrictor).
   - Amrinone may be used if refractory (Amrinone is a phosphodiesterase-3 inhibitor that is a positive inotrope).
   - Intraaortic balloon pump support.
3. *Treat the underlying cause:* *ex.* MI: early angioplasty or thrombolytics.

OBSTRUCTIVE SHOCK

- *OBSTRUCTION OF BLOOD FLOW DUE TO PHYSICAL OBSTRUCTION OF HEART OR GREAT VESSELS.**
- Intrinsic or extrinsic (↑external pressure on the heart decreases the heart's ability to pump blood).

ETIOLOGIES:
1. **Massive pulmonary embolism**: obstruction to pulmonary artery blood flow. Cyanosis, tachycardia, hypotension, VQ mismatch, hemoptysis. ECG: $S_1Q_3T_3$, sinus tachycardia. ABG: PaO_2 <80mmHg, ↑A-a gradient. Low CO, ↑peripheral resistance, ↑CVP.
2. **Pericardial Tamponade:** blood in the pericardial space prevents venous return to the heart, causing obstruction. *Beck's triad*: muffled heart sounds, systemic hypotension & ↑JVP.
3. **Tension pneumothorax**: positive air pressure causes external pressure on the heart. *Hyperresonance to percussion & decreased breath sounds on the affected side. Mediastinal & tracheal shift to the contralateral side*, SQ emphysema, ↑JVP.
4. **Aortic dissection:** proximal dissections.   May also cause hypovolemic shock.

MANAGEMENT
Oxygen, isotonic fluids, inotropic support: dobutamine, epinephrine, intra-aortic balloon pump.
Treat the underlying cause:
   Pulmonary Embolism: heparin, thrombolytics. ±Embolectomy.
   Pericardial tamponade ⇨ pericardiocentesis.
   Tension pneumothorax ⇨ needle decompression.
   Proximal dissections usually require surgical intervention.

DISTRIBUTIVE SHOCK

- *EXCESS VASODILATION & ALTERED DISTRIBUTION OF BLOOD FLOW* (increased venous capacity) with *shunting of blood flow from vital organs* (ex. heart, kidney) *to non-vital tissues* (ex skin, skeletal muscle). **Hallmark: ↓CO, ↓SVR, ↓PCWP.**
- **an <u>important EXCEPTION IS EARLY SEPTIC SHOCK - ASSOCIATED WITH ↑CO & ↓SVR so warm extremities often noted in these patients!</u>** Septic shock is the MC type of distributive shock.

TYPES:

1. SEPTIC SHOCK:

PATHOPHYSIOLOGY: infective organisms activate the immune system ⇨ *host produces systemic inflammatory response* ⇨ cytokines cause prompt peripheral vasodilation ⇨ *↓SVR*),* increased capillary permeability (initiating shock) & end organ thrombosis. These (normally local) responses to infection occur in a systemic fashion, affecting multiple organs.

CLINICAL MANIFESTATIONS: warm shock: hypotension with *WIDE PULSE PRESSURE*,* bounding arterial peripheral pulses. *Only major type of shock associated with ↑CO* (fast capillary refill time; warm, flushed extremities).**

SIRS (Systemic Inflammatory Response Syndrome): at least 2 of the 4 following:
1. <u>Temperature:</u> fever >38°C (100.4° F) or hypothermia <36°C (96.8°F)
2. <u>Pulse:</u> > 90 bpm
3. <u>Respiratory rate:</u> >20 or $PaCO_2$ <32mmHg
4. <u>WBC count:</u> >12,000 cells/hpf or <4,000 cells/hpf

Sepsis = *SIRS + focus of infection. Often associated with ↑LACTATE (>4mmol/L).**
Severe sepsis = *SIRS + MSOF (multi system organ failure).*
Septic shock = *Sepsis + refractory hypotension* despite fluid administration (SBP <90mmHg, MAP <65mmHg or drop in SBP 40mmHg from baseline).

MANAGEMENT:
1. *Broad spectrum IV antibiotics:** (pan culture before initiating). Zosyn + Ceftriaxone or Imipenem. Choose depending on suspected organisms (Gentamicin for Pseudomonas, Vancomycin for MRSA, Clindamycin or Metronidazole for intrabdominal infections, Ceftriaxone in asplenic patients to cover *N. meningitidis & H. influenzae*).
2. *IV fluid Resuscitation: isotonic crystalloids* (Normal saline, Lactated Ringer's)
3. *Vasopressors:* if no response to 2-3L of IV fluids with goal of MAP >60mmHg. ± IV hydrocortisone.

2. ANAPHYLACTIC SHOCK: *IgE-mediated severe systemic hypersensitivity reaction.* History of incest bite/stings, food or drug allergy, recent IV contrast. Symptoms usually begin within 60 minutes of exposure.

PHYSICAL EXAM: pruritus, hives, angioedema ⇨ respiratory distress, stridor, sensation of "lump in throat", hoarseness (life threatening laryngeal edema).

MANAGEMENT: *Epinephrine 1st line* (0.3mg IM of 1:1000 repeat q5-10min as needed). If cardiovascular collapse, give Epinephrine 1mg IV (1:10,000). *Airway management, antihistamines* (Diphenhydramine 25-50mg IV blocks H_1, Ranitidine IV blocks H_2), IV fluids. *Observe patient for 4-6hours* because up to 20% of patients have a biphasic phenomenon (return of symptoms 3-4 hours after the initial reaction).

3. NEUROGENIC SHOCK: due to *acute spinal cord injury*, regional anesthesia.

PATHOPHYSIOLOGY: autonomic sympathetic blockade ⇨ unopposed ↑vagal tone.
⇨ *bradycardia* & hypotension.* Loss of sympathetic tone ⇨ warm, dry skin.
CLINICAL: warm skin, normal or ↓HR, ↓SVR, hypovolemia, *WIDE pulse pressure.*
Management: fluids, pressors +/- corticosteroids.

4. ENDOCRINE SHOCK: ex *adrenal insufficiency (Addisonian crisis).*

Management: *Hydrocortisone 100mg IV** (often unresponsive to fluids & pressors).

	PATHOPHYSIOLOGY	ETIOLOGIES	CO	PCWP	SVR	CLINICAL MANIFESTATIONS
HYPOVOLEMIC	*LOSS OF BLOOD OR FLUID VOLUME* ⇨ ↑PVR & ↑HR to maintain CO.	**Hemorrhage:** GI bleed, AAA rupture etc. **Fluid loss:** GI: vomiting, diarrhea, pancreatitis, severe burns etc.	Decreased	*Decreased*	Increased	• *Pale, cool, mottled skin* • *Prolonged capillary refill* • *Decreased skin turgor, dry mucous membranes* • Usually no severe respiratory distress
CARDIOGENIC	*PRIMARY MYOCARDIAL ABNORMALITY* ⇨ heart unable to maintain CO	• Myocardial Infarction • Myocarditis • Valvular disease • Cardiomyopathies • Arrhythmias	Decreased	*Increased*	Increased	• *Severe respiratory distress* • *Cool clammy skin*
OBSTRUCTIVE	*EXTRINSIC OR INTRINSIC OBSTRUCTION of heart or great vessels*	• Pericardial tamponade • Massive Pulmonary Embolism • Tension Pneumothorax • Aortic dissection	Decreased	*Increased*	Increased	• *Severe respiratory distress* • *Cool clammy skin*
DISTRIBUTIVE 4 types (below)	*MALDISTRIBUTION OF BLOOD & VASODILATION* with shunting of blood away from vital to non vital organs				*Decreased*	
1. SEPTIC	Severe host immune response	Bacteria				
Early (warm)	Vasodilation		*Increased**	↑ or ↓	*Decreased*	• *↑CO*: WARM, FLUSHED EXTREMITIES & skin, brisk capillary refill, bounding pulses, WIDE pulse pressure* • *ONLY SHOCK ASSOC WITH ↑CO**
Late (cool)			Decreased	Decreased	Increased	Cool clammy skin
2. NEUROGENIC	Sympathetic blockade ⇨ unopposed vagal tone on vessels ⇨ vasodilation	Acute spine injury	Decreased	Decreased	Decreased	• *HYPOTENSION without tachycardia** • *± BRADYCARDIA**
3. ANAPHYLACTIC	*IgE mediated* systemic HSN reaction with histamine release ⇨ vasodilation leading to ↑capillary permeability	• Insect bites/stings • Food allergies • Drug allergies • Recent IV contrast	Decreased	Decreased	Decreased	• *Pruritus, hives, ± angioedema* • ± throat fullness, hoarseness, wheezing • Recent h/o of insect bite/sting, food, drug or IV contrast
4. HYPOADRENAL	Decreased corticosteroid & mineralocorticoid activity	Adrenal insufficiency (Addisonian crisis)	Decreased	Decreased	Decreased	• *Low serum glucose.* • *Hypotension refractory to fluids & pressors*

SVR = Systemic Vascular Resistance   CO = Cardiac Output   PCWP = Pulmonary Capillary Wedge Pressure

CARDIOLOGY REFERENCES

Gage BF, Van walraven C, Pearce L, et al. Selecting patients with atrial fibrillation for anticoagulation: stroke risk stratification in patients taking aspirin. Circulation. 2004;110(16):2287-92.

Elmayergi N, Nguyen T, Hiebert B, et al. A "no-option" left main PCI registry: outcomes and predictors of in hospital mortality-utility of the logistic EuroSCORE. Catheter Cardiovasc Interv. 2013;82(3):361-9.

Validation of Clinical Classification Schemes for Predicting Stroke Results From the National Registry of Atrial Fibrillation. JAMA. 2001;285(22):2864.

Pollack CV, Sites FD, Shofer FS, Sease KL, Hollander JE. Application of the TIMI risk score for unstable angina and non-ST elevation acute coronary syndrome to an unselected emergency department chest pain population. Acad Emerg Med. 2006;13(1):13-8.

Janda SP, Tan N. Thrombolysis versus primary percutaneous coronary intervention for ST elevation myocardial infarctions at Chilliwack General Hospital. Can J Cardiol. 2009;25(11):e382-4.

Mccord J, Jneid H, Hollander JE, et al. Management of cocaine-associated chest pain and myocardial infarction: a scientific statement from the American Heart Association Acute Cardiac Care Committee of the Council on Clinical Cardiology. Circulation. 2008;117(14):1897-907.

O'connor RE, Brady W, Brooks SC, et al. Part 10: acute coronary syndromes: 2010 American Heart Association Guidelines for Cardiopulmonary Resuscitation and Emergency Cardiovascular Care. Circulation. 2010;122(18 Suppl 3):S787-817.

Hunt SA, Abraham WT, Chin MH, et al. ACC/AHA 2005 Guideline Update for the Diagnosis and Management of Chronic Heart Failure in the Adult: a report of the American College of Cardiology/American Heart Association Task Force on Practice Guidelines (Writing Committee to Update the 2001 Guidelines for the Evaluation and Management of Heart Failure): developed in collaboration with the American College of Chest Physicians and the International Society for Heart and Lung Transplantation: endorsed by the Heart Rhythm Society. Circulation. 2005;112(12):e154-235.

The Diagnosis of Rheumatic Fever. Journal of the American Medical Association. 1944;126(8):481.

2014 Evidence-Based Guideline for the Management of High Blood Pressure in Adults: Report From the Panel Members Appointed to the Eighth Joint National Committee (JNC 8). JAMA.

Durack DT, Lukes AS, Bright DK. New criteria for diagnosis of infective endocarditis: utilization of specific echocardiographic findings. Duke Endocarditis Service. Am J Med. 1994;96(3):200-9.

Li JS, Sexton DJ, Mick N, et al. Proposed modifications to the Duke criteria for the diagnosis of infective endocarditis. Clin Infect Dis. 2000;30(4):633-8.

Brewster DC, Cronenwett JL, Hallett JW, et al. Guidelines for the treatment of abdominal aortic aneurysms. Report of a subcommittee of the Joint Council of the American Association for Vascular Surgery and Society for Vascular Surgery. J Vasc Surg. 2003;37(5):1106-17.

Guyatt GH, Akl EA, Crowther M, Gutterman DD, Schuünemann HJ. Executive summary: Antithrombotic Therapy and Prevention of Thrombosis, 9th ed: American College of Chest Physicians Evidence-Based Clinical Practice Guidelines. Chest. 2012;141(2 Suppl):7S-47S.

Wells PS, Anderson DR, Rodger M, et al. Excluding pulmonary embolism at the bedside without diagnostic imaging: management of patients with suspected pulmonary embolism presenting to the emergency department by using a simple clinical model and d-dimer. Ann Intern Med. 2001;135(2):98-107.

The role of the emergency pharmacist in trauma resuscitation
Scarponcini T.R. Edwards C.J. Rudis M.I. Jasiak K.D. Hays D.P.
(2011) *Journal of Pharmacy Practice*, 24 (2), pp. 146-159.

Ross H, Howlett J, Arnold JM, et al. Treating the right patient at the right time: access to heart failure care. Can J Cardiol. 2006;22(9):749-54.

Field LC, Guldan GJ, Finley AC. Echocardiography in the intensive care unit. Semin Cardiothorac Vasc Anesth. 2011;15(1-2):25-39.

The TIMI Risk Score for Unstable Angina/Non–ST Elevation MI: A Method for Prognostication and Therapeutic Decision Making. JAMA. 2000;284(7):835.

CARDIOLOGY PHOTO CREDITS

CHAPTER 2 – PULMONARY DISORDERS

LUNG FUNCTION

- Lungs exchange oxygen & carbon dioxide between the alveoli of the lungs & alveolar capillaries.
  1. **Conducting zone**: trachea, primary bronchus & terminal conducting bronchioles. Functions to warm air, trap foreign matter from entering the alveoli & conduct air to the respiratory zone.

  2. **Respiratory Zone**: terminal respiratory bronchioles & alveoli.

  3. **Alveoli**: participates in gas exchange. Diffusion capacity is based on ❶ the surface area of the alveoli ❷ a thin diffusing area & ❸ the partial pressure & concentration of the gases. Patency of the alveoli is determined by surfactant (surfactant reduces surface tension).

V/Q MISMATCH

1. **LOW V:Q RATIO.** *Low ventilation with increased or normal perfusion.* The low ventilation impairs pulmonary gas exchange ⇨ ↓arterial partial pressure of oxygen (↓PaO_2). Carbon dioxide excretion is impaired as well, leading to ↑arteriole $PaCO_2$. Normally, the rise in $PaCO_2$ leads to respiratory stimulation ⇨ ↑alveolar ventilation to increase the V:Q ratio towards one.
   - **Physiologic Low V:Q ratio**: found at the bases of the lungs. Due to gravity, the bases of the lungs receive BOTH greater perfusion and more ventilation (in comparison to the apices of the lungs). Although the bases receive more of both, perfusion exceeds ventilation.

   - **Pathologic Low V:Q**: ex. *asthma, chronic bronchitis & acute pulmonary edema*. In these conditions, the hypoxemic *response to ↓PaO_2 is local* **hypoxic vasoconstriction** ⇨ **pulmonary hypertension** (if persistent). The right ventricle has to pump against higher pressures to pump into the pulmonary arteries ⇨ RVH & right atrial enlargement. Over time, this will lead to *right heart failure (cor pulmonale).* An area with no ventilation but perfusion is termed a *"shunt".* **This is why chronic bronchitis is classically associated with cor pulmonale if untreated & why the only medical treatment to reduce mortality in COPD is oxygen** (O_2 reduces hypoxic vasoconstriction).

2. **HIGH V:Q RATIO.** an area with decreased perfusion in comparison to ventilation.
   - **Physiologic High V:Q:** apices of the lungs.
   - **Clinical correlation**: *reactivation TB tends to occur in the (upper) apices of the lungs* (due to the relatively higher O_2 content of the lung tissue in the apices).

   - **Pathologic High V:Q** : *emphysema, pulmonary embolism or foreign body* in the airways of children. In emphysema, there is good ventilation, so the PaO_2 is relatively normal or mildly decreased & is not usually associated with a large increase in $PaCO_2$. But, because there is an overall decrease in blood flow, this ventilation is wasted as it fails to oxygenate blood. Areas with no perfusion & normal ventilation is *"dead space".*

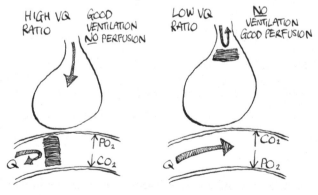

MECHANICS OF BREATHING

- During quiet breathing, inspiration accounts for most of the work of breathing. Expiration is usually a passive process (due to elastic recoil of the lung resuming its original shape). *90% of the normal work of breathing is due to contraction of the diaphragm* (diaphragm contraction increases lung volumes & lowers air pressure to move air into the lungs).
- The work of breathing during inspiration is based on 3 main factors: ❶ tissue compliance ❷ airway resistance & ❸ tissue resistance.

CONTROL OF RESPIRATION

Ventilation is strictly regulated primarily by changes in $PaCO_2$ (partial pressure of carbon dioxide). Blood levels of PaO_2 become important in severe hypoxic conditions.
Ventilation is controlled by:

1. **CENTRAL CHEMORECEPTORS** *in the medulla* indirectly respond to changes in the serum pH via $PaCO_2$ in the CSF. H^+ ions are unable to cross the blood-brain barrier but carbon dioxide can ⇨ ↑$PaCO_2$ in the CSF. This ↑CSF $PaCO_2$ (reflective of the ↓*pH in serum*) activates the medulla ⇨ phrenic nerve stimulation ⇨ ↑rate/depth of breathing (to ↓$PaCO_2$ back to normal).

2. **PERIPHERAL CHEMORECEPTORS** in the *carotid bodies* (near the carotid sinus & via CN IX) and in the *aortic bodies* (via cranial nerve X) *primarily respond directly to ↑$PaCO_2$ (↓pH)* in the arterial blood. ↑$PaCO_2$ stimulates the afferent neurons affecting the medulla ⇨ ↑rate & depth of breathing (to lower $PaCO_2$). Peripheral chemoreceptors are sensitive to ↓arterial PaO_2 but only with significant PaO_2 decline ($PaO_2 < 60$ mm Hg).

<u>Clinical correlation:</u> *Diabetic ketoacidosis stimulates the respiratory centers, causing Kussmaul's respirations (continuous deep breathing in an attempt to blow off excess CO_2).*

DEFENSES OF THE LUNG

- **ALVEOLAR CELLS:**
  <u>Type II cells</u> produce surfactant (maintains the patency of the alveoli at end expiration).
  <u>Type I cells:</u> make up supporting tissue & allows for extravasation of macrophages if needed.

- **MUCOCILIARY ESCALATOR:** covers the nose, bronchi & most of the bronchioles. *"Muco"* goblet cells produce mucus that traps bacteria & foreign debris in inhaled air. The *"cilia"* (hairs) constantly beat upwards to prevent bacteria & foreign debris from entering the alveoli.

- **ALVEOLAR MACROPHAGES:** innate immune lung defense protects the lungs from bacteria & foreign debris that reaches the alveoli. Alveolar macrophages ingest particles/organisms through phagocytosis, destroying them or walling them off. Some organisms may overcome this defense, evading macrophage destruction. Some examples are ❶the capsules of encapsulated organisms make it difficult for macrophages to attach, ❷Pseudomonas (slime layer capsule that makes it difficult for macrophages to penetrate) & ❸ mycolic acid layer of M. tuberculosis protects it from macrophage ingestion by allowing Mycobacterium to live within the macrophages. Chlamydia can evade the phagozyme, avoiding lysozyme destruction.

- **MAST CELLS:** initiate inflammation, repair of the lung & host immunity against bacteria.

- **POLYMORPHONUCLEAR NEUTROPHILS:** usually not present in the alveoli but can be present temporarily during lung infections. Often seen in smokers & chronic inflammatory conditions.

- <u>**Irritant receptors:**</u> cause bronchospasm to reduced harmful substances from entering the alveoli.

LUNG VOLUMES:

- **Tidal volume (TV):** the volume of air moved into or out of the lungs during quiet breathing.

- **Residual Volume (RV):** the volume of air remaining in the lungs after maximal expiration. This residual volume functions to maintain alveolar patency especially during end expiration.

- **Expiratory reserve volume (ERV):** the volume of air that can be further exhaled at the end of normal expiration.

- **Inspiratory reserve volume (IRV):** the volume of air that can be further inhaled at the end of normal inspiration.

- **Vital Capacity (VC):** maximum volume of air that can be exhaled following maximum inspiration (IRV + TV + ERV).

- **Total Lung Capacity (TLC):** the volume in the lungs at maximum inspiration (VC + RV).

- **Functional residual capacity (FRC):** volume of gas in the lungs at normal tidal volume end expiration (ERV + RV). This is the air in which gas exchange takes place.
    - ↑FRC seen in disorders with hyperinflation (due to loss of elastic recoil, PEEP).
    - ↓FRC seen in restrictive lung diseases.

- **FEV_1 Forced Expiratory Volume in 1 second**: the volume of air that has been exhaled at the end of the first second of forced expiration.

- **Forced Vital Capacity (FVC):** measurement of the volume of air that can be expelled from a maximally inflated lung, with the patient breathing as hard & fast as possible.

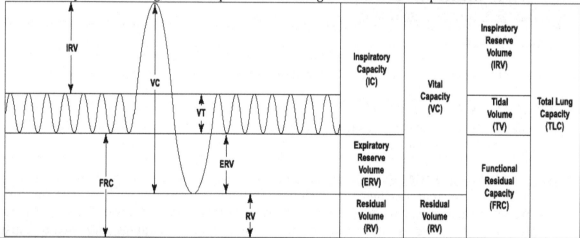

4 MAIN ATYPICAL SOUNDS

1. **WHEEZING:** high-pitched, *whistling, continuous*, musical sound (*usually louder during expiration* compared to inspiration) *produced by narrowed/obstructed airways.* Seen with obstructive lung diseases (asthma, COPD), bronchiectasis, bronchiolitis, lung cancer, sleep apnea, CHF, GERD, anaphylaxis, foreign body etc.
2. **RHONCHI:** continuous, rumbling (rattling), coarse, *low-pitched sounds* (sounds like snoring) that *may clear with cough* or suctioning. Rhonchi are caused by increased secretions or obstruction in the bronchial airways.
3. **CRACKLES (RALES):** *discontinuous* high-pitched sounds *heard during inspiration* (usually not cleared by cough). Due to the "popping" open of collapsed alveoli & small airways (from fluid, exudates or lack of aeration). Seen with pneumonia, atelectasis, bronchitis, bronchiectasis, pulmonary edema & pulmonary fibrosis.
4. **STRIDOR:** monophonic sound usually loudest over the anterior neck due to *narrowing of the larynx or anywhere over the trachea.* Can be heard during inspiration, expiration or throughout the respiratory cycle.

ASTHMA

REVERSIBLE *hyperirritability* of the tracheobronchial tree ⇨ *airway inflammation & bronchoconstriction.*
MC chronic childhood disease (~10%). ½ develop <10y of age; another ⅓ by 40y. *Atopy is a risk factor.**

SAMTER'S TRIAD: ❶ *asthma* ❷ *nasal polyps* ❸ *ASA/NSAID allergy.* *Associated with atopic dermatitis.*

PATHOPHYSIOLOGY 3 main components:
1. **AIRWAY HYPERREACTIVITY:** endogenous & exogenous stimuli. Early IgE-mediated ⇨ T cell later on.
   - **EXTRINSIC (ALLERGIC):*** *allergen triggers* include pollen, ragweed, dander, dust, mold, aerosols, tobacco, smoke, air pollution, etc. MC in children/adolescents (80%). Associated with ↑*IgE.*

   - **INTRINSIC (IDIOSYNCRATIC):** *nonallergic triggers: infection (ex. viral URI/sinusitis), pharmacologic* (β-blockers, Aspirin, NSAIDs, ACEI) *occupational, exercise, emotional, cold air.* MC <3y & >30y.

2. **BRONCHOCONSTRICTION:** *airway narrowing* 2ʳʸ to smooth muscle constriction, bronchial wall edema, thick mucus secretion, collagen deposition, smooth muscle/mucosal hypertrophy, mucus plugging & airway remodeling. This bronchoconstriction leads to air trapping:
   Obstruction: ↓*expiratory airflow,* ↑*airway resistance* (↑work of breathing) & V/Q mismatch.

3. **INFLAMMATION:** 2ʳʸ to cellular infiltration (T lymphocytes, neutrophils, eosinophils) & their pro-inflammatory cytokines (ex. leukotrienes); ↑Histamine released from mast cells (IgE-mediated).

CLINICAL MANIFESTATIONS
A. **History** *classic triad:* ❶ *dyspnea* ❷ *wheezing* ❸*cough (esp @ night).** ±chest tightness, prolonged expiration, fatigue. Clues to severity: steroid use, previous intubations/ICU/hospital admissions.

B. **Physical Examination:**
   1. *prolonged expiration with wheezing, hyperresonance* to percussion, decreased breath sounds, tachycardia, tachypnea, use of accessory muscles.

   2. *Severe asthma & status asthmaticus*: inability to speak in full sentences, PEFR <40% predicted, *altered mental status* (ominous), *pulsus paradoxus (inspiratory ↓SBP >10)*, cyanosis, "tripod" position, *"silent chest"* (no air exchange), tachycardia, severe tachypnea.

DIAGNOSTIC STUDIES
A. **PULMONARY FUNCTION TEST:** *gold standard** - *REVERSIBLE obstruction* (↓FEV₁, ↓FEV₁/FVC).

B. **Bronchoprovocation:** ❶ *Methacholine challenge test* (≥20% decrease in FEV₁) + ❷ Bronchodilator challenge test [≥12% ↑ in FEV₁ (≥200cc)] or ❸ Exercise challenge test (≥15% ↓ in FEV₁).
   Indication: used if pulmonary function testing nondiagnostic. Histamine may also be used.

C. **Peak Expiratory Flow Rate (PEFR):** *best & most objective way to assess asthma exacerbation severity & patient response in ED.** PEFR >15% from initial attempt = response to treatment. Best to obtain baseline prior to treatment. Normal 400-600. Best used for monitoring patients.

D. **Pulse Oximetry:** *O₂ sat <90% indicative of respiratory distress.* Also used in infants.
E. ABG: to assess hypoxia & hypercapnia. During attacks, respiratory drive is stimulated so patients hyperventilate (↓CO₂). *Pseudonormalization/↑CO₂ may indicate impending respiratory failure!**
F. CXR: usually not helpful but may help to rule out other etiologies. Usually normal. ±Hyperinflation.

EMERGENCY DISPOSITION OF ACUTE EXACERBATION
A. Admission criteria: PEFR <50% predicted (PEFR <15% initial value/200cc/or, FEV<1L); ER visit within 3 days of exacerbation, status asthmaticus, posttreatment failure, AMS, etc.
B. Discharge criteria: PEFR >70% predicted, PEFR >15% initial, subjective improvement, clear lungs with good air movement, adequate follow up within 24-72h, response sustained 1 hour after treatment.

MANAGEMENT OF ASTHMA

QUICK RELIEF FOR ACUTE EXACERBATION (RESCUE DRUGS)

β₂ AGONISTS SHORT-ACTING (SABA) *1st line treatment for acute.* Most effective & fastest (2-5min).*
• **Albuterol*** (Proventil), Levalbuterol (Xopenex), **Terbutaline** (Brethine), **Epinephrine**
   1. <u>MOA:</u> *bronchodilator* (especially *peripherally*), decreases bronchospasm, inhibits the release of bronchospastic mediators, increases ciliary movement, ↓'es airway edema & resistance.
   2. <u>Administration:</u> MDI, nebulizer. **Nebulizers MC used in ED** (MDI ±slightly more efficacious). Generally given every 20 minutes x3 doses (or continuous) with reevaluation after 3 doses.
   3. <u>S/E:</u> *β₋₁ cross reactivity: tachycardia/arrhythmias, muscle tremors, CNS stimulation*, hypokalemia.

ANTICHOLINERGICS (ANTIMUSCARINICS)
• **Ipratropium** (Atrovent)
   1. <u>MOA:</u> *central bronchodilator* (inhibits vagal-mediated bronchoconstriction) & inhibits nasal mucosal secretions. ⊕ *synergy between β₂ agonists & anticholinergics.* Most useful in the 1st hour.
   2. <u>S/E:</u> *thirst, blurred vision, dry mouth, urinary retention, dysphagia, acute glaucoma, BPH.**

CORTICOSTEROIDS
• **Prednisone, Methylprednisolone** (Solumedrol); **Prednisolone** (Prelone)
   1. <u>MOA:</u> *anti-inflammatory. All but the mildest exacerbations should be discharged on a short course of oral corticosteroids* (ex. 3-5 days) unless contraindicated. **Steroids decrease relapse** & reverse the late pathophysiology. Short courses don't need tapering (unless on chronic steroids, or recent treatment with repeated short courses in a short period). Onset of action 4-8 hours for both oral & IV.
   2. <u>S/E:</u> *immunosuppression, catabolic, hyperglycemia, fluid retention, osteoporosis, growth delays.**

LONG-TERM (CHRONIC, CONTROL) MAINTENANCE

INHALED CORTICOSTEROIDS (ICS)
• **Beclomethasone** (Beclovent); **Flunisolide** (Aerobid), **Triamcinolone** (Azmacort);
   1. ***Drug of choice for long term, persistent (chronic maintenance)!*** Effective long-term control with very low incidence of systemic side effects. <u>MOA:</u> cytokine & inflammation inhibition.
   2. <u>S/E:</u> *thrush (using spacer & rinsing mouth after inhaler use decreases risk of thrush).**

LONG-ACTING β₂ AGONISTS (LAB₂A)
Salmeterol (Serevent); ICS/LAB₂A Combo: Symbicort (Budenoside/**Formoterol**), Advair diskus (Fluticasone/Salmeterol)
   1. ***Bronchodilator*** that prevents symptoms **(especially nocturnal asthma).**
   2. <u>Ind:</u> *long-acting β₂ agonists added to steroids* (or other long term asthma medications) **ONLY if persistent asthma is not controlled with ICS alone** (the option of increasing the ICS dose = addition of LABA). **Once asthma control maintained (>3 months), step down off LAB₂A is recommended.**
   3. <u>CI:</u> *NOT a rescue drug (NOT used in acute exacerbations)!* LAB₂A should not be used alone.

MAST CELL MODIFIERS
• **Cromolyn** (Intal), **Nedocromil** (Tilade)
   1. <u>MOA:</u> inhibits mast cell & leukotriene-mediated degranulation. Used as prophylaxis only.
   2. Improves lung function, ↓airway reactivity (**inhibits acute phase response to cold air, exercise,*** *sulfites). Minimal side effects* (throat irritation). Effective prophylaxis may take several weeks.

LEUKOTRIENE MODIFIERS/RECEPTOR ANTAGONISTS (LTRA)
• **Montelukast** (Singulair), **Zafirlukast** (Accolate), **Zileuton** (Zyflo)
   1. <u>MOA:</u> blocks leukotriene-mediated neutrophil migration, capillary permeability, smooth muscle contraction via leukotriene receptor inhibition. Zileuton does so via 5-lipoxygenase inhibition.
   2. <u>Ind:</u> *Useful in asthmatics with <u>allergic rhinitis/aspirin induced asthma*</u>.* Prophylaxis only.
   3. <u>S/E:</u> Minimal side effects (*increased LFTs*, headache, GI myalgias).

THEOPHYLLINE

1. **MOA:** methylxanthine (similar to caffeine) - *bronchodilator that improves respiratory muscle endurance,* phosphodiesterase inhibitor which inhibits leukotriene synthesis & inflammation. Not used often due to narrow therapeutic index (TI). Smoking decreases Theophylline levels so *higher doses of Theophylline are needed in smokers.** It is a nonselective adenosine receptor antagonist (may have affect on the heart).
2. **Ind:** long-term asthma prophylaxis in selected patients. *NOT used in acute asthma exacerbations!*
3. **S/E:** *MC nervousness, nausea, vomiting, anorexia, headache,* diuresis, tachycardia, CNS/respiratory stimulant. Many drug interactions. *Narrow TI: (toxicity causes arrhythmias, seizures).*

ADJUNCTS

IV MAGNESIUM: *bronchodilator* ($\downarrow Ca^{+2}$-mediated smooth muscle contraction). Ind: severe asthma.

HELIOX: decreases airway resistance because helium + oxygen is lighter than room air.

KETAMINE: IV anesthetic that has sedative, analgesic & bronchodilator effects. May be useful as an induction/sedation agent in young otherwise healthy population of intubated patients.

OMALIZUMAB: *anti-IgE antibody* (inhibits IgE inflammation). *Used in severe, uncontrolled asthma.*

CLASSIFICATION OF ASTHMA SEVERITY				
	INTERMITTENT	**PERSISTENT**		
		MILD	**MODERATE**	**SEVERE**
Symptoms	≤2 x /day ≤2/ week	>2days/week (but not daily)	Daily	Throughout the day
SAB₂A use for sx	≤2x/day ≤2x/week	>2days/week (but not >1x/day)	Daily	Several times a day
Nighttime awakenings	≤2x/month	3-4 x/month	>1x/week (but not nightly)	Often Usually nightly
Interference c normal activity	None	Minor limitation	Some limitation	Extremely limited
Lung Function	• Normal FEV1 between exacerbations • FEV1 >80% predicted • FEV1/FVC normal	• FEV1 ≥80% predicted • FEV1/FVC normal	• *FEV1 60 – 80%* *predicted** • FEV1/FVC reduced by 5%	• *FEV1 <60%* *predicted** FEV1/FVC reduced >5%
Recommended Management	• Inhaled SABA as needed	• Inhaled SABA as needed + *Low-dose ICS**	• *Low ICS + LABA* or • *Increase ICS dose (medium)* or • Add LTRA	• High dose ICS + LABA • ± Omalizumab (Anti-IgE drug)
Exacerbations requiring PO steroids	0-1/year	≥2/year		

* ICS=Inhaled Corticosteroid; LABA=Long Acting β₂ Agonist; SA = short, LTRA + Leukotriene Receptor Antagonists

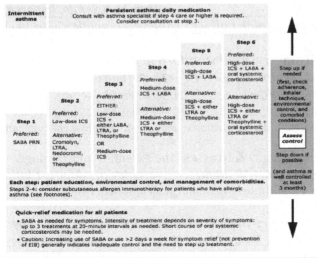

*Step down if symptoms controlled >3 months**

CHRONIC OBSTRUCTIVE PULMONARY DISEASE (COPD)

- **COPD:** *progressive, <u>largely irreversible airflow obstruction</u>* due to ❶ *loss of elastic recoil* & ❷ *increased airway resistance.* COPD includes: ❶ EMPHYSEMA & ❷ CHRONIC BRONCHITIS.
- *Common >55y.* Chronic bronchitis usually episodic; Emphysema usually has a steady decline.
- *Both usually coexist with one being more dominant.*

RISK FACTORS

- CIGARETTE SMOKING/EXPOSURE *most important risk** (90%). Only 15% of smokers develop COPD.

- *<u>α-1</u>* ANTITRYPSIN DEFICIENCY: *only <u>genetic disease linked to COPD</u> in <u>younger patients <40y.</u>* α-1 antitrypsin protects elastin in the lungs from damage by WBCs.* α-1 antitrypsin deficiency associated with panlobular emphysema. **Smoking** associated with **centrilobular emphysema.**
- Occupational/environmental exposures, recurrent airway infections.

PATHOPHYSIOLOGY OF COPD

A. **EMPHYSEMA** *abnormal, permanent <u>enlargement of the terminal airspaces</u>** (pathologic diagnosis).
  1. Smoking ⇨ chronic inflammation & decreased protective enzymes (α-1 antitrypsin) while increasing damaging enzymes (↑elastase release from macrophages & neutrophils) ⇨ alveolar capillary & alveolar wall destruction (decreased gas exchange surface area) ⇨ *<u>loss of elastic recoil</u>* (airway collapse, expiration becomes an active process) & *↑<u>compliance</u>* ⇨ *airway obstruction (↑air trapping).*

B. **CHRONIC BRONCHITIS** *<u>productive cough ≥3 months x 2 consecutive years.</u>** Chronic airway inflammation ⇨hypersecretion of mucus, airway narrowing, *↑airway resistance* leading to *airway obstruction.* Mucus plugging & mucociliary escalator destruction ⇨ patients become *<u>prone to microbial infections</u>.**

	EMPHYSEMA	CHRONIC BRONCHITIS
CLINICAL MANIFESTATIONS	*Dyspnea MC symptom.** Accessory muscle use, tachypnea, prolonged expiration. Mild cough.	*Productive cough hallmark** symptom, prolonged expiration.
PHYSICAL EXAMINATION	**HYPERINFLATION:** *hyperresonance* to percussion, *↓/absent breath sounds, ↓fremitus, barrel chest (↑AP diameter)** quiet chest. *Pursed lip breathing.**	*Rales (crackles), rhonchi, wheezing* ±change in location with cough. *±Signs of cor pulmonale* (peripheral edema, cyanosis)*
ABG/LABS	Respiratory alkalosis. Can develop respiratory acidosis in acute exacerbations.	*Respiratory acidosis.** *↑Hct/RBC** (chronic hypoxia stimulates erythropoiesis)
V/Q MISMATCH	*Matched V/Q defects* *Mild hypoxemia,* often CO_2 is normal	*Severe V/Q mismatch, severe hypoxemia, hypercapnia**
APPEARANCE	*Cachectic, pursed lip breathing- "pink puffers"*	*Obese & cyanotic - "blue bloaters"*

DIAGNOSTIC STUDIES

A. **Pulmonary Function Testing (PFT)/Spirometry:** *gold standard in diagnosing COPD.** *FEV_1 is an important factor of prognosis & mortality.* *FEV_1 <1L ⇨ ↑mortality.*
  1. **OBSTRUCTION:** *↓FEV_1; ↓FVC; ↓FEV_1/FVC <70%;* (↓DLCO in emphysema).
  2. **HYPERINFLATION:** *↑lung volumes: ↑RV, TLC, RV/TLC, ↑FRC* (RV = Residual Volume, TLC = Total Lung Capacity, FRC = Functional Residual capacity). Hyperinflation especially with Emphysema-dominant.

B. **CXR/CT scan** CT helpful in diagnosing emphysema & to assess the extent of lung damage.
  - **Emphysema:** *hyperinflation: flat diaphragm, ↑AP diameter, ↓vascular markings; ± bullae.*
  - **Chronic Bronchitis:** *↑AP diameter, ↑vascular markings, enlarged right heart border.*

C. **ECG:** *cor pulmonale = longstanding pulmonary hypertension* ⇨ *right ventricular hypertrophy, right atrial enlargement, right axis deviation & R-sided heart failure.* Cor pulmonale is especially seen with chronic bronchitis. ± *Atrial fibrillation, flutter, <u>Multifocal Atrial Tachycardia.</u>**

EXACERBATION TRIGGERS
> ➤ Pollutants, bronchospasm, cardiopulmonary dz. Meds: decongestants, β-blockers, sedatives.
> ➤ *Infections:* bronchitis & pneumonia (ex. viral, *S pneumoniae, H. influenzae, M. catarrhalis).*

MANAGEMENT OF COPD

*Smoking cessation is the most important step in the management of COPD!**

❶ BRONCHODILATORS

***combo therapy with anticholinergics + β₂ agonists shows greater response than used alone!*
Ind: treatment of choice in stable COPD with respiratory symptoms (decreases exacerbations).
1. **ANTICHOLINERGICS: Tiotropium** (Spiriva) inhaled long-acting; *Ipratropium* (Atrovent)
   Indications: *anticholinergics preferred over short acting β₂ agonists in COPD.**
   MOA: blocks acetylcholine-mediated bronchoconstriction ⇨ bronchodilation.
   S/E: *dry mouth, thirst, blurred vision, urinary retention,* difficulty swallowing.
   CI: *BPH, glaucoma** (anticholinergics increase urinary retention & pupillary dilation).

2. **β-₂ AGONISTS: Albuterol** (Proventil); **Terbutaline** (Brethine). **Salmeterol** (long-acting).
   MOA: . β-₂ receptor activation ⇨ bronchodilation.
   S/E: *β-₁ cross reactivity: tachycardia/arrhythmias, muscle tremor, CNS stimulation.*
   CI: severe CAD;   Caution in patients with DM (can cause hyperglycemia), hyperthyroidism.

3. **THEOPHYLLINE:** bronchodilator only used in refractory cases. *Narrow TI: monitor serum levels to prevent nausea, palpations, arrhythmias or seizures from toxic levels* (esp >20mg/L). Lower doses: CHF, hepatic disease; *higher doses needed in smokers** (smoking decreases levels).

❷CORTICOSTEROIDS: *inhaled corticosteroids not considered monotherapy.* May be added to long acting bronchodilators (ex. Salmeterol +Fluticasone) if responsive to steroids after a trial of ICS.
   S/E: osteoporosis, thrush, ↑infections, catabolic, hyperglycemia, fluid retention, renal calculi.

❸OXYGEN: *only medical therapy proven to ↓mortality!** (decreases pulmonary HTN/cor pulmonale by decreasing hypoxia-mediated pulmonary vasoconstriction).
   Ind: *Use if* 1) ⊕ *cor pulmonale,** 2) *O₂ sat <88%* or 3) *PaO₂ <55mm Hg.*
   Goal is O₂ sat >90% at rest via nasal cannula or noninvasive ventilation (CPAP, BiPAP).

PEVENTION OF EXACERBATIONS
1. *Smoking cessation: single most important intervention for COPD!** In nonsmokers, the normal rate of decline in FEV₁ after age 35y is 20-30ml/year (60ml/year in smokers).
   - Smoking cessation for >1 year can get decline close to 2x that of nonsmokers.
2. **Vaccinations:** pneumococcal. Influenza every fall (± prevent infectious exacerbations)
3. **Pulmonary Rehab:** improves quality of life, subjective dyspnea & exercise tolerance.
4. **Surgery:**
   - Lung reduction surgery: improves dyspnea by removing damaged lung, which allows the remaining lung to expand & function more efficiently.
   - Lung transplantation. Replacement of α-1 antitrypsin in some patients.

	COPD STAGING AND RECOMMENDED THERAPIES by GOLD Criteria		
	Stage	**PFT % predicted**	**Therapy**
FEV₁/FVC < 70 %	I: mild	FEV₁ ≥ 80%	• *Bronchodilators (short-acting)* • ↓Risk factors: influenza & pneumococcal vaccines.
	II: moderate	FEV₁ 50 – 79%	Above + *long acting dilator.*
	III: severe	FEV₁ 30 – 50%	Above + pulmonary rehab, *Steroids if ↑exacerbations.*
	IV: very severe	*Cor pulmonale,** *respiratory failure, heart failure,* FEV₁<30%	Above + *O₂ therapy.**

Antibiotics are used in ABECB (Acute Bacterial Exacerbations of Chronic Bronchitis) if ❶ increased sputum ❷ change in sputum quality &/or ❸ CXR evidence of infection.

Azithromycin has been shown to have anti-inflammatory properties in the lung.

COPD RADIOLOGIC FINDINGS

NORMAL PA CXR

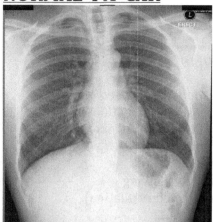

Note roundness of
  the diaphragms.

EMPHYSEMA

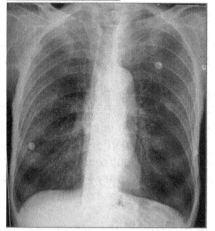

1. *Enlarged lung fields, flattened diaphragms.*
2. *Trapped air* (darker lung areas).
3. *Decreased vascular markings.*
4. *Bullae* seen (right side).

CHRONIC BRONCHITIS

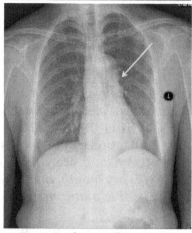

1. *Increased vascular markings, normal diaphragms.*
2. Prominent pulmonary artery & pulmonary hypertension (arrow), horizontal heart.
3. Right heart enlargement.

NORMAL LATERAL CXR

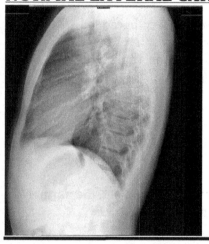

EMPHYSEMA

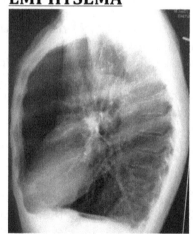

EMPHYSEMA LATERAL CXR:
1. *barrel chest*
2. *increased AP diameter*

NORMAL CT SCAN

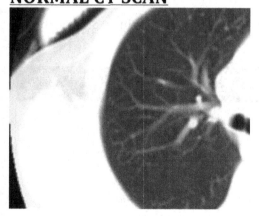

EMPHYSEMA

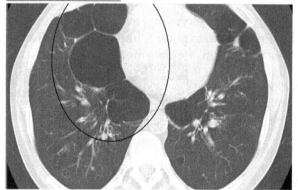

Emphysema: *bullae* (circular areas of darkness), which signifies airspace loss.

BRONCHIECTASIS

- **IRREVERSIBLE** _bronchial dilation_ 2^{ry} to **transmural inflammation** of medium-sized bronchi ⇨ destruction of muscular & elastic tissues of the bronchial wall. The inflamed airways collapse easily ⇨ _obstruction_ of airflow & _**impaired clearance of mucus secretions**_ ⇨ _lung infections._

ETIOLOGIES
1. **Recurrent/chronic lung infections:** _H. influenza MC cause of bronchiectasis if not due to Cystic Fibrosis*_ (35%); _**Pseudomonas MC cause if due to Cystic Fibrosis***_ (31%), M. catarrhalis, Staph aureus, S. pneumoniae, Mycobacterium (TB/atypical/MAC); Viral; Aspergillus.
2. Hereditary: _**Cystic Fibrosis MC cause of bronchiectasis in US,***_ α-1 antitrypsin deficiency.
3. Obstruction: foreign body aspiration, tumors, severe mucus impaction.

CLINICAL MANIFESTATIONS
1. _**Daily chronic cough with thick, mucopurulent, foul-smelling sputum***_ (±separated into 3 layers). Pleuritic chest pain. Patients often develop _recurrent pneumonia._

2. _**Hemoptysis***_ (50-70%). Due to erosion into the bronchial arteries (under systemic pressure). Usually mild. _**Bronchiectasis MC cause of massive hemoptysis.***_
   (Acute Bronchitis & Lung carcinoma MC causes of hemoptysis in general).

3. Persistent crackles at the bases common. Dyspnea, wheezing, rhonchi, clubbing.

DIAGNOSIS
1. **HIGH RESOLUTION CT SCAN:** _**study of choice:***_ _airway dilation, lack of tapering of the bronchi, bronchial wall thickening ("TRAM-TRACK" appearance),*_ mucopurulent plugs, consolidations.
   - Signet ring sign = pulmonary artery coupled with a dilated bronchus.

2. **PFT:** _**obstructive pattern:**_ ↓FEV$_1$; ↓FVC; ↓FEV$_1$/FVC <70%.

3. CXR: nonspecific findings: ± crowded bronchial markings (peribronchial fibrosis), small cysts at the lung bases, linear atelectasis, irregular opacities. _"Tram-track"_ (wall thickening) specific finding.
4. Sputum gram stain & culture. Neutrophilia in the sputum is common.
5. Bronchoscopy: sometimes necessary to evaluate hemoptysis, remove retained secretions and rule out obstructive airway lesions.

PROBLEMATIC PATHOGENS
1. **PSEUDOMONAS:** _**MC organism if bronchiectasis is due to Cystic Fibrosis.***_

2. **Mycobacterium Avium Complex (MAC).** **Management:** _**Clarithromycin + Ethambutol.***_
3. **Aspergillus:** allergic bronchopneumonia. _**Thick, brown sputum.**_
   Management: _**Corticosteroids + Itraconazole.**_ Surgical if symptomatic aspergilloma.

MANAGEMENT
1. _**Antibiotics: cornerstone of treatment.***_ Empiric (Ampicillin, Amoxicillin, Trimethoprim-sulfamethoxazole); Pseudomonal coverage: Fluoroquinolone, Piperacillin/tazobactam, aminoglycoside, cephalosporin). Antibiotic cycling may be used. Azithromycin has anti-inflammatory properties.
2. _**Mucus management/chest physiotherapy:**_ bronchodilators, anti-inflammatory agents; surgery, embolization for bleeding.
3. Surgery: resection (or transplantation) in severe or complicated cases.

CYSTIC FIBROSIS

- Autosomal recessive inherited disorder of defective Cystic Fibrosis Transmembrane Receptor (CFTR) protein. This defect **prevents chloride transport** (water movement out of the cell) ⇨ **_buildup of thick, viscous, mucus in the lungs, pancreas, liver, intestines_** & reproductive tracts ⇨ **_obstructive lung disease_** & **_exocrine gland dysfunction_** (ex. pancreatic insufficiency).

- ↑ **_incidence_** in **_Caucasians, N. Europeans_** (1:3,000 live births). Median age of survival 36.8y.

CLINICAL MANIFESTATIONS
<u>Classic scenario:</u> **_young_** with **_bronchiectasis, pancreatic insufficiency, growth delays & infertility._**
1. <u>GASTROINTESTINAL:</u>
    - **_meconium ileus at birth*_** (due to obstruction of intestine with meconium).
      Suspect CF if a full term infant presents with a meconium ileus.

    - **_Pancreatic insufficiency_** ⇨ ↓**_fat absorption_** ⇨ **_steatorrhea, bulky pale/foul-smelling stools,_** weight loss, **_Vitamin A, D, E & K deficiency._** Pancreatitis, *CF-induced Diabetes Mellitus.* Biliary disease. Children may present with failure to thrive.

2. **PULMONARY:** **_recurrent respiratory infections (especially Pseudomonas & Staph aureus),_** productive cough, dyspnea, chest pain, wheezing, **_chronic sinusitis.*_**
3. <u>Infertility</u> (95%). Heat exhaustion (abnormal sweating). Osteopenia. Malignancies of the GI tract.

DIAGNOSIS
1. Elevated sweat chloride test: **_primary test done.*_** ≥60 mmol/L on two occasions after administration of Pilocarpine (Pilocarpine is a cholinergic drug that induces sweating).

2. **CXR:** **_bronchiectasis*_** (CF most common cause of bronchiectasis in US); **_hyperinflation_** *of the lungs.*

3. **PFTs:** **_obstructive (often irreversible)._** May be a mixed with a restrictive pattern.

4. <u>DNA analysis:</u> definitive test (especially if sweat testing is negative). Genotyping.

5. <u>Sputum cultures:</u> often grow *Pseudomonas aeruginosa, Haemophilus influenzae,* or Staph aureus.

MANAGEMENT
❶ **_Airway clearance treatment:_** bronchodilators, mucolytics, antibiotics, decongestants.

❷ **_Pancreatic enzyme replacement, supplementation of fat soluble vitamins (A,D, E & K)._**
❸ Lung & pancreatic transplantation. Vaccinations (ex. pneumococcal, influenza).

	OBSTRUCTIVE DISORDERS	RESTRICTIVE DISORDERS

PULMONARY FUNCTION TESTS (PFT)	**_INCREASED lung volumes*_**
	    Hyperinflation: ↑*TLC, RV, RV/TLC, FRC*
	
	   Obstruction: ↓*FEV1, ↓FVC; ↓FEV1/ FVC*
		DECREASED lung volumes*
		   ↓*TLC, RV, RV/TLC, FRC, FVC*
		
		   Normal or ↑FEV$_1$,/FVC

COMPLIANCE	↑ *compliance with Emphysema*	↓ *compliance*
EXAMPLES	• Asthma • COPD (Chronic Bronchitis, Emphysema) • Bronchiectasis • Cystic Fibrosis • Coal Workers Pneumoconiosis often presents with an obstructive pattern	• Sarcoidosis • Pneumoconiosis • Idiopathic Pulmonary Fibrosis • ↓Muscular effort: Myasthenia Gravis, Polio • Scoliosis, Mesothelioma

BRONCHIECTASIS

NORMAL CXR

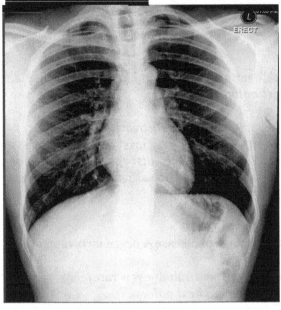

BRONCHIECTASIS

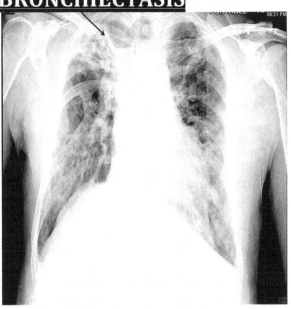

Bronchiectasis: irregular opacities, crowded bronchial markings, "tram track" markings.*

NORMAL CT SCAN

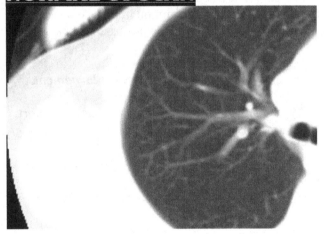

BRONCHIECTASIS

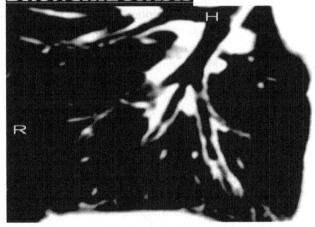

Bronchiectasis: *proximal airway dilation** with *thick walls* & *lack of airway tapering** giving a *"tram-track" appearance,** consolidation.

Signet ring sign: pulmonary artery coupled with a dilated bronchus (white arrow).

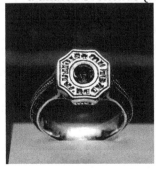

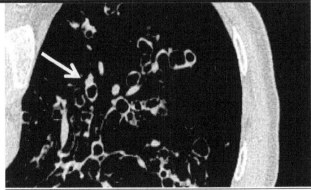

SARCOIDOSIS

- Chronic multisystemic, inflammatory, granulomatous disorder of unknown etiology.
- **Increased prevalence in <u>Afro-Americans, Northern Europeans, females.*</u>** Onset usually **<u>20-40y</u>**.
- Disordered <u>immune</u> regulation in <u>genetically</u> predisposed individuals exposed to certain <u>environmental</u> antigens.

PATHOPHYSIOLOGY

- **Exaggerated T cell response** to a variety of antigens or self-antigens ⇨ <u>central immune activation</u> & <u>peripheral immune depression</u>. T cell accumulation ⇨ **granuloma formation**.

- **Granuloma** = mass of immune cells formed by *macrophages, epithelioid cells (activated macrophages) & multinucleated giant cells* surrounded by a rim of lymphocytes (especially T_4), mast cells & fibroblasts (fibrin deposition) ⇨ ± fibrosis. **These granulomas take up space, disrupting the normal structure &/or function** of the tissues they form in, resulting in the clinical manifestations seen. Granulomas may eventually resolve or undergo fibrosis.

CLINICAL MANIFESTATIONS

- **50% asymptomatic** *(found incidentally on CXR).* Varies with stage of disease & organ involvement.

- *Most complications are pulmonary* (eye 2nd MC although with treatment, blindness is rare).
  1. **Pulmonary:** (90%). **Dry (nonproductive) cough, dyspnea & chest pain**.
  2. **Lymphadenopathy:** painless intrathoracic lymphadenopathy (*hilar nodes, ± paratracheal*).
  3. **Skin:** (25%) **2nd most common organ involved with sarcoidosis.**
     - **ERYTHEMA NODOSUM:*** bilateral tender red nodules on the anterior legs (usually resolves spontaneously in 2-4 weeks). Not specific for sarcoidosis (ex. may be seen with Coccidioidomycosis). ↑**incidence in Northern Europeans** (not common in Afro-Americans).
     - **LUPUS PERNIO pathognomonic:*** violaceous, raised discoloration of the nose, ear, cheek & chin (resembles frost bite).
     - <u>Maculopapular rash</u>: most common dermatologic manifestation of sarcoidosis.
     - Subcutaneous nodules & waxy nodular lesions may be seen. **Parotid gland enlargement.**
  4. **Visual:** (20%)
     - **ANTERIOR UVEITIS:** (inflammation of iris/ciliary body) ⇨ **blurred vision,*** ocular discomfort, photophobia, ciliary flush, floaters. *Ophthalmic exams indicated in all patients.*
     - <u>Conjunctivitis</u>: tearing, erythema. May develop glaucoma, cataracts & blindness.
  5. **Myocardial:** arrhythmias (2ry to conduction system involvement), cardiomyopathies.
  6. **Rheumatologic:** arthralgias, fever, malaise, weight loss, hepatosplenomegaly.
  7. **Neurologic** 5%: cranial nerve palsies (especially facial nerve/CN 7), diabetes insipidus, hypothalamic/pituitary lesions.

DIAGNOSIS

- Based on ❶ compatible clinical/radiologic findings ❷ NCGs ❸ exclusion of other diseases.
  A. **Tissue Biopsy:** NONCASEATING GRANULOMAS* (NCG) *classic nonspecific histological finding.* <u>Noncaseating = no central necrosis</u> in the granuloma. Mainly multinucleated giant cells, T cells. Common biopsy sites include the skin & lymph nodes. Transbronchial biopsy is also high yield.

  B. **CXR:** BILATERAL HILAR LYMPHADENOPATHY* (BHL) *classic!* Right paratracheal also common. CXR is almost always abnormal. **Interstitial lung disease (ILD)** – *reticular* opacities ±fine, ground glass appearance. ± *eggshell nodal calcifications.* Stages of sarcoidosis on CXR:
  Stage I: BHL (no sx or mild pulmonary sx).   **Stage III:** ILD only.
  Stage II: BHL + ILD (moderate pulmonary sx).   **Stage IV:** fibrosis (volume loss/restrictive disease).
  C. **PFT:** **restrictive (seen with advanced disease);** ± Normal or obstructive. **MC finding is isolated** $\downarrow DL_{co}$ (diffusing capacity of the lungs for carbon monoxide).
    - *PFTs primarily used to monitor response to treatment.*
    RESTRICTIVE PATTERN: normal or ↑FEV_1/FVC,* normal/ ↓FVC, ↓lung volumes:* ↓VC, RV, FRC, TLC.

D. <u>**CT scan (high resolution):**</u> hilar/mediastinal lymphadenopathy, nodules, ground glass opacities, parenchymal infiltration. Fibrosis associated with poor prognosis.

E. <u>**Gallium scan:**</u> ↑uptake in affected areas. Parotid/salivary glands tracer localization = *"panda sign".*

F. <u>**Bronchoalveolar lavage:**</u> used to rule out infectious causes. Sarcoid: ↑***CD4:CD8*** (↑CD4, ↓CD8)

LABORATORY STUDIES

1. ↑***ACE**** (40-80%). The granulomas secrete <u>A</u>ngiotensin <u>C</u>onverting <u>E</u>nzyme (may be a cytokine involved in granuloma maintenance). ACE levels usually diminish with clinical improvement (not reliable).
2. ***<u>Hypercalciuria</u>*/Hypercalcemia:** 2ry to granuloma: macrophage-driven ↑1,25 vitamin D production.
3. ***Eosinophilia,*** leukopenia.
4. ***Cutaneous anergy:**** 70% have diminished skin test reactivity to common skin allergens (peripheral immune suppression as a result of central immune system activation). ±False negative PPD.
5. ↑IgG (hypergammaglobulinemia), ↑ESR (erythrocyte sedimentation rate).

MANAGEMENT

1. **OBSERVATION:** *majority of patients have spontaneous remission within 2 years* & *require no treatment.* May follow up with periodic evaluations, CXR & PFTs.

2. **ORAL CORTICOSTEROIDS:** *treatment of choice when treatment is needed*.* **MOA:** reduces granuloma formation & fibrosis. ACE levels usually fall with clinical improvement after corticosteroids.
   Indications: worsening symptoms, deteriorating lung function, progressive radiologic decline. Must rule out tuberculosis & infectious etiologies before initiating corticosteroid treatment.

3. <u>Methotrexate:</u> may be used as a corticosteroid alternative or corticosteroid-refractory disease.

4. **<u>Hydroxychloroquine</u>:** may be good for chronic disfiguring skin lesions.

5. NSAIDs for musculoskeletal symptoms & erythema nodosum; Single lung transplant in severe cases.

➢ ***Prognosis good overall. 40% spontaneously resolve; 40% improve with treatment; 20% progress to irreversible lung injury.***
➢ Good prognosis: Stage I, erythema nodosum.
➢ ***Interstitial lung disease & lupus pernio associated with poorer prognosis.***

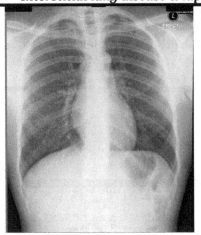

Normal Chest X ray

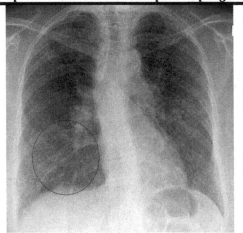

Sarcoidosis:
bilateral hilar lymphadenopathy
above the heart.

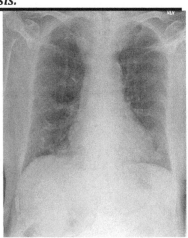

Sarcoidosis:
interstitial fibrosis

SARCOIDOSIS

CLASSIC SARCOID PRESENTATION: *young patient with respiratory & constitutional symptoms, blurred vision & erythema nodosum!** Recognize that pattern!

SARCOIDOSIS
SKIN MANIFESTATIONS (25%)
- *Lupus Pernio:* **Most spp derm manifestation**
  pathognomonic: violaceous, raised discoloration of nose, ear, cheek & chin (resembles frost bite).

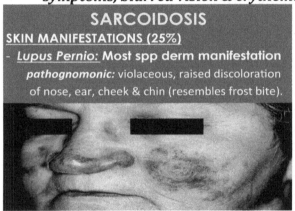

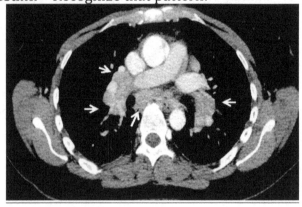

Sarcoidosis: Notice the *hilar lymphadenopathy*; areas of fibrosis and interstitial involvement (arrows)

ERYTHEMA NODOSUM

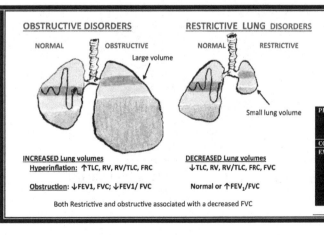

Erythema nodosum: extremely tender nodules that develop on the shins (usually bilateral). Idiopathic inflammatory skin condition commonly associated with use of certain medications (ex. OCPs), Infection: streptococcal, TB, sarcoid, fungal (ex. Coccidioidomycosis), inflammatory bowel disease, leukemia. Generally self-limiting & resolves spontaneously within a few weeks (with excellent prognosis). Not specific to sarcoidosis.

LÖFGREN'S SYNDROME: triad:
❶ *Erythema Nodosum*
❷ *Bilateral hilar lymphadenopathy*
❸ *Polyarthralgias + fever*
- Common presentation of sarcoidosis in **Northern Europeans** (not common in African-Americans).
Associated with a good prognosis and spontaneous remission.

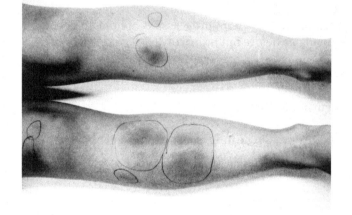

OBSTRUCTIVE DISORDERS

NORMAL   OBSTRUCTIVE
Large volume

INCREASED Lung volumes
Hyperinflation: ↑TLC, RV, RV/TLC, FRC

Obstruction: ↓FEV1, FVC; ↓FEV1/ FVC

Both Restrictive and obstructive associated with a decreased FVC

RESTRICTIVE LUNG DISORDERS

NORMAL   RESTRICTIVE

Small lung volume

DECREASED Lung volumes
↓TLC, RV, RV/TLC, FRC, FVC

Normal or ↑FEV₁/FVC

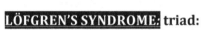

	OBSTRUCTIVE DISORDERS	RESTRICTIVE DISORDERS
PFT'S	*INCREASED Lung volumes** Hyperinflation: ↑TLC, RV, RV/TLC, FRC* Obstruction: ↓FEV1, ↓FVC; ↓FEV1/ FVC*	*DECREASED Lung volumes** ↓TLC, RV, RV/TLC, FRC, FVC Normal or ↑FEV$_b$/FVC*
COMPLIANCE	↑ *compliance with Emphysema**	↓ *compliance**
EXAMPLES	• Asthma • COPD (Chronic Bronchitis, Emphysema) • Bronchiectasis • Cystic Fibrosis • Coal Workers Pneumoconiosis often presents with obstructive pattern	• Sarcoidosis • Pneumoconiosis • Idiopathic Pulmonary Fibrosis • ↓Muscular effort: Myasthenia Gravis, Polio • Scoliosis, Mesothelioma

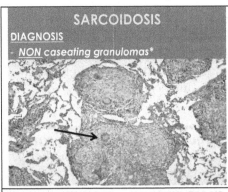

SARCOIDOSIS
DIAGNOSIS
- *NON caseating granulomas**

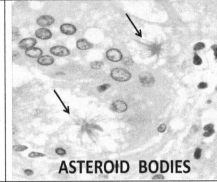

ASTEROID BODIES

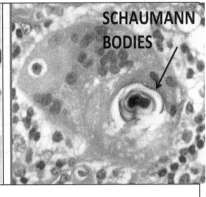

SCHAUMANN BODIES

NONCASEATING GRANULOMAS: *classic histologic finding* (not specific for sarcoid). Giant cells (arrow)	Granulomas consists of: - <u>T cells</u> in the periphery. May have a rim of fibrosis. - **Epithelioid macrophages**: enlarged, activated macrophages that resemble epithelial cells. - **Langerhans Giant cells**: fused epithelioid cells with a horseshoe appearance. Giant cells may contain asteroid bodies: star shaped areas or Schaumann bodies: protein & calcium deposition.

IDIOPATHIC FIBROSING INTERSTITIAL PNEUMONIA (PULMONARY FIBROSIS)

- *Chronic progressive interstitial scarring (fibrosis)* from persistent inflammation (chronic alveolitis) ⇨ loss of pulmonary function with restrictive component. Unknown etiology.
- *MC in men 40-50y.* MC in smokers. Usually limited to lungs. Survival <10y at time of diagnosis.

CLINICAL MANIFESTATIONS: dyspnea and/or nonproductive cough (usually gradual onset).

PHYSICAL EXAMINATION: fine bibasilar inspiratory crackles, *clubbing of the fingers,* ±cyanosis.

DIAGNOSIS: CXR/CT scan: *diffuse reticular opacities (honeycombing),* ground glass opacities.*
Biopsy: *honeycombing (large cystic airspaces from cystic fibrotic alveolitis).*

PFT: *RESTRICTIVE DISEASE*: decreased lung volumes (↓TLC, RV), ↓DLCO. Normal or ↑ FEV_1/FVC.*

MANAGEMENT: No effective treatment. Strategies include: smoking cessation, oxygen, corticosteroids in some acute exacerbations. *Lung transplant only cure* (poor prognosis without transplant).

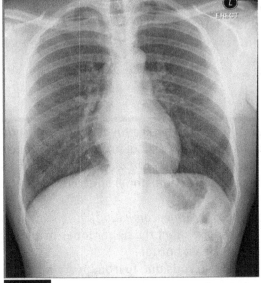

Normal

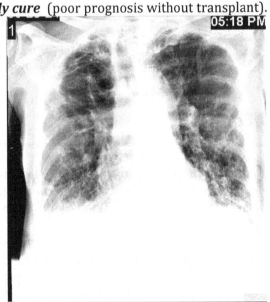

IDIOPATHIC PULMONARY FIBROSIS

PNEUMOCONIOSES/ENVIRONMENTAL LUNG DISEASES

PNEUMOCONIOSIS: chronic fibrotic lung disease secondary to *inhalation of mineral dust.*
- Mineral dust is ingested by alveolar macrophages, triggering inflammation & release of chemical mediators ⇨ parenchymal fibrosis ⇨ restrictive lung disease & ↓lung compliance.

SILICOSIS

- *Silica dust inhalation (mining, quarry work with granite/slate/quartz, pottery sandblasting).**
CLINICAL MANIFESTATIONS: often asymptomatic, ± dyspnea on exertion, nonproductive cough.
  - DIAGNOSIS
    - CXR: multiple small (<10mm) round *nodular** opacities *primarily in the upper lobes.* Bilateral nodular densities progress from the periphery to the hilum. ⊕ *EGG SHELL CALCIFICATIONS* of the hilar & mediastinal nodes* (only seen in 5%). Lung Biopsy
  - MANAGEMENT: No proven treatment. Supportive: bronchodilators, O₂, vaccinations (influenza, pneumococcal), ± corticosteroids (for silicosis alveolitis), rehabilitation.

COAL WORKER'S PNEUMOCONIOSIS (black lung disease)

- Caused by inhalation of dust from coal or carbon mines. Management is supportive (see silicosis).
- CXR: *small upper lobe nodules** & *HYPERINFLATION** resembling centrilobar emphysema (similar to smoking-related emphysema). *May have obstructive pattern on PFT.**
- CAPLAN SYNDROME: *coal worker's pneumoconiosis + Rheumatoid Arthritis.**

BERYLLIOSIS

- *Electronics, aerospace, ceramics, tool & dye manufacturing,* fluorescent light bulbs.*
- CLINICAL MANIFESTATIONS: similar to silicosis, dyspnea, cough, arthralgia, weight loss, fever.
- CXR: normal 50%, hilar lymphadenopathy, increased interstitial lung markings.
- DIAGNOSIS: ⊕ exposure, ⊕ beryllium lymphocyte proliferation test & noncaseating granulomas on biopsy. Associated with ↑risk of lung, stomach, colon cancers.
- MANAGEMENT: *Corticosteroids,* O₂, supportive. ±Methotrexate if Corticosteroids are unsuccessful.

BYSSINOSIS

"Brown lung disease" or "Monday fever" due to *cotton exposure** in the textile industry.
CLINICAL MANIFESTATIONS: dyspnea, wheezing, cough, chest tightness. The symptoms tend to get worse at the beginning of the work week, then improve later in the week or on the weekend ("Monday fever").

ASBESTOSIS

- Seen 15-20 years after long-term exposure to asbestos *(destruction/renovation of old buildings, insulation, ship building, pipe fitters).** Smoking increases the risk of bronchogenic cancer.
↑RISK: ❶ *bronchogenic carcinoma* MC* ❷ *malignant mesothelioma of the pleura* (rare but specific).
CLINICAL MANIFESTATIONS: similar to silicosis (± dyspnea on exertion, nonproductive cough).

CXR: *PLEURAL PLAQUES* (pleural thickening), interstitial fibrosis (honeycomb lung).*
- *AFFECTS LOWER LOBES* primarily* (coal workers & silicosis affect the upper lobes primarily).
- ± "shaggy heart sign" (blurring of the diaphragm & the heart border).
BIOPSY: may show *linear asbestos bodies* in lung tissues (brown rods due to iron/protein deposits).
MANAGEMENT: no specific treatment available. Supportive (see silicosis).

HYPERSENSITIVITY PNEUMONITIS / EXTRINSIC ALLERGIC ALVEOLITIS

PNEUMONITIS: *generalized lung inflammation of the alveoli & respiratory bronchioles due to organic dusts, molds, foreign proteins & chemicals.*

- MC seen in 30s – 50s.
- **PATHOPHYSIOLOGY:** *inflammatory reaction to an ORGANIC ANTIGEN* ⇨ sensitization to the antigen. Subsequent, heavy exposure ⇨ neutrophil activation in small airways & alveoli with mononuclear cell invasion. Release of proteolytic enzymes contributes to the hypersensitivity reaction.

DISEASE	ANTIGEN	SOURCE
FARMER'S LUNG CATTLE WORKER'S LUNG	Thermophilic actinomycetes (gram positive bacteria), Saccharopolyspora rectivirgula, Micropolyspora faeni	Moldy hay
VENTILATION WORKER'S LUNG	Thermophilic actinomycetes, Mycobacterium Avium Complex	Water related contamination: humidifiers, air conditioners, heating/cooling systems
BIRD BREEDER'S LUNG	Avian proteins	Bird feces, feathers, or serum proteins of bird
SEQUOIOSIS	Graphium Auerobasidium	Sawdust from moldy redwood (seen in lumbar mill workers).
"SAW MILL WORKER" LUNG	Other fungi	
METAL WORKER'S LUNG	Mycobacterium immunogenium	Contaminated metalworking fluids
MUSHROOM LUNG	Actinomycetes	Moldy spores
GRAIN WORKER'S LUNG	Sitophilus granaries	Exposure to wheat infested c weevils
CHEMICAL WORKER'S LUNG	Diisocyanate chemical	Manufacture of plastics, polyurethane

CLINICAL MANIFESTATIONS

1. ACUTE HYPERSENSITIVITY PNEUMONITIS: *rapid onset: fevers, chills*, dyspnea, productive cough, chest tightness, malaise *occurring 4-8 hours after prolonged exposure to antigen. Inspiratory crackles on physical exam.*
   <u>Biopsy:</u> micronodular interstitial involvement with poorly formed noncaseating granulomas. May be normal.

2. **SUB ACUTE (INTERMITTENT):** *gradual development* of *dyspnea, productive cough,* anorexia, weight loss, pleuritis. Similar to acute but longer duration & less severe (*usually no fevers, chills*). Associated c more organized granulomas. <u>CXR:</u> micronodular opacities especially in the lower lung fields. **Biopsy:** noncaseating granulomas (more organized than in acute) may be fibrotic.

3. **CHRONIC HYPERSENSITIVITY PNEUMONITIS:** progressive worsening of symptoms. No history of acute episodes. Slow onset of progressive dyspnea, weight loss, clubbing, tachypnea. Associated with only partial recovery after agent exposure is eliminated.

<u>DIAGNOSIS:</u>
1. **CXR:** Acute: diffuse micronodular interstitial pattern. Subacute & chronic: micronodular opacities especially in the lower lung fields.
2. **PFT's:** *restrictive component, ↓DL$_{CO}$,* hypoxemia. CBC: leukocytosis with left shift. Positive hypersensitivity panel

<u>MANAGEMENT</u>
1. *Avoidance of allergen, Corticosteroids*

PSITTACOSIS (PARROT FEVER)
- Caused by bacterium ***Chlamydophila psittaci*** from infected birds (ex. parrots, ducks).

CLINICAL MANIFESTATIONS: *atypical pneumonia*, dry cough, fever, myalgias, ***headache.***

MANAGEMENT: *Tetracyclines 1st line.* Macrolides 2nd line. Chloramphenicol.

SILO FILLER DISEASE

- **HYPERSENSITIVITY PNEUMONITIS** from **NITROGEN DIOXIDE GAS EXPOSURE RELEASED FROM PLANT MATTER** stored in silos as they ferment (especially at the chute & base of the silo). The gas is converted to nitric acid in the lungs when inhaled. Also seen with combustion exposure (ex fires, diesel fume).

CLINICAL MANIFESTATIONS
- Cough, dyspnea, fatigue, cardiopulmonary edema. May develop bronchiolitis obliterans.

MANAGEMENT
- Occupational reduction of exposure - not entering recently filled silos for 2 weeks, entering at the top of the silo, use of respiratory N95 masks.

DIFFERENTIAL DIAGNOSIS
- Farmer's lung (allergic alveolitis/pneumonitis specifically due to moldy hay exposure).

DISEASES OF THE PLEURA
MESOTHELIOMA

- ***Tumor originating from the pleura*** (80%), peritoneum (2nd MC), tunica vaginalis or pericardium. ¾ are malignant. ***80% due to CHRONIC ASBESTOS EXPOSURE.*** *** Poor prognosis if malignant.***

CLINICAL MANIFESTATIONS
- Pleural mesothelioma: pleuritic chest pain, dyspnea, fever, night sweats, weight loss, hemoptysis.

DIAGNOSIS
- Pleural biopsy via video-assisted thoracoscopy (VATS). *Bloody pleural effusions are common.*

MANAGEMENT
1. Localized: pleurectomy (surgical resection with margins).
2. Diffuse – resection, radiation and/or chemotherapy.

COSTOCHONDRITIS & TIETZE SYNDROME

- *ACUTE INFLAMMATION OF THE **COSTOCHONDRAL, COSTOSTERNAL OR STERNOCLAVICULAR JOINTS.***
- Common after viral infection or musculoskeletal trauma (physical strain, excessive coughing etc.).

CLINICAL MANIFESTATIONS
- ***"Pleuritic" chest pain:*** *intermittent sharp, stabbing pain that is **worse with inspiration. Worse with coughing or certain movements of the upper limbs or torso.*** May radiate to the shoulder.

PHYSICAL EXAMINATION
- *LOCALIZED PAIN & TENDERNESS ON PALPATION* especially at the 2nd – 5th costochondral junctions.
  - Costochondritis: ***no palpable edema.*** Usually multiple areas of tenderness. Palpation reproduces the pain. Costochondritis is much more common than Tietze syndrome.
  - Tietze Syndrome: ⊕ ***localized palpable edema (swelling),**** heat & erythema.
    - MC affects the 2nd & 3rd costochondral junctions.

PLEURAL EFFUSION

- *abnormal accumulation of fluid* in the pleural space *(not a disease itself but a sign of a disease)*.
  - EMPYEMA: grossly purulent/turbulent effusion (direct infection of the pleural space).
  - PARAPNEUMONIC: *noninfected* pleural effusion secondary to bacterial pneumonia.
  - HEMOTHORAX: *gross blood* (ex. chest trauma or malignancy).
  - CHYLOTHORAX: ↑lymph. Associated with persistent turbidity after centrifuge (if not ⇨ empyemic).

TRANSUDATE:

- circulatory system fluid due to *either ↑HYDROSTATIC &/OR ↓ONCOTIC PRESSURE.*
- **ETIOLOGIES:** *CHF is the MC cause of transudate effusion (>90%);* nephrotic syndrome, cirrhosis*, hypoalbuminemia, atelectasis. Pulmonary embolism is usually exudative (but may be transudative).

EXUDATE:

- Occurs when *local factors* **increase vascular permeability** (ex. INFECTION/INFLAMMATION).*
- An exudate is fluid that filters from the circulatory system into areas of inflammation: contains ↑plasma proteins, WBCs, platelets, ± RBCs.

CLINICAL MANIFESTATIONS

Asymptomatic. If symptomatic, usually complain of *dyspnea, "pleuritic" chest pain, cough.*

PHYSICAL EXAMINATION

- ↓*TACTILE FREMITUS,* ↓*BREATH SOUNDS, DULLNESS TO PERCUSSION;** ±*pleural friction rub.*
- In extreme cases it may cause lung collapse or mediastinal shift to the contralateral side.

DIAGNOSIS

1. **CXR:**
   - **PA/lateral:** >175cc can obscure the lateral costophrenic sulcus. 500cc (for the diaphragm) **blunting of costophrenic angles*** (⊕ **menisci sign**) ± *loculations* (due to pleural adhesions)
   - *LATERAL DECUBITUS FILMS BEST:** detects smaller effusions, differentiates loculations & empyema from new effusions or scarring.*

2. **Thoracentesis:** *test of choice.* Send pleural fluid for chemistry, cell count, cultures & cytology. LIGHT'S CRITERIA *are **exclusive to** EXUDATES:* the presence of ANY of the 3 = exudative:
   - Pleural fluid protein: serum **protein >0.5**
   - Pleural fluid LDH: serum **LDH >0.6** OR
   - *Pleural fluid LDH > $^2/_3$ upper limit of normal LDH*

3. **CT scan:** used to confirm empyema.

MANAGEMENT:

1. *Treat underlying condition.* Diuretics, sodium restriction.

2. **Thoracentesis: gold standard.** Diagnostic &/or therapeutic. Don't remove >1.5 liters during any one procedure.

3. **Chest tube pleural fluid drainage:** *if empyema (pleural fluid pH <7.2, glucose <40mg/dL, positive gram stain of pleural fluid).** May inject with streptokinase to facilitate drainage.

4. Pleurodesis: if malignant effusions or chronic. Options used to obliterate the pleural space include *talc (MC used), doxycycline,* minocycline. Bleomycin not used as often due to its toxicity.

PLEURAL EFFUSION

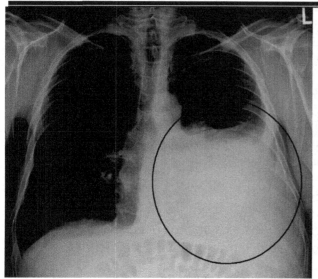

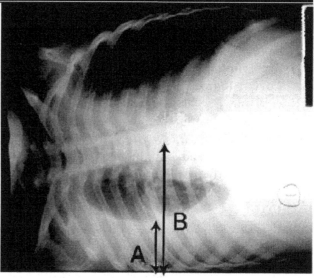

Pleural Effusion PA Film: notice the clear costophrenic angle on the right side with ***blunting of the costophrenic angle*** on the left side.

Pleural Effusion (Lateral Decubitus Film): layering of the fluid.

PNEUMOTHORAX

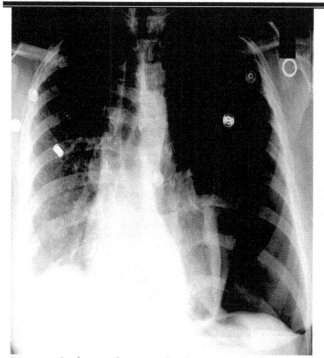

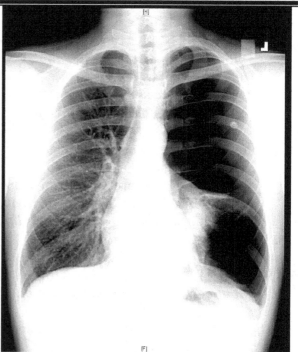

Linear shadow of visceral pleura with ***decreased peripheral lung markings on the left side***

L-sided tension PTX: ***mediastinal shift*** to the right side.

PNEUMOTHORAX

- Air in the pleural space. *Increasingly positive pleural pressure causes collapse of the lung.*

TYPES OF PNEUMOTHORAX

A. **SPONTANEOUS:**
   Atraumatic & idiopathic. Due to **bleb rupture** (bleb = thin-walled air containing space).

   1. **PRIMARY:** *NO underlying lung disease.*
      Mainly affects tall, thin men 20-40y, smokers, ⊕ *family history* of pneumothorax.

   2. **SECONDARY:** ⊕ *underlying lung disease* *without trauma* (ex. *COPD, asthma*).

B. **TRAUMATIC:**
   - **iatrogenic:** during CPR, thoracentesis, PEEP (ventilation), subclavian line placement.
   - other trauma: ex. car accidents, etc.

C. **TENSION:** any type of pneumothorax in which the **positive air pressure pushes lungs, trachea, great vessels & heart to** the **CONTRALATERAL SIDE.*** Immediately life threatening. MC seen during trauma, mechanical ventilation or resuscitative efforts.

Catamenial PTX: *occurs during menstruation* (ectopic endometrial tissue in the pleura).

CLINICAL MANIFESTATIONS

1. *Chest pain:* usually *pleuritic, unilateral, non exertional* & sudden in onset; *Dyspnea.*

2. **PHYSICAL EXAMINATION:**
   - ↑*HYPERRESONANCE to percussion,* ↓*fremitus,* ↓*breath sounds* (over the affected side).

   - Unequal respiratory expansion, tachycardia, tachypnea.

   - **Tension Pneumothorax:** ↑*JVP, pulsus paradoxus, hypotension.*

DIAGNOSIS:

1. **CXR with EXPIRATORY VIEW** *preferred:*
   - ↓*peripheral lung markings* (due to collapsed lung tissue).
   - ± *companion lines* *(visceral pleural line running parallel with the ribs).*
   - deep sulcus sign on supine chest radiograph (air collection basally & anteriorly).

MANAGEMENT:

1. **Observation:** *in primary spontaneous if small (<15-20%* the diameter of the hemithorax or ≤2-3cm between the chest wall & lung on CXR). Observe at least 6 hours with repeat CXR to affirm no progression + 24-48 hour follow up. Often spontaneously resolves within 10 days.
   - Oxygen shown to ↑*air resorption* 3-4x faster than 1.25% every day.

2. **Chest tube placement (thoracostomy):** *if large or severe symptoms.*

3. **Needle Aspiration:** *if tension pneumothorax* *followed by chest tube placement.* Needle placed in *2nd intercostal space* (2nd ICS) *@ midclavicular line* (MCL) of the affected side.

- *Avoid pressure changes: ex. high altitudes, smoking, unpressurized aircraft & scuba diving.*

PULMONARY NODULES

Nodule: small round/coin-shaped or oval, well-circumscribed lesion < 3 cm.
Pulmonary mass if >3 cm.

ETIOLOGIES
- **Granulomatous infections:** *tuberculosis (common cause)*, histoplasmosis, coccidioidomycosis.
- **Tumors:** benign or malignant.
- **Inflammation:** Rheumatoid Arthritis, Sarcoidosis, Wegener's granulomatosis.
- **Mediatinal tumors:** *thymoma MC mediastinal tumor.*

	BENIGN	MALIGNANT
SHAPE	Round, smooth	Irregular, speculated
GROWTH	Slow	Rapid (may double in 4 months)
CALCIUM DEPOSITION	Calcifications usually seen in benign lesions	
CAVITARY	Cavitary usually seen in benign lesions	Cavitary with thickened walls

DIAGNOSIS
- Observation: if low malignant probability (<5%) ex. age <50y no smoking history etc. Active surveillance. Lesions that remain the same size tend to be benign (often a tuberculous granuloma). CT scan may be used to assess the lesion initially & evaluate surrounding tissues.

- Transthoracic needle aspiration or bronchoscopy: intermediate probability (5-60%). Needle aspiration is often used for peripheral lesions whereas bronchoscopy used for central lesions.

- Resection with biopsy: preferred if high probability of malignancy (>60%).

BRONCHIAL CARCINOID TUMORS

- *Rare neuroendocrine (enterochromaffin cell)* tumors characterized by ***slow growth, low METS.***
  GI tract is the MC site of carcinoid tumors. Lung is the 2nd MC site.
- Bronchial carcinoid tumors are usually ***well differentiated*** low-grade malignancies.

- *May secrete serotonin, ACTH, ADH, melanocyte stimulating hormone.* MC <60y.

CLINICAL MANIFESTATIONS
1. *Asymptomatic* 25-40%. ±Focal wheezing, cough, recurrent pneumonia, hemoptysis.

2. ±SIADH, Cushing's syndrome, obstruction.

3. ***Carcinoid syndrome: (diarrhea due to ↑serotonin)***; ↑bradykinin & histamine ⇨ flushing, tachycardia, bronchoconstriction (wheezing), hemodynamic instability (ex. hypotension) & acidosis. Classic but rare (seen in <10% of patients).

DIAGNOSIS:
1. **Bronchoscopy:** *"pink to purple well-vascularized central tumor."**
2. Tumor localization: CT scan & Octreotide scintography.

MANAGEMENT
1. Surgical excision definitive management.
   Often resistant to radiation and chemotherapy.

2. Octreotide may be used to reduce symptoms (↓'es secretion of the active hormones).

BRONCHOGENIC CARCINOMA

MC cause of cancer <u>deaths</u> in men and women. Commonly presents in 50s -60s.

- **<u>Cigarette smoking MC cause</u>*** *(includes 2nd hand).* 85% of lung cancer is seen in smokers (exception is bronchioloalveolar). Asbestosis 2nd MC cause.

- **Greatest tendency to <u>METS</u> to the <u>brain, bone, liver, lymph nodes & adrenals</u>.**

A. **NON SMALL CELL CARCINOMA (85%):**
   1. **ADENOCARCINOMA** – 35%. **MC type in smokers, women & nonsmokers.*** Typically **peripheral.*** Arises from the mucous glands. Tends to metastasize to distant areas.
      - **Bronchioloalveolar:** a rare low-grade subtype (has the best prognosis). Classically presents with voluminous sputum & an interstitial lung pattern on CXR.

   2. **SQUAMOUS CELL** – 20%. Bronchial in origin. Because it is typically **<u>C</u>entrally located,*** it may be picked up on sputum cytology May cause hemoptysis. Associated with **<u>C</u>avitary lesions*** (central necrosis), **hyper<u>C</u>alcemia,* & <u>P</u>ancoast syndrome.*** Think "CCCP."

   3. **LARGE CELL (ANAPLASTIC) CARCINOMA** – 10%. **Very aggressive.**

B. **SMALL CELL (OAT CELL) CARCINOMA (13%):** typically **metastasize early*** ⇨ METS usually found on presentation. Typically central, aggressive & because there is METS at presentation, **surgery is usually not the treatment of choice.**

CLINICAL MANIFESTATIONS
1. Asymptomatic, cough, hemoptysis, dyspnea, anorexia, weight loss. Trousseau's syndrome.
2. **SVC syndrome:** dilated neck veins, facial plethora, prominent chest veins. MC with small cell.
3. **Hypercalcemia: especially with squamous cell.***
4. *SIADH/Hyponatremia - MC with small cell.*
5. Gynecomastia MC with adenocarcinoma.
6. **Cushing's syndrome:** ectopic ACTH production. MC with small cell.
7. *Lambert-Eaton Syndrome* associated with small cell. Antibodies against calcium-gated channels @ the neuromuscular junction ⇨ weakness similar to myasthenia gravis but in *Lambert-Eaton, the weakness IMPROVES with continued use* (unlike in MG where it worsens with use).*
8. **Pancoast Syndrome:** *tumors at the superior sulcus* ⇨ ❶ *shoulder pain* ❷ *Horner's syndrome* (miosis, ptosis, anhydrosis) due to *cervical cranial sympathetic compression.* ❸ *atrophy of hand/arm muscles.*

DIAGNOSIS
1. **CXR & CT scan:** often seen on CXR but not used for screening. CT used for staging.
2. **Sputum cytology:** may be useful for **central lesions** (ex. squamous, small cell).
3. **Bronchoscopy:** useful for **central lesions.**
4. Pleural fluid analysis.
5. <u>Transthoracic needle biopsy</u>: useful for peripheral lesions. CT or fluoroscopy guided.
6. Mediastinoscopy.

MANAGEMENT
1. **NON SMALL CELL: surgical resection** treatment of choice* esp if localized to the chest.

2. **SMALL CELL: chemotherapy treatment of choice*** (with or without radiotherapy).*

ASBESTOSIS
- PLEURAL PLAQUES*

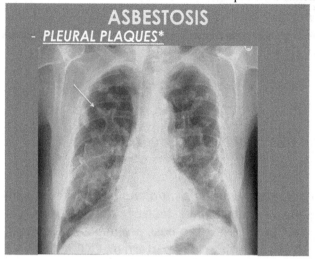

SILICOSIS
- EGGSHELL CALCIFICATIONS*

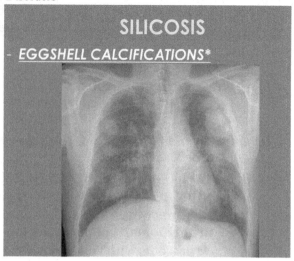

NON SMALL LUNG CA
- PANCOAST TUMOR*: apical

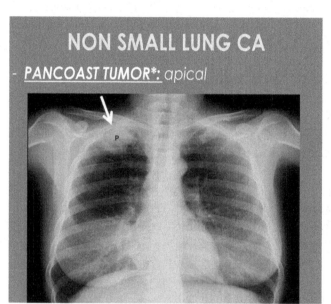

HORNER'S SYNDROME

- especially with NSCLC (esp squamous cell) of superior sulcus: ❶ Shoulder pain ❷ Horner's syndrome (miosis, ptosis, anhydrosis) due to cervical cranial sympathetic compression ❸ atrophy of hand/arm muscles.

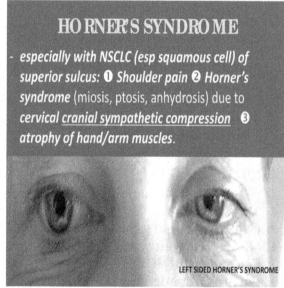

LEFT SIDED HORNER'S SYNDROME

LUNG CANCER

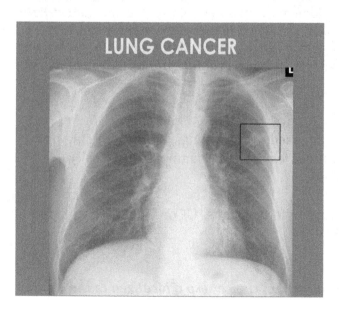

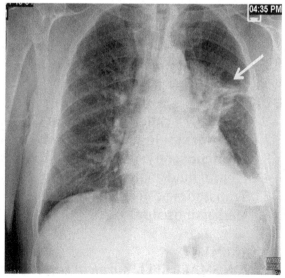

PULMONARY EMBOLISM (PE)

Thrombus in the pulmonary artery or its branches. Not a disease itself but a complication of a DVT.
- 95% PEs arise from DVTs in the lower extremities above the knee (ex. iliofemoral) or pelvis.
  Other causes include: fat emboli from long bone fractures & air emboli (from central lines).
- Most people who die from PE die from subsequent PEs (not the initial one).

CLINICAL MANIFESTATIONS
Dyspnea MC symptom; tachypnea MC sign.* Patients may be asymptomatic.
  A. **History** classic triad: ❶ *dyspnea* (80%), ❷ *pleuritic chest pain* (70%) & ❸ *hemoptysis.* *Classic presentation: post-op patient with sudden tachypnea (70%),* tachycardia. *± cough* or *hemoptysis. If massive PE ⇨ ±syncope, hypotension, pulseless electrical activity.*
    - Factor V Leiden MC predisposing condition.*
  B. **Physical exam**
    1. *The pulmonary exam is usually normal.* May have rales or a pleural friction rub.
    2. ⊕ Homan's sign (calf pain with dorsiflexion is a classic but nonspecific sign).

DIAGNOSTIC STUDIES
  1. *Helical CT scan (CT-PA): best initial test for suspected PE.* More sensitive for proximal emboli. ⊕ if intraluminal defect is seen. May demonstrate other etiologies. Negative CT & US ⇨ <2% rate of PE after follow up (except if high clinical suspicion, then ~5%).
  2. **V/Q scan:** low probability only rules out PE in patients with low clinical suspicion.
  3. *Pulmonary angiography: gold standard.* Ordered if **high suspicion & negative CT or VQ scan.***
  4. **Doppler Ultrasound:** 70% patients with PE will be ⊕ for a lower extremity DVT. Can miss pelvic DVTs. Serial ultrasounds may be performed to increase diagnostic specificity.

ANCILLARY EVALUATION TESTS
  1. **CXR:** most often normal. *A normal CXR in the setting of hypoxia is highly suspicious for PE!*
     ± pleural effusion, atelectasis or abrupt cutoff of vessels. *Classic (but rare) signs:*
       - **WESTERMARK'S SIGN:** avascular markings distal to the area of the embolus.
       - **HAMPTON'S HUMP:** wedge-shaped infiltrate (represents infarction).
  2. **ECG:** *sinus tachycardia & nonspp ST/T changes MC.** S1Q3T3 most specific for PE:
       - wide deep S in lead I; both an isolated Q as well as T wave inversion in lead III.
  3. **ABG:** *initially respiratory alkalosis* (2ry to hyperventilation) ⇨ *respiratory acidosis may occur with time.* ↑A-a gradient.
  4. **D dimer:** *helpful ONLY if negative & low suspicion for PE** (high sensitivity, poor specificity).

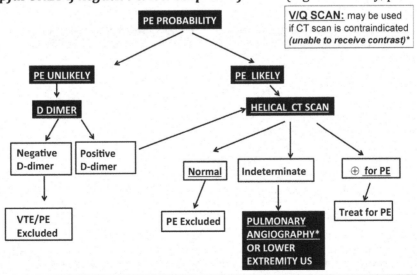

MANAGEMENT OF PULMONARY EMBOLISM

1. ANTICOAGULATION:

LOW MOLECULAR WEIGHT HEPARIN (LMWH)	UNFRACTIONATED HEPARIN (UFH)
• **MOA:** *potentiates antithrombin III* - works more on factor Xa than thrombin (Factor IIa)	• **MOA:** *potentiates antithrombin III, inhibits thrombin & other coagulation factors*
• *SQ injection. Compliant, low-risk patients can be discharged home during bridging therapy.*	• Continuous IV drip – requires hospitalization for bridging therapy.
• *Duration of Action ~12 hours*	• *Duration of action: 1 hour after IV drip is discontinued.*
• *No need to monitor PTT* (weight based – more predictable dosing)	• *Must monitor PTT 1.5-2.5 x normal value.*
• *Protamine Sulfate is the antidote* (not as effective as with UFH)	• *Protamine Sulfate is the antidote.*
• *Lower risk of HIT* (higher anti Xa-IIa ratio means less potential binding with platelets).	• *Heparin Induced Thrombocytopenia (HIT)* – Heparin acts as a hapten (stimulates the immune response when it is attached to platelet factor 4). This complex activates platelets, causing simultaneous thrombocytopenia & thrombosis.
• **CI:** *Renal failure* (Cr >2.0) because LMWH excreted by kidneys, *Thrombocytopenia.*	**Management:** other anticoagulants: ex: Argatroban or Bivalirudin. DO NOT use Warfarin (may develop necrosis).

- **WARFARIN (COUMADIN)** for *at least 3 months.* *

    MOA: *inhibits vitamin K dependent coagulation factors* (EXTRINSIC *pathway*): II, VII, IX, X. Inhibits protein C & S. Should be <u>overlapped with heparin for at least 5 days</u> AND INR 2.0 to 3.0 @ least 24 hours.

- **NOVEL ANTICOAGULANTS:** LMWH followed by Dabigatran (direct thrombin inhibitor) or Edoxaban (Factor Xa inhibitor) can be used instead of Warfarin therapy and may be preferred.

2. IVC FILTER: hemodynamically *stable patients in whom anticoagulation is contraindicated or is unsuccessful.* * No long-term reduction in mortality.

3. THROMBOLYSIS OF CLOT: Streptokinase, Urokinase, Alteplase

Ind: *massive PE, hemodynamically unstable PE.* Resolves emboli within 24 hours. Thrombolysis usually preferred over embolectomy.

CI: CVA or internal bleed within 2 months. Relative: uncontrolled HTN, surgery/trauma within 6 weeks.

4. THROMBECTOMY/EMBOLECTOMY: unstable/massive PE if thrombolysis is contraindicated or ineffective.

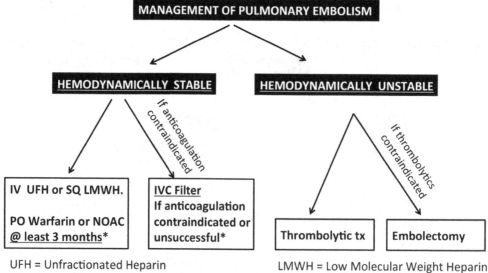

PE PROPHYLAXIS

The single most important step in managing PE. Prophylaxis is warranted preoperatively in patients undergoing surgery with prolonged immobilization, pregnant women, h/o prior DVT/PE.

- **Early ambulation:** low risk, minor procedures in patients <40y.
- **Elastic stockings/pneumatic compression devices/venodyne boots:** moderate risk.
- **Low molecular weight heparin:** patients undergoing orthopedic or neurosurgery, trauma.

CXR FINDINGS IN PULMONARY EMBOLISM

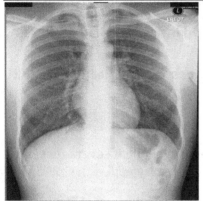

Normal CXR: *MC finding in PE**

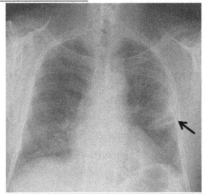

Hampton's Hump:
Wedge-shaped infiltrate/infarction (arrow). Classic (not common)

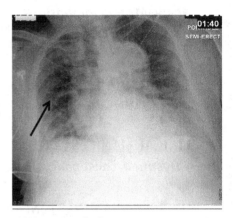

Westermark sign:
avascular markings distal to the area of the embolus. Classic (not common)

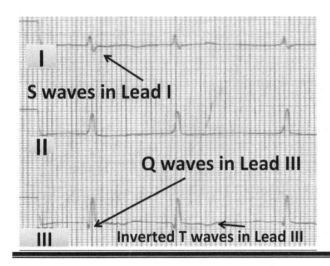

S waves in Lead I

Q waves in Lead III

Inverted T waves in Lead III

ECG FINDINGS:

❶ *Sinus Tachycardia and nonspecific ST/T wave changes MC ECG finding.**

❷ *S1Q3T3:* more specific:*
  - Deep S in lead I
  - Pathological Q wave & T wave inversion in lead III.

S1Q3T3 due to the presence of <u>cor pulmonale</u> with a large pulmonary embolus. Classic (not common).

PERC Criteria
<u>P</u>ulmonary <u>E</u>mbolism <u>R</u>ule Out <u>C</u>riteria
If all of the following is negative, you can effectively rule out PE if there is low suspicion for PE:

Age <50y	No recent trauma or surgery
Pulse <100 bpm	No hemoptysis
O2 sat: >95%	No use of exogenous estrogen
No prior PE	No unilateral leg swelling

PULMONARY HYPERTENSION

- Mean pulmonary arterial pressure ≥ 25mm Hg at rest (normal <20) or > 30 mmHg during exercise.

PATHOPHYSIOLOGY: ↑*pulmonary vascular resistance* ⇨ *RVH* ⇨ *R-sided heart failure.*

I:	***Idiopathic pulmonary arterial hypertension (Primary).*** Diagnosis of exclusion.
II:	Pulmonary HTN due to left heart disease
III:	Pulmonary HTN due to hypoxemic or chronic lung disease (ex. COPD)
IV:	Pulmonary HTN due to chronic thromboembolic disease

❶ **PRIMARY:** *idiopathic.** MC in *middle-aged or young women* (mean age of diagnosis 50y). *BMPR2 gene defect.* BMPR2 gene normally inhibits pulmonary vessel smooth muscle growth & vasoconstriction. Pulmonary vasculature is regulated by local mediators. Rare.

❷ **SECONDARY:** *secondary to pulmonary disease (COPD MC cause of 2ry,** sleep apnea, PE). Cardiac, metabolic, or systemic diseases.

CLINICAL MANIFESTATIONS

Dyspnea, chest pain, weakness, fatigue, cyanosis, edema. Exertional syncope if severe disease.

PHYSICAL EXAMINATION:

1. ***Accentuated S_2*** *(due to prominent P_2).* ± fixed or paradoxically split P_2.
2. ***Signs of R-sided heart failure:*** *↑JVP, peripheral edema, ascites.*
3. ±Systolic ejection click, pulmonary regurgitation, right ventricular heave.

DIAGNOSIS:

1. CXR: enlarged pulmonary arteries, interstitial/alveolar edema, signs of heart failure.

2. *ECG:* ***cor pulmonale:*** *RVH, right axis deviation,* right atrial enlargement, right bundle branch block.

3. Echocardiogram: large right ventricle, right atrial hypertrophy ± right to left shunt.

4. ***Right-sided heart catheterization:*** *definitive diagnosis (gold standard).**
    Mean pulmonary artery pressure ≥25mmHg @ rest (or >30 mmHg during exercise).
5. CBC: ***polycythemia*** with ***increased hematocrit.****

MANAGEMENT

1. ***Primary (idiopathic) pulmonary HTN:*** vasoreactivity trial with inhaled nitric oxide, IV adenosine or calcium channel blocker. *If vasoreactive* ⇨ ***calcium channel blockers 1st line for primary pulmonary HTN.**** If not or need additional vasodilator therapy, options include: prostacyclins (ex. *Epoprostenol,* Iloprost), phosphodiesterase-5 inhibitors (ex *Sildenafil,* Tadalafil) & endothelin receptor antagonists (Bosentan) - endothelin-1 receptor blockade causes vasodilation. Oxygen therapy, long-term anticoagulation.
    - Heart-lung transplant definitive management.
2. Type II: treat the underlying disease.
3. Type III: oxygen is the only therapy shown to decrease mortality. Treat the underlying cause.
4. Type IV: anticoagulation first line therapy. Treat the underlying cause.

PNEUMONIA

PATHOPHYSIOLOGY

Microaspiration of oropharyngeal secretions is the most common route of infection!

PATHOGEN	COMMENTS	GRAM STAIN
STREPTOCOCCUS PNEUMONIAE	*MC CAUSE OF COMMUNITY ACQUIRED PNEUMONIA (CAP)* 65%.*	Gram ⊕ cocci in pairs
HAEMOPHILUS INFLUENZAE	• *2nd MC cause of CAP.* • ↑ *with underlying pulmonary disease*:* __COPD,__* *Bronchiectasis, Cystic Fibrosis,** ETOH, diabetes, children <6y, elderly.	Gram negative rods (bacilli) (GNR)
MYCOPLASMA PNEUMONIAE	• *MC CAUSE OF ATYPICAL (WALKING PNEUMONIA)* especially <40y.* • ↑*in school-aged, college students, military recruits.** • **Clinical:** *pharyngitis, ear (BULLOUS MYRINGITIS),** URI symptoms.	*Lacks cell wall* (doesn't respond to Beta Lactams)
CHLAMYDOPHILA PNEUMONIAE	*Atypical. Hoarseness, URI symptoms, **sinusitis.***	Intracellular parasite
LEGIONELLA PNEUMOPHILA	*No person to person transmission.* Outbreaks related to __CONTAMINATED WATER SUPPLIES:__* ex: __air conditioners, cooling towers,__ etc.* • *GI symptoms: anorexia, N/V/D,↑__LFTs, hyponatremia.__** • ↑incidence: elderly, smokers, immunodeficient patients.	Intracellular GNR *(lives in aquatic environment)*
STAPHYLOCOCCUS AUREUS	*Often seen after viral illness ex. Flu.** Hematogenous spread in IVDU, ↑ in immunocompromised & elderly; Usually bilateral with multilobar infiltrates or abscesses.	Gram ⊕ cocci in clusters
KLEBSIELLA PNEUMONIAE	*Severe illness in ETOHics,* debilitated, chronic illness, aspirators. Associated with __CAVITARY__ lesions.**	Gram negative rods (bacilli)
ANAEROBES	*ASPIRATION pneumonia*, severe periodontal disease.* Fetid sputum, pulmonary abscess & empyema. *MC in R lower lobe.**	Peptostreptococcus, bacteroides, fusobacterium
PSEUDOMONAS AERUGINOSA	*Immunocompromised (ex. HIV, neutropenic, s/p transplant)* Structural abnormalities: *Cystic Fibrosis, Bronchiectasis.*	Gram negative rods (produces slime coat)
VIRAL		
RSV & PARAINFLUENZA	*MC viral cause in infants/small children.*	
INFLUENZA	*MC viral cause in adults.*	
CMV	Transplant recipients & patients with AIDS.	
VARICELLA ZOSTER	Severe in adults.	
FUNGAL/PARASITES		
Pneumocystis jirovecii (carinii) **(PCP)**	*Compromised host (fatigue, dry cough, dyspnea on exertion (__usually associated with O₂ DESATURATION WITH AMBULATION__), pleuritic chest pain.*	
Histoplasma capsulatum	*MISSISSIPPI & OHIO RIVER VALLEY** soil contaminated with *BIRD/BAT DROPPINGS.*	
Coccidioides	Found in the soil of southwest United States (in desert areas).	

MICROBIOLOGY OF PNEUMONIA

CLINICAL SETTING	ETIOLOGIES
COMMUNITY ACQUIRED PNEUMONIA (CAP)	*S. pneumoniae* *Mycoplasma, Chlamydophila,* viral (especially in young, healthy patients). *H. influenzae, M. catarrhalis* (especially in patients with COPD). *Legionella* *Klebsiella & other gram negative rods* (especially in ETOHics). *S. aureus*
HOSPITAL ACQUIRED	*__Gram negative rods:__ PSEUDOMONAS*, E. coli, Klebsiella, Enterobacter, Serratia, Acinetobacter. Also of concern is S. Aureus (especially MRSA).**
IMMUNOCOMPROMISED	Cover for the same organisms as hospital acquired. Added coverage against: PCP, fungi, Nocardia, atypical mycobacterium and viruses such as HSV & CMV.
ASPIRATION	**PNEUMONITIS:** due to aspiration of acidic gastric contents. **PNEUMONIA:** due to inhalation of oropharyngeal microbes. *± abscess.* Outpatients: typical oral flora (Strep, Staph, *anaerobes*). Inpatients or chronically ill: *gram negative rods* & S. aureus.

Hospitalize if multilobar, ⊕ neutropenia or patients have comorbidities that may complicate treatment.
Chlamydia pneumoniae = Clamydophila pneumoniae

COMMUNITY ACQUIRED PNEUMONIA: ❶ *acquired OUTSIDE of the hospital setting* & patient is not a resident of a long-term care facility (ex. nursing home) OR ❷ patient that was ambulatory prior to admission who develops pneumonia *within 48 hours of initial hospital admission*.

HOSPITAL ACQUIRED (NOSOCOMIAL) PNEUMONIA: pneumonia occurring *>48 hours after hospital admission.** Often caused by *Pseudomonas, MRSA* & other organisms found in the hospital.

	TYPICAL PNEUMONIA	ATYPICAL PNEUMONIA
ORGANISMS	*S. pneumoniae* H. influenzae Klebsiella pneumoniae S. Aureus	*Mycoplasma pneumoniae* Chlamydophila pneumoniae Legionella pneumophila Viruses
CHEST X RAY	Lobar pneumonia	Diffuse, patchy interstitial or reticulonodular infiltrates.
CLINICAL MANIFESTATIONS	• sudden onset of fever • productive cough c purulent sputum • pleuritic chest pain • *Rigors (especially S. pneumoniae)** • tachycardia, tachypnea	• Low grade fever • Dry, nonproductive cough • *Extrapulmonary symptoms:* myalgias, malaise, sore throat, headache, N/V/D.
PHYSICAL EXAMINATION	**Signs of consolidation:*** • *bronchial breath sounds* • *dullness on percussion* • *↑TACTILE FREMITUS, EGOPHONY* • Inspiratory rales (crackles)	*Often normal.* ±crackles, rhonchi. Signs of consolidation usually absent.

*****Elderly or confused patients:** may not present with respiratory symptoms, fever or increased WBC count. May present with depressed mental functioning/AMS.

ATYPICAL ORGANISMS

CHLAMYDOPHILA ⇨ hoarseness, fever ⇨ respiratory symptoms after a few days. Send IgM, IgG titers.

MYCOPLASMA ⇨ ear pain, *BULLOUS MYRINGITIS,** erythematous pharynx or tympanic membranes. Persistent nonproductive cough. Send *serum cold agglutinins* as part of the diagnostic workup.

LEGIONELLA ⇨ *associated with GI sx, ↑LFTs, hyponatremia.** Send Legionella urine antigen ±PCR.

DIAGNOSTIC WORKUP OF PNEUMONIA

A. **CXR/CT SCAN** CXR resolution may lag behind clinical improvement for weeks. A pleural effusion may be present (usually exudative).
  1. Abscess formation ⇨ *S. aureus*, *Klebsiella*, anaerobes.
  2. *Upper lobe (especially R upper lobe) with bulging fissure, cavitations* ⇨ *Klebsiella*.

B. **SPUTUM (gram stain/culture):** utility debated. Gross sputum may reveal clues to pathogen:
  1. *Rusty (blood-tinged)* ⇨ *Strep pneumoniae*   3. green sputum ⇨ H. flu, Pseudomonas

  2. *Currant jelly* ⇨ *Klebsiella*   4. foul smelling ⇨ anaerobes

C. **PHYSICAL EXAMINATION**

	PERCUSSION	FREMITUS	BREATH SOUNDS
PNEUMONIA	Dullness	**INCREASED***	**Bronchial, EGOPHONY***
PLEURAL EFFUSION	Dullness	Decreased	Decreased
PNEUMOTHORAX or OBSTRUCTIVE LUNG DISEASE	**HYPERRESONANCE***	Decreased	Decreased

ANTIBIOTIC MANAGEMENT OF PNEUMONIA	
CLINICAL SCENARIO	**EMPIRIC TREATMENT GUIDELINES**
COMMUNITY-ACQUIRED, OUTPATIENT	*Macrolide or Doxycycline first line.** Fluoroquinolones only used first line if comorbid conditions/recent antibiotic use.
COMMUNITY-ACQUIRED, INPATIENT	*[β lactam + macrolide (or Doxycycline)] OR broad spectrum FQ*
COMMUNITY-ACQUIRED IN *ICU*	*β lactam + macrolide OR β lactam + broad spectrum FQ* *If documented β-lactam allergy: FQ, ± Aztreonam (or Clindamycin + Aztreonam)
HOSPITAL ACQUIRED *(pseudomonas infection risk)**	*Anti-PSEUDOMONAL β lactam & anti-PSEUDOMONAL AG or FQ* - Add *Vancomycin* or Linezolid *if MRSA is suspected.** - Add *Levofloxacin* or *Azithromycin* if *Legionella* is suspected. - Add Trimethoprim/sulfamethoxazole ±corticosteroids if PCP suspected. **If documented β-lactam allergy:* Fluoroquinolone ± Clindamycin. Aztreonam, Aminoglycoside
ASPIRATION *(anaerobes)*	Clindamycin or Metronidazole or Amoxicillin/clavulanic acid

Inpatients therapy is IV antibiotics. Change to oral when clinically responding, able to take PO.
1. **β-lactams:** *Ceftriaxone* (Rocephin); Cefotaxime, Ampicillin/sulbactam (Unasyn) or Ertapenem (Invanz).
2. **Anti-Pseudomonal β-lactams:** *Piperacillin/tazobactam* (Zosyn), *Cefepime* (Maxipime); Imipenem (Primaxin), Meropenem (Merrem), Ceftazidime.
3. **Macrolides:** Clarithromycin, Azithromycin.
4. **Respiratory FQ (fluoroquinolone):** *Levofloxacin* (Levaquin), *Moxifloxacin* (Avelox); Gemifloxacin (Factive).
   Please note that *Ciprofloxacin is NOT a respiratory fluoroquinolone* (may be used for Pseudomonas or Legionella)
5. **Aminoglycosides (AG):** *Amikacin, Gentamicin, Tobramycin.*
• Supplemental oxygen, IV fluids, respiratory isolation (if suspect tuberculosis).

PNEUMOCOCCAL VACCINE

PCV13 Pneumococcal Conjugate Vaccine (Prevnar): contains 13 serotypal antigenic polysaccharides. Used in ***childhood vaccination.****
- Healthy children <24 months are given 4 doses: 2, 4, 6, and at 12-15 months of age.
- High-risk children ≥2y of age, should also receive a single dose of PPSV23 at least 8 weeks after they have completed immunization series of PCV13.

PPSV23 Pneumococcal Polysaccharide Vaccine (Pneumovax): - contains capsular *polysaccharides* of 23 of the MC pneumococcal serotypes. Indications:
- *Age ≥ 65 years.* If they received a dose prior to 65, they should receive a dose at 65y if ≥5 years have elapsed since the prior dose.
- *Age ≥2-64 with chronic diseases:* cardiac, pulmonary, diabetes, ETOH, liver disease, chronic care facility , immunocompromised (HIV, malignancy, chronic renal disease, chemotherapy, asplenia, transplant recipients, sickle cell). Single revaccination if ≥5y elapsed since 1st dose.
S/E: 1/3 develop mild local pain, erythema @ site, fever, myalgias.
CI: anaphylaxis to prior dose, used with caution in patients with severe illness.
Influenza vaccine given yearly as well.

SILHOUETTE SIGN

Borders of the heart lost when similar density (pneumonia) lies adjacent. Helps localize lung lesions.

Right heart border → R middle lobe

Left heart border → Lingular

R hemidiaphragm → R lower lobe

L hemidiaphragm → L lower lobe

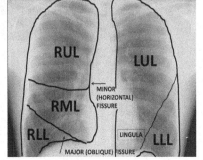

NORMAL CXR – PA VIEW

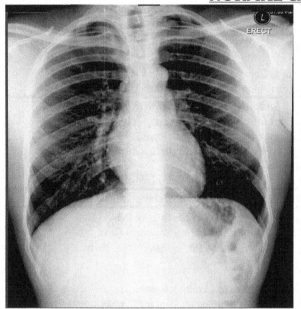 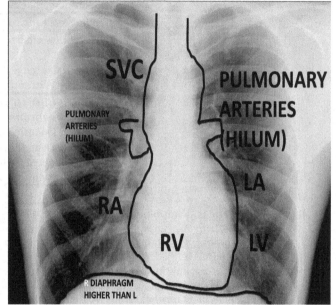

NORMAL CXR – LATERAL VIEW

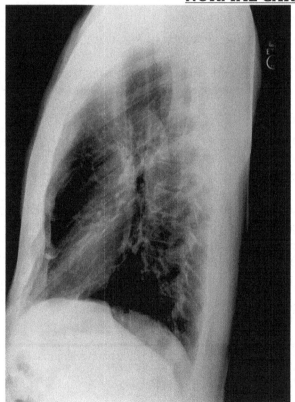 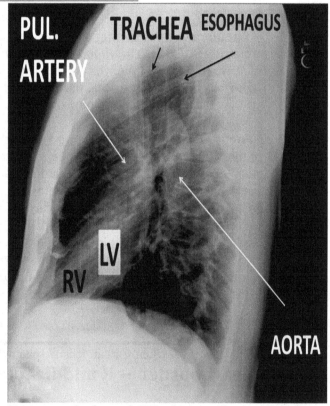

Notice on the lateral CXR, the vertebrae get darker as you descend and the heart has retrocardiac and anterior dark areas.

NORMAL CXR

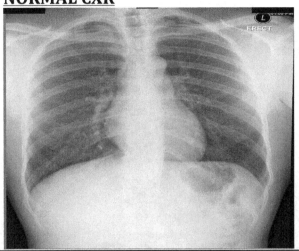

MULTILOBAR PNEUMONIA

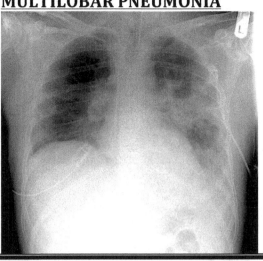

MYCOPLASMA PNEUMONIA

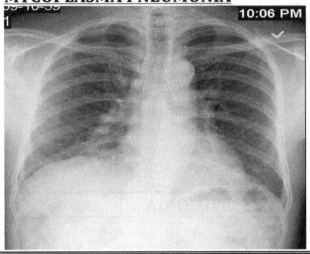

LEFT LOWER LOBE PNEUMONIA

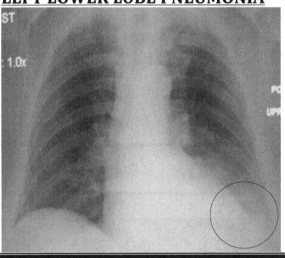

LINGULAR PNEUMONIA

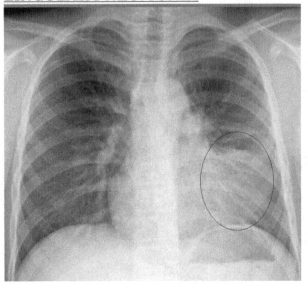

Lingular PNA obscures the <u>left heart border.</u>*

RIGHT MIDDLE LOBE PNEUMONIA

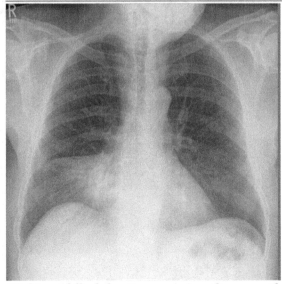

Right middle lobe Pneumonia: <u>obscures the right heart border.</u>* Right diaphragm is clear.

BRONCHIECTASIS

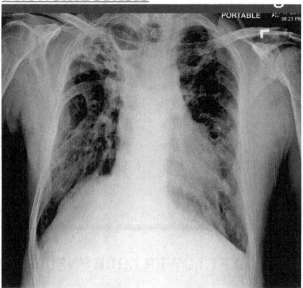

Bronchiectasis with cavitary lesion (air-fluid level in the R apex) of the lung with multiple interstitial markings.

PCP PNEUMONIA

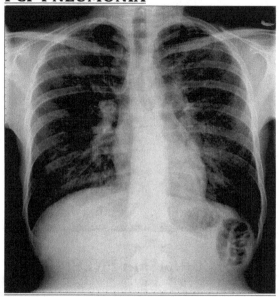

PCP Pneumonia: May have normal CXR 10-40% of cases. When ⊕, CXR findings classically show **bilateral diffuse symmetric finely granular opacities/reticular-interstitial airspace disease** 80% Often with central location (can resemble non cardiogenic pulmonary edema).

LEFT UPPER LOBE PNEUMONIA

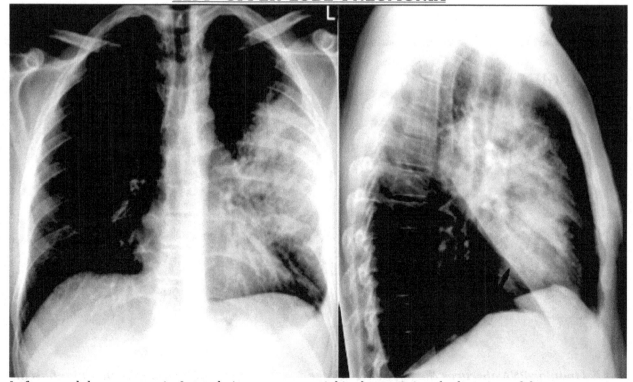

Left upper lobe pneumonia. Lateral views are essential in determining the location of the pneumonia.

TUBERCULOSIS

- Chronic infection with *Mycobacterium tuberculosis* leading to **granuloma formation**.
- High mortality rates in untreated smear positive (50-80%). <5% mortality when treated.

HIGH RISK POPULATIONS
↑risk of exposure: close contacts of patients with active TB, health care workers.
↑risk of TB infection: immigrants from high-prevalence areas, homeless.
↑risk active TB once infected: immunodeficiency (***HIV*** ⊕, CRI, DM, IVDA, ETOHics, malignancy).

PATHOPHYSIOLOGY
- Inhalation of airborne droplets ⇨ Mycobacterium reaches the alveoli & are ingested by alveolar macrophages. Mtb may remain viable within the macrophage or bypass the immune system.

OUTCOMES OF INFECTION WITH TUBERCULOSIS
1. PRIMARY TB: the outcome of initial infection (usually self-limiting).
    - **Primary Rapidly Progressive TB:** active initial infection with clinical progression ⇨ these patients are contagious! Common in children (especially <4y) in endemic areas.

2. CHRONIC (LATENT) INFECTION: *~90% control* initial primary infection via **granuloma formation**. These granulomas may become ***CASEATING*** * (central necrosis, acidic with low oxygen, making it hostile for Mtb to grow). Usually become ***PPD*** ⊕ *2-4 weeks after infection. Patients with Latent TB infection are NOT contagious!* *

3. SECONDARY (REACTIVATION) TB: *reactivation of latent TB with waning immune defenses** (elderly, HIV, steroid use, malignancy). 5-10% lifetime incidence. *MC* localized in **apex/upper lobes with cavitary lesions** (↑O_2 content of lung apices). **These patients are contagious!**

CLINICAL MANIFESTATIONS OF ACTIVE TUBERCULOSIS
1. **Pulmonary TB:**
    pulmonary sx: chronic, productive cough, chest pain (often pleuritic). *Hemoptysis if advanced.*
    constitutional sx: night sweats, fever/chills, fatigue, anorexia, weight loss.
    - **Physical exam:** *signs of consolidation,* rales or rhonchi near apices/involved areas, dullness. May have normal exam.
2. **Extra-pulmonary TB:** can affect any organ. ***Vertebral (Pott's disease); Lymph nodes (scrofula);*** TB meningitis, pericarditis, peritonitis, joints, kidney, adrenal or cutaneous involvement.

3. **TB & HIV infection:** *HIV 7-10% yearly chance of reactivation* of latent infection.

TB SCREENING FOR INFECTION
Purified Protein Derivative (PPD): *examine 48-72h for TRANSVERSE INDURATION (redness not considered positive).*

REACTION SIZE	PERSONS CONSIDERED TO HAVE ⊕ TEST
≥5 mm	- *HIV* ⊕ *or immunosuppressed* (ex. Prednisone 15mg/day >1 month). - *Close contacts of patients with active TB.* - *CXR consistent with old/healed TB (calcified granuloma).*
≥10 mm	- *All other high-risk populations/high prevalence populations.* - Recent conversion = ↑induration by >10 mm in the past 2 years.
≥15 mm	Everyone else (no known risk factors for TB)
False negative	**Anergy** *(HIV, sarcoidosis)*, **Faulty application** (if given SQ instead of TD), acute TB (normally takes 2-10 weeks to convert), acute non-TB infections, malignancy.
False ⊕	**Improper reading, cross reaction with an atypical** (ex Mycobacterium avium complex), **within 2-10yrs of BCG vaccination** (although usually <10mm).
Booster effect	Infected person's immune system "forgets" about TB until years later when testing "reminds" the immune system. Next PPD will be ⊕ because of initial infection (years ago) NOT because recently converted. Confirmed by 2-step PPD testing.

DIAGNOSTIC STUDIES IN SUSPECTED CASES OF ACTIVE TB

1. **Acid-fast Smear & sputum culture x 3 days.** TB ruled out after 3 negative smears.
   *AFB cultures gold standard.** Early AM gastric specimens if unable to give sputum.

2. **CXR:** ❶ indicated to *exclude active TB (ex. newly ⊕ PPD)* ❷ *used as yearly screening in patients with known positive PPD to r/o active TB.* ± be normal or show variety of patterns:
   - **Reactivation:** *apical (upper lobe)* fibrocavitary disease.
   - **Primary TB**: *middle/lower lobe* consolidation.
   - **Miliary TB:** CXR shows small *__millet-seed__* like nodular lesions (2-4mm).
   - TB pleurisy: pleural effusion caused by tuberculosis infection.
   - Granuloma: residual evidence of healed primary TB. Ghon's complex: calcified primary focus + lymph node. Ranke's complex: healed fibrocalcific Ghon complex seen on CXR.

3. **Interferon Gamma Release Assay:** blood test with improved specificity, no reader bias, no booster phenomenon & not affected by prior BCG vaccination. Ex. Quantiferon-TB Gold assay.

TREATMENT OF ACTIVE TB INFECTION

- *INITIAL 4 DRUG REGIMEN* (x2mos). *TOTAL TREATMENT DURATION OF ACTIVE IS 6 MONTHS** (or 3 months after negative sputum culture). If culture shows sensitivity to both INH & RIF ⇨ stop ETH or STM. PZA usually discontinued after 2 months regardless of sensitivity results.
- *"RIPE" or "RIPS": Rifampin + INH + Pyrazinamide + Ethambutol* (or *Streptomycin*)
- Respiratory precautions/isolation. *No longer considered infectious 2 weeks after initiation of therapy.* Directly observed therapy (DOT) for patients at high risk for noncompliance.
- INH prophylaxis given to children <4y with exposure to contacts with active disease.

FIRST LINE ANTI-TUBERCULOUS MEDICATIONS		
DRUG	**ADVERSE EFFECTS**	**CONSIDERATIONS**
RIFAMPIN (RIF)	*Thrombocytopenia,** flu-like symptoms. *Orange colored secretions** (ex tears, urine). GI upset, hypersensitivity, fever, hepatitis.	**MOA:** inhibits RNA synthesis **CI:** in patients taking protease inhibitors, NNRTIs
ISONIAZID (INH)	*Hepatitis* (especially ↑35y of age).* *Peripheral neuropathy.** Drug-induced lupus, rash. Abdominal pain, high anion gap acidosis. Cytochrome P450 inhibition.	**MOA:** inhibits mycolic acid synthesis *Peripheral neuropathy prevented by pyridoxine (B$_6$).** Baseline LFTs recommended.
PYRAZINAMIDE (PZA)	*Hepatitis & hyperuricemia.* GI symptoms, arthritis. *Photosensitive dermatologic rash.*	Can be given after 1st trimester. *Caution in gout or liver disease.**
ETHAMBUTOL (EMB)	*Optic neuritis** ⇨ scotoma, color perception problems (red-green), visual changes.* *Peripheral neuropathy*, GI symptoms, rash.	
STREPTOMYCIN (STM)	*Ototoxicity (CN 8), nephrotoxicity.**	Streptomycin is an aminoglycoside.

2nd line treatment: Amikacin, Ciprofloxacin, Moxifloxacin.

TREATMENT OF LATENT TB INFECTION (LTBI)	
SCENARIO	**REGIMEN**
Likely INH sensitive	*INH + Pyridoxine (Vitamin B6) x 9 months.** Alternatives: RIF x 4 months or INH+ Rifapentine (DOT).
HIV ⊕	*INH + Pyridoxine (Vitamin B6) x 12 months.**
Contact case INH-resistant	RIF + PZA x 4 months (consult with ID specialist).

Latent TB diagnosis must meet *3 criteria*: ❶ *asymptomatic* person who is ❷PPD ⊕ & ❸ *NO evidence of active infection on CXR/CT scan (these patients are NOT contagious).*
- Treatment of latent tuberculosis infection reduces risk of reactivation TB in the future.

NORMAL CXR

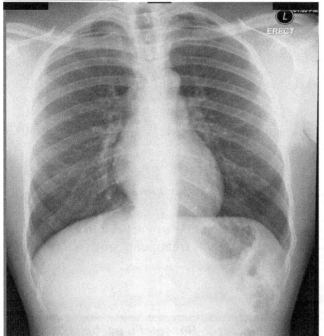

MILIARY TUBERCULOSIS

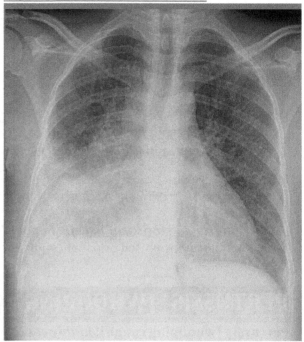

CLASSIC MILIARY TB: *diffuse millet seed size* infiltrates throughout the lung fields.

CLASSIC PRIMARY TB

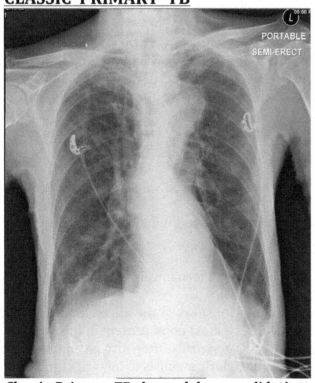

Classic Primary TB: lower lobe consolidation. Right-sided hilar consolidation also seen here.

CLASSIC REACTIVATION TB

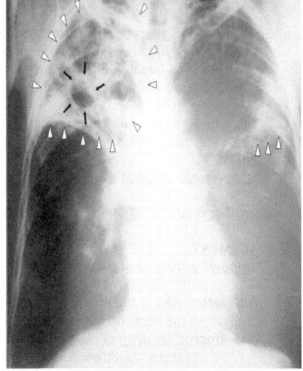

CLASSIC REACTIVATION TB: infiltrates and *cavitation* in the *upper lobe/apices.*

ACUTE BRONCHITIS

ACUTE BRONCHITIS: *inflammation of trachea/bronchi* (conducting airways). *Often follows URI.*

MC caused by viruses:* *adenovirus,* parainfluenza, influenza, coronavirus, coxsackie, rhinovirus, respiratory syncytial virus. Bacterial: *S. pneumoniae, H. influenzae, M. catarrhalis, Mycoplasma.*

CLINICAL MANIFESTATIONS:
- **Hallmark is cough*** (± productive, ± last 1-3 weeks). ±Symptoms similar to pneumonia.

DIAGNOSIS
1. Diagnosis is usually clinical without the need for imaging. If pneumonia is suspected, order a CXR.
2. **Chest radiograph:** *usually normal or nonspecific.***

MANAGEMENT
1. **Symptomatic treatment of choice:*** fluids, rest, ±bronchodilators. *± antitussives only in adults.*

2. **Antibiotics no statistical benefit in healthy patients.*** Antibiotics ± beneficial in elderly, COPD, immunocompromised or patients not responsive to conservative treatment, cough >7-10 days.

PERTUSSIS (WHOOPING COUGH)

Pertussis (whooping cough): *highly contagious infection* 2ry to *Bordetella pertussis.*
- Rarely seen due to widespread vaccination. Gram negative coccobaccillus. MC seen in children <2y.

CLINICAL MANIFESTATIONS
7-10 day incubation period. *catarrhal phase* ⇨ *paroxysmal phase* ⇨ *convalescent phase.*
1. **Catarrhal phase:** URI symptoms lasting 1-2 weeks. Most contagious during this phase.

2. **Paroxysmal phase:** *severe paroxysmal coughing fits* with *inspiratory whooping sound after cough fits.*** *± Post coughing emesis.* Coughing fits may occur spontaneously or can be provoked by laughing, yawning, etc. Often lasts 2-4 weeks. ±Scattered rhonchi. May develop subconjunctival hemorrhage from the increased pressure due to the coughing fits.

3. **Convalescent phase:** resolution of the cough (coughing stage may last for up to 6 weeks).

DIAGNOSIS
1. PCR of Nasopharyngeal swab: *gold standard.* Performed in the first 3 weeks of symptom onset.

2. **Lymphocytosis*** - 60-80% lymphocytes on differential. WBC count may be as high as 50,000.

MANAGEMENT
1. **Supportive treatment mainstay:*** oxygenation, nebulizers, mechanical ventilation as needed.

2. **Antibiotics** used in the management to decrease contagiousness of the affected patient (only shortens the duration within the 1st 7 days of sx onset – most don't present in this stage).
   - **Macrolides drug of choice*** (Erythromycin, *Azithromycin*). Often also given to exposed contacts. Azithromycin may ↑risk of infantile pyloric stenosis in infants <1 month.
   - *Trimethoprim-sulfamethoxazole 2nd line* if allergic to macrolides.

COMPLICATIONS: include *pneumonia*, encephalopathy, otitis media, sinusitis and seizures. ↑mortality in infants due to apnea/cerebral hypoxia associated with coughing fits.

BRONCHIOLITIS

Bronchiolitis: *inflammation of the bronchioles.*

TYPES OF BRONCHIOLITIS

1. **ACUTE BRONCHIOLITIS:** *MC seen in children 2 months - 2 years old after viral infection (esp RSV, Adenovirus).* Due to neutrophil infiltration of the bronchioles. The inflammatory process causes bronchiole narrowing. Fibrosis is not usually seen with acute bronchiolitis.

2. **BRONCHIOLITIS OBLITERANS (CONSTRICTIVE)**
   - Patchy chronic inflammation & fibrosis of the bronchioles ⇨ collapse/obliteration of the bronchioles. Granulation tissue in the bronchiole lumen ⇨ obstructive lung disease. Mosaic pattern on CT scan.
   - MC seen with post lung transplant rejection, inhalation injuries (ex silo filler's dz), drug reactions, RA. **Mgmt:** high-dose Corticosteroids & immunosuppression. Lung transplant definitive treatment.

3. **CRYPTOGENIC ORGANIZING PNEUMONIA (COP)**
   - Formerly known as Bronchiolitis Obliterans with Organizing Pneumonia (BOOP).
   - Persistent alveolar exudates ⇨ inflammation & scarring *(fibrosis) of the **bronchioles AND alveoli**.* Resembles pneumonia on CXR but does not respond to antibiotics. CXR findings that persist despite clinical improvement of the patient. Often idiopathic or occurs after pneumonia.
     Management: *Corticosteroids.*

ACUTE BRONCHIOLITIS

Lower respiratory tract infection of the *small airways* ⇨ proliferation/necrosis of the bronchiolar epithelium produces obstruction from the sloughed epithelium, increased mucus plugging, & submucosal edema leading to ***peripheral airway narrowing & variable obstruction.***

- ***RESPIRATORY SYNCYTIAL VIRUS (RSV) MC CAUSE*** (50-70%). **RSV part of paramyxovirus family.**** Other: adenovirus, influenza, parainfluenza; ±mycoplasma pneumonia, chlamydia trachomatis.

- **RISK FACTORS:** *Infants <2y MC affected (esp ~2 mos).* <6months in age, exposure to cigarettes, lack of breastfeeding, premature (<37 weeks gestation) & crowded conditions. MC in fall & spring.

- **COMPLICATIONS:** *otitis media with S. pneumoniae MC acute cx (asthma MC cx later in life).**

CLINICAL MANIFESTATIONS: *fever, URI symptoms 1-2 days* ⇨ *respiratory distress** (wheezing, tachypnea, nasal flaring, cyanosis, retractions ±rales).

DIAGNOSIS: CXR: hyperinflation, peribronchial cuffing, etc. Nasal washings using monoclonal Ab testing. *Pulse ox single best predictor of disease in children* (<96% ⇨ admit to hospital).

MANAGEMENT:

1. ***Supportive: humidified O_2 mainstay of treatment** - delivered by mask, tent or hood. IV fluids, Acetaminophen/Ibuprofen for fever; Mechanical ventilation if severe.

2. ***Medications play a limited role** ± β-agonists, ±*nebulized racemic* epinephrine (if albuterol not effective); Corticosteroids <u>not</u> indicated unless history of underlying reactive airway disease.

3. ***Ribavirin ± administered if severe lung or heart disease or in immunosuppressed patients.***

PREVENTION: ***Palivizumab prophylaxis may be used in ↑risk groups.** *Hand washing preventative!** RSV is highly contagious & is transmitted via direct contact with secretions and self-inoculation by contaminated hands.

ACUTE EPIGLOTTITIS (SUPRAGLOTTITIS)

Epiglottitis: *inflammation of epiglottis* that may interfere with breathing *(medical emergency).* Mortality usually secondary to asphyxiation.

- ***HAEMOPHILUS INFLUENZAE TYPE B (Hib) MC*** (reduced incidence due to Hib vaccination). May rarely be caused by Streptococcus pneumoniae, S. aureus, GABHS (Streptococcal pyogenes).
- Non Hib seen more commonly seen in adults (especially in patients with crack, cocaine use).

- MC in children 3 months – 6 years. Males 2x MC. Occurs in any season. DM risk factor in adults.

CLINICAL MANIFESTATIONS

1. ***"3 D's" – Dysphagia, D̲ROOLING* & D̲istress.*** Fever, ***odynophagia, inspiratory stridor***, dyspnea, hoarseness, muffled voice, ***tripoding:*** sitting leaned forward with the elbow on the lap.

2. Suspect in a patient with rapidly developing pharyngitis, muffled voice & odynophagia out of proportion to physical findings.

DIAGNOSIS

1. ***Laryngoscopy: definitive diagnosis.*** Provides direct visualization but may provoke spasm. Cherry-red epiglottis with swelling.

2. **Lateral Cervical radiograph:** *THUMB* (or THUMBPRINT) *sign:* swollen, enlarged epiglottis.

3. ***If high suspicion, D̲O N̲OT attempt to visualize the epiglottis with a tongue depressor in children.*** May be attempted in adults.

MANAGEMENT:

❶ ***Maintaining the airway & supportive management is the mainstay of treatment:***
   - Place child in a comfortable position and keep the child calm to avoid airway issues.
   - Dexamethasone to reduce airway edema.
   - Tracheal intubation to protect the airway in severe cases.

❷ *Antibiotics: 2nd/3rd gen cephalosporins:* Ceftriaxone or Cefotaxime.
   ±add Penicillin, Ampicillin or anti-staphylococcal coverage.

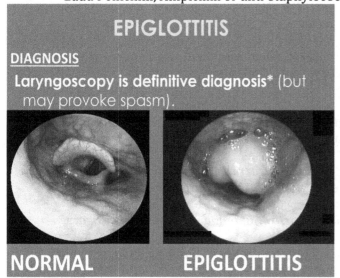

EPIGLOTTITIS

DIAGNOSIS

Laryngoscopy is definitive diagnosis* (but may provoke spasm).

NORMAL   EPIGLOTTITIS

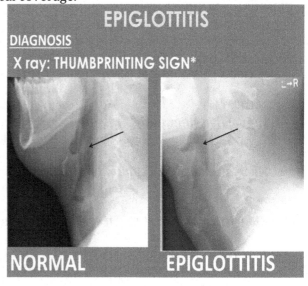

EPIGLOTTITIS

DIAGNOSIS

X ray: THUMBPRINTING SIGN*

NORMAL   EPIGLOTTITIS

LARYNGOTRACHEITIS (CROUP)

Inflammation MC 2ry to acute viral infection of the UPPER AIRWAY (larynx, subglottis, trachea) ⇨
  subglottic larynx/trachea swelling* ⇨ stridor, "BARKING" cough, hoarseness.

- *PARAINFLUENZA VIRUS type 1 MC CAUSE,** adenovirus RSV, rhinovirus etc.   Diphtheria rare.
- 15% of children experience croup in childhood *(MC 6 months – 6 years).* MC in fall/winter.

CLINICAL MANIFESTATIONS
  ❶ *"Barking" cough* (seal-like, harsh).*
  ❷ *stridor* both *inspiratory* & expiratory (worsened by crying or agitating the child).
  ❸ *hoarseness* due to laryngitis.
  ❹ *dyspnea (especially worse at night).* ±URI symptoms* either preceding or concurrent, fever.

DIAGNOSIS:
  1. Clinical diagnosis (once epiglottitis & foreign body aspiration are excluded).
  2. Frontal **cervical radiograph: STEEPLE SIGN*** (*subglottic narrowing of trachea)* - 50%.

MANAGEMENT
  1. **Mild** (no stridor at rest, no respiratory distress): *cool humidified air mist, hydration. Dexamethasone provides significant relief* as early as 6 hours after single dose (oral or IM). Supplemental O_2 in patients with O_2 sat <92%. Patients can be discharged home.

  2. **Moderate** (stridor at rest with mild to moderate retractions): Dexamethasone PO or IM + supportive treatment. ±nebulized Epinephrine. Should be observed for 3-4 hours after clinical intervention. May be discharged home if improvement is seen.

  3. **Severe** (stridor at rest with marked retractions): *Dexamethasone + nebulized epinephrine & hospitalization.*

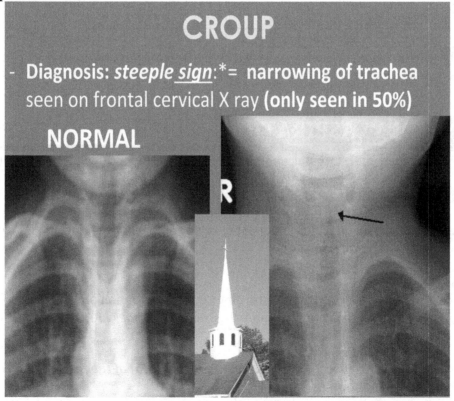

CROUP
- Diagnosis: *steeple sign*:*= narrowing of trachea seen on frontal cervical X ray **(only seen in 50%)**
NORMAL

INFLUENZA

- Acute respiratory illness caused by Influenza A or B viruses. Part of the Orthomyxovirus family.
- *A is associated with more severe, extensive outbreaks.*
- Spreads primarily via airborne respiratory secretions. Outbreaks occur mainly in fall/winter.

CLINICAL MANIFESTATIONS:
1. *Usually **abrupt** onset* of a wide range of symptoms: headache, fever, chills, malaise, URI symptoms, pharyngitis, pneumonia. *Myalgias MC seen in legs & lumbosacral area.*

DIAGNOSIS: usually clinical. Rapid influenza test (nasal swab) or viral culture may be performed.

MANAGEMENT
1. *Supportive mainstay of treatment in healthy patients* (ex. acetaminophen or salicylates, rest).

2. *Antivirals usually only needed in patients with high risk of complications or if hospitalized.* *Best if initiated **within 48 hours of the onset of symptoms.***
    A. **Antivirals vs Influenza A & B (including H1N1) - Neuraminidase inhibitors**
        - *__Oseltamivir (Tamiflu)__* oral. S/E: nausea, vomiting.
        - Zanamivir (Relenza) diskhaler
        - Ribavirin nucleoside analog works against both (especially with aerosol administration).
    B. Antivirals vs. Influenza A *widespread resistance. Not commonly used.*
        1. Amantadine (Symmetrel) S/E: CNS, jitteriness, anxiety, insomnia, difficulty concentrating.
        2. Rimantadine (Flumadine) less side effects than Amantadine.

PREVENTION
Influenza vaccine given annually (usually in October or November).
1. **INFLUENZA TRIVALENT VACCINE:** *CI: eggs, gelatin or thimerosal allergies;** caution if severely ill.

• ≥65 years of age (≥50y advocated by some sources)	• Residents of nursing home/long term care facilities
• Underlying chronic medical conditions ex. Asthma, COPD, sickle cell, heart, DM	• Healthcare workers; immunocompromised
• Contacts of patients infected with influenza	• Women who are pregnant/will be in influenza season

2. **INTRANASAL:** *(live attenuated)* not routinely used. Ind: *healthy patients 2-49* years of age.
   CI: >50y, pregnancy, *immunocompromised,* DM, chronic lung or heart dz, egg allergy, h/o Guillain-Barré.

FOREIGN BODY ASPIRATION

- Risk factors: altered mental status, alcoholism, impaired cough/swallowing reflex, dementia.

- *__MC on the right side__** (due to wider, more vertical & shorter right main bronchus). Position may influence location: Supine: MC in superior segment of the right lower lobe. Sitting/standing: MC in posterobasal segment of the right lower lobe. Lying on right side: MC in right middle lobe or posterior segment of the right upper lobe.

CLINICAL MANIFESTATIONS
- Coughing, choking, wheezing or hemoptysis. May develop aspiration pneumonia.
- Gastric aspiration may cause acute respiratory distress syndrome (ARDS).

DIAGNOSIS
1. **Bronchoscopy: *provides direct visualization of and removal of the foreign object.***
2. CXR: regional hyperinflation.

ACUTE RESPIRATORY DISTRESS SYNDROME

Life threatening <u>acute hypoxemic respiratory failure</u> (organ failure from prolonged hypoxemia).

MC develops in <u>critically ill patients</u> (most develop ARDS while already in the hospital for another reason).
<u>Acute</u>* = hrs to days after inciting event (ex. **<u>sepsis MC*</u>**, severe trauma, aspiration of gastric contents etc.)

PATHOPHYSIOLOGY

- Inflammatory lung injury due to <u>pro-inflammatory cytokines</u> ⇨ <u>diffuse alveolar damage</u> ⇨ **↑*<u>permeability of alveolar-capillary barrier</u>*** ⇨ **pulmonary edema** & alveolar fluid influx, loss of surfactant & vascular endothelial damage ⇨ ↓blood oxygenation.

CLINICAL MANIFESTATIONS:

Acute dyspnea & hypoxemia. Multi-organ failure if severe.

DIAGNOSIS:

3 main components: ❶ severe refractory hypoxemia is HALLMARK of ARDS* ❷ bilateral pulmonary infiltrates on CXR & ❸ the absence of cardiogenic pulmonary edema/CHF (PCWP <18mm Hg).

1. **ABG:** PaO_2/FIO_2 ratio ≤200 mmHg that is **not responsive to 100% O_2 (refractory hypoxemia)***

HYPOXEMIA	PaO_2/FIO_2 ratio (mmHg)	VENTILATION
Mild:	200 – 300	PEEP or CPAP ≥5cm H_2O (formerly Acute Lung Injury).
Moderate:	100 - 200	PEEP ≥5 cm H_2O
Severe:	< 100	PEEP ≥5 cm H_2O

2. **CXR:** *<u>diffuse bilateral pulmonary infiltrates*</u> ⇨ white out pattern* (CXR resembles CHF).
   - *<u>ARDS characteristically spares the costophrenic angles.</u>**

ADULT RESPIRATORY DISTRESS SYNDROME
Pulmonary Capillary Wedge Pressure:
- *CXR of ARDS & cardiogenic pulmonary edema looks the same*
- *PCWP <18mmHg→ ARDS**
- *PCWP >18mmHg→ Cardio Pul. Edema*

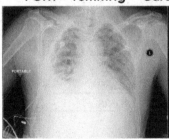 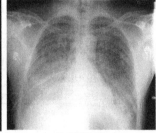

Cardiogenic Pulmonary Edema   **ARDS**

3. **Cardiac catheterization of pulmonary artery (Swan-Ganz):** *pulmonary capillary wedge pressure (PCWP) <18mmHg.** PCWP differentiates ARDS from cardiogenic pulmonary edema. Normal 12-18mmHg.
   - *<u>Low/normal PCWP in ARDS.</u>** Normal left atrial pressure in ARDS.
   - high PCWP in cardiogenic pulmonary edema (>18mmHg).

MANAGEMENT:

1. *<u>Noninvasive or mechanical ventilation & treat the underlying cause:</u>*
   - CPAP with full face mask. Attempt to keep O_2 saturation >90%
   - **Positive End Expiratory Pressure (PEEP):** prevents airway collapse @ end expiration, increases FRC, decreases shunting & expands the alveoli for increased diffusion. Used to maintain PaO_2 >55 mmHg (attempt to maintain FIO_2 <60 to prevent oxygen toxicity).

SLEEP APNEA

- **RISK FACTORS:** *obesity strong risk factor,** Age: MC in 6th & 7th decades. Men more common.

TYPES

1. **Central sleep apnea:** reduced CNS respiratory drive leads to decreased respiratory effort.

2. **Obstructive sleep apnea:** physical airway obstruction (may be due to external airway compression, decreased pharyngeal muscle tone, increased tonsillar size or deviated septum).

CLINICAL MANIFESTATIONS

1. Snoring, unrestful sleep (which may lead to chronic daytime sleepiness). Nocturnal choking.
2. **Physical examination:** large neck circumference, crowded oropharynx, micrognathia.

DIAGNOSIS

1. **In-laboratory polysomnography:** *first line diagnostic test.**
   ≥15 events/hr: obstructive or mixed apneas, hypopneas, respiratory effort arousals etc.

2. Labs: polycythemia (due to chronic hypoxemia) may be seen.
3. Epworth sleepiness scale: used to quantify patient's perception of fatigue and sleep.

MANAGEMENT

1. *CPAP: continuous positive airway pressure mainstay of therapy in adults.**
2. Behavioral: weight loss, exercise, abstaining from alcohol, changes in sleep positioning.
3. Oral appliances can be tried if CPAP is unsuccessful or as an alternative.
4. Surgical correction. Tracheostomy is considered the definitive treatment for obstructive sleep apnea. Other interventions include: nasal septoplasty & uvulopalatopharyngoplasty.

Complications include: pulmonary hypertension, arrhythmias.

NORMAL BREATH SOUNDS

BRONCHIAL	Loud high-pitch sounds heard over trachea and larynx (manubrium).	*Expiration (longer) > inspiration*
BRONCHOVESICULAR	Medium-pitched sounds heard over the primary bronchus and posteriorly between the scapula.	Expiration = Inspiration
VESICULAR	Soft, gentle sounds over all the areas.	Inspiration > expiration

ABNORMAL BREATHING

1. **CHEYNE-STOKES:** *cyclic breathing in response to __hypercapnia.__** Smooth increases in respirations & then gradual decrease in respirations with a period of apnea 15-60 seconds.
   Due to *decreased brain blood flow* slowing the impulses to the respiratory center.

2. **BIOT'S BREATHING:** *irregular respirations (quick shallow breaths of equal depth)* with *irregular periods of apnea* (usually of equal depth in comparison to Cheyne-Stokes breathing).
   *Can be seen with damage to the __medulla oblongata or opioid use.__**

3. **KUSSMAUL'S RESPIRATION:** (hyperpnea): *deep, rapid, continuous respirations** as a result of *metabolic acidosis* - deep breaths with large tidal volumes (body's attempt to compensate by blowing off excess CO_2). No expiratory pause (no stopping between inhalation & exhalation).

1. **LUNGS:** *CO_2 regulation* via respiratory rate (min-hours). *Acidosis stimulates ↑respiration* (to blow off excess CO_2). *Alkalosis depresses respiration* (to retain CO_2).
2. **KIDNEYS:**
   - *generates new HCO_3^- by eliminating H^+* from body (adds one HCO_3^- for every H^+ secreted)
   - *reabsorbs virtually all filtered HCO_3^-:* at the *proximal tubule*.
     _↑HCO_3^- reabsorption seen with ↑PCO_2, hypovolemia, hypokalemia.

Anion Gap Metabolic Acidosis	Non-Gap Metabolic Acidosis	Acute Respiratory Acidosis	Metabolic Alkalosis	Respiratory Alkalosis
"MUDPILERS"	**"HARDUPS"**	*anything that causes hypoventilation, i.e.:* "CHAMPP"	**"CLEVER PD"**	**"CHAMPS"**
Methanol	Hyperalimentation		Contraction	*anything that causes hyperventilation, i.e.:*
Uremia	Acetazolamide		Licorice*	
DKA/Alcoholic KA	Renal Tubular Acidosis	Endo* (Ex Conn's, Cushing's)		
Propylene glycol	Diarrhea	CNS depression (drugs/CVA)		CNS disease
Isoniazid, Infection	Uretero-Pelvic Shunt		Vomiting	Hypoxia
Lactic Acidosis	Post-Hypocapnia	Hemo/Pneumothorax	Excess Alkali*	Anxiety
Ethylene Glycol	Spironolactone	Airway Obstruction	Refeeding Alkalosis*	Mech Ventilators
Rhabdo/Renal Failure		Myopathy	Post-hypercapnia	Progesterone
Salicylates		Pneumonia	Diuretics*	Salicylates/Sepsis
		Pulmonary Edema		
Too much acid or little Bicarbonate	*Too much acid or little Bicarbonate*	*Anything that decreases respiration*	*Little acid or too much bicarbonate*	*Anything that causes hyperventilation*

HIGH ANION GAP METABOLIC ACIDOSIS

↑*Anion Gap acidosis:* the acid in blood dissociates into H^+ & an anion not routinely measured (the H^+ is buffered by HCO_3^- leaving the unmeasured anion to accumulate in serum, creating the AG)

$$HUa + NaHCO_3 \Rightarrow NaUa + H_2CO_3 \Rightarrow CO_2 + H_2O$$

NORMAL GAP METABOLIC ACIDOSIS (HYPERCHLOREMIC)

Normal Gap Acidosis: lost HCO_3^- is replaced by Cl^- (a measured anion) so there is no change in AG but there is an accumulation of Cl^- concentration. In other cases (diarrhea, type II RTA) there is loss of $NaHCO_3$ and the kidney tries to preserve volume by retaining NaCl (same overall sequelae).

$$HCl + NaHCO_3 \Rightarrow NaCl + H_2CO_3 \Rightarrow CO_2 + H_2O$$

METABOLIC ALKALOSIS

- ↑*HCO_3^- (serum) with ↑pH* requires generating & maintenance factors.

ETIOLOGIES (GENERATING FACTORS)

1. **Loss of H^+ from GI tract/kidneys:** *vomiting/NG suction (loss of gastric HCl* that is perpetuated by EFCV depletion), chronic diarrhea (also perpetuated by EFCV depletion), loop diuretics.
2. **Exogenous alkali or contraction alkalosis:** diuresis ⇨ excretion of HCO_3^- poor fluid ⇨EFCV "contracts" around stable level of HCO_3^- ⇨ ↑HCO_3^- concentration.
3. **Post hypercapnia:** rapid correction of respiratory hypercapnia (ex mechanical ventilation) ⇨ transient excess HCO_3^- until kidney can excrete it.

RESPIRATORY ACIDOSIS

Anything that decreases respiration.
1. **Acute Respiratory failure:** *CNS depression* (opioids, sedatives, trauma), cardiopulmonary arrest, pneumonia.
2. **Chronic respiratory failure:** COPD, obesity, neuromuscular disorders (ex. Myasthenia gravis, Guillain-Barré syndrome etc).

RESPIRATORY ALKALOSIS

1. **Hyperventilation:** CNS disorders, pain, anxiety, salicylates, progesterone, pregnancy, hepatic failure, stimulation of pulmonary receptors (pneumonia, asthma).

SIMPLIFIED 3-STEP APPROACH TO ACID BASE DISORDERS

<u>Normal Values:</u> Na: 135-145; Cl: 105, HCO_3^-: 24 (22-26); P_{CO2} = 40 (35-45); AG 10-12; pH = 7.35-7.45, PO_2: 80-100

Step 1: <u>Identify the most *apparent* disorder</u> ✓pH
pH normally 7.35 – 7.45. If in normal range, still check PCO_2 & HCO_3. If abnormal, a disorder may be present.
If pH > 7.45 ⇨ Alkalosis
If pH < 7.35 ⇨ Acidosis

Step 2: <u>Look at P_{CO2} is it normal, low or high??</u>
Normal P_{CO2} 35-45
- **If P_{CO2} *is in going in the opposite direction as the pH, then the 1ry disorder is respiratory.***
- Think **RO**ME (In primary **R**espiratory disorders, P_{CO2} & pH are in **O**pposite directions).
- <u>Respiratory compensation:</u> in primary metabolic disorders, if the P_{CO2} is going in the same direction as the pH, then there is partial respiratory compensation (full compensation if the pH is normal).

Step 3: *<u>Look at [HCO₃⁻] it normal, low or high?</u>*
Normal [HCO₃⁻] 22-26
- *If [HCO₃⁻] is in going in the same direction as the pH, then the 1ry disorder is metabolic.*
- Think RO**ME** (In primary **M**etabolic disorders, HCO_3 & pH are in the same/**E**qual direction).
- <u>Metabolic compensation:</u> in primary respiratory disorders, if the [HCO₃⁻] is going in the opposite direction as the pH, then there is a partial metabolic compensation (full compensation if the pH is normal).

Perform step 4 & 5 ONLY if the primary disorder is metabolic acidosis.

Step 4: If metabolic acidosis is present, calculate the anion gap.
Anion gap (AG) = Na - (Cl⁻ + HCO3⁻)   Normal anion gap 10 - 12

Step 5: If a high anion gap is present in step 4, perform step 5 - calculate the **Delta Ratio** to look for the presence of additional disorders.
(Measured AG – 12)/(24 – measured bicarbonate)

[Measured anion gap – Normal AG (use 12)]

Normal Bicarb (use 24) – measured HCO3

- If 1-2   ⇨   pure elevated anion gap metabolic acidosis only.
- <1   ⇨   normal anion gap metabolic acidosis is also present.
- >2   ⇨   metabolic alkalosis or compensated chronic respiratory acidosis is also present.

EXAMPLE 1: 21 year old with Type I DM presents with nausea vomiting, fruity breath.

pH: 7.29   paCO2: 22   HCO3: 13   Na: 134 Cl: 91 HCO3: 12

CASE 1: pH: 7.45   paCO2: 56   HCO3: 37

CASE 2: pH: 7.29   paCO2: 58   HCO3: 22

CASE 3: pH: 7.32   paCO2: 34   HCO3: 14   Na: 135 Cl: 109 HCO3: 14

CASE 4: pH: 7.49   paCO2: 42   HCO3: 36

CASE 5: pH: 7.36   paCO2: 58   HCO3: 29

CASE 6: pH: 7.25   paCO2: 25   HCO3: 10   Na: 140 Cl: 77 HCO3: 10

CASE 7: pH: 7.48   paCO2: 28   HCO3: 18

CASE 8: pH: 7.28   paCO2: 26   HCO3: 11   Na: 129 Cl: 100 HCO3: 10

EXAMPLE 1 explained: 21 year old with Type I DM presents with nausea vomiting, fruity breath.

Na: 134	Cl: 91	BUN: 29	pH: 7.29	pCO2: 22
K: 5.8	HCO3: 13	Cr: 1.6	HCO3: 12	glucose: 780

Step 1: **Identify the most *apparent* disorder** ✓pH

pH normally 7.35 – 7.45. **pH = 7.29** ↓⇨ *Acidosis*

Step 2: **Look at P_{CO2} is it normal, low or high??**

Normal P_{CO2} 35–45. **pCO2: 22**↓   Normal $[HCO_3^-]$ 22-26. **HCO3: 12**↓

- Think RO**ME** (In primary **M**etabolic disorders, HCO_3 & pH are in the same/**E**qual direction)
    = *primary metabolic acidosis.*
- In primary metabolic disorders, if the P_{CO2} is going in the same direction as pH (which it is in this example), then there is partial respiratory compensation.

Perform step 4 & 5 ONLY if a metabolic acidosis is the primary disorder (which it is in this example)

Step 4: If metabolic acidosis is present, calculate the anion gap.

 AG = Na - (Cl- + HCO3-)   Normal anion gap 10 – 12. 134 – (91 + 13) = 30 = ↑*AG acidosis*

Step 5: If high anion gap is present, calculate the **Delta Ratio** to look for the presence of additional disorders.

(Measured AG – 12)/(24 – measured bicarbonate) (30-12)/(24-13) = **1.64**

- If 1-2 = *pure elevated anion gap metabolic acidosis = final answer* (probably DKA in this case).

ANSWERS

Case 1: Primary Metabolic Alkalosis with full respiratory compensation (normal pH)

Case 2: Primary Respiratory Acidosis uncompensated (since HCO3 is normal)

Case 3: Normal Gap Metabolic Acidosis with partial respiratory compensation.

Case 4: Primary Metabolic Alkalosis uncompensated (since PCO2 is normal)

Case 5: Primary Respiratory Acidosis with full metabolic compensation (normal pH)

Case 6: Mixed disorder: Primary elevated anion gap acidosis + metabolic alkalosis (delta >2).

Case 7: Primary Respiratory Alkalosis with partial metabolic compensation.

Case 8: Primary high anion gap metabolic acidosis with partial respiratory compensation + concurrent non anion gap acidosis (since delta <1)

PULMONARY CHAPTER REFERENCES

Light RW, Macgregor MI, Luchsinger PC, Ball WC. Pleural effusions: the diagnostic separation of transudates and exudates. Ann Intern Med. 1972;77(4):507-13.

Lim WS, Baudouin SV, George RC, et al. BTS guidelines for the management of community acquired pneumonia in adults: update 2009. Thorax. 2009;64 Suppl 3:iii1-55.

Haber RJ. A practical approach to acid-base disorders. West J Med. 1991;155(2):146-51.

Asthma Gudelines. Available at: http://www.nhlbi.nih.gov/guidelines/asthma/asthgdln.

Gold Criteria. Available at: http://www.goldcopd.org/uploads/users/files/GOLD_Report_2013_Feb20#14. Accessed February 21, 2014.

Available at: http://www.ncbi.nlm.nih.gov/books/NBK7232/pdf/TOC. Accessed February 12, 2014.

Sarcodosis. Available at: http://carta.anthropogeny.org/moca/topics/sarcoidosis. Accessed February 22, 2014.

Cherry JD. Clinical practice. Croup. N Engl J Med. 2008;358(4):384-91.

Green H, Paul M, Vidal L, Leibovici L. Prophylaxis for Pneumocystis pneumonia (PCP) in non-HIV immunocompromised patients. Cochrane Database Syst Rev. 2007;(3):CD005590.

Nair GB, Niederman MS. Community-acquired pneumonia: an unfinished battle. Med Clin North Am. 2011;95(6):1143-61.

Grundy S, Bentley A, Tschopp JM. Primary spontaneous pneumothorax: a diffuse disease of the pleura. Respiration. 2012;83(3):185-9.

Porcel JM, Light RW. Pleural effusions due to pulmonary embolism. Curr Opin Pulm Med. 2008;14(4):337-42.

Ashrafian H, Athanasiou T, Yap J, Desouza AC. Two-chamber intracardiac mesothelioma. Asian Cardiovasc Thorac Ann. 2005;13(2):184-6.

Proulx AM, Zryd TW. Costochondritis: diagnosis and treatment. Am Fam Physician. 2009;80(6):617-20.

Ohtani Y, Saiki S, Kitaichi M, et al. Chronic bird fancier's lung: histopathological and clinical correlation. An application of the 2002 ATS/ERS consensus classification of the idiopathic interstitial pneumonias. Thorax. 2005;60(8):665-71.

O'reilly KM, Mclaughlin AM, Beckett WS, Sime PJ. Asbestos-related lung disease. Am Fam Physician. 2007;75(5):683-8. Hollander AG. Byssinosis. Dis Chest. 1953;24(6):674-8.

Castranova V, Vallyathan V. Silicosis and coal workers' pneumoconiosis. Environ Health Perspect. 2000;108 Suppl 4:675-84.

Meltzer EB, Noble PW. Idiopathic pulmonary fibrosis. Orphanet J Rare Dis. 2008;3:8.

Elborn JS, Johnston B, Allen F, Clarke J, Mcgarry J, Varghese G. Inhaled steroids in patients with bronchiectasis. Respir Med. 1992;86(2):121-4.

O'malley CA. Infection control in cystic fibrosis: cohorting, cross-contamination, and the respiratory therapist. Respir Care. 2009;54(5):641-57.

Tønnesen P. Smoking cessation and COPD. Eur Respir Rev. 2013;22(127):37-43.

Ahluwalia SK, Matsui EC. The indoor environment and its effects on childhood asthma. Curr Opin Allergy Clin Immunol. 2011;11(2):137-43.

PULMONARY PHOTO CREDITS

Chapter 2 – Pulmonary Disorders

CHAPTER 3 – GASTROINTESTINAL & NUTRITIONAL DISORDERS

GI BASICS INTRODUCTION

THE STOMACH FUNCTIONS TO MECHANICALLY & CHEMICALLY DIGEST FOOD

MECHANICAL: strong movements of the stomach muscles mix & help to mechanically break down food.

CHEMICAL: hydrochloric acid & pepsin assist in the chemical breakdown of food.
- **Hydrochloric acid:** *secreted by the parietal cells* has many functions, including:
  ❶ *dissolving food* (solvent), ❷ *activating pepsin* (for protein digestion), ❸ *stimulating the duodenal release of* other digestive enzymes & ❹ *killing harmful bacteria in food.*

- **Pepsin:** digests proteins into small, absorbable peptides. The prehormone pepsinogen is *secreted by the chief cells* (to prevent autodigestion). Pepsinogen is converted to pepsin (active form) in the acidic environment of the gastric lumen (due to the presence of hydrochloric acid).

HORMONAL REGULATION OF DIGESTION

PARIETAL CELLS ARE STIMULATED BY 3 HORMONES:
1. **Gastrin:** *stimulates stomach acid secretion & motility.* G cells secrete gastrin, which causes the enterochromaffin-like cells (ECL) to secrete histamine ⇨ parietal cell secretion of hydrochloric acid.

2. **Histamine:** produced by ECL cells in response to gastrin. *Histamine stimulates the parietal cells to secrete hydrochloric acid.* H_2 blockers are meds are used to reduce acid secretion.

3. **Acetylcholine:** *directly stimulates the parietal cells to secrete hydrochloric acid.* The parasympathetic system (primarily via the vagus nerve) *increases gastrointestinal activity (secretion & motility).*
   Acetylcholine is known as the "rest & digest" neurotransmitter.

NEGATIVE FEEDBACK
Somatostatin produced by the pancreatic delta (D-cells) act as negative feedback, *inhibiting the secretion of gastrin,* insulin, glucagon, pancreatic enzymes & inhibiting gallbladder contraction.

MUCUS LAYER PROTECTION

- mucus production
- bicarbonate production

LARGE INTESTINE RESPONSIBLE FOR WATER ABSORPTION

The large intestine consists of the cecum & the colon. The 3 main functions are to:
1. Absorb the remaining water from undigested food (main function).

2. Transport undigested food for removal via feces – contains Haustra.

3. Absorb certain vitamins produced by bacteria: ex. vitamin K, biotin.

THE DUODENUM RESPONSIBLE FOR MOST OF SMALL INTESTINE ABSORPTION

The duodenum is responsible for most of the chemical digestion by the small intestine & regulates the rate of gastric emptying. The duodenum receives the chyme from the stomach, analyzes it & releases the appropriate amount of hormones to continue the digestive process.

1. **SECRETIN:** *released by the duodenum.* Secretin inhibits parietal cell gastric acid production & causes the pancreas to release bicarbonate (to buffer the acid from the chyme leaving the stomach that is entering the duodenum).
   - **Clinical correlation:** In the evaluation of hypergastrinemia, the administration of secretin (secretin test) will lead to reduced gastrin levels except for in Zollinger-Ellison syndrome *(ZES is associated with no suppression of gastrin levels with the Secretin test).*

2. **CHOLECYSTOKININ (CCK):**
   - aids in the breakdown of fats & proteins by *stimulating pancreatic release of digestive enzymes* (trypsin, amylase & lipase).

   - *increases bicarbonate release.* Bicarbonate neutralizes the acid from the stomach. The pancreatic enzymes work maximally in the basic environment provided by the release of bicarbonate.

   - *stimulates gallbladder contraction & bile release.* Bile salts help to emulsify fats into smaller micelles (to make the breakdown of fats by lipase more effective).
      Clinical correlation: *biliary colic is usually worse after a fatty meal* (due to *CCK-mediated* contraction of the gallbladder & the release of bile).

THE PANCREAS FUNCTION AS BOTH AN EXOCRINE & ENDOCRINE GLAND

EXOCRINE GLAND: *acinar cells* produce substances that drain into the duodenum:
1. **Bicarbonate**: neutralizes gastric acid in the duodenum & activates enzymes (such as protease, amylase & lipase). Bicarbonate secretion is stimulated by secretin.

2. **Proteases:** (trypsinogen, chymotrypsinogen) precursors to enzymes that break down proteins. Proteases are released in an inactive form to prevent autodigestion of the GI tract.

3. **Amylase**: breaks down starches into simple sugars.
4. **Lipase:** breaks down fats into fatty acids (with the help of bile salts which ↑ the surface area).

ENDOCRINE GLAND: islets of Langerhans:
1. **insulin** (produced by beta cells): decreases blood glucose levels.
2. **glucagon** (produced by alpha cells): increases blood glucose levels.

3. **somatostatin** (produced by delta cells): *suppresses the release of GI hormones*: CCK, gastrin, secretin, vasoactive intestinal peptide, insulin, glucagon & pancreatic enzymes. In the CNS, somatostatin inhibits growth hormone production.
   Clinical correlation: *Octreotide (somatostatin analog) is used in the medical management of growth-hormone producing tumors (acromegaly, gigantism), some pituitary tumors,* as well as *flushing & diarrhea associated with carcinoid syndrome & VIP secreting tumors. Also used for bleeding esophageal varices* (Octreotide decreases splanchnic circulation). Octreotide imaging may be used to localize neuroendocrine tumors (ex. carcinoid tumors, Zollinger-Ellison syndrome).

COMMON TESTS USED IN GASTROENTEROLOGY

ABDOMINAL RADIOGRAPHS (AXR):
1. **Ind:** evaluates the stomach, liver, spleen as well as both large & small intestines. Can be used as part of the evaluation of abdominal pain. Used to assess for radiopaque stones (ex. calcium oxalate, calcium phosphate & struvite stones), assesses for foreign bodies, assess for free air (if perforation is suspected) or confirm placement of tubes (such as nasogastric tubes).

UPPER ENDOSCOPY (ESOPHAGOGASTRODUODENOSCOPY – EGD):
1. **Endoscopy:** flexible fiber optic tube (endoscope) with a camera on the end. Used to evaluate the upper GI tract (esophagus, stomach & duodenum).
2. **Indications:** evaluate ulcers, diagnose & treat some of the causes of upper GI bleeding, biopsy lesions, evaluate reflux, remove foreign objects in the upper GI tract & evaluate patients with swallowing difficulties.
3. **Diagnostic test of choice:** *Mallory-Weiss tears, peptic ulcer disease, suspected malignancies.*

UPPER GI SERIES (BARIUM SWALLOW, ESOPHAGRAM):
1. **Upper GI series:** specialized radiograph to evaluate the upper GI tract (esophagus, stomach & duodenum). Barium is radiopaque (helpful to outline structures). Fluoroscopy is a video form used to evaluate movement. Sometimes a "double contrast" study is done where air is also given to further delineate structures. In a "small bowel follow through", radiographs are taken at intervals to follow barium's path through the small intestine (ex. terminal ileum).
2. **Indications:** evaluate esophageal motility disorders/webs/rings, evaluate peristalsis, patients with difficulty swallowing, look for scars or strictures & evaluate lesions in the upper GI tract.
3. **Contraindications:** not used if perforation suspected (barium is an irritant outside of the structures of the GI tract). Water-soluble contrast (ex. Gastrografin) can be used if perforation is suspected.
4. **Diagnostic test of choice:** *UGI series with small bowel follow through* is the *test of choice for evaluating a patient with acute Crohn disease.* UGI series good for esophageal webs.

LOWER GI SERIES (BARIUM ENEMA):
1. **Barium enema:** used to evaluate the colorectal area. A double contrast enema may be done as well.
2. **Indications:** often helpful for evaluating inflammatory bowel disease, may show evidence of polyps, evaluate diverticulosis, colon cancer, diagnose & treat intussusception & evaluate for colitis.
3. **Contraindications:** *not used if bowel perforation suspected,* contraindicated in acute ulcerative colitis (may cause toxic megacolon).*

COLONOSCOPY:
1. **Colonoscopy:** a fiber optic tube is passed via the anus to evaluate the entire colorectal area.
2. **Flexible Sigmoidoscopy:** limited form that goes only to the sigmoid area (distal area of the colon).
3. **Indications:** diagnose & treat some of the causes of lower GI bleed, biopsy suspicious lesions, evaluate inflammatory bowel diseases (ulcerative colitis, Crohn disease), other forms of colitis as well as remove colonic polyps for evaluation & treatment.

ENDOSCOPIC RETROGRADE CHOLANGIOPANCREATOGRAPHY (ERCP):
1. **ERCP:** Upper GI endoscopy + radiographs to diagnose & treat disorders of the bile ducts or the pancreatic ducts (ex gallstones, tumors, infection, cholangitis).
2. **Complications:** pancreatitis, perforation & hemorrhage.

ESOPHAGEAL MANOMETRY (ESOPHAGEAL MOTILITY STUDY)
1. **Esophageal Manometry:** used to monitor pressure changes especially of the lower esophageal sphincter & the upper esophageal sphincter. A catheter is placed via the nasal cavity.
2. **Indications:** motility disorders, evaluate peristalsis in patients with difficulty swallowing.
3. **Diagnostic test of choice:** *achalasia, nutcracker esophagus.* May be used to diagnose GERD.

ESOPHAGITIS

ETIOLOGIES
❶*GERD MC cause,* ❷ *infectious in immunocompromised* (ex. *Candida, CMV, HSV*); radiation therapy, medication or corrosive ingestion, eosinophilic (associated with food allergies, atopic disease).

RISK FACTORS: pregnancy, smoking, obesity, ETOH use, chocolate, spicy foods,
   Medications: NSAIDs, beta blockers, calcium channel blockers, bisphosphonates.

CLINICAL MANIFESTATIONS
 - Odynophagia (painful swallowing), dysphagia (difficulty swallowing), retrosternal chest pain.

DIAGNOSIS: *upper endoscopy* allows for direct visualization. Double-contrast Esophagram.

MANAGEMENT: treat the underlying cause.

INFECTIOUS ESOPHAGITIS

ETIOLOGIES: *infectious esophagitis MC in IMMUNOCOMPROMISED PATIENTS.** *Candida, CMV, HSV*.

CLINICAL MANIFESTATIONS: *odynophagia** *hallmark*, dysphagia, retrosternal chest pain.

DISEASE	ENDOSCOPIC FINDINGS	1ST LINE MANAGEMENT	2ND LINE
CANDIDA	*linear yellow-white plaques**	*PO Fluconazole**	Voriconazole, Caspofungin
CMV	*large superficial shallow ulcers**	*Ganciclovir**	Valganciclovir, Foscarnet
HSV	*small, deep ulcers**	*Acyclovir**	Foscarnet

EOSINOPHILIC ESOPHAGITIS

• *Allergic, inflammatory eosinophilic infiltration* of the esophageal epithelium. MC seen in children.
ETIOLOGIES
   MC associated with *atopic disease* (ex. food allergies, non food allergies, asthma, eczema, etc.).

CLINICAL MANIFESTATIONS: *dysphagia* (especially solids), ± reflux or feeding difficulties in children.

DIAGNOSIS: Endoscopy: normal, ±*multiple corrugated rings** on the esophagus, ±white exudates.

MANAGEMENT
 1. Remove foods that incite allergic response. Inhaled topical corticosteroids (<u>without</u> using spacer).

PILL-INDUCED ESOPHAGITIS

ETIOLOGIES: MC due to prolonged pill contact with the esophagus (ex. patients with prolonged supination after pill ingestion). MC seen with NSAIDs, *bisphosphonates,* potassium chloride, iron pills, vitamin C, beta blockers & calcium channel blockers.

CLINICAL MANIFESTATIONS: odynophagia, dysphagia.
DIAGNOSIS: <u>Endoscopy:</u> small, well-defined ulcers of varying depths.

MANAGEMENT: take pills with at least 4 ounces of water, avoid recumbency for at least 30-60 minutes after pill ingestion.

CAUSTIC (CORROSIVE) ESOPHAGITIS

ETIOLOGIES: ingestion of corrosive substances: alkali (drain cleaner, lye, bleach) or acids.

CLINICAL MANIFESTATIONS: odynophagia, dysphagia, hematemesis, dyspnea.

DIAGNOSIS: endoscopy is used to determine the extent of damage & look for complications:
ex. esophageal perforation, stricture & esophageal fistula.

MANAGEMENT: supportive, pain medications, IV fluids.

GASTROESOPHAGEAL REFLUX DISEASE (GERD)

• **_Transient relaxation of LES_** (incompetency) ⇨ gastric acid reflux ⇨ esophageal mucosal injury.

PATHOPHYSIOLOGY: multifactorial: ↑gastric acid, **_incompetent Lower Esophageal Sphincter (LES),_** esophageal motility disorders & delayed gastric emptying, ±Hiatal hernia.

COMPLICATIONS: ❶esophagitis ❷stricture ❸Barrett's esophagus & ❹esophageal _adenocarcinoma._
BARRETT'S: **_esophageal squamous epithelium replaced by precancerous metaplastic columnar cells_** from the cardia of the stomach (more used to the acidic environment but don't belong there).

CLINICAL MANIFESTATIONS
Typical symptoms: _HEARTBURN (PYROSIS) hallmark* often retrosternal & postprandial_ (MC 30-60 minutes after eating, **_increased with supine position*_** & often relieved with antacids; **_regurgitation_** (water brash, sour taste in the mouth), **_dysphagia,_** cough at night (acid aspiration into the lungs causes lung irritation/cough).

Atypical symptoms: hoarseness, aspiration pneumonia, "asthma" (bronchospasm from acid contact with the lung), **_noncardiac chest pain_** _(most common cause of noncardiac chest pain),_ weight loss.

"ALARM" symptoms: **_dysphagia, odynophagia, weight loss, bleeding_** (suspect malignancy or cx).

DIAGNOSIS:
1. _Clinical diagnosis based on history_ (especially if presenting with classic, simple symptoms).

2. **_Endoscopy_**_: **often used 1st***_ if persistent symptoms or complications of GERD (ex. malignancy etc).

3. **Esophageal Manometry:** **_↓LES pressure.*_** May be used if upper endoscopy is normal.

4. **_24h ambulatory pH monitoring: gold standard.*_** Only needed if symptoms are persistent.

MANAGEMENT OF GASTROESOPHAGEAL REFLUX DISEASE
Stage 1: Lifestyle Modifications: elevation of the head of the bed by six inches, _avoid recumbency for three hours after eating_, eating small meals, avoiding certain foods (ex. fatty/spicy, citrus, chocolate, caffeinated products, peppermint), decrease fat & ETOH intake, weight loss, smoking cessation.

Stage 2: "As Needed" Pharmacological Therapy: antacids & OTC **_H₂ receptor antagonists._***
If alarm or atypical symptoms (see above), **_upper endoscopy is the next appropriate step.*_**

Stage 3: Initiation of Scheduled Pharmacologic Therapy: H₂RA, PPI & prokinetic agents (Cisapride).
Proton pump inhibitors drug of choice in moderate-severe disease.* Nissen fundoplication if refractory.

ACHALASIA

ETIOLOGY: idiopathic proximal *loss of Auerbach's plexus** ⇨ *INCREASED LES PRESSURE.** MC in 5th decade.

PATHOPHYSIOLOGY: *failure of LES relaxation (↑LES tone)** ⇨ *obstruction* & *lack of peristalsis.*
Auerbach's plexus = esophageal wall ganglion cells which normally produce nitric oxide, leading to smooth muscle relaxation of the lower esophageal sphincter (LES). Without inhibitory nitric oxide ⇨↑LES tone. Esophageal dilation may occur if left untreated.

CLINICAL MANIFESTATIONS: *dysphagia to BOTH solids & liquids,* malnutrition, weight loss, dehydration, regurgitation of undigested food, chest pain, cough. Symptoms usually between 25-60y.

DIAGNOSIS:
1. **Esophageal Manometry:** *gold standard.** Shows *increased LES pressure* >40mmHg, ↓peristalsis.

2. **Double-contrast esophagram:** "*BIRD'S BEAK APPEARANCE of LES*"* *(LES narrowing)* with proximal esophageal dilation, loss of peristalsis distally. Manometry is more definitive than esophagram.
3. **Endoscopy:** may be needed to rule out esophageal carcinoma or other etiologies.

MANAGEMENT: *decrease LES pressure:* botulinum toxin injection lasts 6-12 months, nitrates, calcium channel blockers, pneumatic dilation of LES. Esophagomyomectomy (GERD common complication).

DIFFERENTIAL DIAGNOSIS:
1. **DIFFUSE ESOPHAGEAL SPASM:** strong non-peristaltic esophageal contractions.
   CLINICAL: *stabbing, chest pain worse with hot or cold liquids/foods.** (pain similar to angina).
   DIAGNOSIS: *Esophagram* shows *"corkscrew"** esophagus. Endoscopy, Manometry.
   MANAGEMENT: nitrates, calcium channel blockers.

2. **ZENKER'S DIVERTICULUM** *pharyngoesophageal diverticulum.* **Clinical:** *Dysphagia,* sense of "lump" in the neck, neck mass, regurgitation of food, cough, halitosis (old, trapped food in pouch).

NUTCRACKER ESOPHAGUS

ETIOLOGY: unknown cause. May be associated with GERD. *Excessive contractions during peristalsis.*
CLINICAL MANIFESTATIONS: dysphagia (liquids/solids), chest pain. May be asymptomatic.

DIAGNOSIS: Manometry: *increased pressure during peristalsis.** Normal EGD/esophagram.

MANAGEMENT: lower esophageal pressure (calcium channel blockers, nitrates, botox, sildenafil).

ZENKER'S DIVERTICULUM

• *Pharyngoesophageal pouch (false diverticulum – only involves the mucosa).* Weakness at the junction between *cricopharyngeus muscle* & lower inferior constrictor ⇨ *herniation*/outpouching.

CLINICAL MANIFESTATIONS: *dysphagia,* regurgitation of undigested food, cough, feeling as if there is a lump in neck (neck mass), choking sensation, halitosis (due to food retention in the pouch).

DIAGNOSIS:
1. **Barium Esophagram:** collection of dye behind esophagus @ pharyngoesophageal junction.

MANAGEMENT: diverticulectomy, cricopharyngeal myotomy. Observation if small & asymptomatic.

BOERHAAVE SYNDROME

- **_Full thickness rupture_** of the **_distal esophagus._** Associated with **_repeated, forceful vomiting_** (ex. Bulimia) or iatrogenic perforation of the esophagus during endoscopy.

CLINICAL MANIFESTATIONS
Retrosternal chest pain worse with deep breathing & swallowing,* hematemesis.
    Physical: _crepitus on chest auscultation_ due to **_pneumomediastinum*_** (air in the mediastinum).

DIAGNOSIS
1. **Chest CT scan/CXR**: pneumomediastinum, esophageal thickening. Left-sided hydropneumothorax.
2. **Contrast esophagram**: **_definitive diagnostic study_**. $\oplus$ leakage. Gastrografin swallow preferred.

MANAGEMENT: small & stable: IV fluids, NPO, antibiotics, H_2 blockers. Surgical repair if large/severe.

MALLORY-WEISS SYNDROME (TEARS)

UGI bleeding from <u>_longitudinal mucosal lacerations_</u> _@ the gastroesophageal junction or the gastric cardia._

PATHOPHYSIOLOGY: sudden rise in intragastric pressure or gastric prolapse into the esophagus (ex. **_persistent retching/vomiting after ETOH binge*_** or bulimic vomiting). 5-10% of all acute UGIB.

CLINICAL MANIFESTATIONS: **_retching/vomiting_** $\Rightarrow$ **_hematemesis after an ETOH binge,*_** melena, hematochezia, syncope, abdominal pain, **_hydrophobia._**

DIAGNOSIS: upper endoscopy test of choice: **_superficial longitudinal mucosal erosions._**

MANAGEMENT:
1. **_Supportive_**. Most cases stop bleeding without intervention. Acid suppression promotes healing.
2. Severe bleeding $\Rightarrow$ epinephrine injection, sclerosing agent, band ligation, hemoclipping or balloon tamponade (ex Sengstaken-Blakemore tube or Minnesota tube).

ESOPHAGEAL WEBS & RINGS

ESOPHAGEAL WEB: thin membranes in the mid-upper esophagus. May be congenital or acquired (ex. as a complication of eosinophilic esophagitis).
    Plummer-Vinson Syndrome: ❶ **_dysphagia_** + ❷ **_esophageal webs_** + ❸ **_iron deficiency anemia._**
    Atrophic glossitis, angular cheilitis, koilonychias, splenomegaly. MC in Caucasian women 30-60y

SCHATZKI RING: lower esophageal webs/constrictions @ the squamocolumnar junction.
    MC associated with sliding hiatal hernias but may be a complication of corrosive esophageal injury.

CLINICAL MANIFESTATIONS
1. dysphagia especially to solids.

DIAGNOSIS
1. **_Barium esophagram (swallow): diagnostic test of choice_** (more sensitive than endoscopy).

MANAGEMENT
    Endoscopic dilation of the area if symptomatic without reflux. Antireflux surgery if reflux is present.

ESOPHAGEAL VARICES

- *__Dilation of the gastroesophageal collateral submucosal veins__* as a complication of *__portal vein hypertension__*.

RISK FACTORS: *Cirrhosis MC cause in adults* (portal vein thrombosis MC cause in children).
> 90% of patients with cirrhosis develop esophageal varices, 30% of them bleed (mortality rate 30-50% with 1st bleed). 70% rebleed within 1st year of the initial bleed (1/3 of re-bleeds are fatal).

CLINICAL MANIFESTATIONS: *upper GI bleed* (hematemesis, melena, hematochezia). Causes 5-11% of all upper GI bleeding. May develop signs & symptoms of hypovolemia (from hemorrhaging).

DIAGNOSIS: upper endoscopy: enlarged veins. ⊕ "red wale" markings & cherry red spots ⇨ ↑ risk of bleed.

MANAGEMENT OF ACUTE ACTIVE BLEEDING VARICES:

Stabilize with 2 large bore IV lines, IV fluids, ± blood transfusion. If coagulopathy ⇨ ±FFP, ±vitamin K (if ↑ PT).
❶ *__ENDOSCOPIC INTERVENTION: endoscopic ligation tx of choice__*__* – lower cx/re-bleed rate__*. ± sclerotherapy.

❷ **PHARMACOLOGIC VASOCONSTRICTORS:**
- *__Octreotide: pharmacologic drug of choice in acute bleeding__** or adjunctive with endoscopic treatment.
  - MOA: somatostatin analog that causes vasoconstriction of the portal venous flow, reducing bleeding.
- Vasopressin: decreases portal venous pressure.
  - S/E: vessel constriction in other areas: coronary artery vasospasm, myocardial infarction, bowel ischemia.

❸ BALOON TAMPONADE: Ind: stabilize bleeding not controlled by endoscopic or pharmacologic intervention, fast bleeds or temporary stabilization prior to surgical decompression. Increased risk of complications: esophageal perforation or ulceration, aspiration pneumonia.

❹ **SURGICAL DECOMPRESSION:**
- **Trans jugular Intrahepatic Portosystemic Shunt (TIPS):** indicated if bleeding despite endoscopic or pharmacologic tx, Child Class C & some patients with Child Class B. Cx: *hepatic encephalopathy, infections.*
- Devascularization & embolization: may be used in severe cases or cases of thrombosis.

MANAGEMENT TO PREVENT REBLEEDS:

70% rebleed within the 1st year of the initial bleed (1/3 of re-bleeds are fatal).
❶ *__NONSELECTIVE BETA BLOCKERS: tx of choice in primary prophylaxis to prevent rebleed.__** (ex PROPRANOLOL, NADOLOL).* MOA: reduces portal venous pressure. *__NOT used in acute bleeds__* (because beta blockers blunt the tachycardic response to hypovolemia, reducing cardiac output).

❷ Isosorbide: *long acting nitrate* (vasodilator) that reduces esophageal variceal pressure.

ANTIBIOTIC PROPHYLAXIS

Fluoroquinolones (ex. Norfloxacin) or Ceftriaxone to prevent infectious complications.

HIATAL HERNIA

Protrusion of the upper portion of the stomach into the chest cavity due to a diaphragm tear or weakness.

TYPE I: *"sliding hernia".* *MC type* (95%). GE junction & stomach "slide" into the mediastinum (increases reflux). **Management:** similar to GERD.

TYPE II: "rolling hernia" (paraesophageal) – fundus of stomach protrudes through diaphragm with the GE junction remaining in its anatomic location. May lead to strangulation.
> **Management:** surgical repair of the defect to avoid complications.

ESOPHAGEAL NEOPLASMS

SQUAMOUS CELL:

- *MC cause* of *esophageal cancer worldwide** (~90%). *MC in upper 1/3 of esophagus. Peaks 50-70y.*

  - **RISK FACTORS:** *tobacco/ETOH use,* decreased intake of fruits/vegetables, achalasia, hot beverage ingestion, **exposure of esophagus to noxious stimuli** (dysplasia leads to neoplasia) men, nitrates. ↑incidence in *African-Americans.*   ↓incidence with NSAIDs & coffee consumption.

ADENOCARCINOMA:

- *MC type in US.* MC in *younger patients, obese, Caucasians.* Usually presents early. *MC in lower 1/3*

- *Adenocarcinoma is usually a complication of GERD** leading to *Barrett's esophagus.**

CLINICAL MANIFESTATIONS:
1. *dysphagia to solid food* ⇨ *fluids** *(fluids/soft foods usually tolerated initially),* **odynophagia.**
2. **weight loss, chest pain,** anorexia, cough, hoarseness, reflux, hematemesis, ±Virchow's node.
3. Hypercalcemia in patients with squamous cell (due to PTH-related protein tumor secretion).

DIAGNOSIS: *upper endoscopy with biopsy** *test of choice.* Double-contrast barium esophagram.

MANAGEMENT: esophageal resection, radiation therapy, chemotherapy (ex 5-FU) depending on stage.

DISORDERS OF THE STOMACH

GASTRITIS

GASTRITIS: superficial inflammation/irritation of the stomach mucosa with mucosal injury.
GASTROPATHY: mucosal injury without evidence of inflammation.

ETIOLOGIES: *imbalance between ↑aggressive & ↓protective mechanisms* of the gastric mucosa.
- ❶ Helicobacter pylori: MC cause of gastritis.
- ❷ NSAIDs/Aspirin: 2nd MC cause. Prostaglandin inhibition disrupts the mucosal protective barrier.
- ❸ Acute stress (in critically ill patients).
- Others: heavy alcohol consumption, bile salt reflux, medications, radiation, trauma, corrosives, ischemia, pernicious anemia, portal hypertension.

CLINICAL MANIFESTATIONS: *MC asymptomatic; If symptomatic* ⇨ *epigastric pain,* nausea, vomiting, anorexia. ± Upper GI bleed (hematemesis, melena) but bleeding is usually minimal.

DIAGNOSIS: *Endoscopy gold standard:** thick, edematous erosions <0.5cm; H pylori testing.

MANAGEMENT:
- **H. pylori positive** ⇨ Clarithromycin + Amoxicillin + PPI "CAP". Metronidazole if PCN allergic.

- **H. pylori negative** ⇨ acid suppression: PPI, H₂ blocker, antacids; Sucralfate.

- Pharmacologic prophylaxis for patients at high risk for developing stress-related gastritis:
  IV proton pump inhibitors or H₂ blockers.

PEPTIC ULCER DISEASE (PUD)

2ry to imbalance of ❶ ↓*mucosal protective factors in GU &* ❷ ↑*damaging factors (acid, pepsin) in DU.*

ETIOLOGIES

1. *H. pylori infection: MC cause.**
2. *NSAIDs: 2nd MC cause.* Inhibit prostaglandin-mediated synthesis of protective mucus.
3. Zollinger-Ellison Syndrome: gastrin producing tumor. 1% of all cases of PUD.
4. ETOH, smoking, stress (burns, trauma, surgery, severe medical illness); males, elderly, steroids, malignancy - *suspect GI malignancy (ZES, gastric cancer) in nonhealing GU.**

CLINICAL MANIFESTATIONS:

1. *Dyspepsia** = epigastric pain *(burning, gnawing, hunger like)* 80%. Symptoms usually *worse at night* (11p-2a). May have hypochondrium pain, nausea, vomiting. May be asymptomatic.
   Ulcer-like or acid dyspepsia: relief with food, antacids, &/or anti-secretory agents. Worse before meals or 2-5h after meals, nocturnal symptoms classically associated with DU.*
   Food-provoked dyspepsia: pain 1-2 hours after meals & weight loss associated with GU.

2. **GI Bleed:** *peptic ulcer disease is the MC cause of upper GI bleed.**

DIAGNOSIS

A. **Endoscopy:** *gold standard** - most accurate diagnostic test for PUD. Helpful if active bleeding.
   - *Biopsy to rule out malignancy if GU present.** Even benign appearing gastric ulcers should have multiple biopsies. Used especially in patients with *alarm symptoms:* (>50y, dyspepsia, history of gastic ulcer, anorexia, weight loss, anemia, dysphagia).

B. **Upper GI series:** used in patients unwilling or unable to do endoscopy. *All GU seen must be followed with endoscopy* to *r/o malignancy & document healing* (8-12 weeks afterwards).

HELICOBACTER PYLORI TESTING

1. *Endoscopy with biopsy: gold standard in diagnosing H pylori infection.*
   - ⊕**rapid urease test:** direct staining of the biopsy specimen for H. pylori.
2. ⊕**Urea breath test:** used for testing if endoscopy can't be done but can also be used to confirm eradication after therapy. H. pylori converts labeled urea into labeled carbon dioxide.
3. ⊕**H. Pylori stool antigen (HpSA):** >90% specific. Useful for diagnosing H. pylori & confirming eradication after therapy.
4. ⊕ **serologic antibodies:** only useful in confirming H. pylori infection *(NOT eradication)!** Antibodies can stay elevated long after the eradication of H. pylori.

COMPLICATIONS

1. **BLEEDING:** *melena, hematemesis, dizziness, hematochezia, pallor, weakness, dyspnea, anemia.*
2. **PERFORATION:** *sudden onset severe, diffuse abdominal pain, rigid abdomen, rebound tenderness. Especially anterior DU*
3. **PENETRATION:** *pain radiating to the back. Especially posterior DU. Not relieved with food or antacids.*
4. **OBSTRUCTION:** *vomiting hallmark, crampy abdominal pain, nausea, "succussion splash".*

MANAGEMENT

1. *H pylori eradication:*
   -**Triple therapy:** *Clarithromycin +* *Amoxicillin +* *PPI** *"CAP". Metronidazole if PCN allergic.**
      Alternate treatment: Bismuth subsalicylate + Tetracycline + Metronidazole
   -**Quadruple therapy:** PPI + Bismuth subsalicylate + Tetracycline + Metronidazole

2. **H pylori negative:** PPI; H_2 blocker, Misoprostol, antacids, Bismuth compounds, Sucralfate.
3. Refractory: parietal cell vagotomy. Bilroth II (associated with dumping syndrome).

MEDICAL MANAGEMENT OF PEPTIC ULCER DISEASE (PUD)

MEDICATION	COMMENTS
PROTON PUMP INHIBITORS "AZOLES" - *Omeprazole* (prilosec) - *Lansoprazole* (prevacid) - *Pantoprazole* (protonix) - *Rabeprazole* (aciphex) - *Esomeprazole* (nexium) - *Dexlansoprazole*	*Drug of choice* - most effective drug to treat PUD.* Gastritis, ZES. - 90% healing of duodenal ulcers after 4 weeks & gastric ulcers after 6 weeks. **MOA**: *blocks H^+/K^+ ATP-ase (proton pump) of parietal cell, reducing acid secretion.* More effective than H₂RA but of little clinical difference after 4 weeks in uncomplicated cases. Associated with faster symptom relief & healing. Usually taken **30min before meals.*** Low risk in pregnant patients. **S/E:** diarrhea, headache, hypomagnesemia, **B_{12} deficiency,*** hypocalcemia. **DI:** Omeprazole causes **CP450 inhibition** ⇨ ↑levels of Theophylline, Warfarin, Phenytoin & other drugs.
H₂ RECEPTOR ANTAGONISTS "TIDINES" - *Cimetidine* (Tagamet) - *Ranitidine* (Zantac) - *Famotidine* (Pepcid) - *Nizatadine* (Axid)	**MOA:** *histamine₂ receptor blocker* (indirectly inhibits proton pump) *reducing acid/pepsin secretion* (especially nocturnal). Ranitidine 6x more potent than Cimetidine. Usually taken at night. - 90% healing of duodenal ulcers after 6 weeks & gastric ulcers after 8 weeks. **S/E:** ↑LFTs. Pepcid has few drug interactions. Pepcid, Axid ± cause dyscrasias. Many **drug interactions with Cimetidine: CP450 inhibition** ⇨ ↑levels of theophylline, warfarin, phenytoin & other drugs. <u>CNS:</u> confusion, headache. ***Anti-androgen effects of Cimetidine: gynecomastia, impotence, ↓libido.*** **CI/Caution:** caution if renal/hepatic dysfunction.
MISOPROSTOL	**MOA:** *prostaglandin E_1 analog* that *increases bicarbonate & mucus secretion,* reduces acid production. ***Good for preventing NSAID-induced ulcers* but not for healing already existing ulcers.*** Also used to keep ductus arteriosus patent. **S/E:** diarrhea & GI upset. **CI:** premenopausal women because it is ***abortifacent & causes cervical ripening.***
ANTACIDS	**MOA:** neutralize acid, prevents conversion of pepsinogen to pepsin (active form). **Systemic:** **Calcium carbonate** (Tums). **S/E:** acid rebound, milk alkali syndrome. **Nonsystemic:** **Milk of Magnesia** (± cause *diarrhea*) **Amphogel (AlOH)** (± cause *constipation*, hypophosphatemia) **Maalox: Magnesium + Aluminum hydroxide (AlOH)** **Mylanta (Mg + ALOH + Simethicone)** less S/E.
BISMUTH COMPOUNDS Pepto-Bismol Kaopectate	**MOA:** *antibacterial & cytoprotective* (similar to Sucralfate) **S/E:** *darkening of tongue/stool,* constipation.*
SUCRALFATE Carafate	**MOA:** *cytoprotective* (forms viscous adhesive ulcer coating that promotes healing, protects the stomach mucosa). **Ind:** usually used as an ulcer prophylactic measure than as for treatment of ulcers. **S/E:** metallic taste, constipation, nausea. Antacids may interfere with its action. **Drug Interactions:** *May reduce the bioavailability of H₂RA, PPI's,* fluoroquinolones, when given simultaneously. Take on empty stomach.

	DUODENAL ULCERS (DU)	**GASTRIC ULCERS (GU)**
CAUSATIVE FACTORS	↑ *DAMAGING factors:* *acid, pepsin, H. pylori*	↓ *MUCOSAL PROTECTIVE factors:* ↓*mucus, bicarb, prostaglandins; NSAIDs*
INCIDENCE	• *4x MC. Almost always benign.* • MC in the duodenal bulb.	• *4% malignant.** • MC in the antrum of stomach.
PAIN	• *Better c meals.* Worse 2-5h p meals*	• *Worse c meals** (esp *1-2h after meals*)
AGE	• *MC in younger patients:* 30-55y.	• *MC in older patients:** 55-70y.

ZOLLINGER-ELLISON SYNDROME

- *GASTRINOMAS: gastrin-secreting neuroendocrine tumors* ⇨ gastric acid hypersecretion ⇨ PUD.

- **MC seen in the duodenal wall** (45%), **pancreas** (25%), lymph nodes (5-15%), other sites.
- Seen in only 1% of PUD. ±Solitary or multiple. **>66% malignant.** 30% associated c MEN 1 syndrome.

CLINICAL MANIFESTATIONS
 Multiple peptic ulcers, refractory ulcers, "kissing" ulcers (ulcers on each side of the luminal wall touching each other); abdominal pain, *diarrhea* (↑acidity in the duodenum inactivates the pancreatic enzymes that normally need a basic environment to become active ⇨ malabsorption).

DIAGNOSIS
1. ↑ *FASTING GASTRIN LEVEL:* **best screening test.*** >1,000pg/mL + gastric pH <2.
   H₂ blockers & PPIs can cause ↑gastrin levels so must be discontinued prior to testing.

2. ⊕ **Secretin test:** *↑gastrin release with secretin seen in gastrinomas.* Normally, gastrin release is inhibited by secretin. Other causes of hypergastrinemia are usually inhibited by secretin.

3. ↑basal acid output: due to ↑gastric acid secretion. ↑Chromogranin A (⊕ in neuroendocrine tumors).
4. Somatostatin receptor scintigraphy: gastrinomas have somatostatin receptors so radioactive somatostatin may be helpful in localizing the tumor. MRI.

MANAGEMENT:
1. **Local:** surgical resection of the tumor.

2. **Metastatic disease:** acid reduction (PPIs), surgical resection if ⊕ liver involvement.
   The liver & abdominal lymph nodes are the MC sites for METS.

GASTRIC CARCINOMA

- *Adenocarcinoma MC worldwide (90%).* 4% lymphomas, carcinoid tumors, stromal, sarcomas.
- MC occurs males & >40y. Patients usually present late in the disease.

RISK FACTORS
 H. pylori most important risk factor. Salted, cured, smoked, pickled foods containing nitrites/nitrates* (thought to be converted by H. pylori into noxious compounds); Pernicious anemia, chronic atrophic gastritis, achlorhydria, smoking, ETOH, blood type A, post antrectomy.

CLINICAL MANIFESTATIONS
1. *Dyspepsia, weight loss, early satiety,* abdominal pain/fullness, nausea, post-prandial vomiting, dysphagia, melena, hematemesis. Patients often have *iron deficiency anemia* (bleeding).
2. **Signs of Metastasis:** Supraclavicular LN (Virchow's node), Umbilical LN (Sister Mary Joseph's node), ovarian METS (Krukenburg tumor), palpable nodule on rectal exam (Blumer's shelf). Left axillary lymph node (LN) involvement (Irish sign). May be seen with other GI tumors.

DIAGNOSIS
1. *Upper endoscopy with biopsy*: ulcerative: all layers. Polypoid: solid mass protruding into the lumen. *Linitis plastica:* diffuse thickening of the stomach wall ("leather bottle" appearance) due to cancer infiltration (worse type). Superficial spreading (best prognosis).
   - Gastric lymphoma: stomach is the MC site of extranodal (Non Hodgkin) lymphoma.

MANAGEMENT
 Gastrectomy, radiation & chemotherapy (both adenocarcinoma & lymphoma). Poor prognosis.

DISORDERS OF THE LIVER/GALLBLADDER

BILIRUBIN METABOLISM

1. **PREHEPATIC PHASE:** bilirubin is produced from heme metabolism (~80% by-product of old RBC destruction & 20% from turnover of immature RBCs, myoglobin & cytochromes). Heme is degraded by macrophages in the reticuloendothelial system (especially in the liver & spleen). Heme ⇨ biliverdin (green pigment) ⇨ bilirubin (red-orange). This *unconjugated (indirect) bilirubin is not soluble in water* & is sent to the liver for conjugation & excretion.

2. **INTRAHEPATIC PHASE:** in hepatocytes, the unconjugated bilirubin is *conjugated* with a sugar via the enzyme *glucuronosyltransferase (UGT).* This *conjugated bilirubin is now water soluble (for bile excretion).*

3. **POSTHEPATIC PHASE:** once soluble in the bile, bilirubin is transported through the biliary & cystic ducts to be stored in the gallbladder or enter the intestine. In the intestine, the conjugated bilirubin is converted to urobilinogen, which can go through 3 main pathways: ❶ urobilinogen is oxidized by intestinal bacteria into stercobilin (gives stool a brown color). ❷ a small amount of urobilinogen is converted in the kidney to urobilin & excreted (gives urine its characteristic color) or ❸ a portion of the urobilinogen is recycled back to the liver & bile for reuse (enterohepatic circulation). In diseases where there is excess direct bilirubin, it gets excreted in the urine. *This is why dark urine & light-colored stools are only seen with elevated direct (conjugated) bilirubin.** In hemolysis (a disorder where there is increased INdirect bilirubin), the urine may be dark due to hemoglobinuria not bilirubinemia!

JAUNDICE

Jaundice: *yellowing of the skin, nail beds & sclera* by tissue *bilirubin deposition* as a consequence of hyperbilirubinemia. Not a disease but a sign of a disease.
- Occurs when bilirubin levels >2.5 mg/dL.

ETIOLOGIES
- ↑bilirubin overproduction (ex. hemolysis), ↓hepatic bilirubin uptake, impaired conjugation, biliary obstruction, hepatitis.
- ↑*bilirubin without ↑LFTs* ⇨ suspect *familial bilirubin disorders (Dubin-Johnson Syndrome, Gilbert Syndrome) & hemolysis.*

DUBIN-JOHNSON SYNDROME

- Hereditary conjugated (direct) hyperbilirubinemia due to decreased hepatocyte excretion of conjugated bilirubin (gene mutation MRP2).

CLINICAL MANIFESTATIONS
Usually asymptomatic but may present with generalized constitutional symptoms. Mild icterus

DIAGNOSIS
1. mild *isolated conjugated (direct) hyperbilirubinemia** (often between 2 – 5 mg/dL) but can increase with concurrent illness, pregnancy or OCPs.
2. *grossly black liver on biopsy.**

MANAGEMENT:
- None needed. Think "D"s **D**ubin, **Direct** bilirubinemia, **D**ark liver

Rotor's syndrome: similar to Dubin-Johnson but milder in nature, associated with conjugated & unconjugated hyperbilirubinemia and not associated with grossly black liver on biopsy.

CRIGLER-NAJJAR SYNDROME:

- Hereditary unconjugated (indirect) hyperbilirubinemia. 0.6 – 1.0 per million.

- Glucuronosyltransferase (UGT) is the enzyme needed to convert indirect bilirubin to direct bilirubin.
  - **Type I**: *no UGT activity*.   Autosomal recessive.
  - **Type II** (Arias Syndrome): very little UGT activity ($\leq 10\%$ of normal).

CLINICAL MANIFESTATIONS

1. **Type I:** *neonatal jaundice with severe progression in the 2nd week, leading to kernicterus* (bilirubin-induced encephalopathy) - ↑bilirubin in CNS & basal ganglia ⇨ *hypotonia, deafness, lethargy, oculomotor palsy & death (often by 15 months of age).*

2. **Type II:** usually asymptomatic. Often an incidental finding on routine lab testing.

DIAGNOSIS

1. *Isolated indirect (unconjugated) hyperbilirubinemia** with **normal liver function tests**.*
   Type I: serum indirect bilirubin often between 20-50 mg/dL.
   Type II: serum indirect bilirubin often between 7-10 mg/dL. May increase during illness/fasting.

2. Liver looks normal on biopsy.

MANAGEMENT:

1. **Type I:**
   - *Phototherapy mainstay of treatment.**
   - Plasmapheresis may be used in acute elevations of bilirubin levels (ex. crisis).
   - Liver transplant definitive.

2. **Type II:** treatment usually isn't necessary but if required, **Phenobarbital** has been shown to increase UGT activity.   Type I is not responsive to Phenobarbital.

GILBERT'S SYNDROME

- Hereditary unconjugated (indirect) hyperbilirubinemia. Relatively common (5 – 10% of US population).

PATHOPHYSIOLOGY:

- **Reduced UGT activity** (10-30% of normal) & decreased bilirubin uptake ⇨ ↑indirect bilirubin.

CLINICAL MANIFESTATIONS

1. Most asymptomatic.

2. May develop **transient episodes of jaundice during periods of stress, fasting, ETOH or illness.**

DIAGNOSIS

- usually incidental finding:
   slight ↑**isolated Indirect bilirubin level with normal LFTs.**

MANAGEMENT

- **None needed** because it is a mild, benign disease.

PATTERNS OF LIVER INJURY

❶ **HEPATOCELLULAR DAMAGE:** ↑ALT & AST primarily. ALT more sensitive for liver disease than AST.

❷ **CHOLESTASIS:** *↑levels of alkaline phosphatase with ↑GGT,* * ↑*bilirubin greater than ↑ALT & AST.*

❸ **LIVER "SYNTHETIC" FUNCTION:**
PROTHROMBIN TIME (PT): depends on synthesis of coagulation factors (vitamin K dependent): Factors 2,7,9,10. *PT is an earlier indicator of severe liver injury/prognosis than albumin.* Prolonged PT is seen when 80% of the liver's protein synthesizing ability is lost.

ALBUMIN: useful marker of overall liver protein synthesis. Levels decreases with liver failure.

DISORDERS	LABORATORY PATTERN OF LIVER INJURIES
ETOH HEPATITIS	*AST:ALT>2* ⇨ *alcohol hepatitis** "S = Scotch" (AST levels usually <500). AST is found primarily in the mitochondria. ETOH causes direct mitochondrial injury ⇨ ↑AST
VIRAL/TOXIC/INFLAMMATORY PROCESSES	• *ALT >AST* ⇨ *usually.* Think A<u>L</u>T for <u>L</u>iver. • *AST & ALT >1,000* ⇨ usually *acute* viral hepatitis (A, B & rarely C) • Chronic viral hepatitis B/C/D ⇨ mildly ↑ALT & AST (usually <400)
BILIARY OBSTRUCTION OR INTRAHEPATIC CHOLESTASIS	• ↑*alkaline phosphatase (ALP)* ⇨ ↑*ALP with ↑GGT suggests hepatic source or biliary obstruction.* GGT most sensitive indicator of biliary injury (nonspecific). If ↑ALP without ↑GGT, look for sources other than the liver (ex. bone, gut).
AUTOIMMUNE HEPATITIS	• ↑*ALT >1,000,* ⊕*ANA,* ⊕ *smooth muscle antibodies,** ↑*IgG. Responds to Corticosteroids,* Azathioprine.

CHOLELITHIASIS

Gallstones in the gallbladder (NO inflammation).
• *Cholesterol* (mixed & pure) 90%; Pigmented 10%.
• **Black stones:** *hemolysis* or ETOH cirrhosis.
• **Brown stones:** ↑in Asian population, parasitic/bacterial infections.

RISK FACTORS
5Fs (fat, fair, female, forty, fertile): OCPs (↑estrogen), Native Americans, bile stasis, chronic hemolysis, cirrhosis, infection, rapid weight loss, inflammatory bowel disease, total parenteral nutrition (TPN), *fibrates,* increased triglycerides.

CLINICAL MANIFESTATIONS:
1. MC asymptomatic. May be an incidental finding.

2. *Biliary "colic" = episodic, abrupt RUQ/epigastric pain,* resolves slowly, *lasting 30 minutes to hours.* May be associated with *nausea & precipitated by fatty foods or large meals.*

DIAGNOSIS
Ultrasound: *test of choice.** CT or MRI may also be used.

MANAGEMENT:
1. If asymptomatic: observation. Ursodeoxycholic acid may be used to dissolve the gallstones.
2. *Elective cholecystectomy (usually laparoscopic) in symptomatic patients.*

COMPLICATIONS OF CHOLELITHIASIS
Choledocholithiasis, acute cholangitis & acute cholecystitis.

CHOLEDOCHOLITHIASIS

- **Gallstones in the common bile duct** associated with ductal dilation.
- **Primary:** formation of stones originating within the common bile duct. Less common. Causes include bile stasis (ex. Cystic fibrosis).
- **Secondary:** passage of gallstones from the gallbladder into the common bile duct. **MC cause.**

CLINICAL MANIFESTATIONS
1. Asymptomatic (50%). May be an incidental finding when doing studies for other reasons or during evaluation of abnormal LFTs on routine testing.
2. Biliary colic with RUQ tenderness ±jaundice.

COMPLICATIONS
1. **Acute pancreatitis:** associated with epigastric pain, ↑amylase & lipase.
2. **Acute Cholangitis:** Charcot's triad of fever, RUQ pain & jaundice.

DIAGNOSIS
1. **Transabdominal ultrasound:** often initial test ordered. A negative ultrasound does not rule out the possibility of choledocholithiasis.

2. **ERCP: diagnostic test of choice.*** Used for both diagnostic as well as therapeutic (allows for stone extraction). Often obtained after ultrasound.
3. Magnetic resonance cholangiopancreatography (MRCP) and endoscopic ultrasound (EUS) may be used in patients with intermediate risk (determined by labs & transabdominal ultrasound).

MANAGEMENT
1. **ERCP stone extraction preferred** over laparoscopic choledocholithotomy.

ACUTE CHOLANGITIS

- **Biliary tract infection 2ry to obstruction** (ex. **gallstones**, malignancy).
- MC due to gram negative enteric organisms that ascend from the duodenum - **E. coli (MC)**, *Klebsiella* (2nd MC), *Enterobacter*, B. fragilis. Anaerobes or *Enterococcus* may be additional organisms.

CLINICAL MANIFESTATIONS
1. **CHARCOT'S TRIAD*:** ❶ **fever/chills** ❷ **RUQ pain &** ❸ **jaundice.*** Triad seen in 50-70% cases.

2. **REYNOLDS PENTAD:** Charcot's triad + ❹ **shock** + ❺ **altered mental status.**

DIAGNOSIS
1. **Labs: leukocytosis. Cholestasis: ↑alkaline phosphatase with ↑GGT, ↑bilirubin > ↑ALT & AST.**

2. **Ultrasound, CT scan:** may show dilation of the common bile duct.

3. **Cholangiography: gold standard** via **ERCP** or PTC (percutaneous transhepatic cholangiography) – usually performed once the patent has been afebrile/stable for 48 hours after IV antibiotics.

MANAGEMENT
1. **Antibiotics vs. colonic bacteria:** monotherapy (Ampicillin/sulbactam, Piperacillin/tazobactam) or Ceftriaxone + Metronidazole OR fluoroquinolone + Metronidazole. Ampicillin + Gentamicin.

2. **Common bile duct decompression/stone extraction: via ERCP*** (sphincterotomy).
   PTC (catheter drainage) if unable to do ERCP. Open surgical decompression + T-tube insertion.

ACUTE CHOLECYSTITIS

- *Gall bladder (cystic duct) obstruction by gallstone* ⇨ *inflammation/infection.*

- *E. coli MC** (50-80%)**, Klebsiella, Enterococci**, B. fragilis, Clostridium– **same bacteria in cholangitis.**

CLINICAL MANIFESTATIONS
1. *RUQ/epigastric pain **continuous*** in duration. May be associated with **nausea** & may be *precipitated by fatty foods or large meals.*

2. Guarding, anorexia, jaundice not common (<20%) but may be seen if choledocholithiasis present.

PHYSICAL EXAMINATION
1. *Fever* (often low-grade).

2. *Enlarged, palpable gallbladder* (33%)
   ⊕ *Murphy's sign:** acute RUQ pain/inspiratory arrest with palpation of the gallbladder.

3. ⊕ *Boas sign* = referred pain to right shoulder/subscapular area (phrenic nerve irritation).*
   NOT to be confused with Kehr's sign (which is referred pain to the *left* subscapular area due to phrenic nerve irritation. Kehr's sign can be seen with splenic rupture).

DIAGNOSIS:
1. **Ultrasound:** *initial test of choice:** ±thickened gallbladder (>3mm); distended gallbladder, sludge, gallstones, pericholecystic fluid, ⊕ sonographic Murphy's sign.

2. CT scan: alternative to ultrasound & can detect complications.

3. Abdominal radiographs: 10% of stones seen. Usually an incidental finding on AXR.

4. **Labs:** ↑*WBCs* (*leukocytosis with left shift*). ↑bilirubin, ↑alkaline phosphatase & ↑LFTs.

5. **HIDA scan**: *Gold Standard.** ⊕ **Hida scan = nonvisualization of the gallbladder** in cholecystitis.

MANAGEMENT
1. *NPO, IV fluids, antibiotics* (ex. Ceftriaxone + Metronidazole) ⇨ *cholecystectomy* (usually within 72 hours). Laparoscopic cholecystectomy preferred whenever possible.

2. Cholecystostomy (percutaneous drainage of the gallbladder) if patient is nonoperative.

3. Pain control with NSAIDs or narcotics.

- ACUTE ACALCULOUS CHOLECYSTITIS: *MC occur in the seriously ill* (post op, ICU patients) 2ry to dehydration, prolonged fasting, total parental nutrition, gallbladder stasis, burns, diabetes mellitus. Due to gallbladder sludge (not gallstones).

- CHRONIC CHOLECYSTITIS: *associated with gallstones* may result from repeated bouts of acute/subacute cholecystitis. *Strawberry GB* (interior of gallbladder resembles strawberry secondary to cholesterol submucosal aggregation) ⇨ *porcelain GB (premalignant condition).*

FULMINANT HEPATITIS (ACUTE HEPATIC FAILURE)

- *Rapid liver failure + hepatic encephalopathy (often with coagulopathy).* Acute = within 8 weeks after onset of liver injury in a patient that was healthy prior to the onset of symptoms.

ETIOLOGIES
- *Acetaminophen MC cause* (overuse of medication or overdose), *drug reactions* (ex. Isoniazid, Pyrazinamide, Rifampin, antiepileptics, antibiotics), *viral hepatitis* (A through E), liver ischemia, *Reye syndrome*, Budd-Chiari syndrome, autoimmune hepatitis, fatty liver associated with pregnancy, mushroom poisoning.

CLINICAL MANIFESTATIONS
1. **Encephalopathy:** vomiting, coma, AMS, seizures, *asterixis* (flapping tremor of the hand with wrist extension), hyperreflexia, cerebral edema, increased intracranial pressure. Ammonia is neurotoxic. Increased ammonia due to failure of the liver to excrete ammonia & reduction of the ability of the liver to convert ammonia into urea. Protein breakdown leads to increased ammonia.

2. **Coagulopathy:** due to decreased hepatic production of coagulation factors (which are proteins).
3. Hepatomegaly, jaundice (not usually seen in Reye syndrome).

DIAGNOSIS
1. ↑*AMMONIA** levels in serum, ↑*PT/INR* ≥1.5 (coagulopathy due to decreased liver production of clotting factor proteins). ↑LFTs, *hypoglycemia.*

MANAGEMENT
1. **ENCEPHALOPATHY**
   - *Lactulose: converted into lactic acid by bacteria, neutralizing the ammonia.*
   - *Rifaximin, Neomycin: antibiotics that decrease the bacteria* producing ammonia in the GI tract.
   - *Protein restriction* reduces the breakdown of protein into ammonia.

2. **LIVER TRANSPLANTATION** is the only **definitive treatment.**

REYE SYNDROME: *fulminant hepatitis MC seen in children associated with Aspirin use during viral infections** but may occur without Aspirin use. May develop rash (hands & feet), intractable vomiting, liver damage, encephalopathy, dilated pupils with minimal response to light & multi-organ failure.

VIRAL HEPATITIS

CLINICAL MANIFESTATIONS:
1. **Prodromal phase:** malaise, arthralgia, fatigue, URI sx, anorexia, *decreased smoking*, nausea, vomiting, abdominal pain, loss of appetite, ± acholic stools. *Hepatitis A associated with spiking fever.**
2. **Icteric phase:** *jaundice* (most don't develop this phase). If present, jaundice usually develops once the patient's fever subsides.

- **Chronic Hepatitis: disease >6 months duration.** *Only HBV, HCV, HDV associated c chronicity.** Chronic may lead to end stage liver disease (ESLD) or hepatocellular carcinoma (HCC).*

- **Fulminant:** encephalopathy, coagulopathy, jaundice, edema, ascites, asterixis, hyperreflexia.

LABORATORY VALUES: ↑*ALT* > ↑AST both >500 if acute (<500 if chronic); ± ↑bilirubinemia.

PROGNOSIS: clinical recovery usually within 3-16 weeks; *10% HBV & 80% HCV become chronic.*

HEPATITIS A VIRUS (HAV)

Transmission: *feco-oral.* Outbreaks with contaminated water/food during ***international travel 40%,*** day care workers, men who have sex with men, shellfish.

CLINICAL MANIFESTATIONS:
1. **Children:** usually asymptomatic in children. ***Asymptomatic children <6y MC source for adults.****
2. **Adults:** mild disease in adults.
   - **Prodromal phase:** malaise, arthralgia, fatigue, URI sx, anorexia, nausea, vomiting, ***decreased smoking.*** ***Hepatitis A only viral hepatitis associated with spiking fever.**** Abdominal pain, loss of appetite, hepatomegaly, ± acholic stools.
   - **Icteric phase:** *jaundice* (most patients don't develop this phase). If present, jaundice usually develops once the patient's fever breaks.

DIAGNOSIS: *acute hepatitis:* ⊕ *IgM HAV Ab;*   Past exposure: ⊕ Ig<u>G</u> HAV Ab with negative IgM.

MANAGEMENT: *self-limiting* (symptomatic treatment). Usually recovers within weeks.
Post exposure prophylaxis: *for close contacts: HAV immune globulin.*
Pre exposure prophylaxis: Hepatitis A vaccine may be given to population at high-risk.

HEPATITIS E VIRUS (HEV)

TRANSMISSION: similar to Hepatitis A virus: *feco-oral. Associated with waterborne outbreaks.*

DIAGNOSIS: IgM anti-HEV.

MANAGEMENT: none (self-limiting infection).
Highest mortality during pregnancy* especially *3rd trimester* ⇨ ↑risk of *fulminant hepatitis.*

HEPATITIS C VIRUS (HCV)

Transmission: *parenteral* (ex. IV drug use, ↑risk if received blood transfusion before 1992). Sexual or perinatal not common. Not associated with documented cases through breastfeeding. ***80% of patients with HCV develop chronic infection.**** 20% clear the infection. Fulminant hepatitis rare.

DIAGNOSIS: anti HCV: ⊕ in 6 weeks. Does <u>not</u> imply recovery (may become negative after recovery).

	HCV RNA	Anti-HCV	
acute hepatitis	⊕	±	**HCV RNA more sensitive**
resolved hepatitis	Negative	±	**than HCV antibody**
chronic hepatitis	⊕	⊕	

MANAGEMENT OF CHRONIC HCV:
1. **Pegylated interferon alpa-2b AND ribavirin.** <u>S/E</u> of interferon: psychosis & depression.
2. Newer options: ledipasvir-sofosbuvir, elbasvir-grazoprevir, ombitasvir-paritaprevir-ritonavir plus dasabuvir with or without ribavirin, simeprevir plus sofosbuvir & daclatasvir plus sofosbuvir. Some of the newer treatments may possibly reactivate Hepatitis B so perform HBV testing prior to tx.

Screening for hepatocellular carcinoma (HCC) via serum alpha-fetoprotein & ultrasound.*

HEPATITIS D VIRUS (HDV)

TRANSMISSION: defective virus that ***requires Hepatitis B virus (HbsAg) to cause coinfection or superimposed infection.***
Direct cytopathic effect ⇨ more severe hepatitis, faster progression to cirrhosis.

HEPATITIS B VIRUS (HBV)

TRANSMISSION: parenteral, sexual, perinatal, percutaneous.

❶ ACUTE: 70% subclinical, 30% jaundice. <1% present with fulminant hepatitis.

❷ CHRONIC (~10% adult acquired; >90% perinatally acquired). ↑risk for hepatocellular carcinoma.
- *Chronic asymptomatic carrier:* ⊕HBsAg, ⊕ HBe antibodies with undetectable or low HBV DNA, normal LFTs and normally or minimally abnormal liver on biopsy. *Although they are asymptomatic, they can transmit the infection to others.*

- *Chronic infection:* ⊕ HBsAg, with ↑AST & ALT, ↑HBV DNA and evidence of hepatocellular damage on liver biopsy.

SEROLOGICAL TESTS:
1. **⊕ HBsAg (SURFACE ANTIGEN):**
   1st evidence of HBV infection (before symptoms). *Establishes infection & infectivity.**
   If HBsAg positive >6 months ⇨ chronic infection is established.

2. **⊕ HBsAb (SURFACE ANTIBODY):**
   ❶ *distant resolved infection (recovery)* OR ❷ *vaccination (sole serologic marker).*
   Positive HbsAb in an infected patient signifies immunity & patient is not contagious.
   If no development of antiHBS in 6 months ⇨ chronic infection is established.

3. **⊕ HBcAb (CORE ANTIBODY):**
   IgM: *indicates acute infection* (1st Ab to appear). *± be only acute marker in window period.**
   IgG: *indicates chronic infection or distant resolved infection.*

4. **⊕ HBeAg (ENVELOPE ANTIGEN):** *↑viral replication & ↑infectivity*. >3 months ⇨ ↑likelihood of developing chronic HBV.

5. **⊕ HBeAb (ENVELOPE ANTIBODY):** indicates *waning viral replication, ↓infectivity*.

6. **⊕ HBV DNA:** presence in the serum correlates with active replication in liver.

Diagnosis	HBsAg	anti-HBs	anti-HBc	HBeAg	Anti-Hbe
WINDOW PERIOD	Negative	Negative	*IgM*	Negative	Negative
ACUTE HEPATITIS	*POSITIVE*	Negative	*IgM*	±	±
RECOVERY (RESOLVED)	Negative	*POSITIVE*	*IgG*	Negative	Negative
IMMUNIZATION	Negative	*POSITIVE*	Negative	Negative	Negative
CHRONIC HEPATITIS REPLICATIVE	*POSITIVE*	Negative	*IgG*	*POSITIVE*	Negative
CHRONIC HEPATITIS NONREPLICATIVE	*POSITIVE*	Negative	*IgG*	Negative	*POSITIVE*

MANAGEMENT OF HBV:
1. **Acute:** supportive.

2. **Chronic:** treatment may be indicated if ↑ALT, inflammation on biopsy or ⊕HBeAg.
   - *alpha–interferon 2b, Lamivudine, Adefovir.* Interferon CI in decompensated liver disease.
   - Newer options include: *Tenofovir, Telbivudine, Entecavir (very potent).*

PREVENTION
Hep B vaccine given @ 0, 1 & 6 months. Contraindicated if allergic to Baker's yeast.*

HEPATIC VEIN OBSTRUCTION (BUDD-CHIARI SYNDROME)

- **Hepatic venous outflow obstruction** (*thrombosis or occlusion*) ⇨↓liver drainage (blood backs up into the liver) ⇨ *portal HTN & cirrhosis*. MC in women 20s – 30s.

PRIMARY: *hepatic vein thrombosis (MC)* or

SECONDARY: *hepatic vein or inferior vena cava occlusion* (ex. exogenous tumor compression).

RISK FACTORS
- **idiopathic, hypercoagulable states** (ex. polycythemia vera, myeloproliferative diseases, pregnancy, oral contraceptive use, paroxysmal nocturnal hemoglobinuria, Factor V Leiden, Protein C & S deficiency, malignancy, antiphospholipid syndrome).

CLINICAL MANIFESTATIONS:
1. **Classic triad: ❶ ascites** (84%) **❷ hepatomegaly** (75%) **& ❸ RUQ abdominal pain.** Rapid development of acute liver disease (including jaundice & hepatosplenomegaly).
2. May present as a subacute illness (progressive development of portal hypertension) or as acute fulminant hepatic failure.

DIAGNOSIS
1. **Ultrasound: *screening test of choice.*** Imaging studies (ultrasound, CT scan, MRI) show occlusion of hepatic vein or inferior vena cava. CT or MRI usually performed if US nondiagnostic.
2. Venography gold standard. Performed only if high suspicion and negative noninvasive testing.
3. Liver biopsy: usually not needed. Congestive hepatopathy classically described as "nutmeg liver".

MANAGEMENT
1. **Shunts:** ex TIPS. Decompresses the congested liver, increases liver drainage. Done in mild disease.

2. **Balloon angioplasty with stent:** patients with stenosis or obstruction of the inferior vena cava.

3. Pharmacologic: anticoagulation, thrombolysis (done if acute thrombus <3-4 weeks & not involving the inferior vena cava).

4. **Management of Ascites:** diuretics (removes excess fluid), low sodium diet, large volume paracentesis (for ascites).

HEPATOCELLULAR CARCINOMA (HCC)

- Hepatic malignancies are more commonly secondary to metastasis (ex. lung, breast malignancies).
- Primary liver neoplasm = hepatocellular carcinoma.

RISK FACTORS
- Chronic viral hepatitis (B, C & D), cirrhosis, aflatoxin B_1 exposure (produced by Aspergillus spp).

CLINICAL MANIFESTATIONS
Malaise, weight loss, jaundice, abdominal pain, hepatosplenomegaly.

DIAGNOSIS:
1. **Ultrasound**, CT scan, MRI, hepatic angiogram.
2. ↑ **alpha-fetoprotein.*** Needle biopsy usually avoided (to prevent seeding).

MANAGEMENT: surgical resection if confined to a lobe & not associated with cirrhosis.

CIRRHOSIS

Mostly *__irreversible liver fibrosis with nodular regeneration__* 2ry to chronic liver disease.   These nodules cause ↑'ed portal pressure. Macronodules associated with higher risk of HCC.

ETIOLOGIES: *__ETOH MC cause in US,__* *chronic viral hepatitis (__HCV,__* HBV, HDV); nonalcoholic fatty liver disease* (obesity, DM, & hypertriglyceridemia), *__hemochromatosis,__* autoimmune hepatitis, primary biliary cirrhosis, primary sclerosing cholangitis, drug toxicity.

CLINICAL MANIFESTATIONS:
1. General symptoms: fatigue, weakness, weight loss, muscle cramps, anorexia.

2. **Physical Exam:** *ascites* (abdominal distention by fluid due to ↓oncotic pressure – decrease hepatic production of protein), hepatosplenomegaly, *__gynecomastia__* (liver unable to metabolize estrogen). spider angioma (especially upper body), caput medusa, muscle wasting, bleeding (↓coag factors), hepatosplenomegaly, palmar erythema, jaundice, Dupuytren's contractures.

3. **HEPATIC ENCEPHALOPATHY:** *__confusion & lethargy__* (↓liver clearance of accumulated ammonia from protein breakdown). PE: *__asterixis* (flapping tremor) & fetor hepaticus. ↑ammonia levels.__**
4. **ESOPHAGEAL VARICES:** *__due to portal HTN.__* May progress to end stage liver disease.

5. **Spontaneous bacterial peritonitis** (infection of peritoneal fluid) may cause fever. Peritoneal fluid will reveal cell count (polymorphonuclear neutrophils) ≥250 cells/mm³
SAAG >1.1g/dL (indicating portal HTN as the cause). SAAG = serum ascites albumin gradient.

DIAGNOSIS: ultrasound: determines liver size & evaluate for hepatocellular carcinoma.   Liver biopsy

MANAGEMENT:
1. **ENCEPHALOPATHY:** *__Lactulose or Rifaximin.__* *__Neomycin__* 2nd line. Lactulose is converted by intestinal bacteria into lactic acid, pulling ammonia into gut *(S/E is diarrhea).* Rifaximin & neomycin are antibiotics that ↓'es the ammonia-producing flora.   Protein restriction.

2. **ASCITES:** *Na⁺ restriction* ⇨ diuretics (Spironolactone, Furosemide).   Paracentesis.

3. **PRURITUS:** *__Cholestyramine__** (Questran) is a bile acid sequestrant that reduces bile salts in the skin, leading to less irritation from the bile salts.
4. Liver transplant: definitive management. Screening for HCC = *__ultrasound + alpha-fetoprotein__**

CIRRHOSIS STAGING CHILD-PUGH CLASSIFICATION

PARAMETERS	1 POINT	2 POINTS	3 POINTS
Total Bilirubin (mg/dL)	<2	2-3	>3
Serum albumin (g/dL)	>3.5	2.8 – 3.5	<2.8
PT INR	<1.7	1.71 – 2.30	>2.30
Ascites	None	Mild	Moderate to severe
Hepatic Encephalopathy	None	Grade I-II (or suppressed with medication)	Grade III-IV or refractory

POINTS	CLASS	1 YEAR SURVIVAL	2 YEAR SURVIVAL
5-6	A	100%	85%
7-9	B	81%	57%
10-15	C	45%	35%

MODEL FOR END STAGE LIVER DISEASE : *slightly more accurate way to measure 3 month mortality*
MELD = 3.78×ln[serum bilirubin (mg/dL)] + 11.2×ln[INR] + 9.57×ln[serum creatinine (mg/dL)] + 6.43

PRIMARY BILIARY CIRRHOSIS (PBC)

- Idiopathic autoimmune d/o of **INTRAhepatic small bile ducts** ⇨ *↓bile salt excretion, cirrhosis & ESLD*
- *MC MIDDLE-AGED WOMEN (40-60y).** *Seen exclusively in adults.*

CLINICAL MANIFESTATIONS
1. Most are asymptomatic - incidental finding of high alkaline phosphatase (↑ALP).
2. *Fatigue (usually 1st symptom), pruritus* (55%), *RUQ discomfort, hepatomegaly, jaundice.*

DIAGNOSIS
1. **Cholestatic pattern:** ↑ALP with ↑GGT.* *GGT often strikingly elevated >* ↑ALT, AST, bilirubin
2. ⊕ *ANTI-MITOCHONDRIAL ANTIBODY hallmark** (98%). Liver biopsy: definitive diagnosis.

MANAGEMENT:
1. *Ursodeoxycholic acid 1st line** (reduces progression)
   MOA: protects cholangiocytes from the toxic effect of bile acids & stabilizes hepatic inflammation.
2. *Cholestyramine & UV light for Pruritus*: Cholestyramine is a bile acid sequestrant that reduces bile salts in the skin, leading to less irritation from the bile salts.

PRIMARY SCLEROSING CHOLANGITIS (PSC)

*Autoimmune, progressive cholestasis, **diffuse fibrosis of INTRAhepatic & EXTRAhepatic ducts.***
- *MC ASSOCIATED WITH INFLAMMATORY BOWEL DISEASE - 90% have **ulcerative colitis,** ±Crohn.*
- MC in **men 20-40y,** ±children. Rare disease. *↑risk of developing cholangiocarcinoma.*

CLINICAL MANIFESTATIONS: *jaundice, pruritus,* fatigue, RUQ pain, *hepatomegaly, splenomegaly.*

DIAGNOSIS
1. **Cholestatic pattern:** ↑ALP (3-5x normal) *with* ↑GGT. ↑ALT/AST, ↑bilirubin. ↑IgM. ⊕ *P-ANCA.**
2. **ERCP:** *gold standard.*

MANAGEMENT: Liver transplant definitive. Stricture dilation to relieve symptoms. Meds not beneficial.

WILSON'S DISEASE   (HEPATOLENTICULAR DEGENERATION)

- *Free COPPER ACCUMULATION IN LIVER, BRAIN, KIDNEY, CORNEA* due to rare autosomal recessive disorder (ATP7B mutation) ⇨ inadequate bile excretion of copper + increased small intestine absorption of copper ⇨ copper deposition in tissues, leading to cellular damage.

CLINICAL MANIFESTATIONS
1. CNS copper deposits ⇨ basal ganglia deposition: Parkinson-like symptoms (bradykinesia, tremor, rigidity), dementia. Personality & behavioral changes. *Arthralgias* from deposition in the joints.
2. *Liver disease:* hepatitis, hepatosplenomegaly, cirrhosis, hemolytic anemia.
3. *Corneal copper deposits* ⇨ *KAYSER-FLEISCHER RINGS** (brown or green pigment in the cornea).

DIAGNOSIS:
1. *↓ceruloplasmin* (the serum carrier molecule for copper), *↑urinary copper excretion.*

MANAGEMENT
1. **D-Pencillamine**: chelates copper (pyridoxine/Vitamin B6 given to prevent depletion). Trientene.
2. **Zinc:** enhances fecal copper excretion & blocks intestinal copper absorption. Used as 2nd line treatment, in patients intolerant of chelating therapy or for maintenance therapy.
3. Ammonium tetrathiomolybdate: increases urinary copper excretion by binding to copper.

ACUTE PANCREATITIS

ETIOLOGIES
Gallstones & ETOH 2 MC causes* ❶ *gallstones* (40%) ❷*ETOH abuse* (35%). *ETOH MC in men (acute-on-chronic pancreatitis);* Meds (thiazides, protease inhibitors, estrogen, didanosine, valproic acid etc.); Iatrogenic (ERCP), malignancy, *scorpion bite,* idiopathic, trauma, cystic fibrosis. *Mumps in children.*

PATHOPHYSIOLOGY:
Acinar cell injury ⇨ *intracellular activation of pancreatic enzymes* ⇨ *autodigestion of pancreas* ⇨ edema, interstitial hemorrhage, coagulation & cellular fat necrosis (due to breakdown).

CLINICAL MANIFESTATIONS:
1. *Epigastric pain: constant, boring* (frequently *radiating to back** or other quadrant). Pain ± exacerbated if supine, eating & walking *relieved with leaning forward,* sitting or fetal position.*

2. Nausea, vomiting & fever common symptoms.
3. **Physical exam**: ±epigastric tenderness, ↓bowel sounds 2ry to adynamic ileus, *tachycardia*. Dehydration/shock if severe.
   Necrotizing, hemorrhagic: *Cullen's:* periumbilical ecchymosis; *Grey Turner*: flank ecchymosis.

DIAGNOSTIC STUDIES
A. <u>Laboratory Values:</u> leukocytosis, ↑glucose, ↑bilirubin, ↑*triglycerides*
   1. **Lipase:** *more specific than amylase** ↑7-14d. Decreased hematocrit if hemorrhagic.
   2. **Amylase:** *>3x ULN suggestive* but levels ≠ severity & not spp for pancreatitis. ↑3-5 days.
   3. **ALT:** ↑*3-fold highly suggestive of gallstone pancreatitis.*
   4. **Hypocalcemia**: necrotic fat binds to calcium, lowering serum calcium levels (saponification).

B. **Abdominal CT:** *diagnostic test of choice.** Ranson's criteria used for prognosis.

C. **Abdominal US:** assess to rule out gallstones, bile duct dilation, ascites, pseudocysts.

D. **Abdominal radiograph:** ±*"sentinel loop"* = localized ileus* – dilated small bowel in LUQ. *Colon cutoff sign:* abrupt collapse of the colon near the pancreas. Pancreatic calcification suggestive of chronic pancreatitis. ±left-sided, exudative pleural effusion.

MANAGEMENT OF ACUTE PANCREATITIS
• 90% recover without complications in 3-7d & require supportive measures only *"rest the pancreas".*
   1. **Supportive:** *NPO, IV fluid resuscitation* (± need up to 10L/day); *analgesia* with Meperidine (Demerol), Morphine may be associated with ↑spasm of the sphincter of Oddi.

   2. **Antibiotics:** *NOT* used routinely. If severe, necrotizing ⇨ *broad spectrum (ex Imipenem).*
   3. ERCP: if biliary sepsis suspected. ERCP only effective in obstructive jaundice.

RANSONS CRITERIA: used to determine prognosis. APACHE score also used.

ADMISSION		WITHIN 48 HOURS	
Glucose	>200mg/dL	Calcium	<8.0 mg/dL
Age	>55 years	Hematocrit fall	>10%
LDH	>350 IU/L	Oxygen	P_{O2} <60 mmHg
AST	>250 IU/dL	BUN	>5 mg/dL p IV fluids
WBC	>16,000/μL	Base deficit	>4 mEq/L
		Sequestration of fluid	> 6L

Interpretation of Ranson's Criteria	
If the score ≥ 3, severe pancreatitis likely.	Score 0 to 2 = 2% mortality
If the score < 3, severe pancreatitis is unlikely	Score 3 to 4 = 15% mortality
	Score 5 to 6 = 40% mortality
	Score 7 to 8 : 100% mortality

CHRONIC PANCREATITIS

• Chronic inflammation causing parenchymal destruction, fibrosis & calcification resulting in *loss of exocrine & sometimes endocrine function.* 2% will develop pancreatic cancer.

ETIOLOGIES
❶ *ETOH abuse (70%),* ❷ *idiopathic* (15%), hypocalcemia, hyperlipidemia, islet cell tumors, familial, trauma, iatrogenic, gallstones not significant as in acute. *Cystic fibrosis MC cause of chronic pancreatitis in children.*

CLINICAL MANIFESTATIONS:
Triad of ❶ *calcifications* ❷ *steatorrhea &* ❸ *Diabetes mellitus* is hallmark* but seen in only $^1/_3$ of pts. Weight loss. Epigastric and/or back pain may be atypical or completely absent.

DIAGNOSIS: AXR: <u>CALCIFIED PANCREAS.</u>* *Amylase/lipase usually not elevated.* Endoscopic US sensitive.

MANAGEMENT: *oral pancreatic enzyme replacement,* ETOH abstinence, pain control.

PANCREATIC CARCINOMA

RISK FACTORS: *smoking,* >60y, chronic pancreatitis, ETOH, DM, males, obesity, African Americans.*

HISTOLOGY:
1. *Adenocarcinoma: ductal MC* (>90%),* islet cell 5-10%.
      70% found in head of pancreas (20% body; 10% tail). 5y survival rate <5% (Avg 6 months).
2. Ampullary & duodenal carcinomas
3. Cystoadenoma & cystocarcinoma: slow growing, better prognosis. Treated aggressively.

CLINICAL MANIFESTATIONS
Usually have metastasis by the time of presentation (lymph nodes ⊕ 90%). Commonly METS to the regional lymph nodes & the liver.
1. *Abdominal pain* ⇨ *back*. May be relieved with sitting up & leaning forward. Tumors in body/tail produce symptoms later than in the head so usually more advanced at diagnosis. New onset DM.

2. *Painless jaundice* classic* (80%) 2ry to common bile duct obstruction; *weight loss* (>75%).

3. *Pruritus* (due to ↑bile salts in skin), anorexia, acholic stools & dark urine (due to common bile duct obstruction). <u>Trousseau's malignancy sign</u> = migratory phlebitis associated with malignancy.

4. **Physical Examination:** *Courvoisier's sign* = palpable, NONtender, distended gallbladder* associated with jaundice* (common bile duct obstruction) associated with pancreatic cancer.

DIAGNOSIS
1. **CT Scan:** *initial diagnostic test of choice.* ERCP most sensitive test.

2. **Laboratory Evaluation:** ↑*tumor markers: CEA, CA 19-9.*

MANAGEMENT:
1. *Whipple procedure:* radical pancreaticoduodenal resection (the gastroduodenal artery supplies both the pancreas & duodenum). Done if the cancer is confined to the head, or duodenal area.
2. Tail: distal resection
3. **Advanced or inoperative:** *ERCP with stent placement as palliative tx for intractable itching.*

MECKEL'S (ILEAL) DIVERTICULUM

- ***Persistent portion of embryonic vitteline duct (yolk stalk).****
- ***Rule of 2's:*** 2% of population; 2 feet from ileocecal valve, 2% symptomatic, 2 inches in length, 2 types of ectopic tissue (gastric or pancreatic), 2 years MC age at clinical presentation, 2x MC in boys.

CLINICAL MANIFESTATIONS
Ectopic pancreatic or gastric tissue may secrete digestive hormones ⇨ bleeding.

1. ***Usually asymptomatic*** – may be seen incidentally during abdominal surgery for other causes.

2. ***Painless rectal bleeding**** **or ulceration.** The pain, if present, is usually periumbilical but radiates to the right lower quadrant.
3. May cause intussusception, volvulus or obstruction. May cause diverticulitis in adults.

DIAGNOSIS: Meckel's scan looks for ectopic gastric tissue in the ileal area.
MANAGEMENT: surgical excision if symptomatic.

SMALL BOWEL OBSTRUCTION

ETIOLOGIES
- ***post-surgical adhesions MC (60%);**** incarcerated hernias (2nd MC), Crohn disease, malignancy, intussusception. Malignancy is the MC cause of large bowel obstruction.

CONSIDERATIONS
1. Closed loop vs. open loop: in closed loop, the lumen is occluded at two points, which can reduce the blood supply, causing strangulation, necrosis & peritonitis.
2. Complete vs. partial: with complete, the patient usually has severe obstipation (unable to have bowel movements or pass gas).
3. Distal vs. partial: distal presents more with abdominal distention & less vomiting.

CLINICAL MANIFESTATIONS 4 hallmark symptoms "CAVO":
❶ ***Cramping abdominal pain*** - the pain usually starts out mild & intermittent before progressing to severe & constant. Severe pain may be indicative of strangulation.

❷ ***Abdominal distention.*** The more distal the more prominent. ±Dehydration & electrolyte disorders.

❸ ***Vomiting:*** may be bilious if proximal. Nausea/vomiting usually follows the abdominal pain.

❹ ***Obstipation*** (absence of stool/flatus) – usually a late finding. Diarrhea is an early finding.

PHYSICAL EXAMINATION
- Abdominal distention. Hyperactive bowel sounds in early obstruction - ***high-pitched tinkles on auscultation & visible peristalsis**** ⇨ hypoactive bowel sounds heard in late obstruction.

DIAGNOSIS
-**Abdominal radiograph:** ***air fluid levels in step ladder pattern,**** ***dilated bowel loops.*** Minimal gas in colon if complete. AXR is first line imaging. May use UGI series with small bowel follow through.

MANAGEMENT
- **Nonstrangulated** ⇨ ***NPO (bowel rest), IV fluids,*** bowel decompression (via NG tube suction).
- **Strangulated** ⇨ surgical intervention.

PARALYTIC (ADYNAMIC) ILEUS

- **_Decreased peristalsis WITHOUT structural obstruction_** – non mechanical factors affect the motor activity of the GI tract.

ETIOLOGIES
1. *Postoperative state* (ex. recent abdominal surgery), medications (ex. *opiates*), metabolic (ex. *hypokalemia*, hypercalcemia), severe medical illness, metabolic (hypothyroidism, diabetes).

CLINICAL MANIFESTATIONS
1. Symptoms similar to small bowel obstruction (abdominal pain, nausea, vomiting, obstipation & abdominal distention). Patient may not be able to tolerate an oral diet.
2. Decreased to no bowel sounds (unlike early SBO that is classically associated with high-pitched sounds). No peritoneal signs.

DIAGNOSIS
1. **Plain abdominal radiographs:** *first line imaging* -* uniformly distended loops of small & large bowel (due to air) as well as air in the rectum with no transition zone.
2. CT scan or upper GI series may be performed if high suspicion and negative abdominal films.

MANAGEMENT
1. NPO or dietary restriction (sips of clear fluids with progression to liquid diet or parenteral feeds in some patients). NG suction (if moderate vomiting). Electrolyte & fluid repletion. Treat underlying cause (ex. discontinuing opioids & using other medications for pain).

OGILVIE'S SYNDROME

- **_Colonic pseudo-obstruction_** (acute dilation of the colon in the absence of any mechanical obstruction). *MC involves the cecum & the right hemicolon.* MC in men, >60y.

ETIOLOGIES
May occur after surgery, elderly, severely ill patients, metabolic imbalances, nonoperative trauma or medications (ex. opiates, anticholinergic drugs).

CLINICAL MANIFESTATIONS
1. *Abdominal distention hallmark.* Abdominal pain, nausea, vomiting & constipation.
2. Physical examination: distended abdomen, positive tympany with normal bowel sounds.

DIAGNOSIS
1. **Abdominal radiographs**: dilated right colon from the cecum with cutoff @ splenic flexure.
2. Abdominal CT scan or contrast enema: proximal right colonic dilation.

MANAGEMENT
1. Conservative: (IV fluid & electrolyte repletion) if colon dilation <12 cm & absence of severe sx.
2. Neostigmine in patients at risk for perforation (ex. cecal diameter >12 cm) or if they failed conservative therapy after 48 hours. Neostigmine may cause medical colonic decompression.
3. Decompression: initially with NG suction or enemas if they fail conservative tx & Neostigmine. Surgical decompression (cecostomy or colostomy) used if all the other therapies fail.

CELIAC DISEASE (SPRUE)

PATHOPHYSIOLOGY: *small bowel* <u>AUTOIMMUNE</u> *inflammation 2ry to α-gliadin in GLUTEN* ⇨ loss of villi* & *absorptive area ⇨ impaired fat absorption.* ↑*incidence: females, European descent (Irish & Finnish).*

CLINICAL MANIFESTATIONS
1. *Malabsorption: diarrhea*, abdominal pain/distention, bloating, steatorrhea, ± growth delays.
2. *DERMATITIS HERPETIFORMIS:** pruritic, papulovesicular rash on extensor surfaces, neck, trunk & scalp.

DIAGNOSIS: ⊕ *ENDOMYSIAL IgA Ab* & TRANSGLUTAMINASE Ab;* Small bowel biopsy definitive diagnosis.**

MANAGEMENT: *gluten free diet (avoid wheat, rye, barley). Oats, rice & corn don't cause celiac disease.* Vitamin supplementation. Corticosteroids may be needed if refractory to conservative treatment.

LACTOSE INTOLERANCE

- Inability to digest lactose due to low levels of lactase enzyme that normally declines in adulthood especially in African Americans, Asians & South American populations.
CLINICAL MANIFESTATIONS: loose stools, abdominal pain, flatulence & borborygmi after ingestion of milk or milk-containing products.

DIAGNOSIS: *HYDROGEN BREATH TEST (test of choice).** Hydrogen produced when colonic bacteria ferment the undigested lactose. *Usually performed after a trial of a lactose-free diet.*

MANAGEMENT: Lactase enzyme preparations; Lactaid (prehydrolyzed milk); Lactose free diet.

DIVERTICULAR DISEASE

- **DIVERTICULA:** outpouchings due to herniation of the mucosa into the wall of the colon along natural openings at the vasa recta of the colon.
  Sigmoid colon MC area* (due to high intraluminal pressure). Onset usually >40y.

- **DIVERTICULOSIS:** uninflamed diverticula. *Associated with low fiber diet,* constipation & obesity.* *Usually asymptomatic but diverticulosis is MC cause of acute lower GI bleeding.**

- **DIVERTICULITIS:** *inflamed diverticula 2ry to obstruction/infection (fecaliths) ⇨ distention.*

CLINICAL MANIFESTATIONS OF DIVERTICULITIS: *fever, LLQ abdominal pain MC** (may have changes in bowel habits), nausea, vomiting, diarrhea, constipation, flatulence & bloating.

DIAGNOSIS: *CT scan test of choice.** Barium enema not done in acute phase. ↑*WBCs*, ⊕ Guaiac.

MANAGEMENT
  DIVERTICULITIS: *clear liquid diet, antibiotics: ex. Ciprofloxacin or Bactrim + Metronidazole.**

  DIVERTICULOSIS: high fiber diet, fiber supplements. Bleeding stops in 90% (±vasopressin if it doesn't).

VOLVULUS

Twisting of any part of the bowel @ its mesenteric attachment site. *MC sigmoid colon** & cecum.
CLINICAL: obstructive symptoms: abdominal pain, distention, nausea, vomiting, fever, tachycardia.
MANAGEMENT: *endoscopic decompression initial tx of choice.** Surgical correction 2nd line.

APPENDICITIS

- Obstruction of the appendix: *ex.* fecalith, lymphoid hyperplasia, inflammation, malignancy or foreign body.

CLINICAL MANIFESTATIONS
  Anorexia & periumbilical/epigastric pain ⇨ *followed by RLQ pain, nausea & vomiting* (vomiting usually occurs after the pain). MC 10y -30y.

PHYSICAL EXAM: rebound tenderness, rigidity & guarding. Retrocecal appendix may have atypical sx.
  Rovsing sign: RLQ pain with LLQ palpation.
  Obturator sign: RLQ pain with internal & external hip rotation with flexed knee.
  Psoas sign: RLQ pain with right hip flexion/extension (raise leg against resistance).
  McBurney's point tenderness: point $1/3$ the distance from the anterior sup. iliac spine & navel

DIAGNOSIS: CT scan, Ultrasound; *Leukocytosis.*
Management: appendectomy.

IRRITABLE BOWEL SYNDROME

- Chronic, functional idiopathic disorder with <u>NO</u> organic cause. **Hallmark: *abdominal pain associated with altered defecation/bowel habits*** (diarrhea, constipation or alternation between the two). ***Pain often relieved with defecation.**** Onset MC in late teens, early 20s. MC in women.

PATHOPHYSIOLOGY OF IBS
  1. **Abnormal motility:** chemical imbalance in the intestine (including serotonin & acetylcholine) causing abnormal motility & spasm ⇨ abdominal pain. Altered gut microbiota.
  2. **Visceral hypersensitivity** patients have lowered pain thresholds to intestinal distention.
  3. **Psychosocial interactions** & altered central nervous system processing.

ROME IV CRITERIA FOR IRRITABLE BOWEL SYNDROME
Diagnostic Criteria
  Recurrent abdominal pain on average at least 1 day/week in the last 3 months associated with at least 2 of the following 3:
    ❶ *related to defecation*
    ❷ *onset associated with* **change in stool frequency**
    ❸ *onset associated with* **change in stool form (appearance)**

ALARM SYMPTOMS IN IBS
  - Evidence of GI bleeding: occult blood in stool, rectal bleeding, anemia
  - Anorexia or weight loss, fever, nocturnal symptoms, family history of GI cancer, IBD or celiac sprue.
  - Persistent diarrhea causing dehydration; severe constipation or fecal impaction; Onset >45y.

MANAGEMENT OF IRRITABLE BOWEL SYNDROME
- **Lifestyle Changes:** *smoking cessation, low fat/unprocessed food diet.* Avoid beverages containing sorbitol or fructose (ex. apples, raisins), avoid cruciferous vegetables. Sleep, exercise.

- **Diarrhea symptoms:** Anticholinergics/spasm (ex *Dicyclomine*), antidiarrheal (ex *Loperamide*).

- **Constipation symptoms:** prokinetics, bulk-forming laxatives, saline or osmotic laxatives. Lubiprostone – activates intestinal chloride transporter ⇨ ↑intestine fluid & motility.

- TCA (Amitriptyline) or serotonin receptor agonists for intractable pain.

CHRONIC MESENTERIC ISCHEMIA

- Ischemic bowel disease: **mesenteric atherosclerosis of the GI tract** ⇨ inadequate perfusion especially @ splenic flexure during **post-prandial states.*** There is usually some collateral flow.

CLINICAL MANIFESTATIONS:
  chronic dull abdominal pain WORSE AFTER MEALS "intestinal angina,"* weight loss (anorexia).*

DIAGNOSIS Angiogram confirms the diagnosis. **Colonoscopy:** muscle atrophy with loss of villi.

MANAGEMENT: bowel rest. Surgical revascularization (angioplasty with stenting or bypass).

ACUTE MESENTERIC ISCHEMIA

- Ischemic bowel disease: **sudden decrease of mesenterial blood supply to the bowel** ⇨ inadequate perfusion especially @ splenic flexure (because of less collateral blood perfusion).

ETIOLOGIES
  MC due to occlusion: embolus (ex. A fib, MI), **thrombus** (atherosclerosis). **Nonocclusive causes** include shock (decreased blood flow) & cocaine (due to vasospasm). Venous thrombosis.

CLINICAL MANIFESTATIONS: "*SEVERE **abdominal pain out of proportion to physical findings**"* usually poorly localized pain. Nausea, vomiting, diarrhea. Peritonitis & shock in advanced disease.

DIAGNOSIS
  - **Angiogram definitive dx.*** Colonoscopy: patchy, necrotic areas. ↑WBC count, lactic acidosis.

MANAGEMENT: surgical revascularization* (angioplasty with stenting or bypass).
  Surgical resection if the bowel is not salvageable.

ISCHEMIC COLITIS

• MC due to systemic hypotension or atherosclerosis involving the superior & mesenteric arteries.
• MC at "watershed" areas with decreased collaterals (ex. splenic flexure & rectosigmoid junction).
CLINICAL MANIFESTATIONS
  Left lower quadrant pain with tenderness, BLOODY DIARRHEA* (due to sloughing of the colon).

DIAGNOSIS: colonoscopy: segmental ischemic changes in areas of low perfusion (splenic flexure).
MANAGEMENT: restore perfusion & observe for signs of perforation.

TOXIC MEGACOLON

- Nonobstructive, extreme **colon dilation >6cm + signs of systemic toxicity.***
ETIOLOGIES: UC, Crohn, pseudomembranous colitis, infectious, radiation, ischemic.

CLINICAL MANIFESTATIONS
  Fever, abdominal pain, diarrhea, nausea, vomiting, rectal bleeding, tenesmus, electrolyte disorders.

PHYSICAL EXAM: abdominal tenderness, rigidity, tachycardia, dehydration, hypotension, AMS.

DIAGNOSIS: abdominal radiographs: large **dilated colon >6 cm.**

MANAGEMENT: bowel decompression, bowel rest, NG tube, broad-spectrum antibiotics.
  Electrolyte repletion. Colostomy reserved for refractory cases.

INFLAMMATORY BOWEL DISEASE (IBD)

- **Etiology:** idiopathic (most likely immune reaction to GI tract flora).   MC in Caucasians. 15-35y

	ULCERATIVE COLITIS (UC)	CROHN DISEASE (CD)
AREA AFFECTED	• *Limited to colon* (begins in rectum* with CONTIGUOUS SPREAD PROXIMALLY* to colon. • *RECTUM ALWAYS INVOLVED*	• *ANY SEGMENT OF THE GI TRACT** from *mouth to anus.* • *MC in TERMINAL ILEUM** ⇨ *RLQ pain*
DEPTH	• Mucosa & submucosa only	• *TRANSMURAL**
CLINICAL MANIFESTATIONS	• *Abdominal pain: LLQ MC,* colicky* • *Tenesmus,* urgency* • *BLOODY DIARRHEA hallmark** (stools c mucus/pus), hematochezia MC in UC.*	• *Abdominal Pain: RLQ pain MC** (crampy) & weight loss more common with Crohn* • *Diarrhea with no visible blood** usually
COMPLICATIONS	• *Primary Sclerosing Cholangitis, Colon ca, Toxic megacolon (More common in UC).* • *Smoking decreases risk for UC.**	• *Perianal dz*:* fistulas, strictures, abscesses, GRANULOMAS.* • Malabsorption: Fe & B_{12} *deficiency*
COLONOSCOPY	• **Uniform inflammation** ±ulceration in rectum and/or colon. • *PSEUDOPOLYPS.**	• *"SKIP LESIONS"** = normal areas interspersed between inflamed areas, COBBLESTONE *appearance.**
BARIUM STUDIES	*"STOVEPIPE SIGN"** (loss of haustral markings).	• *"STRING SIGN":** barium flow through narrowed inflamed/scarred area due to transmural strictures.
LABS	• ⊕ *P-ANCA* (more common in UC)*	• ⊕ *ASCA* (Ab vs Saccharomyces cerevisiae)
SURGERY	• *Curative*	• Noncurative

Both UC & CD: *arthritis (seronegative spondyloarthropathies*, ankylosing spondylitis), episcleritis; uveitis
Systemic: fever, sweats, weight loss, malaise, fatigue.   Skin: Erythema nodosum, Pyoderma gangrenosum

DIAGNOSIS in ACUTE Disease:

Crohn: Upper GI series with small bowel follow through usually the test of choice in ACUTE disease.

UC: Flex sigmoidoscopy test of choice in acute disease. *Colonoscopy CI in acute colitis* ⇨ *± cause perforation.   Barium enema CI in acute colitis* (may cause toxic megacolon).

MANAGEMENT

- *Aminosalicylates (sulfasalazine, mesalamine)* ⇨ *corticosteroids* ⇨ *immune modifying agents* (Azathioprine, 6-Mercaptoprine, Cyclosporine). ASAs more helpful in ulcerative colitis.
  1. **5-AMINOSALICYLIC ACIDS (5-ASA): MOA:** anti-inflammatory agent. Good for flares & remission.
     - **Oral Mesalamine** (Asacol HD) especially active in terminal small bowel & colon. Long acting (Pentasa) works throughout the entire small intestine and colon. *Best for maintenance.*
     - **Topical Mesalamine:** *rectal suppositories & enemas* (ex Rowasa). Topical mesalamines are effective in the distal colon.
     - **Sulfasalazine – *works primarily in the colon*** (UC). S/E: higher side effect profile c sulfasalazine (hepatitis, pancreatitis, allergic reaction, fever, rash).   Give folic acid with sulfasalazine.

  2. **CORTICOSTEROIDS:** *rapid acting antiinflammatory drugs used for acute flares only.* Oral (Prednisone, Methylprednisolone) & topical (rectal suppositories, foams & enemas). Long term risks include osteoporosis, increased infections, weight gain, edema, cataracts.

  3. **IMMUNE MODIFYING AGENTS:** steroid-sparing: 6-mercaptopurine, Azathioprine & Methotrexate.

  4. **ANTI-TNF AGENTS:** inhibits proinflammatory cytokines (Adalimumab, Infliximab, Certolizumab). Anti-integrins (Natalizumab).

COLON POLYPS

1. ***Pseudopolyps/Inflammatory:*** due to IBD (ex UC/Crohn) ***not considered cancerous.***
2. **Hyperplastic:** *low risk for malignancy*.

3. ***Adenomatous polyps:*** Average is ***10-20y before becoming cancerous (esp >1cm).***
   - ***Tubular adenoma***: nonpedunculated (MC & least risk of the 3 types of adenomatous polyps).
   - Tubulovillous (mixture). Intermediate risk.
   - ***Villous adenoma: highest risk of becoming cancerous***. Tends to be sessile.

COLORECTAL CANCER (CRC)

- 3rd MC cause of cancer-related death in the US.
PATHOPHYSIOLOGY: *progression of adenomatous polyp into malignancy (adenocarcinoma)* usually occurs within 10-20 years. MC site of metastatic spread is the ***liver*** (lungs, lymph nodes).

RISK FACTORS
- Genetics: ***Familial adenomatous polyposis*** (genetic mutation on the APC gene- 100% develop colon cancer by age 40y – greatest risk factor so prophylactic colectomy best for survival). Lynch syndrome (Hereditary nonpolyposis colorectal cancer) has 40% risk of colon cancer development as well as endometrial, ovarian, small intestine, brain & skin. ***Peutz-Jehgers: autosomal dominant ⇨ hamartomatous polyps, mucocutaneous hyperpigmentation (lips, oral mucosa, hands).****
- ***Age >50y*** (peaks 65y), Ulcerative colitis > Crohn dz; adenomatous polyps, ***diet (low fiber, high in red/processed meat,*** animal fat); smoking, ETOH, African-Americans, family history of CRC.

CLINICAL MANIFESTATIONS
Iron deficiency anemia, rectal bleeding, abdominal pain, change in bowel habits, ***CRC MC cause of large bowel obstruction in adults.*** Ascites, abdominal masses & hepatomegaly in advanced disease.
   - **RIGHT-SIDED (PROXIMAL):** lesions tend to ***bleed*** (anemia/⊕fecal occult blood) & cause diarrhea.

   - **LEFT-SIDE (DISTAL):** ***bowel obstruction, present later***, ⊕ changes in stool diameter, hematochezia.

DIAGNOSIS
1. **Colonoscopy with biopsy:** *diagnostic test of choice.*
2. **Barium enema:** ***apple core lesion classic.**** Lesions seen on barium enema need f/u colonoscopy.
3. **↑CEA. *CEA levels also monitored during treatment.*** CBC: anemia (***iron deficiency classic***).

MANAGEMENT:
   - Localized (stage I – III): surgical resection.
   - Stage III & metastatic: ***chemotherapy mainstay of treatment* ex. 5FU/****Fluorouracil.*

COLON CANCER SCREENING	Fecal Occult Blood test	COLONOSCOPY
Average Risk	*Annually @ 50y*	*Colonoscopy q 10y (or flex sig q5y)* up to 75y
1st degree relative >60y	*Annually @ 40y*	*Colonoscopy q 10y*
1st degree relative <60y	*Annually @ 40y* (or 10y before the age relative was diagnosed)	*Colonoscopy q 5y*

USPSTF guidelines recommends any of the 3 approaches: ❶ **High Sensitivity Fecal occult blood testing:** annually ❷ **Colonoscopy** every 10y from age 50-75 (individualized after 75) ❸ **Flexible sigmoidoscopy** every 5 years along with fecal occult blood testing every 3 years.
Lynch: screening begin @20-25y colonoscopy q1-2y; FAP: initiate screen at age 10-12 with flexible sig.

PROGNOSIS: preop CEA >5, ulcerative growth patterns are associated with worse prognosis.

INGUINAL HERNIAS

- Protrusion of the contents of the abdominal cavity through the inguinal canal.
- Indirect & direct are determined by their relation to the inferior epigastric vessels.

TYPES

1. **INDIRECT INGUINAL:** protrudes at the internal inguinal ring. The origin of the sac is LATERAL to the inferior epigastric artery. Often congenital due to a ***persistent patent process vaginalis*** an increase in abdominal pressure may force the intestines through the internal ring into the inguinal canal & may follow the testicle tract into the scrotum. *MC in young children & young adults. Most common overall type of hernias in men & women* (but MC occurs in men). Right sided more common.

2. **DIRECT INGUINAL:** protrude MEDIAL to the inferior epigastric vessels within Hesselbach's triangle, defined as ***"RIP"*** *R̲ectus Abdominis* (medial), *I̲nferior epigastric vessels* (lateral) & *P̲oupart's ligament* (inferiorly). Due to weakness in the floor of the inguinal canal. ***Does not reach the scrotum.***

CLINICAL MANIFESTATIONS

1. <u>Asymptomatic:</u> swelling or fullness at the hernia site. Enlarges with increased intrabdominal pressure and/or standing. *May develop scrotal swelling with indirect hernias.*
2. **Incarcerated:** *painful, enlargement of an irreducible hernia* (unable to return the hernia contents back into the abdominal cavity). ± nausea & vomiting if bowel obstruction present
3. **Strangulated:** *ischemic** incarcerated hernias with ***systemic toxicity**** (irreducible hernia with compromised blood supply). Severe painful bowel movement (may refrain defecation).

MANAGEMENT

Inguinal hernias often require surgical repair. Strangulated are surgical emergencies.

FEMORAL HERNIAS

- Protrusion of the contents of the abdominal cavity through the femoral canal below the inguinal ligament. *MC seen in women.**
- Often become incarcerated or strangulated compared to inguinal so surgical repair often done.

UMBILICAL HERNIAS

- Through the umbilical fibromuscular ring. Congenital (failure of umbilical ring closure).
- Usually due to loosening of the tissue around the ring in adults.

MANAGEMENT

1. Observation: usually resolves by 2 years of age.
2. Surgical repair if still persistent in children >5 years old to avoid incarceration or strangulation.

INCISIONAL (VENTRAL) HERNIAS

- Herniation through weakness in the abdominal wall.
- Incisional hernias occur MC with vertical incisions and in obese patients.

OBTURATOR HERNIAS

- Rare hernia through the pelvic floor in which abdominal/pelvic contents protrude through the obturator foramen. MC in women (especially multiparous) or women with significant weight loss.

HEMORRHOIDS

- Engorgement of venous plexus originating from:
    - superior hemorrhoid vein (internal hemorrhoids) proximal to the dentate line.
    - inferior hemorrhoid veins (external hemorrhoids) distal to the dentate line.

- **RISK FACTORS:** increased venous pressure: straining during defecation (ex. constipation), pregnancy, obesity, prolonged sitting, cirrhosis with portal hypertension.

CLASSIFICATION OF INTERNAL based on the degree of prolapse from the anal canal:

I	does not prolapse (confined to anal canal). May bleed with defecation.
II	prolapses with defecation or straining but spontaneously reduce.
III	prolapses with defecation or straining, requires manual reduction.
IV	Irreducible & may strangulate.

CLINICAL MANIFESTATIONS

1. INTERNAL Hemorrhoids:
- *intermittent rectal bleeding MC,* hematochezia (***bright red blood per rectum)*** - seen on toilet paper, coating the stool or dispersed in toilet water. ± rectal itching & fullness, mucus discharge.
- Rectal pain with internal suggests complication. Uncomplicated internal are usually neither tender nor palpable (unless they are thrombosed). Purple nodules may be seen with prolapse.

2. EXTERNAL Hemorrhoids:
- *perianal pain* aggravated with defecation* (covered by pain-sensitive skin). ± tender palpable mass. May have skin tags. Thrombosis may be precipitated by cough, heavy lifting.

DIAGNOSIS
1. Visual inspection, digital rectal examination, fecal occult blood testing.
2. Proctosigmoidoscopy, colonoscopy in patients with hematochezia to r/o proximal sigmoid disease.

MANAGEMENT
1. **Conservative treatment:** high-fiber diet, increased fluids. Warm Sitz baths & topical rectal corticosteroids (± analgesics like lidocaine) may be used for pruritus & discomfort/thrombosis.

2. **Procedures:** if failed conservative management, debilitating pain, strangulation or stage IV. Options include rubber band ligation (MC used), sclerotherapy or infrared coagulation.

3. Hemorrhoidectomy: for all stage IV or those not responsive to the aforementioned therapies.

ANORECTAL ABSCESS & FISTULAS

ABSCESS: often results from bacterial infection of anal ducts/glands. MC Staph aureus, E. coli, Bacteroides, Proteus, Streptococcus. *MC in posterior rectal wall.*

FISTULA: open tract between two epithelium-lined areas. Seen especially with deeper abscesses.

CLINICAL MANIFESTATIONS
- **Abscess:** anorectal swelling, rectal pain that is worse with sitting, coughing & defecation.
- **Fistula:** may cause anal discharge & pain

- **MANAGEMENT:** *I & D (incision & drainage) **followed by WASH** –
    Warm-water cleansing, **A**nalgesics, **S**itz baths, **H**igh-fiber diet.

ANAL FISSURES

- *Painful linear tear/crack** in the distal anal canal (initially only involving the epithelium but may involve the full thickness of the mucosa if untreated).

ETIOLOGIES:
- Low-fiber diets, passage of large, hard stools or other anal trauma.

CLINICAL MANIFESTATIONS:
- *severe painful rectal pain & bowel movements* causing *patient to refrain from having BM*, leading to *constipation, bright red blood per rectum.* ± mucoid discharge.

PHYSICAL EXAM:
- *skin tags* seen in chronic. *MC at posterior midline** (99% men, 90% women).

MANAGEMENT:
1. *>80% resolve spontaneously. Supportive measures:* warm water Sitz baths, analgesics, high fiber diet, increased water intake. Stool softeners, laxatives & mineral oil.
2. Second line treatment: topical vasodilators: Nitroglycerin (S/E: headache & dizziness); Nifedipine ointment.

PILONIDAL CYST/ABSCESS/SACROCOCCYGEAL FISTULA

• Tender abscess with drainage on or near the *gluteal cleft* near the midline of the coccyx or sacrum with small *midline pits.*
• MC in white males, obese, hirsute patients, prolonged sitting & local trauma. Rare over the age of 40y.

MANAGEMENT
Incision & drainage. Excision of pilonidal sinus & tracts recommended if recurrent.

PHENYLKETONURIA

• Autosomal recessive disorder of amino acid metabolism. ↓ability to metabolize the amino acid phenylalanine into tyrosine due to deficiency in the enzyme phenylalanine hydroxylase (PAH)⇨ *accumulation of phenylalanine* in body fluids/plasma ⇨ *phenylketone neurotoxicity.**
• Normally screened for @ 24 weeks gestation. Irreversible if not detected by 3 years old.

CLINICAL MANIFESTATIONS:
• Presents after birth with *vomiting, mental delays*, irritability, convulsions, eczema, ↑deep tendon reflexes. Children often *blonde, blue-eyed with fair skin.**

DIAGNOSIS:
urine with *musty (mousy) odor** (from phenylacetic acid).

MANAGEMENT
1. *Lifetime dietary restriction of phenylalanine* + increase tyrosine supplementation. Phenylalanine levels are followed at regular intervals in neonates & less often in older children/adults. Some adults show improvement in behavior, symptoms & sequelae when treated with a phenylalanine-restricted diet.
2. Foods high in phenylalanine: *milk, cheese, nuts, fish, chicken, meats, eggs, legumes, aspartame (found in diet sodas).*

VITAMIN A

- **Vitamin A Function:** vision, immune function, embryo development, hematopoiesis, skin and cellular health (epithelial cell differentiation).
- **Sources:** found in the kidney, liver, egg yolk, butter, green leafy vegetables.

- **Deficiency risk factors:** patients with liver disease, ETOHics, fat free diets.

CLINICAL MANIFESTATIONS OF VITAMIN A DEFICIENCY
1. *visual changes (especially __night blindness__),* xerophthalmia (dry eyes).
2. impaired immunity (poor wound healing), dry skin, poor bone growth, taste loss.
3. *__squamous metaplasia__* (conjunctiva, respiratory epithelium, urinary tract).
   - *__Bitot's spots:__* white spots on the conjunctiva due to squamous metaplasia of the corneal epithelium.

VITAMIN A EXCESS
Teratogenicity, alopecia, ataxia, visual changes skin disorders, hepatotoxicity.

VITAMIN C (ASCORBIC ACID) DEFICIENCY

- **RISK FACTORS:** diets lacking raw citrus fruits & green vegetables (excess heat denatures vitamin C), smoking, alcoholism, malnourished individuals, elderly.

CLINICAL MANIFESTATIONS
Scurvy 3 "H"s
1. *__H yperkeratosis:__* hyperkeratotic follicular papules (often surrounded by hemorrhage).

2. *__H emorrhage: vascular fragility__* (due to abnormal collagen production) with *__recurrent hemorrhages in gums, skin (perifollicular)__* *__& joints.__* *__Impaired wound healing.__*

3. *__H ematologic:__* anemia, glossitis, malaise, weakness. Increased bleeding time.

VITAMIN D DEFICIENCY

Fortified milk & sun exposure are excellent sources of vitamin D.

VITAMIN D DEFICIENCY
1. RICKETS (children): *__softening of the bones__* leading to bowing deformities (ex bowed legs), fractures, costochondral thickening ("rachitic rosary"), dental problems, muscle weakness & developmental delays.

2. OSTEOMALACIA (adults):
   diffuse body pains, muscle weakness & fractures. *__Looser lines__* (radiolucencies on X ray).

MANAGEMENT:
Ergocalciferol (Vitamin D).

VITAMIN B DEFICIENCY

THIAMINE (B1) DEFICIENCY:

- ***ETOH MC cause in US,**** decreased thiamine intake (ex. non-enriched rice or cereal).
1. **BERIBERI:**
   - "Dry": ***nervous system changes:*** paresthesias, demyelination ⇨ peripheral neuropathy. Symmetric impairment of sensory, motor & reflexes. Anorexia, muscle cramps & wasting.
   - "Wet": ***high output heart failure, dilated cardiomyopathy.***

2. **WERNICKE'S ENCEPHALOPATHY TRIAD:*** "AGO" ❶ ***Ataxia*** *(difficulty walking & balance)* ❷ ***Global confusion*** ❸ ***Ophthalmoplegia*** *(paralysis or abnormalities of the ocular muscles).*

3. **KORSAKOFF'S DEMENTIA:** *memory loss (esp. short term), confabulation.   Irreversible.*

RIBOFLAVIN (B2) DEFICIENCY:

- ***Oral-Ocular-Genital syndrome.****
  - **Oral:** lesions of mouth, ***magenta colored tongue, angular cheilitis,*** pharyngitis.
  - **Ocular:** photophobia, corneal lesions.
  - **Genital:** scrotal dermatitis.

NIACIN/NICOTINIC ACID (B3) DEFICIENCY:

- Often due to diets high in corn (lacks niacin & tryptophan) or diets which lack tryptophan.
- ***PELLAGRA "3 D's":**** ***diarrhea, dementia & dermatitis.****

PYRIDOXINE (B6) DEFICIENCY:

ETIOLOGIES: chronic alcoholism, ***isoniazid,*** oral contraceptives.
- **Neurologic:** ***peripheral neuropathy,**** seizures, headache.
- Stomatitis, cheilosis, glossitis, flaky skin, anemia.

B12 (COBALAMIN) DEFICIENCY:

Animal foods primary natural source of B_{12}. Stomach acids release B_{12} from food & binds it to intrinsic factor for later absorption in the ***terminal ileum.***
ETIOLOGIES
1. ***Pernicious Anemia:*** *autoimmune destruction/loss of gastric parietal cells** that secrete intrinsic factor ⇨ B_{12} deficiency.* **Diagnosis:** Antibody testing, ***Schilling test.***

2. ***Strict vegans*** (lack of animal sources in the diet if B_{12} not supplemented).

3. ***Malabsorption: ETOHism,*** diseases affecting the ileum (*ex. **Celiac disease, Crohn**).

4. ↓intrinsic factor production: *acid-reducing drugs (PPIs & H_2RA reduces absorption), gastric bypass surgery. atrophic gastritis.*

CLINICAL MANIFESTATIONS
1. ***neurologic symptoms:**** ***paresthesias, gait abnormalities, memory loss, dementia*** (due to degeneration of the posterolateral spinal cord).   **GI:** anorexia, diarrhea, glossitis.
2. ***Macrocytic anemia (↑MCV) with hypersegmented neutrophils.****

MANAGEMENT: Intramuscular or oral B_{12}. Intramuscular B_{12} for pernicious anemia.

MANAGEMENT OF DIARRHEA

❶ IV FLUID REPLETION
Mainstay of management of gastroenteritis. *PO preferred.* Sports drinks, broths, IV saline. Pedialyte, Ceralyte.

❷ DIET
- *Bland low-residue diet* usually best tolerated (crackers, boiled vegetables, yogurts, soup). Ex: "BRAT" diet Bananas, Applesauce Rice Toast.

❸ ANTI-MOTILITY AGENTS
- **Ind:** Patients <65y with moderate to severe signs of volume depletion.
- **CI:** *DO NOT give anti-motility drugs to patients with invasive diarrhea!* *(may cause toxicity).*

ANTI-DIARRHEALS	COMMENTS
BISMUTH SUBSALICYLATE Pepto-Bismol Kaopectate	**MOA:** *antimicrobial properties* against bacterial & viral pathogens, *Salicylate: anti-secretory & anti-inflammatory properties.* **Ind:** *safe in patients with dysentery* = significant fever, bloody diarrhea. **S/E:** *dark colored stools, darkening of tongue.* **CI:** children with viral illness (salicylate associated with ↑risk of Reye syndrome). **Reye:** *hepatoencephalopathy associated with ASA/salicylate use after viral illness* ⇨ *↑ICP (vomiting, stupor, coma, death), hepatomegaly & fulminant liver failure.* **Mgmt of Reye:** supportive care, ±lower ICP with mannitol.
OPIOID AGONISTS *Diphenoxylate*/Atropine (Lomotil) *Loperamide* (Immodium)	**MOA:** binds to gut wall opioid receptors, inhibiting peristalsis (subtherapeutic Atropine added to discourage opioid overdose or misuse). **S/E:** *CNS (central opiate effects),* anticholinergic side effects. N/V/abdominal pain. *Remember opiates often cause constipation so they slow GI transit.* **Ind:** *noninvasive diarrhea* (fever is absent or low grade & non bloody). **MOA:** binds gut wall *opioid receptors,* inhibiting peristalsis, ↑anal sphincter tone **S/E:** *avoid in patients c acute dysentery* (bloody stools, high fever) or colitis.
ANTICHOLINERGICS *Phenobarbital/Hyoscyamine/ Atropine/ Scopolamine* (Donnatal)	**MOA:** *anticholinergic* (Hyoscyamine, Atropine, Scopolamine) inhibits acetylcholine-related GI motility, relaxes GI muscles (*antispasmodic*), decreases gastric secretions; Phenobarbital slows down GI motility.

❹ ANTIEMETICS: vomiting usually due to imbalance of serotonin, acetylcholine, dopamine & histamine

Ondansetron (Zofran) *Granisetron* *Dolasetron*	**MOA:** *blocks serotonin receptors* (5-HT3) both peripherally & centrally in the chemoreceptor trigger zone. **S/E:** neurologic: headache, fatigue, sedation. GI bloating, diarrhea, constipation. Cardiac: prolonged QT interval, cardiac arrhythmias.
DOPAMINE BLOCKERS *Prochlorperazine* (Compazine) *Promethazine* (Phenergan) *Metoclopramide* (Reglan)	**MOA:** *blocks CNS dopamine receptors ($D_1 D_2$).* Mild antihistaminic/muscarinic. Metoclopramide is also a prokinetic agent (increases GI motility). **S/E:** *QT prolongation, anticholinergic & antihistamine S/E (ex drowsiness),* hypotension, hyperprolactinemia. **Extrapyramidal Sx (EPS):** *rigidity, bradykinesia, tremor, akathisia* (restlessness) include: 1. ***Dystonic Reactions (Dyskinesia):*** reversible EPS hours-days after initiation → intermittent, spasmodic, sustained involuntary contractions (trismus, protrusions of tongue, forced jaw opening, facial grimacing, difficulty speaking, torticollis)* **Mgmt:** *Diphenhydramine IV* or add anticholinergic agent (ex Benztropine). 2. Parkinsonism: (due to ↓dopamine in nigrostriatal pathways) – rigidity, tremor

NOROVIRUS

• **MC overall cause of gastroenteritis in adults in N. America*** *(often associated with **outbreaks ex. cruise ships, hospitals, restaurants).*** Vomiting predominant symptom in most noninvasive diarrhea.*

ROTAVIRUS

MC cause of diarrhea in children* (70%).

NONINVASIVE (ENTEROTOXIN) INFECTIOUS DIARRHEA

• **NONINVASIVE: vomiting, watery, voluminous (involves small intestine), no fecal WBCs or blood.**

STAPHYLOCOCCUS AUREUS

• *Short incubation period **within 6h*** (due to heat-stable enterotoxin). Food contamination MC source *ex. **dairy products, mayonnaise, meats, eggs.*** **Self-limiting (supportive treatment, fluids).**

• **CLINICAL MANIFESTATIONS:** prominent vomiting, abdominal cramps, headache, diarrhea.

BACILLUS CEREUS

• Very similar course to Staph aureus. ***IP 1-6h.*** MC in contaminated food ***(ex. fried rice).****

• **CLINICAL MANIFESTATIONS:** *vomiting,* cramps, diarrhea. **Management:** supportive, fluids.

VIBRIO CHOLERAE & VIBRIO PARAHEMOLYTICUS

Exotoxin causes hypersecretion of water & chloride ions, leading to severe dehydration.
• **VIBRIO CHOLERAE:** gram-negative rod transmitted via **contaminated food & water. Outbreaks** may occur **during poor sanitation & overcrowding conditions (especially abroad).**

• **VIBRIO PARAHEMOLYTICUS & V. VULNIFICUS:** associated with ***raw shellfish esp in Gulf of Mexico.****

CLINICAL MANIFESTATIONS

1. **Vibrio Cholera & parahemolyticus:** *copious watery diarrhea **"rice water stools" (grey, no fecal odor, blood or pus)*** that may **rapidly produce severe dehydration*** (patients may lose up to 15L/day). If fatal, usually results from hypovolemia.
2. **V. vulnificus:** more associated with **bacteremia & cellulitis** (not diarrhea).

MANAGEMENT:

1. ***Supportive: fluid replacement mainstay.**** Often self-limited.
2. Antibiotics: **tetracyclines,** *fluoroquinolones* or macrolides may shorten the disease course in patients who are severely ill, other comorbid conditions or with high fever.

ENTEROTOXIGENIC E. COLI

*MC cause TRAVELER'S DIARRHEA.** Risks: unpeeled fruits, UNSANITARY DRINKING WATER/ICE.* IP 24-72 hours.

CLINICAL MANIFESTATIONS: abrupt onset of watery diarrhea, abdominal cramping, vomiting.

MANAGEMENT: *Fluids.* ± Bismuths. If severe ⇨ ***±fluoroquinolone;*** Bactrim, Azithromycin.

CLOSTRIDIUM DIFFICILE

• Usually nosocomial/iatrogenic. Organism overgrowth 2ry to alteration of the normal flora (MC after course of antibiotics (especially **Clindamycin***) or chemotherapy.

CLINICAL MANIFESTATIONS: abdominal cramps, diarrhea, fever, tenderness, ***strikingly ↑lymphocytosis.*** **pseudomembranous colitis.** ± cause bowel perforation & **toxic mega colon.**

MANAGEMENT: ***Metronidazole 1st line for mild dz*; Vancomycin PO 2nd line (but 1st line if severe dz).***

INVASIVE INFECTIOUS DIARRHEA

- **INVASIVE:** *high fever,* ⊕ *blood & fecal leukocytes*, not as voluminous (large intestine), mucus.*
- *DO NOT give anti-motility drugs with invasive diarrhea!* (may cause toxicity).*
- Includes: Campylobacter, Shigella, Salmonella, Yersinia, Enterohemorrhagic E coli, Campylobacter.

CAMPYLOBACTER ENTERITIS
- *C. jejuni MC cause of bacterial enteritis in United States.** 3 day average incubation period.
- *C. jejuni MC ANTECEDENT EVENT IN POST-INFECTIOUS GUILLAIN-BARRÉ SYNDROME.**

Sources: contaminated food *(undercooked poultry)*, raw milk, water, dairy cattle.

CLINICAL MANIFESTATIONS
- fever, headache, abdominal pain (±*mimic acute appendicitis).* Diarrhea *initially watery* ⇨ *bloody.*

DIAGNOSIS: stool culture: gram negative *"S, COMMA, OR SEAGULL SHAPED*"* organisms. Blood cultures.

MANAGEMENT: *Fluids.* If severe ⇨ ± *Erythromycin 1st line,** *Fluoroquinolones,* Doxycycline.

SHIGELLA
Fecal/oral contamination. *Highly virulent.* IP 1-7d. S. sonnei MC in US, S flexneri, dysenteriae. Gram-negative

CLINICAL MANIFESTATIONS:
1. *lower abdominal pain*, high fever, tenesmus, *explosive watery diarrhea* ⇨ *mucoid, bloody.**
   Severe cases may lead to toxic megacolon. Cx include reactive arthritis (Reiter's syndrome).
2. Neurologic manifestations especially in young children *(FEBRILE SEIZURES).**

DIAGNOSIS:
1. Stool cultures; Fecal WBC/RBCs. CBC: ± *LEUKEMOID REACTION (WBC >50,000*/μL).
2. **Sigmoidoscopy:** *punctate areas of ulceration.**

MANAGEMENT: *Fluids.* If severe ⇨ ±*Trimethoprim-sulfamethoxazole 1st line,** Fluoroquinolones.

SALMONELLA
- Greater in the summer months (healthy patients need large inoculum). IP 6-48h.
- *MC source: poultry products (dairy, meat, eggs), exotic pets (reptiles ex. turtles).** Feco-oral.

- *High risk groups:* immunocompromised states, *sickle cell disease (↑risk of osteomyelitis with Salmonella),** post splenectomy patients, AIDS, children, elderly.

1. **SALMONELLA GASTROENTERITIS:** *S. typhimurium.* 5-14d IP. Abdominal pain, fever, cramping, vomiting, *mucus + bloody diarrhea.* Usually self-limited.

2. **TYPHOID (ENTERIC) FEVER** *S. typhi.* Prolonged IP >1-2weeks. **CEPHALIC PHASE:** *headache,* constipation, pharyngitis, cough ⇨ crampy abdominal pain, diarrhea *PEA SOUP STOOLS** (brown-green color). *intractable fever, relative bradycardia,** hepatosplenomegaly, blanching *"ROSE SPOTS"** appears in 2nd week. Patients may have ⊕ blood cultures for Salmonella & leukopenia.

MANAGEMENT: *Fluids.* If severe ⇨ ± *Fluoroquinolones,* Ceftriaxone, Trimethoprim-sulfamethoxazole.

ENTEROHEMORRHAGIC E COLI 0157:H7

- **Sources:** ingestion of **_undercooked ground beef, unpasteurized milk/apple cider, day care centers, contaminated water._** Incubation period average 4-9 days. **_Produces cytotoxin._**

CLINICAL MANIFESTATIONS:
Watery diarrhea early on ⇨ bloody, crampy abdominal pain, vomiting. Fever low grade or absent.

MANAGEMENT:
- **_Fluid replacement_** & supportive measures.
- **_Antibiotic use controversial (↑incidence of Hemolytic Uremic Syndrome in children)._***

YERSINIA ENTEROCOLITICA

Sources: contaminated pork, milk, water & tofu

CLINICAL MANIFESTATIONS: fever, abdominal pain **_mimic acute appendicitis_** (can cause **_mesenteric adenitis,_** producing abdominal tenderness, guarding).

MANAGEMENT: _fluid replacement._ If severe ⇨ ±Fluoroquinolones, Trimethoprim-Sulfamethoxazole

	NON-INVASIVE DIARRHEAS	INVASIVE DIARRHEAS
Pathophysiology:	Enterotoxins increase GI secretion of electrolytes ⇨ **_secretory diarrhea_** **_No cell destruction/mucosal invasion._**	**Cytotoxins cause mucosal invasion & cell damage.**
Affected area:	**_Small bowel_** ⇨ **_large voluminous_*** stools.	**_Large bowel_** ⇨ **_many small-volume stools, high fever._**
Vomiting	**_Vomiting predominant symptom._**	Vomiting not as common.
Fecal Blood/WBC/mucus:	**Absent**	⊕ **_Fecal blood/WBCs & mucus._***
Examples	Viral, S. Aureus, B. cereus, V. cholera, Enterotoxigenic E coli	Enterohemorrhagic E coli, Shigella, Salmonella, Yersinia, Campylobacter

PROTOZOAN INFECTIONS

GIARDIA LAMBLIA

Sources: ingestion of **_contaminated water from remote streams/wells_*** aka **_Beaver's fever_** or "**_Backpacker's diarrhea_**". Beavers are reservoirs for the protozoa.
Boil H_2O x 1 minute to kill cysts.

CLINICAL MANIFESTATIONS
1. **_Frothy, greasy, foul diarrhea_*** (no blood or pus) and malabsorption with cramping, bloating.

DIAGNOSIS: trophozoites/cysts in the stool.

MANAGEMENT: _fluids. Metronidazole_*, Tinidazole, Albendazole, Quinacrine; **_Furazolidone in children._***

AMEBIASIS

Sources: _Entamoeba histolytica_ transmitted by fecally contaminated soil/water & feco-oral.
MC seen in travelers to developing nations or in the immigrant population.

CLINICAL MANIFESTATIONS: _GI colitis, dysentery, AMEBIC LIVER ABSCESSES._*
DIAGNOSIS: stool ova & parasites.

MANAGEMENT: _Fluid replacement._
1. **Colitis: _Metronidazole_*** *(Flagyl)* or Tinidazole followed by an intraluminal agent: ex. Paromomycin (anti-parasitic aminoglycoside) or Diloxanide furoate or Diiodohydroxyquin (Iodoquinol).
2. **Abscess:** Metronidazole or Tinidazole + intraluminal antiparasitic followed by Chloroquine. May need drainage if no response to medications after 3 days.

CRYPTOSPORIDIUM
- *MC cause of chronic diarrhea in patients with AIDS.* Feco-oral transmission. No proven efficacious treatment (HAART with immune restoration).

ISOSPORA BELLI
- MC in homosexual men, patients c AIDS. Transmitted feco-oral. **Tx:** Trimethoprim-Sulfamethoxazole

OSMOTIC DIARRHEA

- *MALABSORPTION OF NONABSORBABLE SUBSTANCES* in the intestinal lumen with secondary accumulation of fluid (the increased solutes in GI tract promotes diarrhea by pulling water into the gut).
- *↓diarrhea with fasting, ↑osmotic gap, ↑ fecal fat, deficiency in fat soluble vitamins.*

RAPID TRANSIT OF GI CONTENTS
1. Medications: Lactulose, Sorbitol, Antacids

BACTERIAL OVERGROWTH
1. **Whipple's disease:** caused by *Tropheryma whippelii*
2. **Tropical Sprue:** occurs in the tropics; treatment with antibiotics and folate, B$_{12}$

MALABSORPTION ABNORMALITIES
1. **Celiac Sprue (disease):** reaction to α-gliadin in gluten ⇨ loss of villi & absorptive area.
2. **Pancreatic insufficiency,** bile salt insufficiency.
3. **Lactose Intolerance.**

SECRETORY DIARRHEA

- *Normal osmotic gap, large volume, no change in diarrhea with fasting*.*
    1. **Hormonal:** serotonin (carcinoid syndrome), calcitonin (medullary cancer of thyroid), gastrin (Zollinger-Ellison Syndrome).
    2. **Laxative abuse**

WHIPPLE'S DISEASE

Tropheryma whippelii. MC in farmers around contaminated soil

CLINICAL MANIFESTATIONS:
malabsorption: weight loss, steatorrhea, nutritional deficiency, fever, lymphadenopathy, nondeforming arthritis, neurologic symptoms, *rhythmic motion of eye muscles while chewing.*

DIAGNOSIS
1. **duodenal biopsy:**
    *Periodic acid-Schiff (PAS) -positive macrophages, non acid-fast bacilli, **dilation of lacteals.***

MANAGEMENT:
Penicillin or Tetracycline for 1-2 years.

CONSTIPATION

- Infrequent bowel movements (<2/week), straining, hard stools, feeling of incomplete evacuation).

Etiologies: disordered movement of stool through colon/anus/rectum (usually the proximal GI tract is intact). ***Slow colonic transit:*** idiopathic, motor disorders (colorectal CA, DM, hypothyroid), S/E of many drugs ***ex. verapamil, opioids.*** Outlet delay: Hirschsprung's dz.

DRUG/INTERVENTION	COMMENTS
FIBER	**MOA**: *retains water & improves GI transit.*
BULK FORMING LAXATIVES ***Psyllium*** ***Methylcellulose*** (Citrucel) ***Polycarbophil*** (Fibercon) ***Wheat Dextran*** (Benefiber)	**MOA**: *absorbs water & increases fecal mass* (natural or synthetic polysaccharides or cellulose). Increases the frequency & softens the consistency of stool with minimal effects. Dietary fiber & bulk forming laxatives the most physiologic & effective approach to constipation. **S/E:** flatulence, bloating
OSMOTIC LAXATIVES ***Polyethylene Glycol (PEG)*** - Golytely - Miralax (no e'lytes) ***Lactulose*** ***Sorbitol*** **Saline Laxatives** - ***Milk of Magnesia*** - ***Magnesium Citrate***	**MOA**: *causes H_2O retention in stool (osmotic effect pulls H_2O into gut)* Synthetic disaccharide (sugar) not absorbed (pulls water into gut). **S/E:** bloating, flatulence. Also used in hepatic encephalopathy. Synthetic sugar (cheap). **S/E:** bloating, flatulence. **S/E:** hypermagnesemia (especially with chronic renal disease).
STIMULANT LAXATIVES ***Bisacodyl*** (Dulcolax) ***Senna***	**MOA**: ↑*acetylcholine-regulated GI motility (peristalsis)* & alters electrolyte transport in the mucosa. **S/E:** diarrhea, abdominal pain

SELECTED REFERENCES

Festi D, Scaioli E, Baldi F, et al. Body weight, lifestyle, dietary habits and gastroesophageal reflux disease. World J Gastroenterol. 2009;15(14):1690-701.

Kaltenbach T, Crockett S, Gerson LB. Are lifestyle measures effective in patients with gastroesophageal reflux disease? An evidence-based approach. Arch Intern Med. 2006;166(9):965-71.

Cullen DJ, Hawkey GM, Greenwood DC, et al. Peptic ulcer bleeding in the elderly: relative roles of Helicobacter pylori and non-steroidal anti-inflammatory drugs. Gut. 1997;41(4):459-62.

Larvin M, Mcmahon MJ. APACHE-II score for assessment and monitoring of acute pancreatitis. Lancet. 1989;2(8656):201-5.

Pederzoli P, Bassi C, Vesentini S, Campedelli A. A randomized multicenter clinical trial of antibiotic prophylaxis of septic complications in acute necrotizing pancreatitis with imipenem. Surg Gynecol Obstet. 1993;176(5):480-3.

Drossman DA. The functional gastrointestinal disorders and the Rome III process. Gastroenterology. 2006;130(5):1377-90.

Winawer S, Fletcher R, Rex D, et al. Colorectal cancer screening and surveillance: clinical guidelines and rationale-Update based on new evidence. Gastroenterology. 2003;124(2):544-60.

Hershcovici T, Fass R. Pharmacological management of GERD: where does it stand now?. Trends Pharmacol Sci. 2011;32(4):258-64.

Kahrilas PJ, Shaheen NJ, Vaezi MF, et al. American Gastroenterological Association Medical Position Statement on the management of gastroesophageal reflux disease. Gastroenterology. 2008;135(4):1383-1391, 1391.e1-5.

Enzinger PC, Mayer RJ. Esophageal cancer. N Engl J Med. 2003;349(23):2241-52.

Cholongitas E, Papatheodoridis GV, Vangeli M, Terreni N, Patch D, Burroughs AK. Systematic review: The model for end-stage liver disease--should it replace Child-Pugh's classification for assessing prognosis in cirrhosis?. Aliment Pharmacol Ther. 2005;22(11-12):1079-89.

O'leary JG, Friedman LS. Predicting surgical risk in patients with cirrhosis: from art to science. Gastroenterology. 2007;132(4):1609-11.

O'leary JG, Yachimski PS, Friedman LS. Surgery in the patient with liver disease. Clin Liver Dis. 2009;13(2):211-31.

Kamath PS, Wiesner RH, Malinchoc M, et al. A model to predict survival in patients with end-stage liver disease. Hepatology. 2001;33(2):464-70.

Ranson JH, Rifkind KM, Roses DF, Fink SD, Eng K, Spencer FC. Prognostic signs and the role of operative management in acute pancreatitis. Surg Gynecol Obstet. 1974;139(1):69-81.

Baron TH, Morgan DE. Acute necrotizing pancreatitis. N Engl J Med. 1999;340(18):1412-7.

Cullen DJ, Hawkey GM, Greenwood DC, et al. Peptic ulcer bleeding in the elderly: relative roles of Helicobacter pylori and non-steroidal anti-inflammatory drugs. Gut. 1997;41(4):459-62.

Caroli A, Follador R, Gobbi V, Breda P, Ricci G. [Mallory-Weiss syndrome. Personal experience and review of the literature]. Minerva Dietol Gastroenterol. 1989;35(1):7-12.

Wang L, Li YM, Li L. Meta-analysis of randomized and controlled treatment trials for achalasia. Dig Dis Sci. 2009;54(11):2303-11.

Kato S, Yamamoto R, Yoshimitsu S, et al. Herpes simplex esophagitis in the immunocompetent host. Dis Esophagus. 2005;18(5):340-4.

Lundell LR, Dent J, Bennett JR, et al. Endoscopic assessment of oesophagitis: clinical and functional correlates and further validation of the Los Angeles classification. Gut. 1999;45(2):172-80.

Kurata JH, Nogawa AN. Meta-analysis of risk factors for peptic ulcer. Nonsteroidal antiinflammatory drugs, Helicobacter pylori, and smoking. J Clin Gastroenterol. 1997;24(1):2-17.

Sachs G, Shin JM, Howden CW. Review article: the clinical pharmacology of proton pump inhibitors. Aliment Pharmacol Ther. 2006;23 Suppl 2:2-8.

Jensen RT. Gastrinomas: advances in diagnosis and management. Neuroendocrinology. 2004;80 Suppl 1:23-7.

Ghaneh P, Costello E, Neoptolemos JP. Biology and management of pancreatic cancer. Gut. 2007;56(8):1134-52.

Ducrotté P. [Irritable bowel syndrome: current treatment options]. Presse Med. 2007;36(11 Pt 2):1619-26.

Amoebiasis. Report of a WHO Expert Committee. World Health Organ Tech Rep Ser. 1969;421:1-52.

Dupont HL. Interventions in diarrheas of infants and young children. J Am Vet Med Assoc. 1978;173(5 Pt 2):649-53.

CHAPTER 4 – MUSCULOSKELETAL & RHEUMATOLOGIC DISORDERS

SHOULDER INJURIES

ANTERIOR GLENOHUMERAL SHOULDER DISLOCATION

<u>Mechanism:</u> blow to an abducted, externally rotated arm that is extended.

CLINICAL MANIFESTATIONS: *arm <u>ABDUCTED, EXTERNALLY ROTATED</u>;** Can palpate the humeral head inferiorly (loss of deltoid contour) ⇨ *"squared off shoulder".* *Anterior dislocation MC type.*

DIAGNOSIS: axillary & "Y" view. <u>Humeral head inferior/anterior to the glenoid fossa.</u>
Hill-Sachs lesion- *groove on humeral head* (compression fracture from impact against glenoid).
Bankart lesion – *glenoid inferior rim fracture.*

MANAGEMENT: Reduction. *Must rule out <u>AXILLARY NERVE INJURY (PINPRICK SENSATION OVER THE DELTOID).</u>**

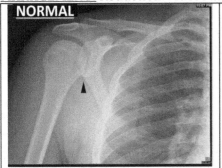 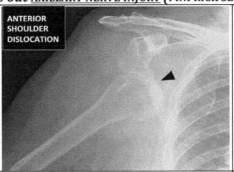 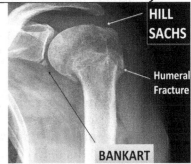

NORMAL AP: humeral head articulates with glenoid (arrowhead). Appears overlapped.	ANTERIOR DISLOCATION: Humeral head **anterior & inferior to glenoid**	HILL-SACHS: Humeral head groove BANKART: **fracture of glenoid rim**

POSTERIOR GLENOHUMERAL SHOULDER DISLOCATION

<u>Mechanism:</u> forced adduction, internal rotation. *MC associated with seizures, electric shock,* trauma.
CLINICAL MANIFESTATIONS: arm *ADDUCTED, INTERNALLY ROTATED;* Anterior shoulder flat, humeral head prominent.
MANAGEMENT: reduction & immobilization.

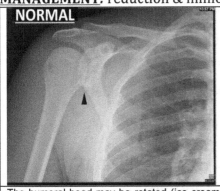 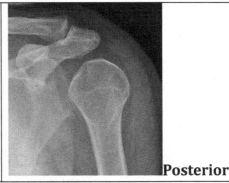 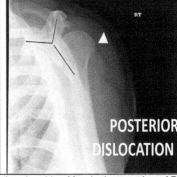

The humeral head may be rotated (ice cream on cone/light bulb appearance) and isn't centered on the glenoid. May look normal on AP view, or may show increased distance from the glenoid rim (normally there is overlap between glenoid rim and the humeral head).

AXILLARY & "Y" VIEW – MOST HELPUL TO DETERMINE ANTERIOR VS. POSTERIOR

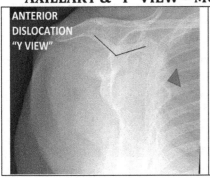 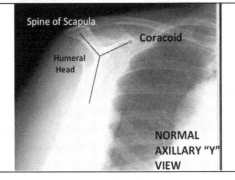 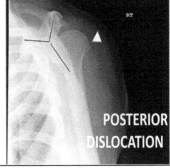

ROTATOR CUFF INJURIES

MOI: chronic erosion, ± trauma. ***SITS*** (***supraspinatus,*** * infraspinatus, teres minor, subscapularis).
Common in athletes or laborers performing repetitive overhead movements. ***Supraspinatus MC.****
- **Tendonitis:** inflammation usually associated with **subacromial bursitis:** MC **adolescents <40y.**

- **Rotator cuff tear:** MC cause of shoulder pain **>40y.** Trauma 50% or chronic overuse.

CLINICAL MANIFESTATIONS
1. ***Anterior deltoid pain with ↓ROM especially c overhead activities, external rotation or abduction***
   (combing hair, reaching for wallet), inability to sleep on the affected side (especially with tears).

2. *Weakness, atrophy & continuous pain most commonly seen with tears.**

PHYSICAL EXAMINATION:
✓ **ROM:** ***passive ROM usually greater than active ROM**** (limited active ROM) of the humerus.
   Pain with abduction >90º suggests tendinopathy.

✓ ***Supraspinatus strength test:*** "empty can" test.

✓ **Impingement tests:** of subscapular nerve/supraspinatus:
   ⊕**Hawkins test:** Elbow/shoulder flexed @90º with ***sharp anterior shoulder pain with internal rotation.***

   ⊕ **Drop arm test:** pain with inability to lift arm above shoulder level or hold it or severe pain
   when slowly lowering the arm after the shoulder is abducted to 90º.

   ⊕ **Neer test:** ***arm fully pronated*** (thumb's down) ***with pain during forward flexion*** (while
   shoulder is held down to prevent shrugging).
   Supraspinatus test: pain with abduction against resistance.

✓ ***Subacromial lidocaine test:*** may help to distinguish tendinopathy from tears.
   Normal strength with pain relief = tendinopathy. Persistent weakness seen with large tears.

MANAGEMENT
1. **Tendinitis:** ***shoulder pendulum/wall climbing exercises***, ice, NSAIDs, stop offending activity.

2. **Tear:** Conservative: rehab, NSAIDs, intraarticular corticosteroids, ROM preservation; Surgery.

ROTATOR CUFF INJURIES

PHYSICAL EXAMINATION

*Impingement of subscapular nerve/supraspinatus between acromial
process & humeral head:*

- ⊕ *Neer test: arm fully pronated (thumb's down) c pain during
  forward flexion (shoulder is held down to prevent shrugging)*

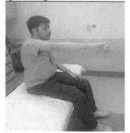
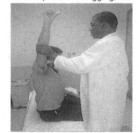

ROTATOR CUFF INJURIES

PHYSICAL EXAMINATION

*Impingement of subscapular nerve/supraspinatus between acromial
process & humeral head:*

- ⊕ *Hawkins test*: Elbow/shoulder flexed @90º c sharp anterior
  shoulder pain on passive internal rotation of humerus*

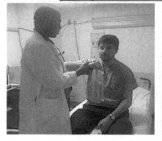
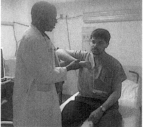

ACROMIOCLAVICULAR JOINT DISLOCATION "shoulder separation"

Mechanism: direct blow to an adducted shoulder.

CLINICAL MANIFESTATIONS: pain with lifting arm, unable to lift arm @ shoulder. ± deformity @AC joint.

DIAGNOSIS: radiograph taken without weights or with weights to reveal mild separations.

SHOULDER SEPARATION

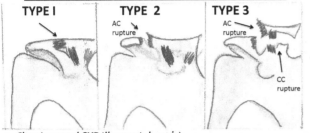

TYPE I   TYPE 2   TYPE 3

AC rupture   AC rupture

CC rupture

- **Class I:** *normal CXR (ligamental sprain)*
- **Class II:** *slight widening (Acromioclavicular ligament ruptured)*
  Coracoclavicular ligament sprained
- **Class III:** *significant widening: rupture of both AC & CC ligaments*
- Class IV: AC & CC rupture + displacement of clavicle into/through trapezius
- Class V: Class IV + disruption of the clavicular attachments

GRADE 2 SHOULDER SEPARATION

- Acromioclavicular (AC) ligament RUPTURED
- Coracoclavicular (CC) ligament sprained

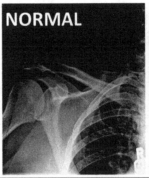
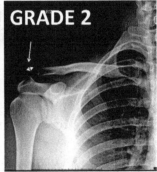

NORMAL   GRADE 2

MANAGEMENT: *brief sling immobilization*, ice, analgesia, & ortho follow up. Type III may need surgery.

PROXIMAL HUMERUS/HUMERAL HEAD FRACTURES

MOI: FOOSH, direct blow to arm. Common site for pathologic fractures in metastatic breast cancer.

CLINICAL MANIFESTATIONS: arm held in adducted position.
   *Check deltoid sensation, (to **rule out <u>brachial plexus or axillary nerve injuries</u>**).**

HUMERAL SHAFT FRACTURES

MOI: FOOSH, direct trauma. ***Must rule out <u>radial nerve injury</u>** (injury may cause **wrist drop**).**

Management: "Sugar tong splint", Coaptation splint, sling/swathe. Ortho follow up in 24-48h.

PROXIMAL HUMERUS FRACTURE
arm usually held in adducted position.
Check deltoid sensation*, brachial plexus injury
± crepitus/ecchymosis

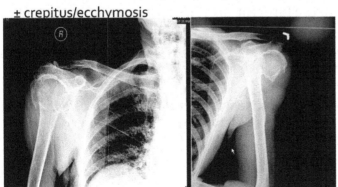

HUMERAL SHAFT FRACTURE
- **MOI:** FOOSH, direct trauma.
- *R/o radial nerve injury (may develop a wrist drop)**

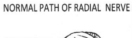
NORMAL PATH OF RADIAL NERVE

AXILLARY NERVE

RADIAL NERVE

ULNAR NERVE

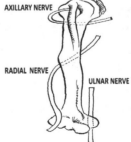
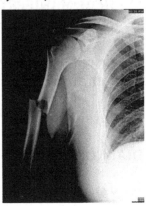

CLAVICLE FRACTURES

- *Most commonly fractured bone in children, adolescents & newborns during birth.***

- <u>MOI:</u> mid-high energy impact to the area. MC in males. In children <2y ⇨ suspect child abuse.

<u>CLINICAL MANIFESTATIONS:</u> pain with ROM, deformity @ site, ±"tenting" of skin, crepitus, may hold arm against the chest to protect against motion.

<u>COMPLICATIONS</u>
pneumothorax, coracoclavicular ligament disruption (distal), hemothorax, brachial plexus injuries.

<u>MANAGEMENT</u>
mid $^1/_3$ ⇨ arm sling 4-6 weeks in adults. Figure-of-eight sling in children

proximal $^1/_3$ ⇨ orthopedic consult.

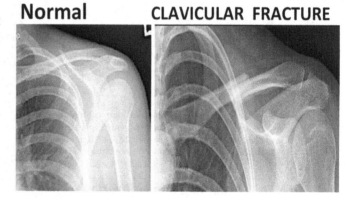

Normal   **CLAVICULAR FRACTURE**

ADHESIVE CAPSULITIS (FROZEN SHOULDER)

- <u>Shoulder stiffness</u> due to inflammation (*especially with DM, hypothyroidism*). MC 40s - 60s

<u>CLINICAL MANIFESTATIONS</u>
1. ***Shoulder pain/stiffness*** lasts 18-24 months, ↓***ROM* (especially with external rotation).** *Stiff-pain cycle.* Pain is usually worse at night. Gradual return of range of motion.
2. **Physical Examination:** resistance on passive range of motion (ROM) only on the affected side.

<u>MANAGEMENT</u>
1. Rehab ROM therapy mainstay of tx. Antiinflammatories, intraarticular steroid injection, heat.

THORACIC OUTLET SYNDROME

- *Idiopathic compression of brachial plexus* (95%), *subclavian vein* (5%) *or subclavian artery* (1%) as they exit the narrowed space between shoulder girdle & 1st rib. MC in women 20-50y.

<u>CLINICAL MANIFESTATIONS:</u>
1. <u>Nerve compression:</u> pain/paresthesias to the forearm, arm &/or ***ulnar side*** of the hand.

2. <u>Vascular compression:</u> swelling /discoloration of the arm *especially with abduction of the arm* (erythema, edema or cyanosis of affected arm).

3. <u>Physical examination:</u> ⊕ *Adson:** loss of radial pulse with head rotated to affected side.*

<u>DIAGNOSIS:</u> MRI

<u>MANAGEMENT</u>
Controversial. Physical therapy 1st line, avoid strenuous activity. Orthopedic consult, ± surgery.

ELBOW & FOREARM INJURIES

SUPRACONDYLAR HUMERUS FRACTURES

MOI: FOOSH with hyperextended elbow (extra-articular). *MC in children 5-10y.*

CLINICAL MANIFESTATIONS

  swelling, tenderness at the elbow, prominent olecranon (with depression proximally).

DIAGNOSIS
- *abnormal anterior humeral line* may be seen on the lateral view if displaced.
- *Nondisplaced* ⇨ *displaced anterior fat pad sign or* ⊕ *posterior fat pad sign** (hemarthrosis).
- ⊕ *anterior/posterior fad pad = supracondylar fracture in children (= radial head fracture in adults).**

COMPLICATIONS: *median nerve & brachial artery injury* ⇨ *Volkmann ischemic contracture**
  (claw-like deformity from ischemia with flexion/contracture of wrist). *Radial nerve injury.*

MANAGEMENT: Nondisplaced ⇨ posterior splint; Displaced ⇨ ORIF; All displaced fractures or severe swelling should be admitted for observation *(immediate orthopedic consult).*

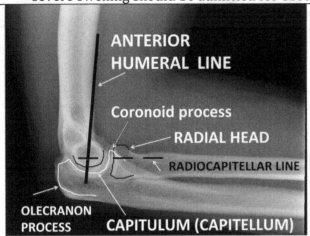

NORMAL LATERAL VIEW: the radial head dissects the capitellum. A line drawn from the anterior humerus should also dissect the capitellum.

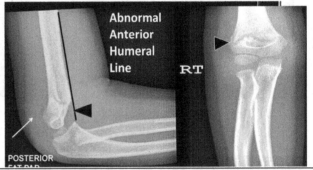

SUPRACONDYLAR FRACTURE

DIAGNOSIS
- *Abnormal anterior humeral line* on lateral view

SUPRACONDYLAR FRACTURE: abnormal anterior humeral line (does not dissect the capitellum). Note the posterior fat pad sign. The fracture site is easily visible on the AP film (arrowhead)

SUPRACONDYLAR FRACTURE

DIAGNOSIS
- ⊕ Anterior or Posterior fat pad sign (hemarthrosis)

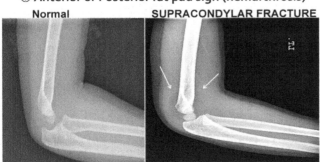

SUPRACONDYLAR FRACTURE:
Sometimes there is a normal anterior humeral line and the only clue is an abnormal anterior or ⊕ posterior fat pad (joint effusion).

Posterior fat pads are always abnormal.

Anterior fat pads may be seen as a normal variant if they are small and almost parallel to the humerus.

RADIAL HEAD FRACTURES

MOI: FOOSH (fall on an outstretched hand). Usually intraarticular.

PHYSICAL EXAMINATION: Lateral (radial) elbow pain, ***inability to fully extend the elbow.***

DIAGNOSIS: notoriously difficult to see.
 fat pad sign: ⊕ ***posterior fat pad or displaced anterior fat pad*** (hemarthrosis).

MANAGEMENT: non displaced ⇨ sling, long arm splint 90º; Displaced ⇨ ORIF.

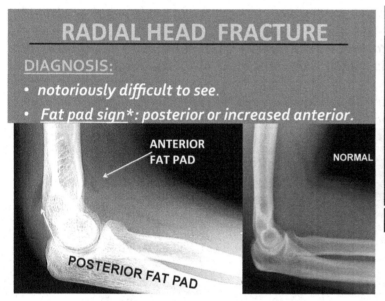
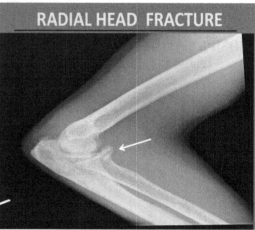

SUPPURATIVE FLEXOR TENOSYNOVITIS

Infection of the flexor tendon synovial sheath of the finger.
 • ***Skin flora: Staph aureus MC***, S. epidermis, GABHS; Others: Pseudomonas or mixed flora.
Mechanism: often due to penetrating trauma or contiguous spread from adjacent tissues.

CLINICAL MANIFESTATIONS
 Pain & swelling especially to the palmar aspect of the affected finger.
 Kanavel's signs (4): **FLEX**or tenosynovitis
 1. **Finger held in flexion.**
 2. **Length of tendon sheath is tender** (tenderness along the tendon sheath).
 3. **Enlarged finger** (fusiform swelling of the finger).
 4. **Xtension of the finger causes pain (*pain with passive extension*).***

DIAGNOSIS
 Radiographs & MRI are often obtained but definitive diagnosis is via aspiration &/or biopsy.

MANAGEMENT
 Incision & drainage with irrigation of the tendon sheath ± debridement & IV antibiotics.

OLECRANON FRACTURES

MOI: direct blow (fall on a flexed elbow).

CLINICAL MANIFESTATIONS:
Pain, swelling, ***inability to extend the elbow.*** The triceps muscle may rupture or pull the proximal fragment superiorly, causing distraction (because it inserts at the olecranon).

COMPLICATIONS: *ulnar nerve dysfunction.**

MANAGEMENT: Reduction. Nondisplaced ⇨ splint (90° flexion); Displaced ORIF.

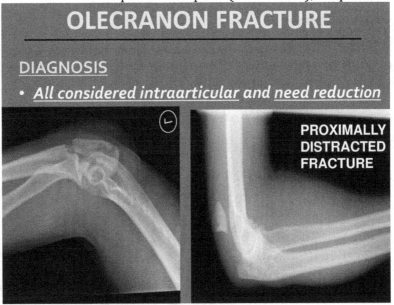

OLECRANON BURSITIS

- Inflammation of the bursa over the bony prominences.

ETIOLOGIES: gout, inflammation, direct trauma (repetitive, microtrauma), infectious.

CLINICAL MANIFESTATIONS: *abrupt "goose egg"* swelling (boggy, red elbow); ± tender or painless. *Limited ROM with flexion.* Evaluate for skin breaks (rule out septic bursitis).

MANAGEMENT: rest, NSAIDs, local steroid injection, padding, avoid repetitive motions.

SEPTIC BURSITIS: bursa aspiration: WBC count >2,000 cells/mm³ may be septic (cell count may be lower). Gram stain & culture helpful when unsure based on cell count.

ULNAR SHAFT (NIGHTSTICK) FRACTURE

MOI: direct blow. May present with localized pain & swelling.
MANAGEMENT:
Nondisplaced distal $^1/_3$ ⇨ short arm cast.
Nondisplaced mid-proximal $^1/_3$ ⇨ long arm cast.
Displaced ⇨ open reduction & internal fixation.

MONTEGGIA FRACTURE

• ***Proximal ulnar shaft fracture with an anterior radial head dislocation.***

MOI: direct blow to the forearm.

CLINICAL MANIFESTATIONS: elbow pain, thumb paresthesias. The dislocated radial head can damage the radial nerve ⇨ ***radial nerve injury*** (may develop a ***wrist drop*)** 17%.

MANAGEMENT: unstable. Open reduction & internal fixation (ORIF).

GALEAZZI FRACTURE

• ***Mid-distal radial shaft fracture with dislocation of DRUJ**** (distal radioulnar joint).
MOI: FOOSH (fall on an outstretched hand) or direct blow.

CLINICAL MANIFESTATIONS: fracture/deformity on the radial side of the wrist. Additionally, the ulnar head will appear prominent at the wrist (because it is dorsally displaced).

MANAGEMENT *UNSTABLE! Needs ORIF.* Long arm splint; Sugar tong splint temporarily.

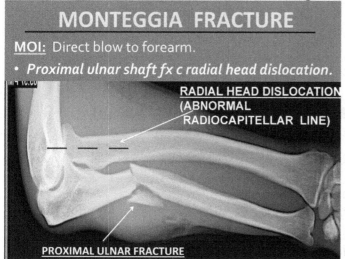

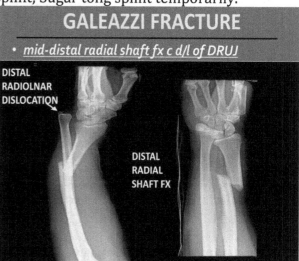

RADIAL HEAD SUBLUXATION (NURSEMAID'S ELBOW)

MOI: *lifting/swinging/pulling a child (MC 2-5y)* while the forearm is pronated & extended ⇨ radial head wedges into the ***stretched annular ligament.***

CLINICAL MANIFESTATIONS: *children present with arm slightly flexed, refuses to use arm* (usually no swelling). Tenderness to palpation of the radial head.

MANAGEMENT: *reduction (pressure on the radial head with supination & flexion).* Observe child for normal function. If child uses the arm after 15 minutes, no radiographs are needed. If no use after 15 minutes ⇨ ±radiographs to rule out fracture or reattempt reduction.

HUTCHINSON FRACTURE: radial styloid fracture (aka Chauffeur's fracture).

LATERAL EPICONDYLITIS (TENNIS ELBOW)

MOI: inflammation of the tendon insertion of ECRB *(extensor carpi radialis brevis muscle)** due to repetitive pronation of the forearm & *excessive wrist extension.*

CLINICAL MANIFESTATIONS:
*Lateral elbow pain especially with gripping, forearm pronation & WRIST EXTENSION against resistance.** ± radiate down the forearm or worsen when lifting objects with forearm prone.

MANAGEMENT: RICE, NSAIDs, physiotherapy, brace; Intraarticular steroid injection.
Surgery if refractory to conservative management.

MEDIAL EPICONDYLITIS (GOLFER'S ELBOW)

MOI: inflammation of the *pronator teres-flexor carpi radialis** due to repetitive stress @ tendon insertion of flexor forearm muscle. MC in golfers, patients who do household chores.

CLINICAL: *tenderness over the medial epicondyle **worse with pulling activities,** reproduced by performing WRIST FLEXION against resistance** with the elbow fully extended.*
MANAGEMENT: similar to lateral epicondylitis (however more difficult to treat).

ELBOW DISLOCATION

MOI: FOOSH with hyperextension (high energy). ***Posterior MC type.****

CLINICAL MANIFESTATIONS: *presents with flexed elbow, marked olecranon prominence,* & inability to extend elbow. Often associated with radial head or coronoid process fracture.
MANAGEMENT: *EMERGENT reduction! Posterior splint* @ 90° x7-10d; Unstable ⇨ ORIF.

COMPLICATIONS: Must r/o *brachial artery & median/ulnar/radial nerve injury!**

NORMAL

POSTERIOR ELBOW DISLOCATION

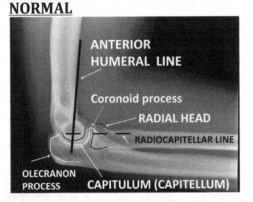
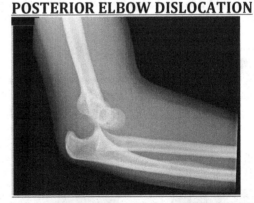

CUBITAL TUNNEL SYNDROME (ULNAR NEUROPATHY)

• *Ulnar nerve compression* at the cubital tunnel along the medial elbow ⇨ *paresthesias/pain along the ULNAR NERVE** distribution (worse with elbow flexion).

PHYSICAL EXAMINATION
⊕ *TINEL'S SIGN AT THE ELBOW;** ⊕ *FROMENT'S SIGN** (ulnar nerve evaluation via adductor pollicus – holds paper & compensates with flexion of IP joint – pinching effect).

MANAGEMENT: Wrist immobilization especially with sleep, NSAIDs, intraarticular steroids (chronic).

WRIST INJURIES

SCAPHOID (NAVICULAR) FRACTURE

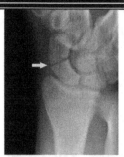

MOI: *FOOSH* on extended wrist. MC carpal fracture (65% occur at the waist).
CLINICAL MANIFESTATIONS: Pain along the radial surface of the wrist with *ANATOMICAL SNUFFBOX TENDERNESS.* *
DIAGNOSIS: fracture may not be evident for up to 2 weeks ⇨ *if snuffbox tenderness, treat as fracture* because ↑*incidence of avascular necrosis* * ⇨ *nonunion* * (blood supply to scaphoid is distal to proximal). MRI.
MANAGEMENT *Thumb spica* * *if nondisplaced or snuffbox tenderness.*
Displaced ⇨ ORIF is the definitive management.

SCAPHOLUNATE DISSOCIATION

Pain on the dorsal radial side of wrist (±click c wrist movement). ⊕ Terry Thomas sign (>3mm space).
MANAGEMENT: radial gutter splint. May need operative repair of the scapholunate ligament.
Order of ↑instability: scapholunate dissociation ⇨ perilunate dislocation ⇨ *lunate dislocation.*

COLLES FRACTURE

• *Distal radius fracture with DORSAL/POSTERIOR ANGULATION.* * 60% also have ulnar styloid fracture. *MC FOOSH with wrist extension.* * ↑postmenopausal (60-70%), Asian, osteoporotic women.

DIAGNOSIS: *"dinner fork deformity".* * On AP, Colles & Smith look alike (need lateral view).
Unstable fractures: if >20º angulation, intraarticular, >1cm shortening or comminuted.
COMPLICATIONS: *EPL extensor pollicus longus tendon rupture MC,* * malunion, joint stiffness, median nerve compression, residual radius shortening, complex regional pain syndrome.
MANAGEMENT: *Sugar tong* splint/cast.* If stable (<20º angulation ⇨ closed reduction).
ORIF if unstable or comminuted.

SMITH FRACTURE

• "Reverse Colles Fracture" *(ventral/anterior) angulation.* * *MC FOOSH* with *wrist flexion.* *

COLLES FRACTURE
DORSAL angulation. *

SMITH FRACTURE
VENTRAL angulation.

BARTON FRACTURE
Intra-articular distal radius fracture with *carpal displacement.* *

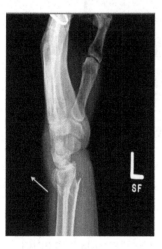
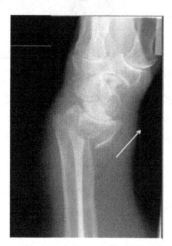
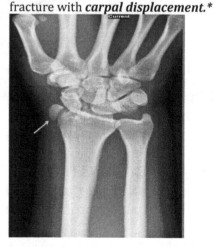

PERILUNATE DISLOCATION

- Lunate doesn't articulate with the capitate (but lunate still articulates with the radius).

PERILUNATE DISLOCATION	PERILUNATE DISLOCATION
Capitate no longer articulates with lunate (us dorsal) Lunate still articulates with radius	Capitate no longer articulates with lunate (us dorsal) Lunate still articulates with radius.
Normal PERILUNATE	Normal PERILUNATE
AP VIEW: capitate does not articulate with the lunate.	**LATERAL VIEW:** note the appearance of the lunate in relation to the capitate.

LUNATE DISLOCATION

- The lunate *doesn't articulate with the both the capitate OR the radius. Emergent consult!*

DIAGNOSIS: AP view: *"piece of pie" sign;* lateral view: *lunate = "spilled teacup" sign.**

MANAGEMENT: *unstable.* Needs ORIF (open reduction internal fixation).

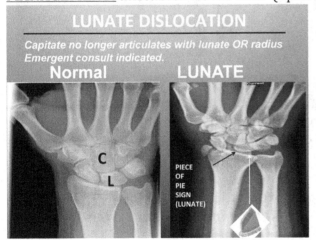

LUNATE DISLOCATION: *"piece of pie sign"* – seen on the AP view.

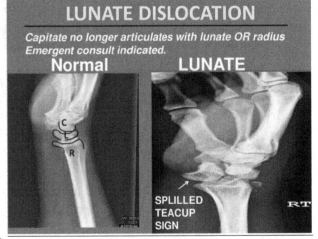

LUNATE DISLOCATION:" spilled teacup" sign" – seen on the lateral view.

LUNATE FRACTURE

- ***Most serious carpal fracture*** since the lunate occupies ²/₃ of the radial articular surface. Radiographs are often negative.

- ***Avascular necrosis of the lunate bone = Kienböck's disease.***
<u>MANAGEMENT:</u> immobilization with orthopedic follow up.

CARPAL FRACTURES

Normal   **LUNATE FRACTURE**   **TRIQUETRUM FRACTURE**

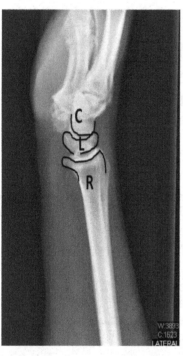 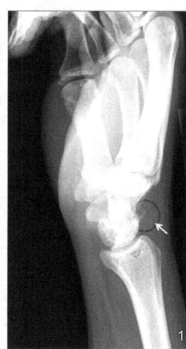 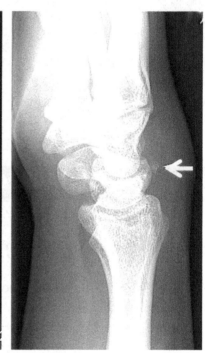

COMPLEX REGIONAL PAIN SYNDROME (CRPS)

- Formerly known as reflex sympathetic dystrophy (RSD). Unknown etiology.
- ***Autonomic dysfunction following bone or soft tissue injuries*** (ex. wrist fracture or post surgery). 30% have no history of injury.

<u>CLINICAL MANIFESTATIONS:</u> MC affects the upper extremities.
  <u>Stage I:</u> ***pain out of proportion to injury. Autonomic nervous system symptoms:*** swelling, extremity color changes, ↑nail & hair growth.

  <u>Stage II:</u> waxy or pale skin, brittle nails, loss of hair.

  <u>Stage III</u>: joint atrophy & contractures.

<u>MANAGEMENT:</u> NSAIDs initial treatment. Anesthetic blocks, physical therapy, oral corticosteroids, tricyclic antidepressants, transcutaneous electric nerve stimulation, etc. ***Vitamin C prophylaxis after fractures may reduce the incidence of CRPS.***

HAND & FINGER INJURIES

MALLET (BASEBALL) FINGER

MOI: *extensor tendon avulsion* after sudden blow to tip of an extended finger with forced flexion.

CLINICAL MANIFESTATIONS: *inability to straighten the distal finger (flexed @ DIP joint).**
Commonly associated with an avulsion fracture of the distal phalanx at the distal insertion of the extensor tendon.

MANAGEMENT *splint the DIP in* <u>UNINTERRUPTED EXTENSION</u> *x 6 weeks vs. surgical pinning.*

MALLET FINGER

- Mechanism: *avulsion of extensor tendon c̄ sudden blow to tip of extended finger c̄ forced flexion. UNABLE TO EXTEND DIP*

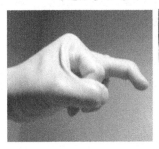

Tear in extensor tendon

MALLET FINGER

- *Commonly associated with avulsion fracture of the distal phalanx (at its distal insertion).*

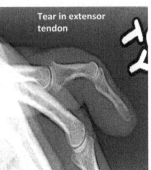

Distal Phalanx Avulsion Fracture

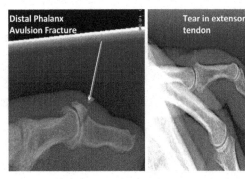

Tear in extensor tendon

BOUTONNIERE DEFORMITY

MOI: sharp force against the tip of a partially extended digit ⇨ hyperflexion at the PIP joint with hyperextension at the DIP. Disruption of extensor tendon at the base of the middle phalanx.

MANAGEMENT: splint PIP in extension x 4-6weeks with hand surgeon follow up.

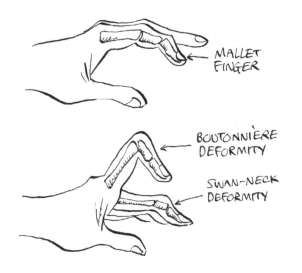

MALLET FINGER

BOUTONNIÈRE DEFORMITY

SWAN-NECK DEFORMITY

MALLET FINGER
Finger flexed at the DIP joint
    unable to extend at the DIP joint

BOUTONNIERE DEFORMITY
Finger flexed @ PIP joint &
    hyperextended @ DIP joint

SWAN NECK DEFORMITY
Finger hyperextended @ PIP joint &
    flexed @ DIP joint

GAMEKEEPER'S (SKIER'S) THUMB

- Sprain or tear of the <u>ULNAR COLLATERAL LIGAMENT</u> *of the thumb* ⇨ *instability of MCP joint.**

- **SKIER'S THUMB**: *acute* condition (ex. after fall); **GAMEKEEPER'S**: *chronic hyperabduction injury.**
  Mechanism: Forced abduction of the thumb (UCL functions to resist against valgus forces).

  CLINICAL MANIFESTATIONS: *thumb far away from the other digits* (especially with *valgus stress* – pulling thumb away from the hand), MCP tenderness, weakness in pinch strength.
  ± *fracture at the base of the proximal phalanx* (if UCL ruptures, it may pull off piece of bone).

  MANAGEMENT: *thumb spica** & referral to hand surgeon (because it *affects pincer function)*.
  Complete rupture: surgical repair.

GAMEKEEPER'S (SKIER'S) THUMB

FORCED
HYPERABDUCTION INJURY

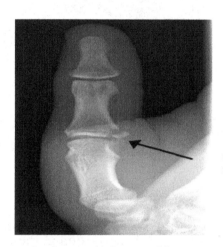

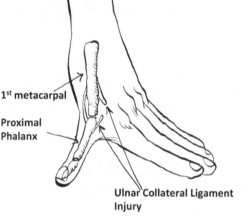

1st metacarpal

Proximal
Phalanx

Ulnar Collateral Ligament
Injury

In some cases, a fracture of the proximal
phalanx on the ulnar side may be seen.

BOXER'S FRACTURE

- *Fracture at the neck of 5th metacarpal* (±4th).*
- ± rotational deformity. ± Loss of the knuckle on exam.

Mechanism: punching with a clenched fist.
  If at the base ⇨ look for associated carpal injuries.

MANAGEMENT
1. <u>ULNAR GUTTER SPLINT</u>* with joints in @ least 60°
   flexion.
   - any fracture > 25-30° angulation should be reduced.
   - ORIF if it remains >40° angulated.

2. **Always check for bite wounds.*** If present treat
   with the appropriate antibiotics
      (ex. Amoxicillin/clavulanic acid).

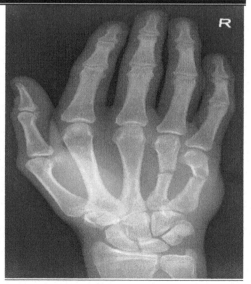

Boxer's fracture of the 5th. 4th
metacarpal fracture also seen here.

BENNETT FRACTURE – DISLOCATION/ROLANDO FRACTURE

BENNETT'S FRACTURE: *intraarticular fracture through the base of 1st metacarpal (MCP) bone* with a large distal fragment dislocated radially & dorsally by the abductor pollicus longus muscle.

ROLANDO'S FRACTURE: *comminuted Bennett's fracture.*

MANAGEMENT *Unstable! Requires ORIF.* **Thumb spica** for temporary stabilization.

BENNETT & ROLANDO FX

- **Bennett's Fracture:** *intraarticular fracture through base of the 1st metacarpal (MCP)*

- **Rolando's fracture:** *COMMINUTED Bennett's fracture.*

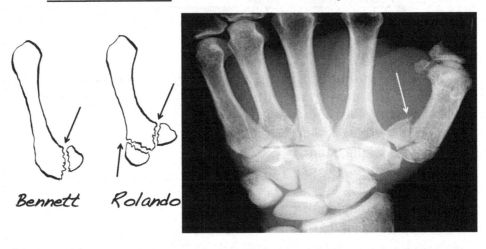

Bennett   Rolando

SALTER- HARRIS CLASSIFICATION OF FRACTURES

- *Growth (Epiphyseal) Plate Fractures. "SALTR" useful mnemonic IN RELATION TO PLATE*

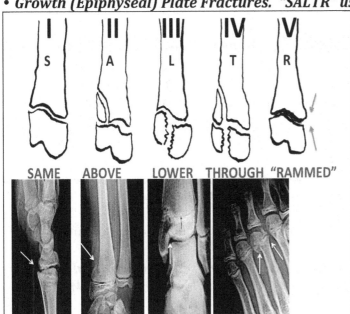

I S — SAME
II A — ABOVE
III L — LOWER
IV T — THROUGH
V R — "RAMMED"

Type I: isolated growth plate fracture (may look normal). Best outcome.

Type II: growth plate fracture + *fracture of the metaphysis (good prognosis).* *MC of all Salter-Harris Fractures.*

Type III: growth plate fracture + *fracture of the epiphysis.* (good prognosis).

Type IV: fracture *extending across the metaphysis, growth plate & epiphysis (needs reduction).*

Type V: *Growth plate compression injury* (may arrest growth). *Worst type!*

de QUERVAIN TENOSYNOVITIS

Stenosing tenosynovitis of the *abductor pollicus longus (APL) & extensor pollicus brevus (EPB).*

MOI: excessive thumb use with repetitive action. Seen in golfers, clerical workers, etc.

CLINICAL MANIFESTATIONS: *pain along the radial aspect of the wrist* radiating to the forearm* especially with thumb extension or gripping. Pain at the radial styloid.

DIAGNOSIS: ⊕ *FINKELSTEIN TEST:* pain with ulnar deviation or thumb extension.*

MANAGEMENT: *Thumb spica splint* (x3weeks); NSAIDs x10-14d, steroid injection, physical therapy.

CARPAL TUNNEL SYNDROME

MEDIAN NERVE **entrapment/compression** at the carpal tunnel. ↑incidence with *Diabetes Mellitus.*

CLINICAL MANIFESTATIONS
Paresthesias, & pain of palmar 1st 3 (& ½ of the 4th) digits underline especially @ night* (because of normal wrist flexion during sleep). Pain may radiate to the neck, shoulder, chest. *Thenar muscle wasting** seen if advanced.
 - *Increased pain: worse @ night** (repeated flexion/extension of wrist).
 - Decreased pain: shaking hands.

DIAGNOSIS
Workup may include electromyography & nerve conduction velocity studies.
 • ⊕ *TINEL'S SIGN:** percussion of the median nerve produces symptoms.

 • ⊕ *PHALEN'S SIGN:** flexion of both wrists for 30-60 seconds reproduces the symptoms.

MANAGEMENT *volar splint* + NSAIDs ⇨ steroid injections. Carpal tunnel surgery in refractory cases.

DIFFERENTIAL DIAGNOSIS: PRONATOR SYNDROME *median nerve compression* in the *proximal forearm.* May develop paresthesias in the same distribution as carpal tunnel. However, *pronator syndrome* associated more with *proximal forearm pain* than wrist/hand pain & *not associated with pain at night* (like seen in carpal tunnel).

DUPUYTREN CONTRACTURE

• MC in men 40-60y. Genetic predisposition (ex. *Northwestern Europeans*), ETOH abuse, DM.

MOI: contractures of the palmar fascia due to nodules/cords ⇨ fixed flexion deformity @ MCP.

CLINICAL MANIFESTATIONS: *nodules over the distal palmar crease or proximal phalanx* (especially ring, little finger).* Nodules often painful. *Fixed flexion deformity @ MCP joint.*

MANAGEMENT: intralesional corticosteroid injection, collagenase injection, Physical therapy; Surgical correction if contracture >30° at the MCP joint or any PIP flexion contracture.

HIP & PELVIS INJURIES

PELVIC FRACTURES

MOI: high-impact injuries (ex. MVA). Acetabular fractures MC occur with associated lower extremity, abdominal or neurologic injuries. May have **perineal ecchymosis**.

MANAGEMENT: ORIF. Weight bearing as tolerated for some pubic rami fractures.
COMPLICATIONS: infection, DVT, sciatic nerve damage, vascular injury (bleeding).

HIP DISLOCATIONS

MECHANISM: *trauma MC cause* (MVA, fall from height). True orthopedic emergency!

COMPLICATIONS: *avascular necrosis** up to 13% (reduced with early closed reduction <6h). *Sciatic nerve injury,* DVT, bleeding.
- **Posterior MC (90%).** Anterior usually secondary to forced hip abduction.

CLINICAL MANIFESTATIONS:
1. **Hip pain with <u>LEG SHORTENED, INTERNALLY ROTATED</u>* & adducted with hip/knee slightly flexed.** Anterior may be externally rotated.

HIP FRACTURES

MOI: minor or indirect trauma in the elderly. High-impact injuries in younger patients.
- MC in osteoporotic women. Common in the elderly & patients with decreased bone mass.
- <u>Femoral Head/Neck Fractures:</u> **high incidence of avascular necrosis with femoral neck fractures.*** High incidence of DVT & pulmonary embolism.
- Intertrochanteric/Subtrochanteric are extracapsular. Femoral head/neck fractures are intracapsular.

CLINICAL MANIFESTATIONS: *hip pain with leg* <u>SHORTENED, EXTERNALLY ROTATED,</u>* *ABDUCTED.*

MANAGEMENT: ORIF. ± Observation if high surgical risk, minimal pain or non ambulatory.

HIP FRACTURES
- Femoral head/neck fractures are INTRACAPSULAR
- Intertrochanteric/Subtrochanteric fractures are EXTRACAPSULAR
- Leg is SHORTENED, EXTERNALLY ROTATED, ABDUCTED

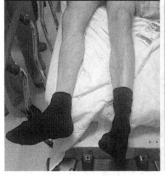
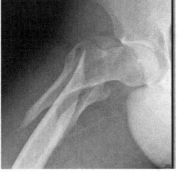

HIP DISLOCATION
- Clinical Manifestations: *pain, posterior* →*LEG SHORTENED, INTERNALLY ROTATED, ADDUCTED C HIP/KNEE SLIGHTLY FLEXED.*

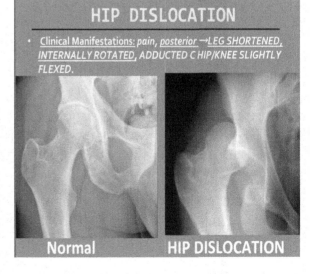

Normal   HIP DISLOCATION

LEGG-CALVÉ-PERTHES DISEASE

- *Idiopathic <u>AVASCULAR OSTEONECROSIS OF THE FEMORAL HEAD IN CHILDREN</u>* due to ischemia of capital femoral epiphysis* in children.

- ***MC in children 4-10y,*** 4x ***MC in boys,*** low incidence in African-Americans.

CLINICAL MANIFESTATIONS:

1. <u>*PAINLESS LIMPING*</u>** x weeks (worsen with continued activity especially at the end of the day).* May have intermittent hip, thigh, knee or groin pain.

2. Restricted range of motion (<u>***LOSS OF ABDUCTION & INTERNAL ROTATION***</u>).*

DIAGNOSIS:

1. <u>hip radiographs</u>:
   - **early:** ↑*density of the femoral head, widening of the cartilage space.*
   - **advanced***: deformity,* <u>*CRESCENT SIGN*</u>*** (microfractures with collapse of the bone).

MANAGEMENT:

1. **Observation**: because it is self-limiting with revascularization within 2y, activity restriction (non weight bearing initially) with orthopedic follow up is initial treatment in most cases. ± protected weight bearing during early stages until reossification is complete. Physical therapy.

2. Pelvic osteotomy may be indicated in some children > 8 years of age, especially lateral pillar B and B/C.

LEGG-CALVÉ-PERTHES DISEASE

- Idiopathic avascular necrosis of the femoral head in children due to <u>ischemia of the femoral epiphysis</u>.

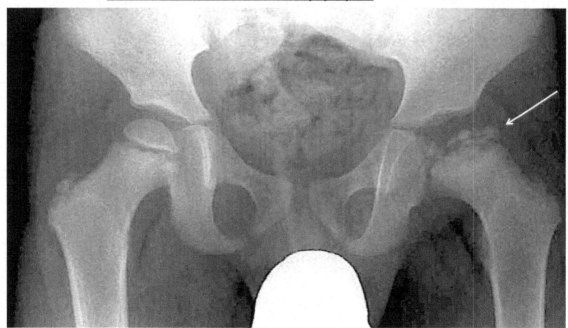

SLIPPED CAPITAL FEMORAL EPIPHYSIS

- Femoral head (epiphysis) slips posterior & inferior at the growth plate.
- *MC in **7-16y, obese, African-American, males** during growth spurt* (due to weakness of the growth plate & hormonal changes at puberty). ***If seen in children before puberty, suspect hormonal/systemic disorders (ex hypothyroidism,****hypopituitarism).*

<u>**CLINICAL MANIFESTATIONS:**</u> ***hip, thigh or knee pain with limp,*** external rotation* *of affected leg.*

MANAGEMENT: non weight-bearing with crutches ⇨ **ORIF** (↑ risk of avascular necrosis).

SLIPPED CAPITAL FEMORAL EPIPHYSIS

- Femoral head epiphysis slips <u>POSTERIOR & INFERIOR</u> @ **growth plate** *(seen here on the left side).*

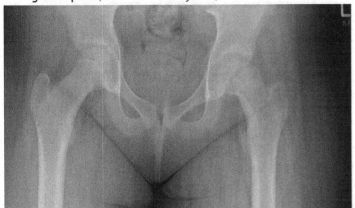
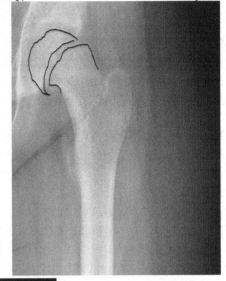

PEDIATRIC FRACTURE TYPES

GREENSTICK FRACTURES

- Incomplete fracture with cortical disruption & periosteal tearing on the convex side of the fracture (intact periosteum on the concave side) ***"bowing".****

TORUS (BUCKLE) FRACTURES

- Incomplete fracture with ***"wrinkling or bump"*** of the metaphyseal-diaphyseal junction (where the dense bone meets the more porous bone) due to axial loading.

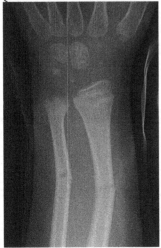
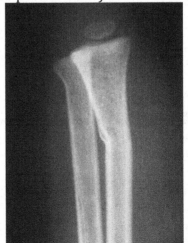

GREENSTICK FRACTURE   **TORUS (BUCKLE) FRACTURE**

KNEE INJURIES

MCL (Medial) & LCL (lateral) COLLATERAL LIGAMENT INJURIES

Mechanism: **MCL:** *vaLgus stress with rotation.* **LCL:** *vaRus stress.*

CLINICAL MANIFESTATIONS: localized pain, swelling, ecchymosis, stiffness.
MANAGEMENT:
1. Grades I (sprains) & II (incomplete tears): *conservative*: pain control, physical therapy to restore range of motion & muscle strength, RICE, NSAIDs, knee immobilizer.
2. Grades III (complete tears): ± surgical repair.

ANTERIOR CRUCIATE LIGAMENT (ACL) INJURIES

- **MC knee ligament injury** (± be associated with meniscal tears). 70% sports-related.
MOI: *NONCONTACT PIVOTING INJURY** (deceleration, hyperextension, internal rotation).

CLINICAL MANIFESTATIONS: associated with **"pop & swelling ⇨ hemarthrosis".** ± **knee buckling**, inability to bear weight. Does not actively extend the knee. MC in women.

PHYSICAL EXAM:
1. **ACL Laxity:** *LACHMAN'S TEST** *most sensitive.* Pivot shift test.
   ANTERIOR DRAWER TEST (least reliable because spasms may stabilize the knee).
2. **± Segond fracture:** avulsion of the lateral tibial condyle with varus stress to the knee. If present, ligamental injuries are most likely present. *Pathognomonic for ACL tear.*
MANAGEMENT: controversial (depends on activity level of the patient). Therapy vs. surgical.
Unhappy (O'Donoghue's) triad: injury to ❶ ACL + ❷medial collateral ligament + ❸ medial meniscus.

POSTERIOR CRUCIATE LIGAMENT (PCL) INJURIES

MOI: *MC associated with dashboard injuries* (anterior force to proximal tibia with knees flexed), direct blow injury or fall on a flexed knee. Usually associated with other ligamentous injuries.
CLINICAL MANIFESTATIONS
Anterior bruising (especially to the anteromedial aspect of proximal tibia). Large effusion.

PHYSICAL EXAMINATION: *Pivot shift test, Posterior drawer test.*
MANAGEMENT: almost always treated operatively (± lead to degenerative changes).

MENISCAL TEARS

MOI: degenerative (squatting, twisting, compression or trauma with femur rotation on the tibia).
- **Medial 3x MC > lateral** (because of more bony attachments).

CLINICAL MANIFESTATIONS: *LOCKING,** *popping, "giving way", EFFUSION AFTER ACTIVITIES.**

PHYSICAL EXAMINATION: ⊕*McMURRAY'S SIGN** (pop or click while the tibia is externally & internally rotated), Apley test, *joint line tenderness*, effusion.
MANAGEMENT: NSAIDs, partial weight bearing until orthopedic follow up. Arthroscopy.

PATELLAR FRACTURE

MOI: *MC direct blow* (fall on a flexed knee, ± forceful quadriceps contraction).
MC in young patients.

CLINICAL MANIFESTATIONS: pain, swelling, deformity. Limited knee extension with pain.
DIAGNOSIS: *sunrise view radiographs** (best view).

MANAGEMENT: Nondisplaced ⇨ knee immobilizer, leg cast x 6 weeks; Displaced ⇨ surgery.

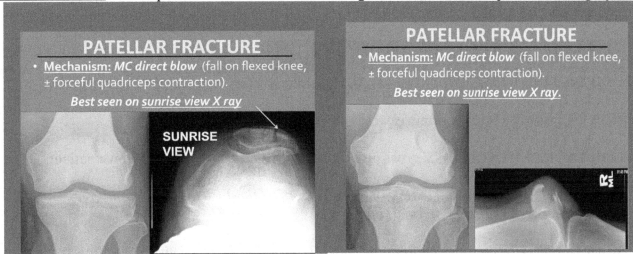

PATELLAR & QUADRICEPS TENDON RUPTURES

MOI: *forceful quadriceps contraction* (fall on a flexed knee, walking up/down stairs).
- *MC males >40y,* history of *systemic disease* (DM, gout, obesity, renal disease).
- Quads > patellar. Quads rupture usually >40; Patellar rupture usually <40y.

CLINICAL MANIFESTATIONS:
1. Sharp proximal knee pain with ambulation, *inability to extend knee/straight leg raise.*
2. **Quadriceps tendon rupture***: patella baja-* palpable *defect above* knee.
3. **Patellar tendon rupture***: patella alta –* palpable *defect below* knee.

MANAGEMENT knee immobilizer, non or partial weight bearing, RICE.
Surgical repair within 7-10 days.

NORMAL KNEE	PATELLAR TENDON RUPTURE	QUADRICEPS TENDON RUPTURE
Lateral View	"Patella Alta" Lateral View	"Patella Baja" - Lateral View

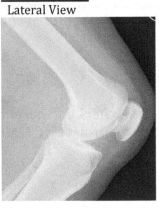
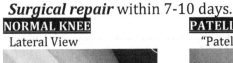
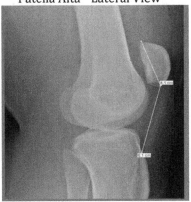

PATELLAR DISLOCATION

MOI: *vaLgus stress* after twisting injury, direct blow. *MC females; Usually <u>laterally.</u>*

PHYSICAL EXAM: ⊕*apprehension sign:* patient exhibits anxiety/forcefully contracts the quadriceps when the examiner pushes laterally. Only performed if patellar is already reduced.

MANAGEMENT *closed reduction:* push anteromedially on the patella while gently extending the leg. Post reduction films. Knee immobilizer (full extension), quads strengthening.

KNEE (Tibial-femoral) DISLOCATIONS

• ***<u>SEVERE LIMB THREATENING EMERGENCY!</u>*** (popliteal artery rupture severe complication).

MOI: high velocity trauma, often associated with multiple trauma.

CLINICAL MANIFESTATIONS: gross deformity, may reduce by itself (so believe patients).

COMPLICATIONS: *<u>popliteal artery injury</u>* in $^1/_3$ of patients ⇨ arteriography.*
    ± Peroneal or tibial nerve injury.

MANAGEMENT *Immediate orthopedic consult.* Prompt reduction via longitudinal traction.

FEMORAL CONDYLE FRACTURES

MOI: *axial loading* (fall from height); direct blow to the femur.

CLINICAL MANIFESTATIONS: pain, swelling, inability to bear weight.

COMPLICATIONS: *<u>peroneal nerve injuries</u> (check 1ˢᵗ web space); popliteal artery injury.*

MANAGEMENT *immediate orthopedic consult!* ORIF. Usually heals poorly.

TIBIAL PLATEAU FRACTURES

MECHANISM: *axial loading/rotation/direct trauma **(MC in children in motor vehicle accidents).** Lateral plateau MC.*

Complications: post degenerative arthritis (>50%); loss of joint congruity.

CLINICAL MANIFESTATIONS: pain, swelling, hemarthrosis. If displaced, ***check for peroneal nerve injury (foot drop).*** ± hard to see on radiographs; may need to confirm with CT/MRI.

MANAGEMENT:
1. Nondisplaced ⇨ conservative tx (non weight bearing cast 6-8 weeks).
2. Displaced ⇨ ORIF (open reduction, internal fixation).

OSGOOD-SCHLATTER DISEASE

- Osteochondritis of the patellar tendon @ tibial tuberosity from ***overuse*** (repetitive stress) or small avulsions (due to quadriceps contraction on the patellar tendon insertion into the tibia).
- *MC cause of chronic knee pain in young, active adolescents.*
- *MC males, 10-15y, athletes with "growth spurts"** (bone growth faster than soft tissue growth, so quadriceps contraction transmitted through patellar tendon to the tuberosity).

CLINICAL MANIFESTATIONS
1. *ACTIVITY-RELATED KNEE PAIN/SWELLING** (running, jumping, kneeling).
2. Painful lump below knee, ***tenderness to the anterior tibial tubercle.***

DIAGNOSIS: radiographs show prominence or heterotopic ossification at the tibial tuberosity.
MANAGEMENT: *RICE, NSAIDs, quadriceps stretching.* Surgery only in refractory cases (if done, usually performed after growth plate has closed).

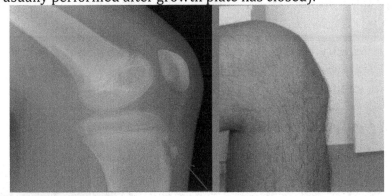

- Lump below the knee.

- Prominent tibial Tuberosity.

Usually resolves with time.

BAKER'S CYST

MOI: *synovial fluid effusion* (ex. from a meniscal tear) *is displaced with cyst formation* (± serve as a protective mechanism).
CLINICAL MANIFESTATIONS: popliteal mass, knee effusion, clicking, buckling, locking of the knee. Not usually painful but ***ruptured cyst*** ⇨ pseudothrombophlebitis syndrome that ***mimics DVT).***
DIAGNOSIS: *ultrasound* helps to identify cysts as well as rule out DVT as a cause for the calf pain.

MANAGEMENT: Conservative: ice, assisted weight bearing, NSAIDs. Intraarticular corticosteroid injection. Surgical excision may be reserved for refractory cases.

PATELLOFEMORAL SYDNROME (CHONDROMALACIA)

MOI: idiopathic softening/fissuring of the patellar articular cartilage. *MC in seen in runners.**

CLINICAL MANIFESTATIONS: *anterior* KNEE PAIN "BEHIND"* OR AROUND THE PATELLA worsened with knee hyperflexion (ex. prolonged sitting), jumping or climbing.

DIAGNOSIS: ⊕ APPREHENSION SIGN* (examiner applies pressure medial – lateral patella with pain or patient refuses test in anticipation of pain).

MANAGEMENT
NSAIDs, rest & rehab (strengthening the vastus medialis obliquus of the quadriceps, weight loss). Elastic knee sleeve for patellar stabilization.

ILIOTIBIAL BAND (ITB) SYNDROME

MOI: inflammation of the iliotibial band bursa due to lack of flexibility of the ITB bursa.
- *MC cause of knee pain in runners,** cyclists (worse with continuous running movement).

CLINICAL MANIFESTATIONS: *LATERAL knee pain** during the onset of running then resolves. Worse with climbing stairs or running downhill.

DIAGNOSIS: ⊕ *OBER TEST:** *pain or resistance to adduction* of the leg parallel to the table in neutral position. *Positive lateral condyle tenderness.**

MANAGEMENT: NSAIDs, physical therapy, corticosteroid injections.

ANKLE & FOOT INJURIES

ANKLE DISLOCATIONS

MOI: major trauma (ex. MVA), high velocity injury. *Posterior MC. ± Peroneal nerve injury.*

CLINICAL MANIFESTATIONS: pain, edema, deformity, inability to bear weight.

MANAGEMENT: *closed reduction + posterior splint.* ± ORIF in severe cases.

ANKLE SPRAINS

85% involve the *collateral ligaments (ANTERIOR TALOFIBULAR MC,* Calcaneofibular). ATFL is the main stabilizer during INVERSION.* Deltoid ligament injury seen with eversion injuries.

CLINICAL MANIFESTATIONS: "pop" ⇨ swelling, pain, inability to bear weight.
x
MANAGEMENT: *RICE, NSAIDs* ⇨ increase ROM & conditioning. Crutches for 1st 2-3 days.
Grade I and II (incomplete tears); Grade III (complete tears).

OTTAWA ANKLE RULES	
ANKLE FILMS	**FOOT FILMS**
Pain along the *lateral malleolus*	*navicular (midfoot) pain*
Pain along the *medial malleolus*	*5th metatarsal pain*
Inability to walk >4 steps at the time of injury & in the ER.	

ACHILLES TENDON RUPTURE

MOI: mechanical overload from eccentric contraction of gastrocsoleus complex.
- 75% occur as a sports-related injury. Common 30-50y. ↑*risk with fluoroquinolone use.**

CLINICAL MANIFESTATIONS: *sudden heel pain after push-off movement, "pop", sudden, sharp calf pain.*
   1. ⊕ *THOMPSON TEST:** *weak, absent plantar flexion* when gastrocnemius is squeezed.

MANAGEMENT: splint initially in mild plantar flexion with subsequent splinting employing gradual dorsiflexion towards neutral. Surgical repair allows for early range of motion.

WEBER ANKLE FRACTURE CLASSIFICATION

Way to classify ankle fractures on the basis of the lateral malleolus (fibular bone).

NORMAL	WEBER A	WEBER B	WEBER C

WEBER A
- Fibular fx BELOW syndesmosis
- Tibiofibular syndesmosis intact
- Deltoid ligament intact
- Usually stable
- ± medial malleolar fracture

WEBER B
- Fibular fx AT LEVEL of syndesmosis
- Tibiofibular syndesmosis intact or mild tear (talofibular joint not widened).
- Deltoid ligament intact or may be torn
- Can be Stable or Unstable

WEBER C
- Fibular fx ABOVE Mortise
- Tibiofibular syndesmosis torn c widening of talofibular joint
- Deltoid ligament damage or
- Medial malleolar fx
- Unstable – requires ORIF

LEVEL OF FIBULAR FRACTURE RELATIVE TO THE SYNDESMOSIS

A- BELOW THE SYNDESMOSIS

B- LEVEL OF SYNDESMOSIS.

C- ABOVE LEVEL OF SYNDESMOSIS

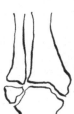

WEBER A

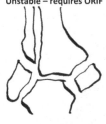

WEBER B

WEBER C

MAISONNEUVE FRACTURE

- ***SPIRAL PROXIMAL FIBULAR FRACTURE*** due to rupture of the *distal talofibular syndesmosis & interosseus membrane as a result of a* **distal medial malleolar fracture and/or deltoid ligament rupture**. Anyone with a distal ankle fracture should have a proximal view to rule out a Maisonneuve fracture.

MAISONNEUVE FRACTURE

PROXIMAL

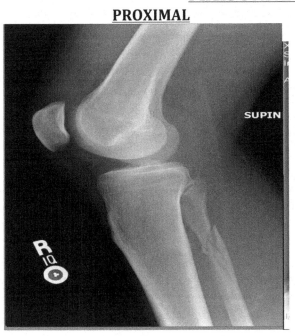

DISTAL

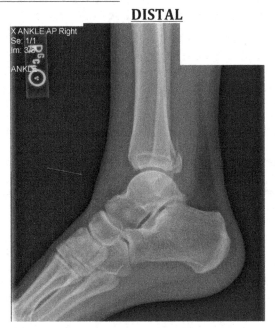

PILON (TIBIAL PLAFOND) FRACTURE

MOI: Fracture of the distal tibia from impact with the talus (axial load), interrupting the ankle joint space ex. high-impact trauma. The fracture extends into the ankle joint.

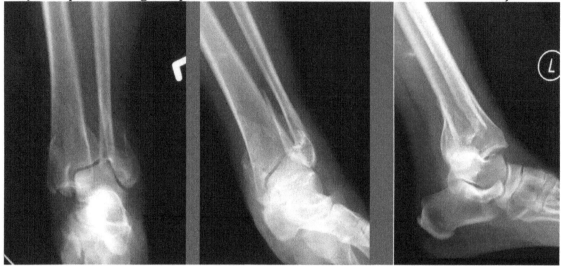

CLINICAL MANIFESTATIONS: severe pain, swelling, deformity.

MANAGEMENT: ORIF (open reduction internal fixation).

STRESS (MARCH) FRACTURE

• Common in athletes & military personnel due to overuse. ***3ᴿᴰ METATARSAL MC.****

CLINICAL MANIFESTATIONS
Early findings: insidious onset of localized aching pain, swelling & tenderness at the end of activities. As it progresses, the patient may have tenderness throughout weight bearing.

DIAGNOSIS: *50% of X-rays will be negative (⊕ with healing).* Bone scan/MRI may be needed.

MANAGEMENT: rest (avoidance of high-impact activities), splint or post-op shoe.

PLANTAR FASCIITIS

MOI: inflammation of the plantar fascia (aponeurosis) due to overuse (especially in patients with flat feet or a heel spur).

CLINICAL MANIFESTATIONS
Heel pain, tenderness of the plantar fascia of the medial foot (±↑ with dorsiflexion of toes).
-   ***Pain usually worse after period of rest (ex. 1ˢᵗ few steps in the morning).****
-   Pain usually decreases throughout the day.

DIAGNOSIS
Radiographs may show a flat foot deformity or a heel spur.

MANAGEMENT: rest, ice, NSAIDs, heel/arch support. Plantar stretching exercises. Corticosteroids used with caution (may cause fascia rupture). Surgery in severe cases.

TARSAL TUNNEL SYNDROME

MOI: *posterior tibial nerve compression* from *overuse, restrictive footwear, edematous states.*

CLINICAL MANIFESTATIONS
   Pain/numbness at the medial malleolus, heel & sole ⇨ can mimic plantar fasciitis *(plantar fasciitis pain decreases throughout day; tarsal tunnel pain increases throughout the day).*
   - *Pain worsens at night and with dorsiflexion. ⊕Tinel sign.*

MANAGEMENT: avoid exacerbating activities. NSAIDs.
   Corticosteroid injection if no improvement. Surgery if conservative measures fail.

BUNION (HALLUX VALGUS)

- Hallux valgus deformity of the bursa *over 1st metatarsal.*
- History of wearing poorly-fitted shoes MC, pes planus (flat feet), rheumatoid arthritis.

CLINICAL MANIFESTATIONS: medial eminence pain with *1st metatarsal lateral deviation.*
MANAGEMENT: comfortable, wide-toed shoes; Surgical if no response to conservative tx.

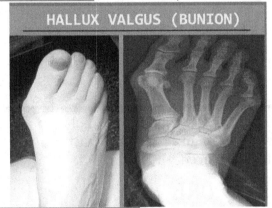

HALLUX VALGUS (BUNION)

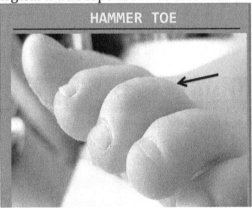

HAMMER TOE

HAMMER TOE

MOI: deformity of PIP joint: *flexion of PIP joint & hyperextension of MTP & DIP joint.*
Seen if 2nd, 3rd or 4th toe is longer than the first, people who wear tight fitting shoes, OA, RA.

CLINICAL MANIFESTATIONS: *PIP pain* (due to contact with shoe). PIP deformity.

CHARCOT'S JOINT (DIABETIC FOOT)

MOI: *joint damage & destruction as a result of peripheral neuropathy* from DM, peripheral vascular disease or other diseases. Repetitive microtrauma to the foot with no sensation & autonomic dysfunction leads to bone resorption & weakening. MC affects the midfoot.

CLINICAL MANIFESTATIONS
   Pain, swelling, alteration of the shape of the foot, ulcer or skin changes.

RADIOGRAPHS: *obliteration of joint space,* scattered chunks of bone in fibrous tissue. ±↑ESR.

MANAGEMENT: rest, non-weight bearing; Surgical.

MORTON'S NEUROMA

MOI: degeneration/proliferation of the plantar digital nerve ⇨ *painful mass near the tarsal heads.* MC in women 25-50y *especially if they wear **tight shoes/high heels/flat feet.***

CLINICAL MANIFESTATIONS
1. ***lancinating pain*** especially with ambulation. ___3rd___ — *3rd metatarsal head MC** ___(±4th).___
   Reproducible pain on palpation, ± palpable mass.
2. May be associated with numbness/paresthesias of the toes.

DIAGNOSIS: MRI may be needed for diagnosis.

MANAGEMENT:
   Wide shoes, glucocorticoid injection (usually curative) ⇨ surgical resection if failed conservative management *(**surgical resection ± cause permanent numbness).***

JONES FRACTURE

• ***Transverse fracture*** through the <u>DIAPHYSIS OF THE 5TH METATARSAL.</u>*

   MANAGEMENT: Non weight bearing x 6-8 weeks, followed by repeat radiographs as it is often complicated by ***nonunion/malunion.**** Frequently requires ORIF/pinning.

PSEUDOJONES FRACTURE

• ***Transverse*** <u>*AVULSION FRACTURE @ BASE (TUBEROSITY) of 5TH METATARSAL*</u> due to plantar flexion with inversion. Much more common and less serious than a true Jones fracture.
   MANAGEMENT: *walking cast* x 2-3 weeks; ORIF if displaced.

JONES   FRACTURE

• <u>JONES:</u> Transverse fx through *DIAPHYSIS of 5th metatarsal*
• <u>PSEUDO JONES:</u> <u>Transverse</u> avulsion fx @ base (tuberosity) of 5th metatarsal

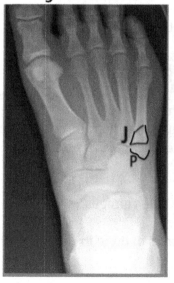 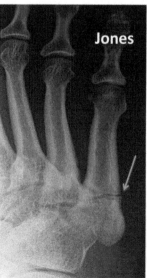 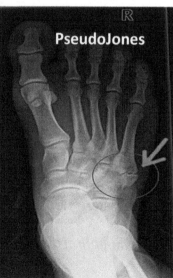

LISFRANC INJURY

- Lisfranc joint: bases of the 1st 3 metatarsal heads & their respective cuneiforms.
- ***Lisfranc Injury:*** disruption between the articulation of the medial cuneiform & the base of the 2nd metatarsal.

Mechanism: varied: rotational (midfoot), severe axial load.

DIAGNOSIS:

1. MC variant is one metatarsal away from the other toes.
2. ***Fleck sign* - fracture at the base of the 2nd metatarsal pathognomonic*** for disruption of the tarsometatarsal ligaments. May be associated with multiple fractures of the metatarsals.

MANAGEMENT: ***ORIF*** followed by non-weight bearing cast for 12 weeks.

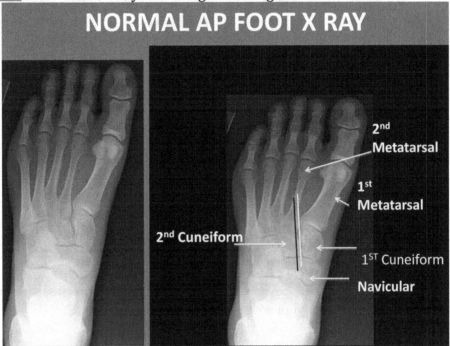

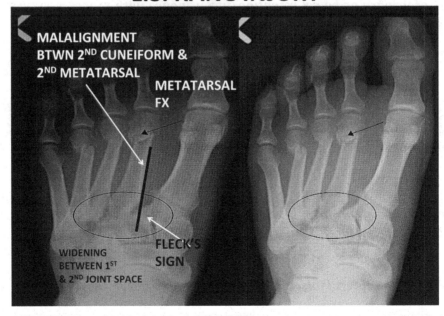

DISORDERS OF THE BACK/SPINE

HERNIATED DISC (NUCLEUS PULPOSUS)

- **Pain in a dermatomal pattern.** ↑pain with coughing, straining, bending, sitting.
- **MC @ L5-S1** (because it is the junction between the mobile & non-mobile spine). Also L4-L5.

CLINICAL MANIFESTATIONS

1. **sciatica:** *BACK PAIN RADIATING TO THE THIGH/BUTTOCK* ⇨ **lower leg** *(below the knee)* **down L5-S1 dermatome** (↑ with Valsalva).

2. **Physical:** ⊕ **straight leg raise,** ± ⊕ **crossover test,** ± *strength, reflex & sensation deficits.*

	L4	L5	S1
Sensory "ALP"	• **ANTERIOR** thigh pain. • Sensory loss to the medial ankle.	• **LATERAL thigh/leg, hip groin** paresthesias & pain. • **Dorsum of the foot:** especially between 1st & 2nd toes.	• **POSTERIOR leg/calf,** gluteus. • **Plantar surface of the foot.**
Weakness	• **ANKLE DORSIFLEXION**	• **BIG TOE EXTENSION (big toe dorsiflexion).** • Walking on heels more difficult than on toes.	• **PLANTAR FLEXION** • Walking on toes more difficult than on heels.
Reflex Diminished	• **LOSS OF KNEE JERK.** • Weak knee extension – quads).	Reflexes usually normal. ± loss of ankle jerk.	• **LOSS OF ANKLE JERK.**

CAUDA EQUINA SYNDROME

- Serious complication of herniated lumbar disc syndrome.
- Massive central herniation compresses several nerve roots of the cauda equina.

CLINICAL MANIFESTATIONS

1. **New onset of urinary or bowel retention/incontinence with** SADDLE ANESTHESIA, **uni/bilateral leg radiation,** DECREASED ANAL SPHINCTER TONE ON RECTAL EXAM* (NO "ANAL WINK").

MANAGEMENT: *Neurosurgical emergency.** Corticosteroids to reduce inflammation.

SPINAL STENOSIS (Pseudoclaudication) (Neurogenic)

- **Narrowing of the spinal canal** with impingement of the nerve roots. **Seen >60y.**

CLINICAL MANIFESTATIONS

1. **BACK PAIN** with paresthesias in one or both extremities. Pain may radiate to the thighs. Pain is:
   - **worsened with extension:** *prolonged standing/walking.*
   - **RELIEVED WITH FLEXION:*** **sitting/walking uphill** (unlike claudication). Lumbar flexion ⇨↑canal volume.

MANAGEMENT: *lumbar epidural injection of corticosteroids,* decompression laminectomy.

LUMBOSACRAL SPRAIN/STRAIN

- Acute strain or tear of the paraspinal muscles, especially after twisting/lifting injuries.

CLINICAL MANIFESTATIONS:
   Back muscle spasms, loss of lordotic curve, ↓ROM, ***NO NEUROLOGIC CHANGES*** (no pain below knee).

MANAGEMENT: ± BRIEF bed rest (≤2 days) if in moderate pain, NSAIDs/analgesics, ± muscle relaxers.

SPINAL COMPRESSION FRACTURES

- "Burst" fractures occur in children from jumping/fall from height. ***Lumbar compression fractures*** in the elderly (osteoporosis), tumor or systemic illness. ***Pathologic fractures in malignancy.***

CLINICAL MANIFESTATIONS: pain & ***POINT TENDERNESS**** *at the level of compression.*

MANAGEMENT: orthopedic & neurosurgery consult. Analgesics; ± kyphoplasty/vertebroplasty.

SCOLIOSIS

- ***LATERAL CURVATURE OF SPINE >10°.*** ***± associated with kyphosis (humpback) or lordosis (sway back).***
- MC begins at 8-10y of age. MC in girls (⊕ family history).
- If associated with café au lait spots, skin tags & axillary freckles ⇨ neurofibromatosis type I.

DIAGNOSIS: ***ADAMS FORWARD BENDING TEST*** ***most sensitive.*** ***COBB'S ANGLE*** measured on AP/lateral films.
MANAGEMENT: observation in most cases; ±Bracing (if 20 – 40°); Surgical correction if >40°.

SPONDYLOLYSIS & SPONDYLOLISTHESIS

- **SPONDYLOLYSIS:** ***pars interarticularis defect*** from either ***failure of fusion or stress fracture,*** often from repetitive hyperextension trauma (ex. football players, gymnasts).
- Often 1st step to spondylolisthesis. MC form of back pain in children & adolescents. MC at L5/S1.

- **SPONDYLOLISTHESIS:** ***forward slipping of a vertebrae on another.**** MC 10-15y (adolescence).

CLINICAL MANIFESTATIONS: lower back pain, ± sciatica symptoms.
   Spondylolisthesis may cause bowel or bladder dysfunction.
MANAGEMENT:
   1. Spondylolysis: symptomatic relief, activity restriction, physical therapy, bracing.
   2. Spondylolisthesis: low grade: treat like spondylolysis;   High grade ⇨ surgical.

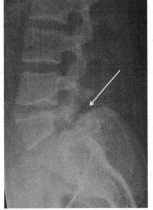

Spondylolysis

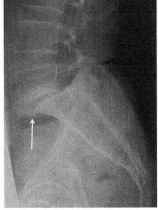

Spondylolisthesis

OSTEOMYELITIS

Inflammation/infection of bone by pyogenic organisms. *MC <20y* & >50y.

RISK FACTORS: Sickle cell dz, DM, immunocompromised, preexisting joint disease, URIs in children.
- ACUTE OSTEOMYELITIS: *MC seen in children (S. AUREUS MC ORGANISM*), GABHS (S. pyogenes).*
  SALMONELLA PATHOGNOMONIC FOR SICKLE CELL DISEASE.*

- CHRONIC (SUBACUTE) OSTEOMYELITIS: *MC in adults* 2^{ry} to open injury/bone surrounding soft tissue (trauma/recent surgery). *S. aureus MC organism* (80%), Staph epidermis (coag negative staph in prosthetic joint infections); Gram negative: Pseudomonas (IVDU), Serratia, E. coli.

SOURCES
1. **Acute hematogenous spread:** *MC route in children.**
2. **Direct Inoculation:** *infection close to bone* s/p trauma, surgery, insertion of a prosthetic joint.
3. Contiguous spread with vascular insufficiency: ex. DM, peripheral vascular disease.

CLINICAL MANIFESTATIONS
1. Gradual onset of symptoms days - weeks; Signs of bacteremia: high fever, chills, malaise.
2. **Local signs:** *inflammation/infection, pain over the involved bone,* ↓ROM in adjacent joint.
3. Refusal to use extremity/bear weight (Hip MC joint in children). Sinus tract drainage in chronic.

DIAGNOSIS
1. **Labs:** ↑WBC, ↑*ESR* (↓'es as it resolves). *If ESR is normal, osteomyelitis is unlikely.* ±↑CRP
2. **MRI:** *most sensitive test in early disease.** CT scan often used for surgical planning.
3. **Radiographs:** evidence of bone infection (but ±not be evident up to 2 weeks after symptom onset).
   - **early:** soft tissue swelling & *PERIOSTEAL REACTION,* lucent areas of cortical destruction.*
   - **advanced/chronic:** *sequestrum** (segments of necrotic bone separated from living bone by granulation tissue), osteolysis, bony destruction. Involucrum = new bone formation.
4. **Radionuclide bone or Gallium scan:** *sensitive in early disease.* Blood cultures are ⊕ in 50%.
5. *Bone Aspiration: Gold Standard.** Bone scan shows ↑activity (but not specific).

MANAGEMENT

ACUTE OSTEOMYELITIS: *Antibiotics 4-6 weeks (at least 2 weeks via IV).* May need debridement.		
Newborn (<4mos)	*Group B Strep,* Gram neg.	Nafcillin or Oxacillin + 3rd generation Cephalosporin
>4mos *Staph. aureus*	*Methicillin Sensitive (MSSA)*	- *Nafcillin or Oxacillin* or *Cefazolin* (Ancef) (Clindamycin or Vancomycin if PCN allergic)
	Methicillin Resistant (MRSA)	*Vancomycin* or Linezolid
Sickle Cell disease	*Salmonella,* S. Aureus	*3rd gen Cephalosporin or FQ* (Cipro* or Levofloxacin)
Puncture wound	*Pseudomonas*	*Ciprofloxacin* or Levofloxacin. Ceftazidime or Cefepime

- **CHRONIC:** more refractory to treatment ⇨ generally treated with ❶ *Surgical debridement* + ❷ *cultures* (antibiotic treatment depends on biopsy *culture* & sensitivities) + ❸Antibiotics (empiric antibiotics usually not recommended in chronic osteomyelitis).

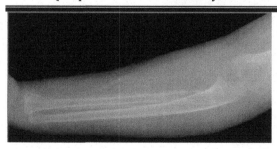

Bony destruction of the tibia & fibula in osteomyelitis.

Periosteal reaction of the radial shaft.

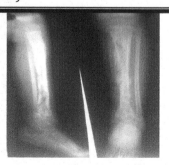

SEPTIC ARTHRITIS

Infection in the joint cavity (usually bacterial). Most dangerous form of acute arthritis.
MEDICAL EMERGENCY (because it can rapidly destroy the joint). Most monomicrobial.

- **Pathogenesis:** ❶ *hematogenous spread,* ❷ *direct inoculation:* trauma, puncture wound or surgery; ❸ *contiguous spread* (ex. from osteoarthritis). May occur after URI or impetigo.
- **Risk Factors:** extremes of age, chronic debilitating disease, immunosuppressive drugs, IVDA. Prosthetic joint/surgery, chronic arthropathies (ex rheumatoid arthritis, gout, osteoarthritis).

MICROBIOLOGY
S. AUREUS MC organism* (40-50%), Neisseria gonorrhoeae (sexually active young adults* – associated with tenosynovitis), ***Streptococci;*** Gram-negative; Staph epidermis if prosthesis; Mycobacteria & fungi less common. ***Neonates – Group B Strep***, S. aureus, H. flu.

CLINICAL MANIFESTATIONS
1. **Joint involvement:** *single, swollen, warm, painful joint (↓ROM), tender to palpation.* (children ± limp or refuse to use limb). ***Knee MC**** (>50%); hip > elbow > ankle, wrists.
2. Constitutional symptoms: ***fever***, chills, diaphoresis, myalgia, malaise, pain.

DIAGNOSIS
1. **Arthrocentesis:** *joint fluid aspirate definitive diagnosis* - WBC >50,000* – primarily PMNs; gram stain & culture; crystals.* Cell count >2,000 is inflammatory range, Normal is usually <500 (mostly monocytes). WBC >1,100 considered positive in prosthetic joints. MRI/CT.

MANAGEMENT
- ***Prompt antibiotics guided by gram stain. ARTHROTOMY with joint drainage.*** 2-4 week course.

GRAM STAIN	ANTIBIOTIC REGIMEN
GRAM POSITIVE COCCI	***Nafcillin (Vancomycin if MRSA suspected).*** Vancomycin or Clindamycin if penicillin-allergic.
GRAM NEGATIVE COCCI OR GONOCOCCUS SUSPECTED	***Ceftriaxone*** *(Gonococcal usually doesn't need arthrotomy).* Ciprofloxacin if penicillin-allergic.
GRAM NEGATIVE RODS	***Ceftriaxone (3rd generation Cephalosporin) +*** ***Anti-Pseudomonal aminoglycoside (ex. Gentamicin).***
NO ORGANISM SEEN	Nafcillin or Vancomycin + Ceftriaxone (±anti-Pseudomonas).

COMPARTMENT SYNDROME

- ***Muscle/nerve ischemia (↓tissue perfusion)*** *when closed muscle compartment pressure > perfusion pressure.*
- **Etiologies:** *trauma: MC after fracture of long bones* (75%), crush injuries, tight casts, tight pressure dressings & thermal burns.

CLINICAL MANIFESTATIONS:
1. ***Pain out of proportion to injury**** (persistent deep/burning), Volkmann's contracture.
2. **Physical Exam:** *PAIN ON PASSIVE STRETCHING EARLIEST INDICATOR,* tense extremities* ("firm/wooden" feeling), paresthesias (30 minutes – 2 hours). Pulselessness & paresis are late findings (however capillary refill is usually preserved).

DIAGNOSIS: ↑*intracompartmental pressure >30-45 mm Hg;* ↑CK/myoglobin.

Δ pressure = Diastolic BP – measured compartment pressure. Delta pressure <20-30 mm Hg

MANAGEMENT: *fasciotomy** to decompress the compartmental pressure.

MALIGNANT BONE TUMORS

OSTEOSARCOMA

- **MC bone malignancy.* MC adolescents** (80% occur <20y). Produces osteoid (immature bone).
- **2nd peak 50-60y** (especially if history of Paget disease of the bone or radiation therapy).
- 90% occur in the metaphysis of long bones (MC in femur ⇨ tibia, humerus).
- **MC METS to the lungs*** (usually the cause of death).

CLINICAL MANIFESTATIONS: *bone pain/joint swelling.* Palpable soft tissue mass.

DIAGNOSIS
1. **Radiographs:** *"HAIR ON END" or "SUN RAY/BURST"* **appearance** of the soft tissue mass. Mixed sclerotic/lytic lesions. Periosteal bone reactions.
2. Codman's triangle: ossification of raised periosteum.
   Codman's triangle may also be seen with Ewing Sarcoma.

MANAGEMENT: limb-sparing resection (if not neovascular); radical amputation (if neovascular). *Chemotherapy as adjuvant treatment.*

Hair On End

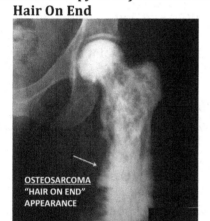

Codman's Triangle

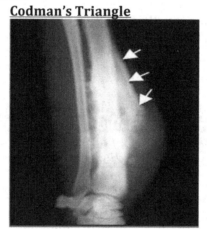

EWING SARCOMA

- Giant cell tumor MC in children. MC in males 5-25y. *Femur (MC) & pelvis are common sites.*

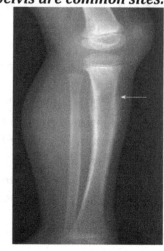

CLINICAL MANIFESTATION
Bone pain, ±palpable mass, may have joint swelling. ± fever.
Bone MC site of metastasis.

DIAGNOSIS
lytic lesion, layered *periosteal reaction "ONION SKIN"** appearance on
radiographs. ± Codman's triangle.

MANAGEMENT
Options include chemotherapy, surgery & radiation therapy.

CHONDROSARCOMA

- *Cancer of the cartilage. MC seen in adults* (40-75y).
- 3rd MC primary malignancy of the bone after myeloma & osteosarcoma.

DIAGNOSIS
Mineralized chondroid matrix with *PUNCTATE OR RING & ARC APPEARANCE* pattern of calcification.

MANAGEMENT
1. **Surgical resection:** all grades and subtypes of nonmetastatic chondrosarcoma.
2. Chemotherapy may be used in select cases of advanced disease.

BENIGN BONE TUMORS

OSTEOCHONDROMA

- *MC benign bone tumor* (seen especially ages **10-20y).   MC in males.*
- Begins in childhood & grows until skeletal maturity. May precede chondrosarcomas.

DIAGNOSIS: *Often PEDUNCULATED, GROWS AWAY FROM GROWTH PLATE* & involves medullary tissue.*

MANAGEMENT: observation.
Resection if it becomes painful or if located in the pelvis (pelvis MC site of malignant transformation).

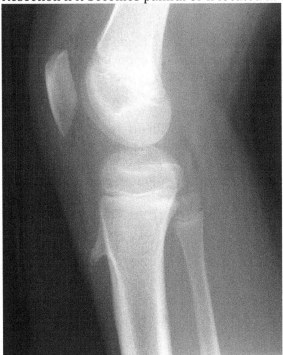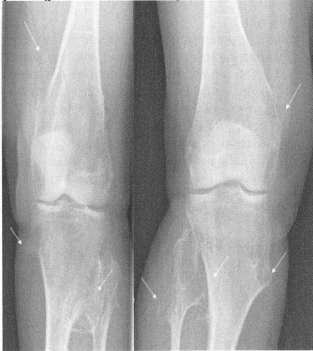

Osteochondroma: often pedunculated, grows away from growth plate & involves medullary tissue
(directly contiguous with marrow space).

PAGET DISEASE OF THE BONE (OSTEITIS DEFORMANS)

- **_Abnormal bone remodeling_** & disorganized osteoid formation. **_MC >40y (elderly)._**
- Mainly persons of **_western European descent._** 40% autosomal dominant.

PATHOPHYSIOLOGY
1. **_Disordered bone remodeling_**: with ❶ ↑**_osteoclast bone resorption_** ⇨ ❷ ↑abnormal trabecular bone formation ⇨ **_larger, weaker, less compact bones_** _more vascular_ & **_prone to fractures._**
2. **_Lytic phase_** (↑**_osteoclast activity_**) ⇨ mixed phase ⇨ **_sclerotic phase_** (↑_osteoblast activity_).

CLINICAL MANIFESTATIONS
1. **Asymptomatic** MC (70-90%). Found incidentally on radiographs or because of an incidentally **_high alkaline phosphatase_*** on routine lab testing.
2. **_Bone pain: MC symptom._*** Pelvis MC, axial skeleton, skull, long bones or femur pain usually due to _stress fractures or_ ↑**_warmth_** _(hypervascularity)._ Secondary osteoarthritis.
3. Soft bones: bowed tibias, kyphosis, frequent fractures with slight trauma.
4. **_Skull involvement: deafness_*** (seen in up to 50% due to compression of CN VIII); _Headache._

DIAGNOSIS
1. **_Labs: markedly_** ↑**_alkaline phosphatase;_*** Normal Ca^{+2} & phosphate. ↑urinary pyridinolines or ↑N-telopeptide (collagen breakdown markers increased during bone resorption).

2. **Radiographs:** _lytic phase: "_**_blade of grass/flame shaped" lucency_** ⇨ mixed phase (lucency + sclerosis) ⇨ sclerotic phase: **_coarsened trabeculae_** (↑_trabecular markings, denser/expanded bones);_ Multiple fissures may be seen along lone bones. **Skull = _COTTON WOOL APPEARANCE._***

MANAGEMENT
Asymptomatic patients require no treatment usually. **_Bisphosphonates_** _& Calcitonin. NSAIDs for pain_
1. **_Bisphosphonates: tx of choice:_*** _PO: Alendronate, Risedronate,_ Etidronate. _IV: **Zoledronic acid, Pamidronate**_
   - **_MOA: inhibit osteoclast activity (decreasing bone resorption & turnover)._** Alendronate & Risedronate inhibit osteoclast & osteoblast activity.
   - **Considerations:** taken with 8 ounces of plain water, 1-2 hours before meals, Aspirin, Ca^{+2}, Mg^{+2}, Al^{+3}, antacids. Alendronate associated with high incidence of **_esophagitis_** so recumbency after dose is discouraged. Alendronate CI if esophageal stricture, dysphagia or hiatal hernia.
   - **Side Effects:** nephrotoxicity, thrombocytopenia, **_atypical femur fractures,_*** **_jaw osteonecrosis._**

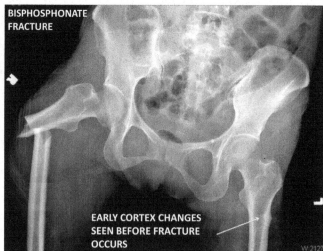

2. **_Calcitonin:_** ↓**_osteoclast activity._** Given SQ or intranasally.

AUTOIMMUNE DISORDERS

SYSTEMIC LUPUS ERYTHEMATOSUS (SLE)

- Chronic systemic, multi-organ autoimmune disorder of connective tissues. Type III HSN.
- **_Young females_** 9:1; **_onset in 20-40s, ↑African-American, Hispanic, Native Americans._**
- Genetic, environmental **_sun exposure,_** infections, hormonal **_(estrogen)._**
- **DRUG INDUCED:** **_Procainamide, Hydralazine, INH, Quinidine._** ⊕ _ANTI-HISTONE ANTIBODIES*_
  Usually resolves with drug discontinuation. Not associated with kidney/CNS damage or alopecia.

CLINICAL MANIFESTATIONS
1. **_Triad of_ ❶_joint pain_** (90%) ❷**_fever_** & ❸**_malar "butterfly rash":_** fixed erythematous rash on cheeks/bridge of nose sparing the nasolabial folds; fatigue. _Serositis **(pericarditis, pleuritis).***_
2. **_Discoid lupus:_ annular,** _erythematous patches on face & scalp that **heals with scarring.**_
3. Systemic: CNS, cardiovascular, **_glomerulonephritis, retinitis, oral ulcers, alopecia.*_**

DIAGNOSIS:
1. ⊕ _ANTI-NUCLEAR AB:_ **ANA best initial test*** (not specific). ⊕ _Rheumatoid Factor._

2. ⊕ _ANTI DOUBLE-STRANDED DNA & ANTI-SMITH AB_ **100% specific for SLE*** (not sensitive).

3. _ANTIPHOSPHOLIPID AB SYNDROME_ **_(APLS): ↑risk of arterial & venous thrombosis.*_**
   - ⊕ **_Anticardiolipin Ab_** associated with **_false_** ⊕ _VDRL/RPR_ (due to cardiolipin present in reagent).
   - **_Lupus Anticoagulant._** _Misnomer because paradoxically ↑'es PT/PTT but assoc c ↑thrombosis._
   - β-2 glycoprotein I Ab. **_Women c APLS may have frequent miscarriages,_** livedo reticularis.

4. CBC: ± anemia, leukopenia, lymphopenia, thrombocytopenia. Associated with HLA-DR.

MANAGEMENT: skin: **_sun protection, Hydroxychloroquine (for lesions)._** Arthritis: **_NSAIDs or acetaminophen._** ±pulse-dose Corticosteroids; cytotoxic drugs (Methotrexate, Cyclophosphamide).

SCLERODERMA (SYSTEMIC SCLEROSIS)

- Systemic connective tissue disorder: **_thickened skin (sclerodactyly),_** lung, heart, kidney & GI tract.

CLINICAL MANIFESTATIONS:
1. **_Tight, shiny, thickened skin (localized or generalized)_** due to fibrous collagen buildup.

2. **LIMITED CUTANEOUS SYSTEMIC SCLEROSIS "CREST SYNDROME":** _**C**alcinosis cutis, **R**aynaud's phenomenon, **E**sophageal motility disorder, **S**clerodactyly (claw hand),* **T**elangiectasia._ MC type (80%).
   - Affects the face, neck as well as **_distal to the elbows & knees.*_** Spares the trunk. ±Pulm HTN.
   - **_Raynaud's phenomenon_** (60-70%): vasospasm-induced tricolor changes of fingers, toes, ears, nose, tongue worsen c cold, smoking or emotional stress. Often starts in teenage years. Affects the face, neck as well as distal elbows & knees. _Calcium Channel blockers tx of choice.*_

3. **DIFFUSE CUTANEOUS SYSTEMIC SCLEROSIS:** skin thickening: **_trunk & proximal extremities.*_**

DIAGNOSIS
1. ⊕ _ANTI-CENTROMERE AB:_ **_associated with Limited/CREST dz* - more specific. Better prognosis._**
2. ⊕ _ANTI-SCL-70 AB:_ **_associated with DIFFUSE dz* & multiple organ involvement._** ⊕ ANA (nonspp).

ACUTE MANAGEMENT: DMARDs, Corticosteroids; **Raynaud's:** **_vasodilators (CCBs,* prostacyclin)._**

SJÖGREN'S SYNDROME

- **Autoimmune** disorder that **attacks _exocrine glands:_* salivary glands** ⇨ **_xerostomia_** *(dry mouth);* **lacrimal glands** ⇨ **_dry eyes_*** (keratoconjunctivitis sicca) & **_parotid enlargement._*** Thyroid gland dysfunction common.

PRIMARY SS (occurs alone); **SECONDARY SS** (associated c other autoimmune disorders – SLE, RA, etc)
- Activation of the immune system possibly triggered by viruses, *aggregation of lymphocytes (ex CD4 cells) in exocrine glands (lymphocytic invasion).* HLA-DR52 seen in 85%.
- ↑**incidence of non-Hodgkin lymphoma**, interstitial nephritis & pneumonitis.

DIAGNOSIS: _ANA: esp antiSS-A (Ro) & antiSS-B (La);_* ⊕_RF,_ ⊕_SCHIRMER TEST*_ (↓tear production).

MANAGEMENT: *artificial tears, Pilocarpine for xerostomia.*
1. **PILOCARPINE: _cholinergic_ drug** *that increases lacrimation & salivation* **(SLUDD-C).**
   S/E: common: diaphoresis, flushing, sweating, bradycardia, diarrhea, N/V, incontinence, blurred vision. *(Salivation, Lacrimation, Urination, Defecation, Digestion, Constriction of pupil).*

2. **CEVIMELINE** (Exovac): **stimulates muscarinic cholinergic receptors.**

FIBROMYALGIA

- _WIDESPREAD MUSCULAR PAIN_ (chronic), fatigue, muscle tenderness, headaches, poor **sleep/memory problems**. May be due to **increase in pain perception** (↑**substance P**).
- **Middle aged women MC** *(9:1)*; ↑incidence with rheumatoid arthritis, lupus & ankylosing spondylitis.

CLINICAL MANIFESTATIONS: diffuse pain (especially in the morning), **extreme fatigue,*** stiffness, painful, tender joints. **Sleep disturbances,*** haziness ("fibro fog"), symptoms may worsen with stress.

DIAGNOSIS:
1. _DIFFUSE PAIN IN 11 OUT OF 18 TRIGGER POINTS_** >3months +** widespread pain.
2. **Muscle biopsy:** _"MOTH-EATEN" APPEARANCE_ of the type I muscle fibers, muscle damage.

MANAGEMENT: exercise (**swimming preferred** - relaxing effect of water on the muscles).
Medical: **TCAs**, Duloxetine (SSNRI), SSRIs, Neurontin. **Pregabalin FDA approved for fibromyalgia.**

POLYMYALGIA RHEUMATICA

- Idiopathic inflammatory condition causing **_synovitis, bursitis & tenosynovitis_** ⇨ **_pain/stiffness_** of the **_proximal joints (shoulder, hip, neck)*_** in patients **_>50y_**.

- **Polymyalgia rheumatica is _CLOSELY RELATED TO GIANT CELL ARTERITIS._***

CLINICAL MANIFESTATIONS
1. **Bilateral proximal joint aching/STIFFNESS* morning stiffness > 30mins of the pelvic, neck & shoulder girdle** ⇨ difficulty with combing hair, putting on a coat, getting out of chair.
2. No severe muscle weakness.

DIAGNOSIS: Clinical dx. ↑ESR, anemia (normochromic normocytic); ±↑platelets (acute phase reactant).

MANAGEMENT: low-dose Corticosteroids* (10-20 mg/day). NSAIDs. Methotrexate.

POLYMYOSITIS (PM) & DERMATOMYOSITIS (DrM)

- *Idiopathic inflammatory muscle disease of proximal limbs, neck, pharynx.* May affect heart, lungs & GI.

CLINICAL MANIFESTATIONS

1. *PROGRESSIVE SYMMETRICAL PROXIMAL MUSCLE WEAKNESS* **(usually painless),** dysphagia, skin rash, polyarthralgias, muscle atrophy (difficulty rising from a chair/climbing stairs, combing hair, problems with overhead movements).

DIAGNOSIS:

- ↑*muscle enzymes: (↑aldolase,* creatine kinase);* ↑ESR, ⊕ muscle biopsy, **abnormal EMG.**
- ⊕ **Anti-Jo 1 Ab: myositis specific antibody** (vs. tRNA synthetase). Associated with **"mechanic hands"** (hyperkeratotic "cracked hands" with "dirty appearance") & **interstitial lung fibrosis.**
- ⊕ **Anti-SRP Ab:** (Signal Recognition Particle Ab). **Almost exclusively seen with PM.** Associated with more prominent muscle weakness/atrophy & cardiac manifestations.

- ⊕ **Anti-Mi-2 Ab: specific for dermatomyositis.**
- **Muscle biopsy:** endomysial involvement (PM);   perifascicular/perivascular involvement (DrM).

Management: high-dose Corticosteroids 1ˢᵗ line.* ± Methotrexate, Azathioprine, IV Immunoglobulin.

DERMATOMYOSITIS:

Pathognomonic: ❶ *HELIOTROPE (BLUE-PURPLE)* **upper eyelid discoloration** ❷ *GOTTRON'S PAPULES:* **raised violaceous scaly eruptions on the knuckles.** Malar rash with erythema (including the nasolabial folds), Photosensitive poikiloderma "shawl or V sign", diffuse alopecia.

DIAGNOSIS: *muscle enzymes: (↑aldolase,* creatine kinase);* ↑ESR,   ↑incidence of malignancy.

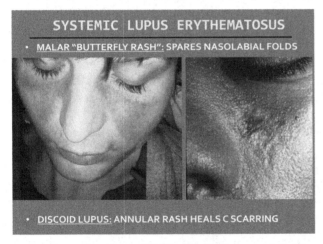

SYSTEMIC LUPUS ERYTHEMATOSUS
- MALAR "BUTTERFLY RASH": SPARES NASOLABIAL FOLDS
- DISCOID LUPUS: ANNULAR RASH HEALS C̄ SCARRING

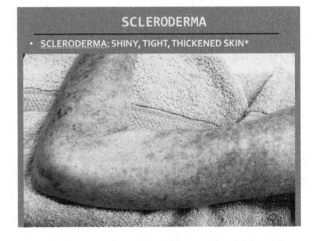

SCLERODERMA
- SCLERODERMA: SHINY, TIGHT, THICKENED SKIN*

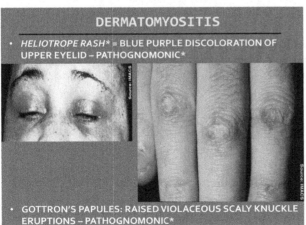

DERMATOMYOSITIS
- HELIOTROPE RASH* = BLUE PURPLE DISCOLORATION OF UPPER EYELID – PATHOGNOMONIC*
- GOTTRON'S PAPULES: RAISED VIOLACEOUS SCALY KNUCKLE ERUPTIONS – PATHOGNOMONIC*

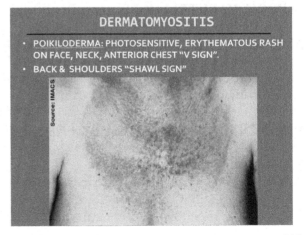

DERMATOMYOSITIS
- POIKILODERMA: PHOTOSENSITIVE, ERYTHEMATOUS RASH ON FACE, NECK, ANTERIOR CHEST "V SIGN".
- BACK & SHOULDERS "SHAWL SIGN"

ARTHRITIS SYNDROMES

GOUT

- **_Uric acid deposition in the soft tissue, joints & bone._** MC due to underexcretion of uric acid (90%).
- Attacks 2ry to **purine-rich foods** (alcohol, liver, seafood, yeasts) causing rapid changes in uric acid concentrations. **Meds: _diuretics (thiazides, loop), ACEI, Pyrazinamide, Ethambutol, Aspirin & ARBs_** _(notable exception is Losartan which decreases uric acid levels)._
- **_MC in men_** _(especially >30y)._ If seen in women, they are usually postmenopausal.

CLINICAL MANIFESTATIONS
1. **_Acute gouty arthritis_** (80% monoarthropathy): severe joint pain, erythema, swelling & stiffness (often extends past the affected joint).
    - **_Podagra (1ST MTP JOINT INVOLVEMENT MC),_** * knees, feet & ankle also common.
2. **_Tophi deposition_** * (chronic arthropathy): collection of solid uric acid in soft tissues (ex. helix of ear, eyelids, Achilles tendon). Usually occurs after 10-20 years of chronic hyperuricemia.
3. Uric acid nephrolithiasis & nephropathy. Uric acid stones associated with low urine volume & acidic pH. May cause glomerulonephritis. May lead to renal failure.

DIAGNOSIS
1. **Arthrocentesis:** shows _NEGATIVELY BIREFRINGENT NEEDLE-SHAPED URATE CRYSTALS._*
2. **Radiographs:** _"MOUSE/RAT BITE" "PUNCHED-OUT" EROSIONS_* with overhanging margins; ± Tophi.
3. Clinical dx. ↑ESR & WBC during acute attacks. Serum uric acid levels don't reflect joint involvement.

ACUTE MANAGEMENT
1. **_NSAIDs drug of choice_** * ex. **_Indomethacin, Naprosyn._** _Avoid Aspirin_ (Aspirin ↑'es serum uric acid).
2. **_Colchicine 2nd line;_** Steroids reserved for severe renal dz or if no response to NSAIDs/Colchicine.

CHRONIC MANAGEMENT (PROPHYLAXIS):
1. **_Allopurinol: reduces uric acid production by_** **_inhibiting xanthine oxidase_** * & increases uric acid excretion. **_S/E: taken with meals to prevent gastric irritation, HSN/SJS._** Caution if renal dz.
2. Febuxostat (Uloric): xanthine oxidase inhibitor that is safer in patients with renal disease.
3. Uricosuric drugs: Probenecid & Sulfinpyrazone promote renal uric acid secretion.
4. **_Colchicine (only med that can be used in acute & chronic gout);_** Vitamin C, Losartan (for HTN).

CALCIUM PYROPHOSPHATE DIHYDRATE DEPOSITION DISEASE

- **_Calcium pyrophosphate deposition in the joints/soft tissue_**: inflammation & bone destruction.
- Often associated with other diseases (ex OA, hyperthyroidism). ↑**_elderly (>60y), females._**

CLINICAL MANIFESTATIONS
1. Asymptomatic.
2. **_PSEUDOGOUT (acute arthritis): red, swollen, tender joint_** (resembles gout). **_Knee MC._** *
3. **_CHONDROCALCINOSIS (cartilage calcification)_** * - **_linear radiodensities seen on radiographs._**
4. Chronic CPPD disease (resembles RA): inflammatory arthritis.
5. OA with CPPD (resembles osteoarthritis).

DIAGNOSIS: arthrocentesis: _POSITIVELY BIREFRINGENT, RHOMBOID-SHAPED CPPD CRYSTALS_* **_(pseudogout)._**

MANAGEMENT
1. **_Pseudogout: intraarticular Corticosteroids 1st line,_** * **_NSAIDs. Colchicine (acute or for prophylaxis)._**
2. Chronic (pseudo-RA): NSAIDs, Colchicine (low dose oral corticosteroids if no response).
3. Pseudo-OA: treat like OA. No treatment needed in patients with asymptomatic CPPD.

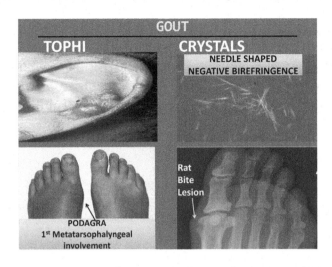

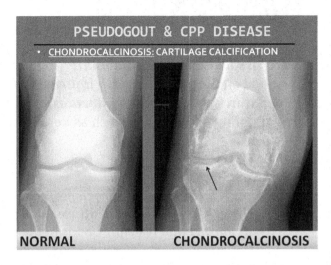

	GOUT	PSEUDOGOUT
PREVALENCE	• 17-20 per 1,000 individuals. • *Mostly adult men* Postmenopausal women.	• <1 per 1,000 individuals. • *Female predominance, elderly*
CRYSTAL CHEMISTRY	*Monosodium urate*	**Calcium pyrophosphate dihydrate**
SYNOVIAL FLUID CRYSTALS	*NEGATIVELY BIREFRINGENT; NEEDLE-SHAPED.*	*WEAKLY POSITIVE; RHOMBOID-SHAPED.*
MOST FREQUENTLY AFFECTED JOINTS	• *First MTP joint MC (Podagra)** 50% initially; 90% eventually. • *80% monoarticular typically lower extremities* (ankle, knees, foot)	• Knees, wrists, MCP joints, elbows, MTP.
RADIOGRAPH FINDINGS	• *"MOUSE BITE" (PUNCHED OUT) EROSIONS**	• *CHONDROCALCINOSIS** - calcification of the cartilage
THERAPEUTIC OPTIONS	**ACUTE ATTACKS:** • *NSAIDs 1st line,* Colchicine* • Corticosteroids **CHRONIC MANAGEMENT:** • **Uric acid-lowering agents** Allopurinol, Febuxostat, Probenecid • Colchicine	**ACUTE ATTACKS:** • *Intraarticular steroids 1st line.** • *NSAIDs, Colchicine* **CHRONIC MANAGEMENT:** • *NSAIDs* • ± Colchicine

Note that the ***medications used in the chronic management of gout are NOT initiated during an acute attack*** *(because it may precipitate an attack).* Colchicine can be used for acute & chronic. Any acute increase OR decrease in serum uric acid levels can cause an acute attack. Note that measuring serum uric acid levels are generally not helpful to determine if the attack is due to gout.

RHABDOMYOLYSIS

- Acute breakdown & necrosis of skeletal muscle.
- *MC associated with immobility* (ex. a patient who sustained a hip fracture that is found lying on the ground), *crush injuries, overexertion (ex marathon runners), seizures, burns.*
- <u>Meds:</u> *ex statins,* niacin, fibrates,* drugs that inhibit the CP450 system (ex. macrolides & nondihydropyridines such as Verapamil & Diltiazem).

DIAGNOSIS
1. <u>LABS:</u>
   - *↑CPK (creatinine phosphokinase) >20,000,** ↑LDH, ALT.
   - *Hyperkalemia** (due to intracellular potassium release from damaged tissues).
   - *Hypocalcemia* (calcium bonds to the damaged muscle).

2. <u>UA:</u> *dark urine* that is ⊕ *for heme but negative for blood (reflecting myoglobinuria).**
3. <u>ECG:</u> to look for signs of hyperkalemia.

MANAGEMENT
1. *IV saline hydration:* 4-6L/day. *Mannitol:* to induce osmotic diuresis. *Bicarbonate to alkalinize the urine. Calcium gluconate if hyperkalemia with significant ECG changes.*
2. <u>COMPLICATIONS:</u> *acute kidney injury (acute tubular necrosis)* due to excess myoglobin kidney deposition. May cause multi-organ failure.

JUVENILE IDIOPATHIC ARTHRITIS (RHEUMATOID)

- Autoimmune mono or polyarthritis in *children <16y (often resolves by puberty). 3 types:*

❶ PAUCI-ARTICULAR *(Oligoarticular):* 50%.
   - <u><5 *joint involvement*</u> in the 1st 6 months. MC large joints (ex. knees, ankle). ± small joints.
   - Type I associated with *iridocyclitis (anterior uveitis).* Often iridocyclitis is asymptomatic (but may cause blindness if not treated). Joint involvement is usually asymmetric.
   - Type II associated with ↑ incidence of ankylosing spondylitis.

❷ SYSTEMIC/ACUTE FEBRILE (STILL'S DISEASE) 20%.
   - *Daily arthritis, <u>DIURNAL HIGH FEVER</u>** within the 1st 6 months. Both small & large joints.
   - <u>*SALMON-COLORED/PINK MIGRATORY RASH:***</u> often accompanies the fever (±Koebner phenomenon)
   - No iridocyclitis but associated with hepatosplenomegaly, hepatitis, lymphadenopathy & serositis (pericardial & pleural effusions).

❸ POLYARTICULAR 30%
   - *Arthritis ≥5 small joints* within the 1st 6 months (usually symmetric). *Most similar to adult rheumatoid arthritis.* Hip involvement is common (may present as a limp).
   - *↑risk of iridocyclitis,* may have low-grade fever. Systemic symptoms not as common.
   - Rheumatoid factor negative disease associated with better prognosis than RF positive patients.

DIAGNOSIS
1. Clinical diagnosis. ↑ESR, CRP; ⊕ANA seen in oligoarticular. ⊕Rheumatoid factor only in 15%.

MANAGEMENT
1. NSAIDs &/or corticosteroids. Methotrexate or Leflunomide. Frequent eye exams to detect iridocyclitis.

OSTEOARTHRITIS (OA)

- Chronic disease due to *__articular cartilage damage & degeneration.__* *Obesity big RF.*
- *MC in __WEIGHT-BEARING JOINTS__* (knees, hips, cervical/lumbar spine, hip).
- *Narrowed joint space* (loss of articular cartilage), *sclerosis &* __OSTEOPHYTE FORMATION.__*
- Chondrocyte inability to repair the damaged cartilage.

CLINICAL MANIFESTATIONS
1. *EVENING JOINT STIFFNESS* decreases with rest, *__worsens throughout the day__* *& with changes in weather.* ↓ROM, crepitus. Absence of inflammatory signs & *"HARD BONY JOINTS".*
2. *"HARD BONY JOINTS"* = OSTEOPHYTES. *Heberden's node* (palpable osteophytes @ DIP joints). *Bouchard's node: PIP osteophytes.* OA of the hands MC in women.

RADIOLOGIC FINDINGS
1. *joint space loss, OSTEOPHYTES,* subchondral bone cysts/sclerosis.

MANAGEMENT: *Acetaminophen preferred initial tx* for OA in elderly c̄ bleed risk & mild-mod dz ⇨ NSAIDs. NSAIDs more effective.* Intraarticular corticosteroid injections, sodium hyaluronate, glucosamine & chondroitin. Knee replacement. Avoid high-impact exercises.

RHEUMATOID ARTHRITIS (RA)

- Chronic inflammatory disease with persistent symmetric polyarthritis, bone erosion, cartilage destruction & joint structure loss (due to destruction by *pannus*).* *T-cell mediated.**
- **Pannus:** *granulation tissue that erodes into cartilage & bone.* ↑**Risk:** *females*, smoking.

CLINICAL MANIFESTATIONS:
1. Prodrome: constitutional *systemic* symptoms: fever, fatigue, weight loss, anorexia. ↓ROM.
2. *SMALL JOINT stiffness:* (MCP, wrist, PIP, knee, MTP, shoulder, ankle) worse with rest.
   *MORNING JOINT STIFFNESS >60 MINUTES __after initiating movement, improves later in day.__**

3. **SYMMETRIC ARTHRITIS:** *swollen, tender, erythematous, "boggy" joint.* Boutonniere *deformity* (flexion @ PIP, hyperextension of DIP); *swan neck deformity* (flexion @ DIP joint hyperextension @ PIP joint. ULNAR DEVIATION* *at MCP joint.* Rheumatoid nodules.

4. FELTY'S SYNDROME: rare. Triad of: *RA + splenomegaly + ↓WBC/repeated infections.**
5. CAPLAN SYNDROME: *pneumoconiosis + RA.**

DIAGNOSIS:
1. ⊕ RHEUMATOID FACTOR: *best initial test* (sensitive, not specific); ↑CRP & ↑ESR. HLA-DRB1 & 4.

2. ⊕ ANTI-CYCYLIC CITRULLINATED PEPTIDE ANTIBODIES: *most specific for RA.**
3. Arthritis ≥3 joints, morning stiffness, disease duration >6 weeks. Anemia of chronic disease.
4. Radiologic findings: *__narrowed joint space (osteopenia/erosions),__** subluxation, deformities, ulnar deviation of the hand.

MANAGEMENT
1. *PROMPT initiation of DMARDs* reduces permanent joint damage* ex. *Methotrexate 1st line.**
   Often used in conjunction with agents for symptom control (NSAIDs or Corticosteroids).

2. *NSAID 1st line for PAIN CONTROL.* Corticosteroids 2nd line if no symptom relief with NSAIDs.*

OVERVIEW OF THE MANAGEMENT OF RHEUMATOID ARTHRITIS

A. ANTIINFLAMMATORY MEDICATIONS FOR SYMPTOM CONTROL

1. **NSAIDs:** analgesic & anti-inflammatory. ***1st line for SYMPTOM CONTROL.* NSAIDs do not affect disease course, so DMARD must ALSO be initiated (DMARDs reduce progression of RA).**
   - **S/E:** GI (gastritis, peptic ulcer disease), renal insufficiency, cardiovascular (↑ bleeding).

2. **CORTICOSTEROIDS: *suppresses inflammation.*** Low-dose oral, IV or intraarticular routes.
   - **S/E:** hyperglycemia, cataracts, weight gain, fluid retention, immunosuppression, hypertension, osteopenia (prevented with Calcium + Vitamin D).

B. DMARDs FOR REDUCTION OF PROGRESSION OF RA

Disease-modifying antirheumatic drugs. 2 classes non biologic (synthetic) and biologic. These drugs *REDUCE/PREVENT JOINT DAMAGE & PRESERVE JOINT FUNCTION.**
   - NON BIOLOGIC: Hydroxychloroquine, Sulfasalazine, Methotrexate, Leflunomide, Minocycline. *Methotrexate or Leflunomide preferred in patients with high disease activity & advanced disease.*
   - BIOLOGIC: produced by recombinant DNA technology, generally target cytokines or their receptors or are directed against surface cell molecules.

NON BIOLOGIC

METHOTREXATE	**MOA:** immunosuppressant, inhibits lymphocyte proliferation (folic antagonist). **S/E: *hepatotoxicity, stomatitis,*** GI sx, *leukopenia* **bone marrow suppression,** neurotoxicity, *interstitial pneumonitis,* renal toxicity. **CI:** pregnancy, severe renal or liver disease.	- ***1st line DMARD in active RA.**** More sustained results over time than other DMARDs. - ↓'es mortality. - Can be used in combination with biologic DMARDs.
LEFLUNOMIDE	Inhibits T cell activation. Prevents new joint erosion.	Alternative if unable to take Methotrexate (similar efficacy).
HYDROXYCHLOROQUINE (Plaquenil)	Inhibits rheumatoid factor & acute phase reactants, immunosuppressive. Can be used when diagnosis is uncertain (mild disease).	***Retinal toxicity**** (funduscopic exam every 6-12 months). Smoking reduces its effects.
SULFASALAZINE	Antiinflammatory that can be used when diagnosis is uncertain & mild disease. Usually reserved for use in patients unable to take Methotrexate or Leflunomide. Not as effective as Methotrexate or Leflunomide.	**S/E:** hepatitis, bone marrow suppression, nausea, G6PD anemia (sulfa drug).

BIOLOGIC

ETANERCEPT (Enbrel)	***TNF inhibitor*** (TNF-3). Long term effects comparable with Methotrexate.	Slows joint damage. Usually one of the 1st line biologic DMARDs.
INFLIXIMAB (Remicade)	***TNF inhibitor.*** Monoclonal antibody to TNF-3. TNF (Tumor Necrosis Factor) is a cytokine central to the inflammatory cascade in RA. *Not recommended to use as monotherapy usually.*	Patients with poor response to methotrexate have a good response to Infliximab or as add on therapy.
ADALIMUMAB (Humira)	***TNF inhibitor*** (TNF-α). Recombinant IgG1 antibody with additive effect when taken with Methotrexate.	
ANAKINRA	Recombinant ***interleukin-1 receptor antagonist.*** Increased activity when given with Methotrexate	Often used when treatment with other DMARDs not effective.
RITUXIMAB	Anti CD20-B cell depleting monoclonal antibody (B cells also play a role in the pathogenesis of RA).	Avoid in patients with acute or chronic infection (±reactivate TB). Infusion reactions.
ABATACEPT	Inhibits T cell activation (There is a T-cell mediated component of RA).	Avoid in patients with acute or chronic infections. Obtain PPD prior to initiating. Increases exacerbations of COPD.

- *All patients on biologic DMARDs should have a PPD to rule out tuberculosis before initiating therapy.**
- Avoid TNF inhibitors in patients with active or chronic infections as well as patients with multiple sclerosis.
- Screen for HBV & HCV with the use of all DMARDs.

DISTINGUISHING BETWEEN RHEUMATOID ARTHRITIS AND OSTEOARTHRITIS

FEATURE	RHEUMATOID ARTHRITIS	OSTEOARTHRITIS
Primary joints affected	*Wrists, MCP, PIP (DIP usually spared)**	*DIP*, thumb (CMC)
Heberden's nodes	Absent	Frequently present
Joint Characteristics	Soft, warm, ***BOGGY***, tender	***HARD & BONY***
Stiffness	• Worse after resting • Morning stiffness • ***MORNING STIFFNESS**** *> 60 minutes**	• Worse after effort • ***Evening stiffness.**** • If morning stiffness present it is usually <60 minutes.
X ray findings	• *OSTEOPENIA** • *SYMMETRIC joint narrowing**	• *OSTEOPHYTES,* Osteosclerosis* • *ASYMMETRIC joint narrowing**
Laboratory findings	*Positive:** RF, anti-CCP Ab, ESR, CRP	*Negative:* RF, anti-CCP Ab, ESR, CRP

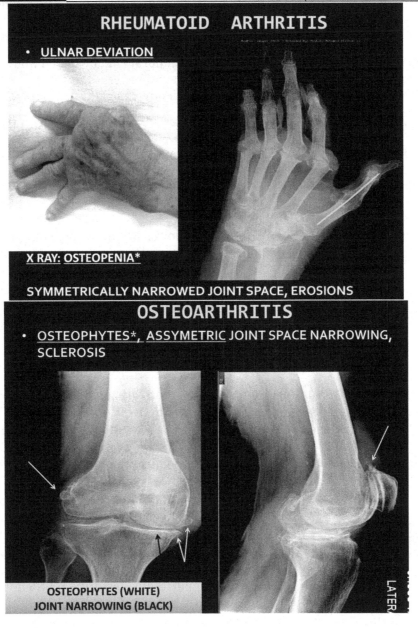

RHEUMATOID ARTHRITIS
• **ULNAR DEVIATION**

X RAY: OSTEOPENIA*

SYMMETRICALLY NARROWED JOINT SPACE, EROSIONS

OSTEOARTHRITIS
• <u>OSTEOPHYTES*, ASSYMETRIC</u> JOINT SPACE NARROWING, SCLEROSIS

OSTEOPHYTES (WHITE)
JOINT NARROWING (BLACK)

LATER

GIANT CELL (TEMPORAL) (CRANIAL) ARTERITIS

- *Same clinical spectrum as Polymyalgia Rheumatica** (which is present in 50% of cases).
- MC seen in women >50y. MC in *NE Europeans.*

ETIOLOGIES
- Idiopathic, ±autoimmune (ex. viral infection causes monocyte activation, inflammatory cytokine production, inflammation & tissue destruction).
- *Vasculitis* of the *extracranial branches of the carotid artery: temporal artery, occipital artery, ophthalmic artery & posterior ciliary artery.*

PATHOPHYSIOLOGY
- Systemic, granulomatous (cell-mediated), chronic vasculitis (inflammation of large & medium arteries) *mostly affecting cranial arteries (head & neck).*   Intimal damage.

CLINICAL MANIFESTATIONS
❶ HEADACHE *MC symptom - new onset, localized. Usually unilateral, temporal & lancinating.*

❷ JAW CLAUDICATION *with mastication -* trismus to jaw <u>immediately</u> after chewing.

❸ ACUTE VISION DISTURBANCES: *amaurosis fugax* (temporary monocular blindness) often heralds visual changes. Diplopia, scotomas, or permanent vision loss due to *1) anterior ischemic optic neuritis MC* 2) central artery occlusion 10% 3) ischemic retinopathy 4) CVA or a combination.

❹ Constitutional sx: fatigue, weight loss, anorexia, fever, night sweats, malaise, pharyngitis.

❺ *Thickened temporal artery (temporal artery/scalp may be tender, pulseless, or normal).*

❻ *Aortic aneurysm (ex. thoracic).*   May have TIA/CVA sx (GCA rarely involves intracranial artery).

DIAGNOSIS
Labs & biopsy are supportive but *GCA is a clinical diagnosis. Blindness MC complication.**
1. ↑*ESR* ≥*100** (average); ↑*CRP.* Normochromic normocytic anemia. Leukocyte usually normal.

2. *Temporal Artery Biopsy:* arteries may have *skip lesions.* If biopsy is positive, it confirms the diagnosis. If negative, temporal arteritis is not fully excluded.
   <u>Biopsy:</u> *mononuclear   lymphocyte   infiltration,   multinucleated   giant   cells* (granulomatous inflammation), *lamina cell degradation.*

MANAGEMENT
1. *High-dose Corticosteroids** 40-60mg/day x 6 weeks with gradual tapering based on sx & ESR. *In patients whom you have a suspicion for GCA, start therapy with Prednisone rather than wait for testing!** Patients dramatically improve within 24-72h after starting treatment.

2. Steroid-sparing antiinflammatories (ex. Methotrexate & Azathioprine) if corticosteroid-refractory.

<u>Hallmark of GCA:</u> *headache, scalp tenderness, jaw claudication, fever, visual changes.**

BEHÇET'S SYNDROME

- Multisystemic autoimmune disorder characterized by *recurrent, painful oral & genital ulcers** (aphthous), erythema nodosum, eye (uveitis, conjunctivitis), arthritis & CNS involvement.

MANAGEMENT: Corticosteroids during flares.

TAKAYASU's ARTERITIS "pulseless disease"

- Chronic large-vessel vasculitis that *affects the AORTA, AORTIC ARCH & PULMONARY ARTERIES.*
- *Women 80-90%. Younger patients (Onset 10-40y).* Highest prevalence in *Asians*.

PATHOPHYSIOLOGY
- Cell-mediated vascular infiltration of all layers of large arteries (inflammation, granuloma formation, giant cell, killer T cell & lymphocyte infiltration).

CLINICAL MANIFESTATIONS
1. **Systemic phase:** (early) : fatigue, arthralgias, myalgias, weight loss, night sweats, low grade fever.
2. *Vascular occlusive phase:* late phase
   - *Vessel stenosis/occlusion/ischemia:* *CORONARY ARTERY (MI);* Common carotid (*TIA, CVA,* headaches, visual changes, syncope); Renal artery (*HTN crisis*, renal failure); Subclavian (arm claudication); Posterior vertebral artery (visual changes, dizziness); Pulmonary artery (dyspnea, hemoptysis). *LOWER EXTREMITY CLAUDICATION.*
   - Aneurysm formation/rupture: aortic dissection/rupture, aortic valve regurgitation.

3. **Physical Examination:** carotid or abdominal *arterial bruits, DIMINISHED PULSES,* *asymmetric BP measurements* >10mmHg, HTN, signs/sx peripheral arterial dz (cool extremities, ↓muscle)

DIAGNOSIS
1. *Angiography: necessary to confirm the diagnosis & determine the extent of disease.*
2. Helical CT scan angiography or MRA may show thickness & edema within arterial wall.
3. ↑ESR/CRP. Normochromic normocytic anemia.

MANAGEMENT
1. *High-dose Corticosteroids* ex. 60mg/day x 6 weeks with gradual tapering .
2. Cytotoxic drugs (chronic active disease): ex. Methotrexate & Azathioprine. ± Revascularization.

KAWASAKI SYNDROME (Mucocutaneous Lymph Node Syndrome)

- *MC in children (especially <5y), boys, Asians (highest risk).* Thought to be an unidentified respiratory agent or viral pathogen with a propensity towards vascular tissue.
- Medium & small vessel necrotizing vasculitis including the *coronary arteries.*

CLINICAL MANIFESTATIONS & DIAGNOSIS:
"warm + CREAM" = fever + 4 of the following 5:
1. **C**onjunctivitis: *bilateral & nonexudative* (± photophobia), involvement spares the limbus.
2. **R**ash: *polymorphous* (erythematous or morbiliform or macular).
3. **E**xtremity (peripheral) *changes:* desquamation (especially perineum), edema, erythema of the palms & soles, induration of the hands & feet, Beau's lines (transverse nail grooves), *arthritis.*
4. **A**denopathy: *cervical lymphadenopathy* (erythematous, nonsuppurative, induration, unilateral).
5. **M**ucous membrane: pharyngeal erythema, *lip swelling & fissures, strawberry tongue.*

COMPLICATIONS: *coronary vessel arteritis: CORONARY ARTERY ANEURYSM,* *MYOCARDIAL INFARCTION,* pericarditis, myocarditis, peripheral arterial occlusion.

DIAGNOSIS
1. ↑ESR/CRP, *leukocytosis, reactive thrombocytosis (↑platelets).* Normochromic normocytic anemia. *Sterile pyuria.* Echocardiogram & angiography may be needed if heart involvement is suspected.

MANAGEMENT: *INTRAVENOUS IMMUNE GLOBULIN + HIGH-DOSE ASPIRIN MAINSTAY OF TREATMENT* (lowers fever, joint pain, & prevents coronary artery thrombosis/aneurysm); Corticosteroids if refractory.

POLYARTERITIS NODOSA (PAN)

- Systemic vasculitis of <u>medium/small arteries</u> ⇨necrotizing inflammatory lesions.
- ↑*association with Hepatitis B.** ↑*microaneurysms* with aneurysmal rupture ⇨ hemorrhage, thrombosis ⇨ organ ischemia or infarction. *Muscular arteries involved.* Type III HSN.

CLINICAL MANIFESTATIONS:
1. **Renal**: *HTN* (due to ↑renin), renal failure.* Usually no glomerulonephritis. No capillaries involved.
2. **Constitutional**: fever, myalgias, arthritis. ***Lungs usually spared.****
3. **CNS: *neuropathy,*** amaurosis fugax, *peripheral neuropathy,* **Mononeuritis multiplex.**
4. **Dermatologic:** *livedo reticularis,* purpura, ulcers, gangrene, nodules, Raynaud's phenomenon.

DIAGNOSIS: ↑*ESR;* angiography. MC seen in men (~45y of age). ***Classic PAN is ANCA negative**** (but *P-ANCA positive in <20% of cases*). <u>Biopsy</u>: necrotizing inflammatory lesions. *No granulomas.* **<u>Renal or Mesenteric angiography</u>: *microaneurysms with abrupt cut-off of small arteries.****

MANAGEMENT: *Corticosteroids (±Cyclophosphamide if refractory).* ±Plasmapheresis if HBV⊕.

EOSINOPHILIC GRANULOMATOSIS WITH POLYANGIITIS (EGPA- CHURG-STRAUSS)

- Systemic small (medium) vasculitis of arteries & veins with ❶ *ASTHMA.**
    ❷ *HYPEREOSINOPHILIA** & ❸ *chronic RHINOSINUSITIS** with necrotizing vasculitis & granulomas.

CLINICAL MANIFESTATIONS
Lung MC involved, Skin 2nd, heart GI tract, liver, peripheral nerves, allergic rhinitis.
1. **Prodromal phase:** *atopic disease, allergic rhinitis, asthma* (98-100%). MC in 2nd/3rd decades.
2. **Eosinophilic phase:** peripheral blood eosinophilia & eosinophilic infiltration of multiple organs *(especially lungs & GI tract).* <u>GI:</u> eosinophilic gastritis: pain, bleeding, colitis (30-60%). **Pulmonary:** dyspnea, infiltrates, pulmonary hemorrhage, nodular disease, pleural effusion.
3. **Vasculitic phase:** life-threatening systemic vasculitis. MC in the 3rd/4th decades.

DIAGNOSIS: *eosinophilia hallmark;** ↑ESR, ↑CRP, ↑BUN/Cr; ⊕ *P-ANCA;** ↑IgE, ⊕Rheumatoid factor.

MANAGEMENT: *Corticosteroids* (may add Cyclophosphamide).

GRANULOMATOSIS WITH POLYANGIITIS (GPA - WEGENER'S)

- Small vessel vasculitis with granulomatous inflammation & necrosis of the ***nose, lungs & kidney.****
CLINICAL MANIFESTATIONS OF GPA:
TRIAD: ❶ *UPPER RESPIRATORY/NOSE SX** ❷ *LOWER RESPIRATORY TRACT SX** & ❸ *GLOMERULONEPHRITIS.**
1. <u>**UPPER RESPIRATORY TRACT/NOSE (ENT) SX:**</u> nasal congestion, ***saddle-nose deformity*** (cartilage involvement), epistaxis, otitis media, mastoiditis, stridor, ***sinusitis often refractory to tx.**** Constitutional: fever, migratory arthralgias, malaise, weight loss. Episcleritis, conjunctivitis.

2. <u>**LOWER RESPIRATORY TRACT (LUNG) SX:**</u> parenchymal involvement ⇨ cough, dyspnea, hemoptysis (pulmonary hemorrhage), wheezing, pulmonary infiltrates, cavitation.

3. <u>**RENAL: GLOMERULONEPHRITIS*:**</u> *rapidly progressing/crescentic.** **Hematuria,** proteinuria.

DIAGNOSIS: ⊕ *C-ANCA.** CXR: infiltrates, nodules, masses or cavities (nonspecific).

MANAGEMENT: *Corticosteroids + Cyclophosphamide. Methotrexate alternative to cyclophosphamide.*

MICROSCOPIC POLYANGIITIS (MPA)

- Small (medium)-vessel vasculitis (NO necrotic or granulomatous inflammation as seen with GPA). *Affects the arterioles, venules & capillaries* (capillary involvement not classically seen with PAN).

CLINICAL MANIFESTATIONS:
1. Constitutional: fever, arthralgias, malaise, weight loss, *palpable (elevated) purpura*.
2. *Lung sx:* cough, dyspnea, hemoptysis (pulmonary hemorrhage). *Mononeuritis multiplex.*
3. *Renal: acute glomerulonephritis (rapidly progressing/crescentic).*

DIAGNOSIS: ⊕*P-ANCA.** CXR: infiltrates, nodules, masses or cavities (nonspecific).

MANAGEMENT: *Corticosteroids plus Cyclophosphamide.*

HENOCH-SCHÖNLEIN PURPURA (HSP)

- *IgA deposition in skin* ⇨ *immune-mediated leukocytoclastic vasculitis. MC after URI symptoms.**
- MC systemic small-vessel vasculitis in children (MC 3-15y). 90% occur in children, ±occur in adults.

CLINICAL MANIFESTATIONS: "**HSP** affects Ig**A**" helpful to remember the 4 cardinal symptoms:
1. **H**ematuria. Azotemia (↑BUN/Creatinine), proteinuria.
2. **S**ynovial: *arthritis/arthralgias.* Knees & ankles MC. Tenderness/swelling (no erythema, warmth).
3. **P**alpable purpura: *MC on lower extremities (NOT due to thrombocytopenia or coagulopathy).*
4. **A**bdominal pain: 2ry to vasculitis of the GI tract. May present with GI bleeding.

DIAGNOSIS
1. Clinical diagnosis
2. **Kidney biopsy*: *mesangial IgA deposits.**
3. *Normal coags** (PT/PTT) *& normal platelets** because *bleeding is due to vasculitis NOT coagulation nor platelet abnormalities.**

MANAGEMENT
   Supportive (self-limited - lasts 1-6 weeks). Bed rest, hydration, NSAIDs for joint pain.

GOODPASTURE'S DISEASE

- Type II HSN: *IgG antibodies against type IV collagen of the alveoli & glomerular basement membrane of the kidney.*

CLINICAL MANIFESTATIONS
   Think **G**ood**P**astures = ❶ **G**lomerulonephritis (rapidly progressing)* + ❷ **P**ulmonary hemorrhage (hemoptysis).*

DIAGNOSIS:
1. **Biopsy:** *linear IgG deposits** in the glomeruli or alveoli* on immunofluorescence.

MANAGEMENT
Think **G**ood**P**astures:
1. **G**lucocorticoids *(Corticosteroids) plus Cyclophosphamide*.
2. **P**lasmapheresis.

	INCIDENCE	PATHOPHYSIOLOGY	CLINICAL	DIAGNOSIS	MANAGEMENT
LARGE VESSEL					
GIANT CELL (TEMPORAL) ARTERITIS	*Older women ≥50y**	*Cranial arteries* - *Temporal & Ophthalmic artery**	• *Headache, visual loss,** jaw claudication • Temporal artery sx	• *Temporal Artery Bx* • *Clinical Dx**	*High-dose corticosteroids*
TAKAYASU ARTERITIS	*MC in young, Asian women <40y**	• *Aorta & aortic arch** • *Pulmonary artery*	• *Vessel aneurysm, occlusion (TIA, CVA, MYOCARDIAL INFARCTION** • *Lower extremity claudication, ↓pulses**	*Angiography*	*High-dose steroids* Methotrexate (MTX) Azathioprine (AZA)
MEDIUM VESSEL	Affects ARTERIOLES				
KAWASAKI'S DISEASE	*MC in Asian children <5y**	Necrotizing vasculitis	*"warm + CREAM"* Coronary aneurysms*	• ↑ESR/CRP, anemia • Clinical dx	*IVIG + Aspirin**
POLYARTERITIS NODOSA (PAN)	Males ~45y ↑Assoc c Hep B Virus*	Necrotizing vasculitis of arterioles. *Capillaries not involved*	CNS, GI, derm, renal *Lungs usually spared.* Renovascular HTN*	• *Angiogram* • *ANCA negative** (⊕P-ANCA <20%) • *No granulomas*	*Corticosteroids* ± MTX, AZA
SMALL VESSEL	Affects ARTERIOLES, CAPILLARIES & VENULES				
GRANULOMATOUS **EOSINOPHILIC GPA (CHURG STRAUSS)**	Males >40y	Necrotizing *granulomatous*	*Upper airway: allergic** *ASTHMA** Skin, Lung MC involved	• *↑EOSINOPHILS**, *asthma* • ⊕*P-ANCA**	*Corticosteroids* Cyclophosphamide (Cyc), AZA
GPA (WEGENERS)	Men = Women Peaks 30-40y	Necrotizing *granulomatous*	TRIAD *1. Upper airway: necrotic** *2. Lower airway dz* *3. Acute Glomerulonephritis*	• ↑ESR/CRP, anemia • ⊕ *C-ANCA**	*Corticosteroids +* *Cyclophosphamide* MTX
NONGRANULOMATOUS **MICROSCOPIC POLYANGIITIS (MPA)**	Males ~50y	*NON granulomatous capillaries, arteries, veins (unlike PAN)*	*Upp airway: unaffected* *Lung sx.* *Acute Glomerulonephritis*	⊕*P-ANCA**	*Steroids + Cyclophosphamide* MTX
HENOCH-SCHÖNLEIN PURPURA (HSP)	*Children 3-15y* *Males MC*	• *Ig-A deposition* vasculitis • *MC after URI**	❶ *Purpura* ❷ *Arthritis* ❸ *Abdominal pain* ❹ *Hematuria*	• *↑Ig-A** • *Normal coags, plts.* • UA: RBC, proteinuria	*Self-limiting –* *supportive mgmt.* ± Prednisone

SERONEGATIVE SPONDYLOARTHROPATHIES

- *YOUNG MALE predominance <40y,** inflammatory arthritis. Patients also develop UVEITIS & SACROILIITIS.*
- ⊕ *HLA-B27* gene susceptibility* & environmental factors (ex. infection).
- *Negative ANA, RF*.* ⊕ *ENTHESITIS** = inflammation where ligaments & tendons insert into bone.
- Includes **"PEAR"**: **P**soriatic arthritis, **E**nteropathic arthritis, **A**nkylosing spondylitis & **R**eactive arthritis.

PSORIATIC ARTHRITIS

- 15-20% of patients with psoriasis develop psoriatic arthritis. MC around 40-50y.
- Psoriasis usually precedes the development of psoriatic arthritis by months to years.

CLINICAL MANIFESTATIONS:
1. *Asymmetric arthritis* may mimic RA but affects the DIP joint, *dactylitis ("sausage" digits)** appearance of the fingers/toes. *Sacroiliac arthritis (sacroiliitis), chronic uveitis.*
2. *Signs of psoriasis: pitting of the nails,* erythematous rash with thick, silvery white scales.

DIAGNOSIS:
1. *X ray: "PENCIL IN CUP" DEFORMITY,** osteolysis, narrowed joint space. ⊕ *HLA-B27, ↑ESR.*

MANAGEMENT: *NSAIDs 1ˢᵗ line,* (Methotrexate drug of choice after NSAIDs) ⇨ TNF-inhibitors.

ENTEROPATHIC ARTHRITIS: associated with IBD: *Crohn, Ulcerative Colitis.*

ANKYLOSING SPONDYLITIS

- Chronic inflammatory arthropathy of the *axial skeleton & sacroiliac joints c progressive stiffness.* MC in young males 15-30y.

CLINICAL MANIFESTATIONS:
1. **Chronic low back pain**: *morning stiffness with ↓ROM.* Back pain may radiate to thighs. *Back STIFFNESS DECREASES WITH EXERCISE/ACTIVITY.** Patient unable to put head down while supine.
2. Peripheral arthritis: *may develop SACROILIITIS** (bilateral),* kyphosis, large-joint arthritis.
3. Extra skeletal: pulmonary fibrosis, aortitis, Achilles enthesitis, sarcoidosis, oral ulcers, uveitis.

DIAGNOSIS
1. *↑ESR,* ⊕ *HLA-B27** inflammatory arthropathy. Negative ANA & Rheumatoid factor.
2. *BAMBOO SPINE** on X ray *= SQUARING (BRIDGING) OF THE VERTEBRAL BODIES,** loss of normal curvature.

MANAGEMENT
1. *NSAIDs,** rest, physical therapy 1ˢᵗ line ⇨ TNF-α inhibitor (ex. Infliximab) ⇨ Steroids.

REACTIVE ARTHRITIS (REITER'S SYNDROME)

- *Autoimmune response* to an infection in another part of the body ❶ *ARTHRITIS: asymmetric inflammation* ❷ *CONJUNCTIVITIS/uveitis* ❸ *URETHRITIS,* cervicitis. MC 20-40y especially males.
- 1-4 weeks p *Chlamydia (MC),* gonorrhea, *GI infections: Salmonella, Shigella, Campylobacter, Yersinia.*

CLINICAL MANIFESTATIONS
1. **Triad:** *conjunctivitis, urethritis & arthritis* (especially lower extremities), sausage toes/fingers.
2. *Keratoderma blennorrhagicum** = hyperkeratotic lesions on palms/soles. Circinate balanitis.

DIAGNOSIS
1. ⊕ *HLA-B27* (80%); CBC: ↑WBC (10,000 - 20,000), ↑ESR, normochromic anemia, ↑IgG.
2. **Synovial fluid:** ↑WBC 1,000–8,000 cells/mm³. *Fluid is bacterial culture negative (aseptic).**

MANAGEMENT: *NSAIDs mainstay of tx.** If no response, Methotrexate ⇨ Sulfasalazine, Steroids. Anti-TNF agents (Etanercept, Infliximab). Antibiotic use during precipitating disease ↓'es incidence.

ANKYLOSING   SPONDYLITIS

- SACROILIITIS, ⊕ HLA-B27, <u>BAMBOO SPINE*</u>

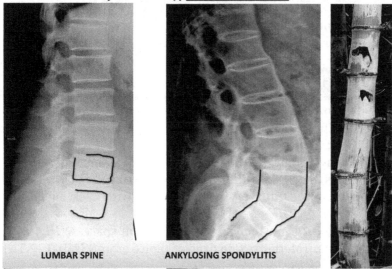

LUMBAR SPINE   ANKYLOSING SPONDYLITIS

PSORIATIC   ARTHRITIS

- <u>SAUSAGE DIGITS*</u>
- <u>X RAYS:</u> PENCIL IN CUP DEFORMITY*

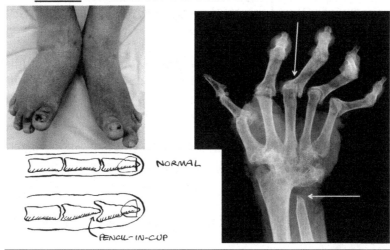

NORMAL

PENCIL-IN-CUP

ARTHOCENTESIS ANALYSIS OF FLUID			
	WBCs (/μL)	MICROSCOPIC	CULTURES
NORMAL	200		
INFLAMMATORY ARTHRITIS			
• GOUT	<50, 000 (mostly PMN)	• *Needle shaped crystals - negatively birefringent** • *Uric Acid Crystals*	Negative
• PSEUDO GOUT	<50, 000 (mostly PMN)	• *Rhomboid-shaped crystals- positively birefringent** • *Calcium Pyrophosphate crystals*	Negative
• REACTIVE ARTHRITIS & OTHER INFLAMMATORY ARTHRITIS	<50, 000 (mostly PMN) PMN = Polymorphonuclear neutrophils		Negative
SEPTIC ARTHRITIS	**≥50,000*** **(>90% PMNs)**	*Bacteria, Cloudy*	*Positive**

P-ANCA

- Perinuclear antineutrophil cytoplasmic antibodies cause the release of lytic enzymes from white blood cells, resulting in inflammation of the blood vessel wall (vasculitis). The protein targeted is myeloperoxidase.
- Diseases: **Microscopic Polyangiitis (MPA), Churg Strauss, Ulcerative Colitis, Primary Sclerosing Cholangitis**.

C-ANCA

- Cytoplasmic antineutrophil cytoplasmic Ab. Protein targeted is proteinase 3. **Wegener's granulomatosis (GPA).**

ESR (ERYTHROCYTE SEDIMENTATION RATE)

- Erythrocyte sedimentation rate. When inflammation is present, high levels of fibrinogen causes RBCs to stick together (Rouleaux formation) causing them to settle faster. Nonspecific marker of inflammation.

CRP (C- REACTIVE PROTEIN)

- Nonspecific marker of inflammation. CRP is released by the liver in response to factors secreted by macrophages, which help to activate the complement system (acute phase reactant).

ANA (ANTI-NUCLEAR ANTIBODY)

- Auto-Ab against the nucleus. Present in low titers in the general population. Increased in **autoimmune diseases.**

TNF (TUMOR NECROSIS FACTOR)

- Group of cytokines that promote the inflammatory response, can cause cell death apoptosis (seen in tumor regression, septic shock and cachexia). Elevated in rheumatoid arthritis, ankylosing spondylitis, psoriasis, Crohn.

Immunoglobulin A (IgA)

- **Critical role in mucosal immunity** (secreted in tears, saliva, respiratory epithelium, GI tract, genitourinary tract).
- Seen in Berger's disease (IgA nephropathy), Henoch-Schönlein Purpura & Celiac disease (IgA endomysial Ab)

ANTIBODIES/AUTO ANTIBODIES	CLASSIC DISEASE ASSOCIATION
ACETYLCHOLINE RECEPTOR	Myasthenia Gravis
β-2 GLYCOPROTEIN 1	Antiphospholipid Antibody Syndrome (SLE)
CARDIOLIPIN	Antiphospholipid Antibody Syndrome (SLE)
CENTROMERE	CREST syndrome (Limited Systemic Sclerosis)
CYCLIC CITRULLINATED PEPTIDE (PROTEIN) – CCP	Specific for Rheumatoid Arthritis. Rheumatoid Factor used for screening but is not specific.
DOUBLE-STRANDED DNA	Systemic Lupus Erythematosus (*specific*, not sensitive)
ENDOMYSIAL	Celiac disease
GLOMERULAR BASEMENT MEMBRANE	Goodpasture's syndrome
HISTONE	Drug-induced Lupus
JO-1	Polymyositis, Dermatomyositis
LA (SS-B)	Sjögren syndrome
LUPUS ANTICOAGULANT	Antiphospholipid Antibody Syndrome (SLE)
Mi-2	Dermatomyositis
MITOCHONDRIAL	Primary Biliary Cirrhosis
MUSK (Muscle specific receptor tyrosine kinase)	Myasthenia Gravis - may be positive in AChR-negative patients with MG.
P-ANCA	Microscopic Polyangiitis (MPA), Churg Strauss Ulcerative Colitis, Primary Sclerosing Cholangitis
RHEUMATOID FACTOR	Rheumatoid Arthritis
RIBONUCLEOPROTEIN (RNP)	Mixed Connective Tissue disease, SLE
RO (SS-A)	Sjögren syndrome, Systemic Lupus Erythematosus
SACCHAROMYCES CEREVISIAE	Crohn disease
SCL-70 (TOPOISOMERASE)	Diffuse Systemic Sclerosis (Scleroderma)
SIGNAL RECOGNITION PROTEIN (SRP)	Polymyositis
SMITH	Systemic Lupus Erythematosus (*specific,* not sensitive)
SMOOTH MUSCLE	Autoimmune hepatitis
THYROGLOBULIN	Hashimoto's thyroiditis, Autoimmune thyroiditis
THYROID PEROXIDASE (TPO)	Hashimoto's thyroiditis, Autoimmune thyroiditis
TOPOISOMERASE (SCL-70)	Diffuse Systemic Sclerosis (Scleroderma)
TRANSGLUTAMINASE	Celiac disease, Dermatitis Herpetiformis
TSH (THYROTROPIN) RECEPTOR	Graves disease
VOLTAGE-GATED CALCIUM CHANNEL	Lambert-Eaton Syndrome

SELECTED REFERENCES

Ezoe M, Naito M, Inoue T. The prevalence of acetabular retroversion among various disorders of the hip. J Bone Joint Surg Am. 2006;88(2):372-9

Cacopardo B, Benanti F, Pinzone MR, Nunnari G. Rheumatoid arthritis following PEG-interferon-alfa-2a plus ribavirin treatment for chronic hepatitis C: a case report and review of the literature. BMC Res Notes. 2013;6(1):437.

Lykissas MG, Mccarthy JJ. Should all unstable slipped capital femoral epiphysis be treated open?. J Pediatr Orthop. 2013;33 Suppl 1(3):S92-8.

Smith TO, Chester R, Pearse EO, Hing CB. Operative versus non-operative management following Rockwood grade III acromioclavicular separation: a meta-analysis of the current evidence base. J Orthop Traumatol. 2011;12(1):19-27.

Shen PH, Lien SB, Shen HC, Lee CH, Wu SS, Lin LC. Long-term functional outcomes after repair of rotator cuff tears correlated with atrophy of the supraspinatus muscles on magnetic resonance images. J Shoulder Elbow Surg. 2008;17(1 Suppl):1S-7S.

Kawasaki Disease. http://sketchymedicine.com/2012/07/kawasaki-disease. Accessed 2/20/2014.

Shankarkumar U, Devraj JP, Ghosh K, Mohanty D. Seronegative spondarthritis and human leucocyte antigen association. Br J Biomed Sci. 2002;59(1):38-41.

Seo P, Stone JH. The antineutrophil cytoplasmic antibody-associated vasculitides. Am J Med. 2004;117(1):39-50.

Milan B, Josip K. [Ocular manifestations of the aortic arch syndrome (pulseless disease; Takayasu's disease)]. Ann Ocul (Paris). 1967;200(11):1168-79.

Henegar C, Pagnoux C, Puéchal X, et al. A paradigm of diagnostic criteria for polyarteritis nodosa: analysis of a series of 949 patients with vasculitides. Arthritis Rheum. 2008;58(5):1528-38.

Van der kraan PM, Van den berg WB. Osteoarthritis in the context of ageing and evolution. Loss of chondrocyte differentiation block during ageing. Ageing Res Rev. 2008;7(2):106-13.

Scott DL, Wolfe F, Huizinga TW. Rheumatoid arthritis. Lancet. 2010;376(9746):1094-108.

Rosenthal AK, Ryan LM. Crystal arthritis: calcium pyrophosphate deposition-nothing 'pseudo' about it!. Nat Rev Rheumatol. 2011;7(5):257-8.

Asherson RA, Cervera R, De groot PG, et al. Catastrophic antiphospholipid syndrome: international consensus statement on classification criteria and treatment guidelines. Lupus. 2003;12(7):530-4.

Meijer JM, Pijpe J, Bootsma H, Vissink A, Kallenberg CG. The future of biologic agents in the treatment of Sjögren's syndrome. Clin Rev Allergy Immunol. 2007;32(3):292-7.

Gelderblom H, Hogendoorn PC, Dijkstra SD, et al. The clinical approach towards chondrosarcoma. Oncologist. 2008;13(3):320-9.

Yashar A, Loder RT, Hensinger RN. Determination of skeletal age in children with Osgood-Schlatter disease by using radiographs of the knee. J Pediatr Orthop. 1995;15(3):298-301.

Joseph B. Prognostic factors and outcome measures in Perthes disease. Orthop Clin North Am. 2011;42(3):303-15, v-vi.

Murrell GA. Treatment of shoulder dislocation: is a sling appropriate?. Med J Aust. 2003;179(7):370-1.

PHOTO CREDITS

By Gilo1969 (Own work) [CC-BY-SA-3.0 (http://creativecommons.org/licenses/by-sa/3.0) or GFDL (http://www.gnu.org/copyleft/fdl.html)], via Wikimedia Commons

Legg Calves Perthes Disease
By J. Lengerke (Praxis Dr. Lengerke) [Public domain], via Wikimedia Commons

Buckle Fracture
© Nevit Dilmen [CC-BY-SA-3.0 (http://creativecommons.org/licenses/by-sa/3.0) or GFDL (http://www.gnu.org/copyleft/fdl.html)], via Wikimedia Commons

Patella Alta
By Hellerhoff (Own work) [CC-BY-SA-3.0 (http://creativecommons.org/licenses/by-sa/3.0)], via Wikimedia Commons

Patella Baja
By Hellerhoff (Own work) [CC-BY-SA-3.0 (http://creativecommons.org/licenses/by-sa/3.0)], via Wikimedia Commons

Osgood Schlatter
By Lucien Monfils (Own work) [GFDL (http://www.gnu.org/copyleft/fdl.html) or CC-BY-SA-3.0-2.5-2.0-1.0 (http://creativecommons.org/licenses/by-sa/3.0)], via Wikimedia Commons

Osgood
By D3aj86 (Own work) [CC-BY-3.0 (http://creativecommons.org/licenses/by/3.0)], via Wikimedia Commons

Hallux Valgus
By Michael Nebel http://de.wikipedia.org/wiki/Benutzer:Jakker [CC-BY-SA-2.0-de (http://creativecommons.org/licenses/by-sa/2.0/de/deed.en)], via Wikimedia Commons

Hallux Valgus
By Cyberprout at fr.wikipedia [CC-BY-SA-1.0 (http://creativecommons.org/licenses/by-sa/1.0)], from Wikimedia Commons

Lisfranc Injury
By James Heilman, MD (Own work) [CC-BY-3.0 (http://creativecommons.org/licenses/by/3.0)], via Wikimedia Commons

Jones Fracture
By Lucien Monfils (Own work) [GFDL (http://www.gnu.org/copyleft/fdl.html) or CC-BY-SA-3.0-2.5-2.0-1.0 (http://creativecommons.org/licenses/by-sa/3.0)], via Wikimedia Commons

Spondylolysis &other films
By Hellerhoff (Own work) [CC-BY-SA-3.0 (http://creativecommons.org/licenses/by-sa/3.0)], via Wikimedia Commons

Hammertoe
By Richard Huber (Own work) [CC-BY-SA-3.0 (http://creativecommons.org/licenses/by-sa/3.0)], via Wikimedia Commons

Normal Foot X ray
By Andrew Magill (Flickr) [CC-BY-2.0 (http://creativecommons.org/licenses/by/2.0)], via Wikimedia Commons

Spondylolisthesis
By Lucien Monfils (Own work) [GFDL (http://www.gnu.org/copyleft/fdl.html) or CC-BY-SA-3.0-2.5-2.0-1.0 (http://creativecommons.org/licenses/by-sa/3.0)], via Wikimedia Commons

Ostoechondroma

By Dr Frank Gaillard. Used With Permission.
http://images.radiopaedia.org/images/137159/aa2551e220f734fece9b37fd38f00e_big_gallery.jpg

Osteomyelitis
Case by Dr. Hani Salam. Copyrighted by radiopaedia.org. Used with permission.

Osteomyelitis
Sarindam7 at the English language Wikipedia [GFDL (http://www.gnu.org/copyleft/fdl.html) or CC-BY-SA-3.0 (http://creativecommons.org/licenses/by-sa/3.0/)], from Wikimedia Commons

Codman's triangle
By User:Ajimsha619 (Own work) [CC-BY-SA-3.0 (http://creativecommons.org/licenses/by-sa/3.0)], via Wikimedia Commons

Osteochondroma
By J Bovee (Orphanet J Rare Dis. 2008 Feb 13;3:3.) [CC-BY-SA-3.0-nl (http://creativecommons.org/licenses/by-sa/3.0/nl/deed.en)], via Wikimedia Commons

Ewing's Sarcoma
By Michael Richardson, M.D. on Oct 25th, 2004; Upload by Christaras A (EN:Wikipedia. IMG EwingSarcomaTibia.jpg) [GFDL (www.gnu.org/copyleft/fdl.html) or CC-BY-SA-3.0 (http://creativecommons.org/licenses/by-sa/3.0/)], via Wikimedia Commons

Dermatomyositis
By Elizabeth M. Dugan, Adam M. Huber, Frederick W. Miller, Lisa G. Rider [CC-BY-SA-3.0 (http://creativecommons.org/licenses/by-sa/3.0)], via Wikimedia Commons

Dermatomyositis
By Elizabeth M. Dugan, Adam M. Huber, Frederick W. Miller, Lisa G. Rider [CC-BY-SA-3.0 (http://creativecommons.org/licenses/by-sa/3.0)], via Wikimedia Commons

Dermatomyositis
By Elizabeth M. Dugan, Adam M. Huber, Frederick W. Miller, Lisa G. Rider [CC-BY-SA-3.0 (http://creativecommons.org/licenses/by-sa/3.0)], via Wikimedia Commons

Pagets disease of skull
By dr Laughlin Dawes (radpod.org) [CC-BY-3.0 (http://creativecommons.org/licenses/by/3.0)], via Wikimedia Commons

Paget's disease CT scan
By Hellerhoff (Own work) [CC-BY-SA-3.0 (http://creativecommons.org/licenses/by-sa/3.0)], via Wikimedia Commons

Osteosarcoma in Paget's disease
From Radiopaedia.org. Used with permission

Scleroderma
By AVM (talk) 02:54, 9 January 2009 (UTC) (Own work) [GFDL (http://www.gnu.org/copyleft/fdl.html) or CC-BY-3.0 (http://creativecommons.org/licenses/by/3.0)], via Wikimedia Commons

Systemic Lupus Erythematosus
By Sarella (Own work) [CC-BY-SA-3.0 (http://creativecommons.org/licenses/by-sa/3.0)], via Wikimedia Commons

Discoid Lupus
By Leonard C. Sperling, M.D., COL, MC, USA, Department of Dermatology, Uniformed Services University [Public domain], via Wikimedia Commons

Uric Acid crystals
By Bobjgalindo (Own work) [GFDL (http://www.gnu.org/copyleft/fdl.html) or CC-BY-SA-3.0-2.5-2.0-1.0 (http://creativecommons.org/licenses/by-sa/3.0)], via Wikimedia Commons

CHAPTER 5 – ENT (EARS, NOSE, THROAT DISORDERS)

ECTROPION

• *Eyelid & lashes turned outward* (due to relaxation of the orbicularis oculi muscle).
• MC seen in the elderly (tends to be bilateral) but can be congenital, infectious, CN 7 palsy.

CLINICAL MANIFESTATIONS
Irritation, ocular dryness, tearing, sagging of the eyelid, ↑sensitivity.

MANAGEMENT: Surgical correction if needed. Lubricating eye drops for symptom relief.

ENTROPION

• *Eyelid & lashes turned inward* (may be caused by spasms of the orbicularis oculi muscle).
• MC seen in the elderly.

CLINICAL MANIFESTATIONS
Eyelashes may cause corneal abrasion/ulcerations, erythema, tearing, ↑sensitivity.

MANAGEMENT: Surgical correction if needed. Lubricating eye drops for symptom relief.

DACROCYSTITIS

• *Infection of the lacrimal sac.* MC *S. aureus*, GABHS, S. epidermis H. Flu & S. pneumo.

CLINICAL MANIFESTATIONS:
Tearing, tenderness, edema & *redness to MEDIAL CANTHAL (NASAL SIDE) OF LOWER LID* (±purulent).

MANAGEMENT acute= *antibiotics*⇨ ±Dacryocystorhinostomy. Clindamycin. Vanco + Ceftriaxone.
chronic: Dacryocystorhinostomy.

BLEPHARITIS

• Inflammation of *both eyelids.* Common in patients with Down syndrome & eczema.
ETIOLOGIES
1. **Anterior:** involves the skin & base of the eyelashes. Less common. 2 types:
   ❶ *Infectious (Staph aureus* or Staph epidermis). Viruses. ❷ *Seborrheic.*

2. **Posterior:** Meibomian gland dysfunction (associated with rosacea & allergic dermatitis).

CLINICAL MANIFESTATIONS
1. Eye irritation/itching.
2. Eyelid: burning, erythema, *crusting, scaling, RED-RIMMING* of the eyelid & eyelash flaking.*
3. ± Entropion or ectropion (especially with posterior).

MANAGEMENT:
1. **Anterior:** *eyelid hygiene:* warm compresses, eyelid scrubbing/washing with baby shampoo.
   ± *antibiotics:* ex. Azithromycin solution or ointment (Erythromycin or Bacitracin).

2. **Posterior:** *eyelid hygiene, regular massage/expression of the Meibomian gland.*
   ± systemic antibiotics in severe or unresponsive cases ex.Tetracyclines or Azithromycin.

HORDEOLUM (STYE)

- Local abscess of the eyelid margin. ***Staph. aureus*** 90-95%.
   External: infection of eyelash follicle or external sebaceous glands ***near the lid margin.***
   Internal: inflammation/infection of the Meibomian gland.

CLINICAL MANIFESTATIONS: focal abscess: ***painful, warm, swollen red lump on eyelid.****

MANAGEMENT:
   1. ***warm compresses mainstay of treatment*** (most eventually point & drain spontaneously).
      ± add topical antibiotic ointment (ex. Erythromycin, Bacitracin) if actively draining.

   2. ***± incision & drainage if no spontaneous drainage after 48 hours.***

CHALAZION

- ***Painless granuloma of the internal Meibomian sebaceous gland⇨ focal eyelid swelling.***
   Chalazions are often larger, firmer, slower growing & less painful than hordeola.

CLINICAL MANIFESTATION
   NONTENDER EYELID SWELLING* on the conjunctival surface of eyelid ⇨ rubbery nodule.

MANAGEMENT
   1. ***eyelid hygiene,**** warm compresses. *Antibiotics usually not necessary.* Injection of corticosteroid or incision + curettage may be necessary in large ones affecting vision.

PTERYGIUM & PINGUECULA

- **PTERYGIUM** elevated, superficial *FLESHY, TRIANGULAR-SHAPED "GROWING"** fibrovascular mass* (MC in inner corner/***nasal side of eye**** & extends laterally).
- ***Associated with ↑UV exposure in sunny climates*** as well as *sand, wind & dust exposure.*

   Management: ***observation for most,*** ± artificial tears. ***Removal only if growth affects vision.***

PINGUECULA: yellow, elevated nodule on the ***nasal side of sclera*** (fat/protein) *DOES NOT GROW!**
   Management: observation in most cases.
      May be excised for cosmetic reasons or if it becomes inflamed.

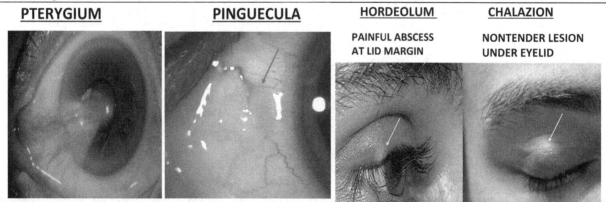

PTERYGIUM	PINGUECULA	HORDEOLUM	CHALAZION
		PAINFUL ABSCESS AT LID MARGIN	NONTENDER LESION UNDER EYELID

GLOBE RUPTURE

- The outer membranes of the eye is disrupted by blunt or **penetrating trauma. Ophtho EMERGENCY!**

CLINICAL MANIFESTATIONS: diplopia, ocular pain (may be painless).

PHYSICAL EXAMINATION
1. Misshapened eye with prolapse of ocular tissue from the sclera or corneal opening.
2. Visual acuity: markedly reduced (may be light perception only).
3. Orbits: **enophthalmos*** (recession of the globe within the orbit) but may have exophthalmos. Foreign bodies may be present. **Severe conjunctival hemorrhage (360° bulbar).**
4. Corneal/Sclera: prolapse of the iris through the cornea, ⊕**Seidel's test*** = parting of fluorescein dye by a clear stream of aqueous humor from the anterior chamber. Obscured red-reflex, **teardrop or irregularly-shaped pupil, hyphema** (blood in anterior eye chamber).

MANAGEMENT
1. **Rigid eye shield*** (protects eye from applied pressure, IMPALED OBJECT SHOULD BE LEFT UNDISTURBED).* **Immediate ophtho consult.** IV Antibiotics. Avoid topical eye solutions.
2. **Hyphema** (blood in anterior chamber): **place at 45°** (keeps RBCs from staining the cornea).

ORBITAL FLOOR "BLOWOUT" FRACTURES

- Fractures to the orbital floor as a result of trauma. May lead to trapping of eye structures.

CLINICAL MANIFESTATIONS:
1. **decreased visual acuity** (trapped orbital tissue).

2. **DIPLOPIA ESPECIALLY WITH UPWARD GAZE*** (if there is **INFERIOR RECTUS MUSCLE** entrapment).*

3. **Orbital emphysema.*** Eyelid swelling after blowing nose – air from the maxillary sinus.

4. Epistaxis. Dyesthesias, hyperalgesia or **anesthesia to the anteromedial cheek** (due to stretching of the **infraorbital nerve**).

DIAGNOSTIC: CT scan test of choice. May show a "teardrop" sign.

MANAGEMENT
1. **Initial: nasal decongestants** (decreases pain), **avoid blowing nose,** corticosteroids (to reduce edema), **antibiotics** (ex. Ampicillin/Sulbactam or Clindamycin).
2. Surgical repair: severe cases, patients with enophthalmos or for persistent diplopia.

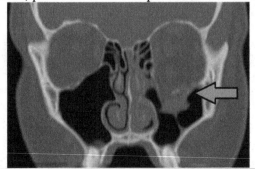

MACULAR DEGENERATION

Risk Factors: *age >50y*, Caucasians, females, smokers.

- **_MC cause of permanent legal blindness & visual loss in the elderly_*** (≥75y).
- The macula is responsible for **_central vision as well as detail & color vision._**

- 2 types:
  ### 1. DRY (ATROPHIC):
    - gradual breakdown of the macula ⇨ gradual blurring of central vision.

    - _DRUSEN_* = **_small, round, yellow-white spots on the outer retina (scattered, diffuse)._**
      Drusen = accumulation of waste products from the retinal pigment epithelium.

  2. **WET (NEOVASCULAR OR EXUDATIVE):** *new, abnormal vessels* grow under the central retina, which leak & bleed ⇨ retinal scarring. Rarer than dry (but progresses more rapidly).

CLINICAL MANIFESTATIONS
  1. **bilateral blurred or loss of CENTRAL VISION** **(including detailed & colored vision).***

  2. *Scotomas* (blind spots, shadows), **metamorphopsia** (straight lines appear bent), *micropsia* (object seen by the affected eye looks smaller than in the unaffected eye).

DIAGNOSIS OF WET
  Fluorescein angiography.

MANAGEMENT
  1. **Dry:** Amsler grid at home to monitor stability. *Zinc, Vitamin A, C & E may slow progression.*

  2. **Wet:**
    - **_Intravitreal anti-angiogenics ex. Bevacizumab_** – inhibits vascular endothelial growth factor (VEGF) ⇨ reduces neovascularization.

    - Laser photocoagulation.

    - Optical Tomography done to monitor treatment response.

MACULAR DEGENERATION

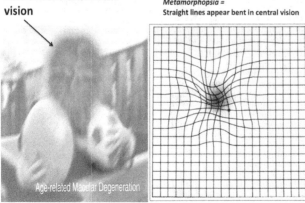

Loss of central & detail vision

AMSLER GRID
Metamorphopsia =
Straight lines appear bent in central vision

Age-related Macular Degeneration

MACULAR DEGENERATION

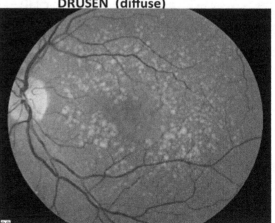

DRUSEN (diffuse)

DIABETIC RETINOPATHY

- **_MC cause of new, permanent vision loss/blindness in 25-74y*_** (MC due to maculopathy).
- **Diabetic Retinopathy:** retinal blood vessel damage ⇨ retinal ischemia, edema. Glycosylation (excess sugar attaches to the collagen of the blood vessels) ⇨ capillary wall breakdown.

1. **NONPROLIFERATIVE (BACKGROUND):** _microaneurysms_ ⇨ _blot & dot hemorrhages, flame-shaped hemorrhages, cotton wool spots, hard exudates,_ retinal vein beading (tortuous/dilated veins), closure of retinal capillaries. **_Not associated with vision loss._**
   - **Cotton Wool Spots:** (soft exudates) = fluffy gray-white spots – nerve layer microinfarctions.
   - **Hard Exudates:** yellow spots with sharp margins often **_circinate_** (due to lipid or lipoprotein deposits from leaky blood vessels). Hard exudates are seen in hypertensive & DM retinopathy.
   - **Blot & dot hemorrhages:** (bleeding into deep retinal layer); **Flame:** nerve fiber layer hemorrhage.
   MANAGEMENT: panlaser treatment. Strict glucose control.

2. **PROLIFERATIVE:** _NEOVASCULARIZATION:* new, abnormal blood vessel growth, vitreous hemorrhage._
   Mgmt: VEGF inhibitors (ex. Bevacizumab), laser photocoagulation treatment, tight glucose control.

3. **MACULOPATHY:** _macular edema or exudates, blurred vision, central vision loss._ Can occur @ any stage.
   Maculopathy is due to macular microaneurysm leakage, causing macular edema & damage. **Mgmt:** Laser.

HYPERTENSIVE RETINOPATHY

- **Hypertensive Retinopathy:** damage to retinal blood vessels from longstanding high blood pressure.
- 4 Grades (I through IV with increasing severity):

I	**Arterial narrowing**: abnormal light reflexes on dilated tortuous arteriole shows up as colors **_Copper wiring*_** = moderate, **_Silver-wiring_** = severe
II	**AV nicking** – venous compression at the arterial-venous junction by ↑arterial pressure.
III	_flame shaped hemorrhages, cotton wool spots_ (soft exudates).
IV	PAPILLEDEMA (MALIGNANT HTN).*

MANAGEMENT: blood pressure control.

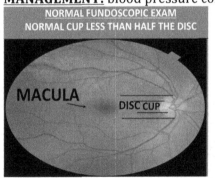

NORMAL FUNDOSCOPIC EXAM
NORMAL CUP LESS THAN HALF THE DISC
MACULA   DISC CUP

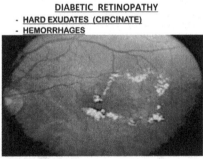

DIABETIC RETINOPATHY
- HARD EXUDATES (CIRCINATE)
- HEMORRHAGES

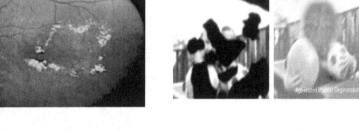

DIABETIC RETINOPATHY

DIABETIC RETINOPATHY   vs.   MACULAR DEGENERATION
- Vitreal Hemorrhages   - Central vision loss

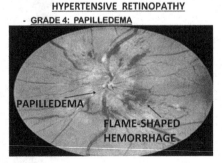

HYPERTENSIVE RETINOPATHY
- GRADE 4: PAPILLEDEMA
PAPILLEDEMA
FLAME-SHAPED HEMORRHAGE

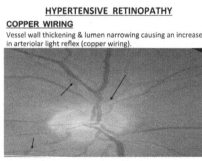

HYPERTENSIVE RETINOPATHY
COPPER WIRING
Vessel wall thickening & lumen narrowing causing an increase in arteriolar light reflex (copper wiring).

RETINAL DETACHMENT

3 Main types:

❶ ***Rhegmatogenous MC type:*** *retinal tear* ⇨ *retinal inner sensory layer detaches from choroid plexus.* MC predisposing factors are myopia (nearsightedness) & cataracts.

❷ Traction = adhesions separate the retina from its base (proliferative DM retinopathy, sickle cell, trauma).

❸ Exudative (serous) = fluid accumulates beneath the retina ⇨ detachment (ex. HTN, CRVO, papilledema).

CLINICAL MANIFESTATIONS
1. ***photopsia (flashing lights)**** with detachment ⇨ ***floaters**** ⇨ *progressive **unilateral** vision loss:* SHADOW *"CURTAIN COMING DOWN" IN PERIPHERY INITIALLY* ⇨ ***loss of central visual field.****
2. *No pain/redness.*

DIAGNOSIS
Funduscopy:
1. retinal tear (detached tissue "flapping" in the vitreous humor).
2. ⊕ ***Shafer's sign**** = clumping of brown-colored pigment cells in the anterior vitreous humor resembling "tobacco dust" (another name for this sign).

MANAGEMENT
1. ***Ophtho emergency:*** keep patient supine while awaiting consult. ***Don't use miotic drops.***
2. Laser, cryotherapy, ocular surgery.

Differential dx: *amaurosis fugax: temporary "curtain" that "lifts up" usually within 1 hour.*

OCULAR FOREIGN BODY & CORNEAL ABRASION

CLINICAL MANIFESTATIONS: foreign body sensation, tearing, red & painful eye.

DIAGNOSIS
1. pain relieved with instillation of ophthalmic analgesic drops.

2. **Fluorescein staining:** ***corneal abrasion = "Ice rink"/linear abrasions*** seen especially if the foreign body is underneath the eyelid (so evert the eyelid to look for it).

MANAGEMENT: *check visual acuity 1st*
1. Foreign body removal: remove with sterile irrigation or moistened sterile cotton swab (needle via slit lamp if experienced). Avoid sending patients home c̄ topical anesthetics!

2. Corneal abrasions: patching not indicated for small abrasions. May patch the eye in some patients with large abrasions (>5 mm) but do not patch longer than 24 hours.
   - ***Do not patch the eye in contact lens wearers/Pseudomonas.**** Place them on fluoroquinolone eye drops (ex. ***Ciprofloxacin***) with close follow ophtho follow up.

3. ***Antibiotic drops:*** for both corneal abrasions & foreign bodies. 24 hour ophtho follow up.
   - topical Erythromycin, Polymyxin/Trimethoprim, Sulfacetamide, Ciprofloxacin.

4. Rust ring: remove rust ring at 24 hours usually with rotating burr by an ophthalmologist.

VIRAL CONJUNCTIVITIS

• *MC Adenovirus. Swimming pool MC source.* * *MC in children.* Highly contagious.

CLINICAL MANIFESTATIONS
Foreign body sensation, erythema & itching. Normal vision. May have accompanying viral symptoms.

PHYSICAL EXAM
PREAURICULAR LYMPHADENOPATHY, * *copious watery discharge*, scanty *mucoid discharge*. Often bilateral. May have *PUNCTATE STAINING* on slit lamp examination.

MANAGEMENT
Supportive (cool compresses, artificial tears). ± antihistamines for itching/redness (ex. Olopatadine).

ALLERGIC CONJUNCTIVITIS

CLINICAL MANIFESTATIONS
Conjunctival erythema (red eyes). May have other allergic symptoms (ex. rhinorrhea etc).

PHYSICAL EXAM
"COBBLESTONE MUCOSA" * appearance to the inner/upper eyelid, itching, tearing, redness, stringy discharge. Usually bilateral. ± *Chemosis* (conjunctival swelling).

MANAGEMENT
1. *Topical Antihistamines (H₁ blockers)*:* *Olopatadine* (Patanol - antihistamine/mast cell stabilizer), *Pheniramine/Naphazoline* (*Naphcon A* - antihistamine/decongestant), Emedastine.
2. Topical NSAID: Ketorolac.
3. Topical corticosteroids. Side effect of long term steroid use ⇨ glaucoma, cataracts, HSV keratitis.

BACTERIAL CONJUNCTIVITIS

• *MC S. aureus, Strep pneumoniae,* H. influenzae. Transmitted by direct contact & autoinoculation.

CLINICAL MANIFESTATIONS
PURULENT DISCHARGE, LID CRUSTING, * usually *no visual changes* (mild pain). *Absence of ciliary injection.* *Fluorescein staining needed to detect corneal abrasions or keratitis.*

MANAGEMENT
1. **Topical antibiotics:**
   - *Erythromycin, Fluoroquinolones (ex. Moxifloxacin), Sulfonamides, Aminoglycosides.*
   - *If contact lens wearer, cover Pseudomonas* (Fluoroquinolone or Aminoglycoside).*

2. If Chlamydia or Gonorrhea, ± admit for IV & topical Abx (ophtho emergency). *No Steroids.* Gonoccccal conjunctivitis: IV Ceftriaxone (± add topical); Chlamydia (Azithromycin).

OPHTHALMIA NEONATORIUM (NEONATAL CONJUNCTIVITIS)

Day 1	Silver nitrate (chemical cause).
Day 2-5	*Gonococcal* most likely cause.
Day 5-7	*Chlamydia* most likely cause.
Day 7-11	*HSV* is the likely cause.

Recommended standard prophylaxis given immediately after birth includes: erythromycin ointment, topical Tetracycline, silver nitrate, or povidone-iodine.

May cause corneal ulceration, opacification & blindness if it develops and left untreated.

CHEMICAL BURNS

Ophtho Emergency! Every minute counts!!! Irrigation must be started ASAP!
- **Alkali Burns:** ***worse than acids (liquefactive necrosis),*** denatures proteins & collagen, causes thrombosis of vessels. Ex: fertilizers, household cleaners, drain cleaners.

- **Acid Burns:** coagulative necrosis (H⁺ precipitates protein barrier). Ex: cleaners, batteries.

MANAGEMENT:
1. ***Immediate irrigation**** *(greatest impact on prognosis).* ***Lactated Ringers**** ***or Normal Saline*** (LR ideal because at a pH of 6 – 7.5, it is closer to the pH of the tears (7.1) than NS (pH 4.5 – 7.0) & is less irritating. Irrigate x30 minutes or @ least 2 liters of fluid.

2. ***Check pH & visual acuity after irrigation.*** Irrigate until pH of the eye is 7.0 – 7.3.

3. **Antibiotics** ***ex. Moxifloxacin*** & Cycloplegic agent (ex 0.25% Atropine drops), ***ophtho f/u.***

ORBITAL (SEPTAL) CELLULITIS

- ***Usually 2ry to sinus infections**** *(Ethmoid 90%).* *S. aureus, S. pneumo, GABHS, H. flu.*
- May be caused by dental/facial infections or bacteremia. MC occurs in children (especially 7-12y).

CLINICAL MANIFESTATIONS
 DECREASED VISION, PAIN WITH OCULAR MOVEMENT,* ***proptosis*** (bulging eye), eyelid erythema & edema.

DIAGNOSIS:
 High resolution CT scan: *infection of the fat & ocular muscles.* MRI.

MANAGEMENT: IV antibiotics ex. Vancomycin, Clindamycin, Cefotaxime, Ampicillin/sulbactam. Amoxicillin if preseptal.

DIFFERENTIAL DIAGNOSIS: PRESEPTAL CELLULITIS: infection of the eyelid & periocular tissue. May have ocular pain & swelling but ***NO visual changes & NO pain with ocular movement.****

STRABISMUS

Misalignment of the eyes. Stable ocular alignment not present until age 2-3 months.
 Esotropia: convergent strabismus - deviated inward ("crossed eyed").
 Exotropia: divergent strabismus (deviated outward).

CLINICAL MANIFESTATIONS
 1. Diplopia, scotomas or amblyopia.

DIAGNOSIS: *Hirschberg corneal light reflex testing (often used as screening test).* Cover-uncover test to determine the angle of strabismus, cover test, convergence testing.

MANAGEMENT
 1. ***Patch therapy:*** normal eye is covered to stimulate & strengthen the affected eye. Eyeglasses.
 2. ***Corrective surgery*** if severe or unresponsive to conservative therapy.
  If not treated before 2 years of age, amblyopia may occur = decreased visual acuity not correctable by refractive means.

KERATITIS (CORNEAL ULCER/INFLAMMATION)

- **Bacterial MC cause**, inflammation. Pseudomonas or acanthamoeba (contact lens wearers).*
- Fungal. Exposure keratitis (ex. Bell palsy). *May rapidly progress & be sight-threatening.*

CLINICAL MANIFESTATIONS
pain, photophobia, reduced vision, tearing, conjunctival erythema.

PHYSICAL EXAM: conjunctival injection/erythema, CILIARY INJECTION (LIMBIC FLUSH),* *corneal ulceration/defect on slit lamp exam,* purulent or watery discharge.
1. **Bacterial Keratitis:** *hazy cornea,* ulcer, stromal abscess, ± hypopyon.
   Mgmt: fluoroquinolone drops (ex. *Moxifloxacin, Gatifloxacin*). **DO NOT PATCH EYE!***

2. **HSV Keratitis:** *dendritic lesions* = branching seen with fluorescein staining.*
   Mgmt: topical antivirals: *Trifluridine*, Vidarabine, Ganciclovir ointment. PO acyclovir.

UVEITIS (IRITIS)

- **Anterior:** inflammation of iris (iritis) or ciliary body (cyclitis).
- **Posterior:** choroid inflammation.

ETIOLOGIES
- **Systemic inflammatory diseases:** may be associated with HLA-B27 spondyloarthropathies, sarcoid, Behçet's disease. **Infectious:** CMV, toxoplasmosis, syphilis, TB; Trauma.
- If recurrent, suspect some underlying inflammatory disease.

CLINICAL MANIFESTATIONS
Anterior: *unilateral ocular pain/redness/photophobia;* excessive tearing (no discharge).
   Anterior usually occurs after blunt trauma.
Posterior: *blurred/decreased vision,* floaters, absent sx of anterior involvement, *no pain.*

PHYSICAL EXAM
1. CILIARY INJECTION (LIMBIC FLUSH),* **consensual photophobia,** ± visual changes.
2. **inflammatory CELLS & FLARE** within the aqueous humor (cells = WBCs. Flare = proteins).

MANAGEMENT
1. **Anterior:** **topical corticosteroids.** Scopolamine. Topical cycloplegics (ex. Cyclopentolate or *Homatropine)* used to relieve the pain from spasms of the muscles controlling the pupil.
2. **Posterior:** **systemic corticosteroids.**

CATARACT

- **Lens opacification (thickening).** Usually bilateral.

- **RISK FACTORS:** **aging** (MC >60y). **cigarette smoking,* corticosteroids,** Diabetes Mellitus, UV light, malnutrition, trauma. *Congenital: ToRCH syndrome (Toxoplasmosis, Rubella, CMV HSV).*

CLINICAL MANIFESTATIONS: blurred/loss of vision over months – years.

PHYSICAL EXAMINATION: absent red reflex, opaque lens. **MANAGEMENT:** surgical.

Differential Dx: RETINOBLASTOMA: *absent red reflex (fundus reflection) + "white pupil".**

PAPILLEDEMA

- *OPTIC NERVE (DISC) SWELLING 2ry to ↑INTRACRANIAL PRESSURE* (classically bilateral).*

ETIOLOGIES
❶*idiopathic intracranial HTN (pseudotumor cerebri),* ❷*space-occupying lesion* (ex. cerebral tumor, abscess) ❸↑CSF production ❹cerebral edema, severe HTN (malignant, grade IV).

CLINICAL MANIFESTATIONS
headache, nausea/vomiting, vision is usually well preserved but may have changes.

DIAGNOSIS:
1. Funduscopy: swollen optic disc with blurred margins.
2. MRI or CT scan of the head 1st to rule out mass effect ⇨ LP (↑ CSF pressure).

MANAGEMENT: *diuretics ex. Acetazolamide* (↓'es production of aqueous humor & CSF).

	PAPILLEDEMA	PAPILLITIS	RETROBULBAR NEURITIS	GLAUCOMA
DEFINITION	Edema of the optic nerve head due to ↑*CSF pressure*	Edema of optic nerve head <u>in</u> the orbit (eye) - *Optic Neuritis*	Edema of optic nerve <u>behind</u> the eye - *Optic Neuritis*	Edema of the optic nerve from ↑*intraocular pressure*
LATERALITY	Bilateral	Unilateral	Unilateral	Acute: Unilateral Chronic: Bilateral
VISUAL DEFICIT	Enlarged blind spot	Range from central scotoma to complete loss of vision	Range from central scotoma - complete loss of vision	Halos around light to blindness
FUNDUSCOPIC	Blurred disc-cup	Blurred disc-cup	Normal	Blurred disc-cup
MARCUS GUNN	Negative	**POSITIVE**	**POSITIVE**	Negative
MANAGEMENT	Reduce ICP	Corticosteroids	Corticosteroids	Reduce IOP

OPTIC NEURITIS (OPTIC NERVE/CN II INFLAMMATION)

- *Acute inflammatory demyelination of the optic nerve.* MC young patients 20-40y.

ETIOLOGIES
*Multiple Sclerosis MC,** Medications: *Ethambutol, Chloramphenicol,* autoimmune.

CLINICAL MANIFESTATIONS
1. *loss of color vision, visual field defects (ex. central scotoma/blind spot), loss of vision* over a few days (usually *unilateral).*

2. Associated with *OCULAR PAIN THAT IS WORSE WITH EYE MOVEMENT.**

PHYSICAL EXAM:
1. *MARCUS-GUNN PUPIL:** relative *afferent pupillary defect* – during swinging-flashlight test *from the unaffected eye into the affected eye, the pupils appear to dilate* (delayed response of affected optic nerve).

2. **Funduscopy:** 2/3 *normal disc/cup (retrobulbar neuritis)* or
   1/3 ⊕*optic disc swelling/blurring (papillitis).* MRI also used in some cases.

MANAGEMENT: IV Methylprednisolone followed by oral corticosteroids. Vision usually returns with tx.

MARCUS GUNN PUPIL (RELATIVE AFFERENT PUPILLARY DEFECT)

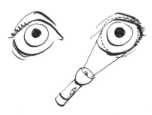
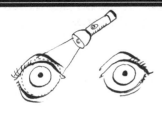

1. ***Optic neuritis MC cause.****
2. Severe retinal disease (ex. CRVO, CRAO, significant retinal detachment).

• During swinging-flashlight test into the unaffected eye, both pupils constrict.

• **MARCUS GUNN:** during swinging-flashlight test ***from the unaffected eye into the affected eye, the pupils appear to dilate*** (due to less than normal constriction).

• <u>R</u>elative <u>A</u>fferent <u>P</u>upillary <u>D</u>efect mnemonic = when you shine a
<u>R</u>ay in the <u>A</u>ffected <u>P</u>upil it <u>D</u>ilates

ARGYLL-ROBERTSON PUPIL

• Near-light dissociation. Pupil ***constricts on accommodation but does not react to bright light.***

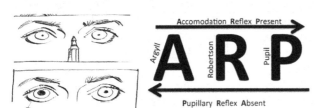

CAUSES OF ARGYLL ROBERTSON PUPIL

• ***Neurosyphilis MC****

• Midbrain lesions
   (ex. Parinaud syndrome)

• Diabetic neuropathy

VISUAL PATHWAY DEFECTS

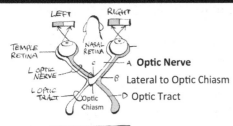

- A **Optic Nerve**
- B Lateral to Optic Chiasm
- D Optic Tract

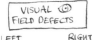

A. <u>TOTAL BLINDNESS OF IPSILATERAL EYE</u>
   If lesion is on **Optic Nerve or Retina***

B. <u>IPSILATERAL NASAL HEMIANOPSIA</u>
   If lesion is **lateral** to the optic chiasm.

C. <u>BITEMPORAL HETERONYMOUS HEMIANOPSIA</u>
   If ***midline optic chiasm lesion
   (ex. pituitary adenoma)****

D. <u>CONTRALATERAL HOMONYMOUS HEMIANOPSIA</u>
   If lesion at **optic tract** or in **occipital lobe stroke**

ACUTE NARROW ANGLE-CLOSURE GLAUCOMA

- ↑intraocular pressure (IOP) ⇨ *optic nerve damage* ⇨ ↓visual acuity. ***Ophtho emergency!***

- **ACUTE ANGLE CLOSURE GLAUCOMA:** ***decreased drainage of aqueous humor*** via trabecular meshwork & canal of Schlemm in *patients with preexisting narrow angle or large lens* – elderly, hyperopes (far-sighted) & Asians. Leading cause of preventable blindness in US.

PRECIPITATING FACTORS
- *MYDRIASIS* (pupillary dilation further closes the angle)
   ex. dim lights, sympathomimetics & anticholinergics.*

CLINICAL MANIFESTATIONS
1. ***severe, sudden*** onset of *UNILATERAL OCULAR PAIN.** *± Nausea/vomiting, headache.*
2. **Vision changes:** intermittent blurring, ***halos around lights,** PERIPHERAL VISION LOSS (TUNNEL).**

PHYSICAL EXAM
Conjunctival erythema, "steamy" cornea* = corneal epithelial edema or cloudiness, shallow chamber, *MID-DILATED, FIXED, NONREACTIVE PUPIL,* **eye feels hard to palpation** (↑IOP).

DIAGNOSIS
1. ↑***Intraocular pressure** by tonometry* (>21mm Hg). ***"Cupping" of optic nerve*** on Funduscopy.

MANAGEMENT:
   2 steps: ❶ *lower IOP* (acetazolamide, ßB, mannitol) ⇨ ❷ *open the angle* (cholinergics).
1. ***Acetazolamide** 1ˢᵗ line -* ↓'es intraocular pressure by ↓***'ing aqueous humor production.***

2. ***Topical beta blocker: (ex. Timolol) reduces IOP pressure without affecting visual acuity.****

3. ***Miotics/cholinergics: (ex. Pilocarpine, Carbachol)*** acetylcholine-induced papillary constriction, reduces intraocular pressure by increasing aqueous humor drainage. Reverses the angle closure (usually started once IOP is being reduced).
   S/E: visual changes, lens opacity.

4. Alpha-2 agonists: (Apraclonidine, Brimonidine) suppress aqueous humor production & ↑outflow.

5. ***Peripheral iridotomy definitive treatment.****   ***Avoid anticholinergics, sympathomimetics.****

ACUTE ANGLE CLOSURE GLAUCOMA
- MID DILATED PUPIL

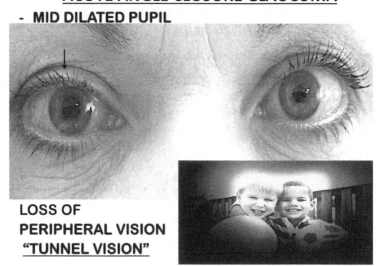

LOSS OF
PERIPHERAL VISION
"TUNNEL VISION"

CHRONIC (OPEN ANGLE) GLAUCOMA

Slow, progressive BILATERAL peripheral vision loss (compared to unilateral vision in acute glaucoma).
- 2nd MC cause of blindness in the world (after cataracts).

RISK FACTORS: African-Americans, age >40y, family history, Diabetes Mellitus (DM).
➢ Open angle: normal anterior chamber. The ↑IOP in chronic open angle glaucoma is due to reduced aqueous drainage through the trabeculum, which eventually damages the optic nerve.

CLINICAL MANIFESTATIONS
1. _GRADUAL BILATERAL PAINLESS peripheral vision loss (tunnel vision)*_ ⇨ central loss. Usually **asymptomatic** until late in the disease course & vision loss is usually the presenting symptom.

2. Physical exam: **cupping of optic discs** (↑cup to disc ratio), notching of the disc rim.

MANAGEMENT
1. _Prostaglandin analogs 1st line_ (ex _Latanoprost_ – greater reduction of IOP), Timolol (ß-blocker), Brimonidine (α -2 agonists), Acetazolamide (carbonic anhydrase inhibitor - reduction of IOP).
2. Laser therapy (Trabeculoplasty) if medical therapy fails. Surgical (Trabeculostomy) last line tx.

AMAUROSIS FUGAX

- Temporary monocular vision loss (lasting minutes) with complete recovery. Due to retinal emboli or ischemia. Can be seen with TIA, Giant cell arteritis, CRAO, SLE & other vasculitic disorders.
- **Vision loss** described as a **temporary "curtain" that resolves ("lifts up")** usually **within 1 hour**.

CENTRAL RETINAL ARTERY OCCLUSION (CRAO)

Retinal artery thrombus or embolus. **MC 50-80y** with _ATHEROSCLEROTIC DISEASE.*_ **Ophtho Emergency!**

MANIFESTATIONS
  ACUTE, SUDDEN MONOCULAR VISION LOSS,* often **preceded by** _AMAUROSIS FUGAX.*_

DIAGNOSIS:
Funduscopy:
  1. _PALE RETINA WITH CHERRY-RED MACULA (red spot)*_ due to obstruction of retinal blood flow.
  2. _"BOX CAR" appearance*_ of the retinal vessels (segmentation). ± emboli (20%). No hemorrhage.

MANAGEMENT: no treatment has been shown truly effective but should be attempted.
  1. Decrease IOP: to prevent anterior chamber involvement ex. Acetazolamide, chamber paracentesis.
  2. Revascularization including placing the patient supine + orbital massage orbit to dislodge clot.

CENTRAL RETINAL VEIN OCCLUSION (CRVO)

- **_Central retinal vein thrombus_** ⇨ fluid backup in retina ⇨ _ACUTE, SUDDEN MONOCULAR VISION LOSS.*_
  Risk factors: HTN, DM, glaucoma, hypercoagulable states.

DIAGNOSIS
  Funduscopy: **extensive retinal hemorrhages** (_"BLOOD & THUNDER" APPEARANCE_),* retinal vein dilation, macular edema, optic disc swelling. ± Relative afferent pupillary defect.

MANAGEMENT: no known effective tx. ± antiinflammatories, steroids, laser photocoagulation. May resolve spontaneously or progress to permanent vision loss.

EAR DISORDERS

OTITIS EXTERNA

- *Aka "Swimmer's ear" – excess H_2O* or *local trauma* changes the normal acidic pH of the ear, causing bacterial overgrowth.
- *Pseudomonas MC,* * Proteus, S. aureus, S. epidermis, GABHS, anaerobes (Peptostreptococcus); Aspergillus.

CLINICAL MANIFESTATIONS
1. 1-2 days of *ear pain, pruritus* in the ear canal (may have recent activity of swimming).
2. *Auricular discharge*, pressure/fullness. Hearing usually preserved.

PHYSICAL EXAM
PAIN ON TRACTION OF THE EAR CANAL/TRAGUS,* external auditory canal erythema/edema/debris.

MANAGEMENT
Protect ear against moisture (drying agents include isopropyl alcohol & acetic acid). Topical Abx:
1. *Ciprofloxacin/dexamethasone (Ofloxacin safe if there is an associated TM perforation).*

2. Aminoglycoside combination: Neomycin/Polytrim-B/Hydrocortisone otic (*not used if TM perforation is suspected* * - aminoglycosides are ototoxic). Amphotericin B if fungal.

MALIGNANT OTITIS EXTERNA:
- *Osteomyelitis at skull base 2ry to Pseudomonas* (MC seen in DM & immunocompromised).**
MANAGEMENT:
IV antispseudomonal Abx: ex. Ceftazidime or Piperacillin + Fluoroquinolones or Aminoglycoside.

MASTOIDITIS

- Inflammation of the mastoid air cells of the temporal bone.

ETIOLOGIES
- *Usually a complication of prolonged or inadequately treated otitis media.* * All patients with acute otitis media have some degree of mastoiditis because the mastoid and middle ear are connected.

CLINICAL MANIFESTATIONS
1. *deep ear pain* (usually worse at night), fever.
2. *mastoid tenderness*, may develop cutaneous abscess (fluctuance).
3. Complications: hearing loss, labyrinthitis, vertigo, CN VII paralysis, brain abscess.

DIAGNOSIS
CT Scan 1st line diagnostic test.

MANAGEMENT
1. *IV antibiotics + middle ear/mastoid drainage hallmark of treatment.* *
   - Ear/Mastoid drainage: *myringotomy* with or without *tympanostomy tube placement.* Tympanocentesis can be performed to obtain a middle ear culture.
   - IV antibiotics: same antibiotics used in acute otitis media (see page 248).

2. *Refractory or complicated mastoiditis $\Rightarrow$ mastoidectomy.* *

ACUTE OTITIS MEDIA (AOM)

- Infection of middle ear, temporal bone & mastoid air cells. **_MC preceded by viral URI._*
- **AOM:** rapid onset + signs/sx of inflammation. <u>OM c̄ effusion</u>: asymptomatic/no inflammation.

- **_4 MC organisms: S. pneumo (MC),* H. influenza, Moraxella catarrhalis, Strep pyogenes_** (same organisms seen in Acute sinusitis). Peak age 6-18 months.

PATHOPHYSIOLOGY
Upper respiratory infection causes Eustachian tube edema ⇨ negative pressure ⇨ transudation of fluid & mucus in the middle ear ⇨ 2ry colonization by bacteria & flora.

RISK FACTORS: **_Eustachian tube (ET) dysfunction, young_** (ET is narrower, shorter & more horizontal), day care, pacifier/bottle use, parental smoking, not being breastfed.

CLINICAL MANIFESTATIONS
1. fever, **_otalgia_** (ear pain), **_ear tugging in infants_**, conductive hearing loss, stuffiness.
2. **_If TM perforation_** ⇨ **_rapid relief of pain + otorrhea_** (usually heals in 1-2 days).

PHYSICAL EXAM
1. **_bulging, erythematous <u>tympanic membrane (TM) with effusion.</u>_** Loss of landmarks.
   <u>DECREASED TYMPANIC MEMBRANE MOBILITY*</u> on pneumatic otoscopy.

2. <u>If bullae on TM</u> ⇨ suspect *Mycoplasma pneumoniae.**

MANAGEMENT:
1. **_Antibiotics: AMOXICILLIN TREATMENT OF CHOICE*_** (10-14 days). **_Cefixime in children._**
   - *2nd line:* Amoxicillin/clavulanic acid (Augmentin) or Cefaclor.
   - *PCN allergic* ⇨ **_Erythromycin-Sulfisoxazole_**, Azithromycin, Trimethoprim/Sulfamethoxazole.

2. <u>Severe/Recurrent cases:</u> Myringotomy (surgical drainage).
      Tympanostomy if recurrent or persistent.
3. <u>Otitis Media with effusion:</u> *observation in most cases.*
- In children with recurrent otitis media ⇨ iron deficiency anemia workup & CT scan.

CHRONIC OTITIS MEDIA

ETIOLOGIES
Complication of acute otitis media, trauma or due to cholesteatoma.
- Pseudomonas, S. aureus 2 MC. Gram negative rods (ex. Proteus), anaerobes, Mycoplasma.

CLINICAL MANIFESTATIONS
1. **_<u>Perforated TM + persistent or recurrent purulent otorrhea</u>*_** ± pain.
2. May have varying degrees of **_conductive hearing loss._** ± cholesteatoma (1ry of 2ry).

MANAGEMENT
1. **Topical antibiotics 1st line treatment:** ex. *Oflaxacin or Ciprofloxacin.*
   Avoid water/moisture/topical aminoglycosides in the ear whenever there is a TM rupture.*
2. Surgical: tympanic membrane repair/reconstruction. Mastoidectomy in severe cases.

EUSTACHIAN TUBE DYSFUNCTION

- Eustachian tube (ET) swelling inhibits ET's autoinsufflation ability ⇨ negative pressure.
- **Often follows viral URI or allergic rhinitis.**

CLINICAL MANIFESTATIONS

Ear fullness, popping of ears, underwater feeling, intermittent sharp ear pain, disequilibrium, fluctuating conductive hearing loss, tinnitus.

DIAGNOSIS: Otoscopic findings usually normal. ± fluid behind TM if acute serous otitis media.

MANAGEMENT

1. **Decongestants:** (↓'es ET edema) **pseudoephedrine, phenylephrine, oxymetazoline nasal spray.**
2. **Autoinsufflation** (swallowing, yawning, blowing against a slightly-pinched nostril).
3. **Intranasal corticosteroids.**

COMPLICATIONS

Patients may develop **Acute serous otitis media** (non-infected fluid in the middle ear), which may become colonized, by bacteria **infectious otitis media** if the blockage is prolonged.

BAROTRAUMA

- **Rapid pressure change ⇨ inability of ET to equalize pressure ⇨ sx similar to ET dysfunction.**
  Ex: taking a flight on an airplane (descent), scuba divers or patients on mechanical ventilation.

CLINICAL MANIFESTATIONS

1. Auricular pain & fullness/hearing loss that persists after the etiologic event.
2. May have bloody discharge if traumatic.
3. Tympanic membrane: ± rupture or petechiae.

MANAGEMENT

1. **Autoinsufflation** (swallowing, yawning). **Decongestants or antihistamines** (↓'es ET edema).

AUDITORY EXAMINATION FINDINGS   AC = air conduction. BC = bone conduction.

Assessed with a tuning fork	WEBER: place on top head	RINNE: place on mastoid by ear
NORMAL	No lateralization	Normal (Positive) AC > BC
SENSORINEURAL LOSS (INNER EAR):	Lateralizes to NORMAL ear*	Normal: AC > BC. Difficulty hearing their own voice & deciphering words.
CONDUCTIVE LOSS (EXT/MIDDLE):	Lateralizes to AFFECTED* ear	BC ≥ AC (Negative)

*sensoriNeural lateralizes to Normal ear + Normal Rinne (think of the **N** for sensori**N**eural).

ETIOLOGIES OF CONDUCTIVE HEARING LOSS:
External or middle ear disorders: defect in sound conduction (ex. obstruction from a foreign body or cerumen impaction), damage to ossicles (otosclerosis, cholesteatoma), mastoiditis, otitis media.
CERUMEN IMPACTION MC CAUSE OF CONDUCTIVE HEARING LOSS.*

ETIOLOGIES OF SENSORINEURAL HEARING LOSS:
Inner ear disorders: ex presbyacusis, chronic loud noise exposure, CNS lesions (ex acoustic neuroma), Labyrinthitis, Meniere syndrome. **PRESBYACUSIS MC CAUSE OF SENSORINEURAL HEARING LOSS.***

CERUMEN IMPACTION

- External auditory canal (EAC) wax impaction. May lead to *conductive hearing loss*, ear fullness.
MANAGEMENT:
1. Cerumen softening: *Hydrogen Peroxide* 3%, *Carbamide peroxide* (Debrox).
2. Aural toilet: irrigation, curette removal of cerumen, suction. Irrigation (if no evidence of TM perforation & water must be at body temperature to prevent vertigo).

TYMPANIC MEMBRANE PERFORATION

- MC occurs due to penetrating or noise trauma (MC occurs at the pars tensa), otitis media.
CLINICAL MANIFESTATIONS
1. Acute ear pain, hearing loss, ± bloody otorrhea. ± Tinnitus & vertigo.

DIAGNOSIS
1. Otoscopic examination: perforated TM. May lead to cholesteatoma development.
2. ± conductive hearing loss (Weber: lateralization to affected ear, Rinne: BC ≥ AC/negative).

MANAGEMENT
1. Most perforated TMs heal spontaneously. Follow up to ensure resolution. ± Surgical repair.
2. *Avoid water/moisture/topical aminoglycosides in the ear whenever there is a TM rupture.*

CHOLESTEATOMA

- *Abnormal keratinized collection of desquamated squamous epithelium* ⇨ mastoid bony erosion.
- MC due to chronic ET dysfunction: chronic negative pressure inverts part of the tympanic membrane ⇨ *granulation tissue that erodes the ossicles over time* ⇨ *conductive hearing loss*.

CLINICAL MANIFESTATIONS
1. *painless otorrhea (brown/yellow discharge with strong odor).* ± develop vertigo/dizziness

DIAGNOSIS
1. **Otoscope: *granulation tissue (cellular debris).*** ± perforation of the tympanic membrane.
2. Peripheral vertigo, *conductive hearing loss* (Weber: lateralization to affected ear, Rinne: BC ≥ AC)

MANAGEMENT: surgical excision of the debris/cholesteatoma & reconstruction of the ossicles.

OTOSCLEROSIS

- Abnormal bony overgrowth of the stapes bone ⇨ *conductive hearing loss* (blocked conduction).

CLINICAL MANIFESTATIONS slowly progressive conductive hearing loss, tinnitus. Vertigo uncommon.
MANAGEMENT: *stapedectomy with prosthesis.* Hearing aid. Cochlear implantation if severe.

FOREIGN BODY IN THE EAR

- MC in children <6y.
CLINICAL MANIFESTATIONS:
Ear pain, drainage, conductive hearing loss. May be asymptomatic.
MANAGEMENT: foreign body removal & assess for tympanic membrane rupture or complications.

VERTIGO

• *False sense of motion* (or exaggerated sense of motion).   2 types:

	PERIPHERAL VERTIGO	CENTRAL VERTIGO
LOCATION OF PROBLEM	**Labyrinth or Vestibular nerve** (which is part of CN VIII/8).	**Brainstem or cerebellar**
ETIOLOGIES	1. BENIGN POSITIONAL VERTIGO (MC) *episodic vertigo, no hearing loss* 2. MENIERE: *episodic vertigo + hearing loss* 3. VESTIBULAR NEURITIS *continuous vertigo, no hearing loss* 4. LABYRINTHITIS: *continuous vertigo + hearing loss* 5. Cholesteatoma	Cerebellopontine tumors Migraine Cerebral vascular disease Multiple sclerosis Vestibular Neuroma
CLINICAL	• *HORIZONTAL nystagmus** (usually beats away from affected side). *Fatigable.** • *Sudden onset of tinnitus & hearing loss usually associated with peripheral compared to central causes.*	• *VERTICAL nystagmus.* Nonfatigable (continuous)** • *Gait problems more severe.* • *Gradual onset.* • *Positive CNS signs.*

MANAGEMENT OF NAUSEA/VOMITING IN PATIENTS WITH VERTIGO:

Nausea & vomiting are caused by sensory conflict mediated by the neurotransmitters *GABA, acetylcholine, histamine, dopamine & serotonin.* Antiemetics work primarily by these transmitters.

1. **ANTIHISTAMINES: *1st line.***   **MOA:** blocks emetic response. Most antihistamines have anticholinergic properties. Ex. ***Meclizine***, Cyclizine, Dimenhydrinate, Diphenhydramine (Benadryl).

2. **DOPAMINE BLOCKERS** (phenothiazines):
   Metoclopramide, Prochlorperazine (Compazine) IM/rectal; ***IV Promethazine*** (Phenergan).
   - **MOA:** *antagonizes dopamine D$_2$ receptors.**   Used to treat severe nausea/vomiting.
   - ***Often given with Benadryl to prevent dystonic reactions.**** *Dopamine inhibition may lead to Parkinsonism symptoms. Anticholinergic property of Benadryl prevents/tx dyskinesias.*

3. **ANTICHOLINERGICS:** *Scopolamine (good for motion sickness & recurrent vertigo).*
   S/E: *dry mouth, blurred vision, urinary retention, constipation.*

4. **BENZODIAZEPINES:** Lorazepam, Diazepam used in refractory patients (potentiates GABA).

BENIGN PAROXYSMAL POSITIONAL VERTIGO

• *Caused by displaced otoliths** (calcium carbonate particles).   *MC cause of vertigo.**

• Normally, otoliths are attached to the hair cells inside the saccule & utricule (attached to the 3 semicircular canals).   Head movements cause displaced otolith movement ⇨ vertigo.

CLINICAL MANIFESTATIONS
1. *Sudden, episodic peripheral vertigo provoked with changes of head positioning.** *Vertigo usually lasts 10-60 seconds.**

2. ⊕ *DIX-HALLPIKE TEST/NYLAN BARANY:** patient placed in supine position with head 30° lower than body. Head quickly turned 90° to one side ⇨ delayed *fatigable horizontal nystagmus*.
   If nystagmus is persistent or non-fatigable, assess for a central cause of vertigo.

MANAGEMENT
1. *EPLEY MANEUVER:** canalith repositioning mainstay of treatment.** Usually resolves with time as the otoliths naturally dissolve & the vertigo episodic/brief ⇨ *medications usually not needed*.

2. **Medications:** *antihistamines*, anticholinergics, benzodiazepines (ex. Lorazepam only short-term).

LABYRINTH: the bony & membranous part of the inner ear. It consists of 2 components:
- ❶ **Cochlea:** responsible for **_hearing_** (converts wave impulses from the middle ear into auditory nerve impulses.
- ❷ **_vestibular system:_** 3 semicircular canals originating in the vestibule responsible for **_balance._**

VESTIBULAR NEURITIS & LABYRINTHITIS

- **VESTIBULAR NEURITIS:** *inflammation of the vestibular portion of CN 8* **_MC AFTER VIRAL INFECTION._** *

- **LABYRINTHITIS:** *= vestibular neuritis + hearing loss/tinnitus** (from cochlear involvement).

CLINICAL MANIFESTATIONS
1. **Vestibular sx: _peripheral vertigo_** (usually **_continuous)_, dizziness, N/V, gait disturbances.** Nystagmus is usually horizontal and rotary (away from the affected side).
2. **Cochlear sx (with labyrinthitis): _hearing loss._** Symptoms usually resolve in weeks.

MANAGEMENT:
*CORTICOSTEROIDS 1ST LINE;** **If symptomatic:** *antihistamines (ex. Meclizine),* benzodiazepines.

MÉNIÈRE'S DISEASE   (IDIOPATHIC ENDOLYMPHATIC HYDROPS)

- *IDIOPATHIC distention of the endolymphatic compartment* of the *inner ear* by *excess fluid* ⇨ increased pressure within the inner ear ⇨ *hearing & balance disorders* characterized by:
  - ❶ *episodic vertigo:* peripheral lasting *minutes - hours* ❷ *tinnitus* ❸ *ear fullness* &
  - ❹ fluctuating *hearing loss** (primarily low-tone hearing loss).

CLINICAL MANIFESTATIONS
1. *Episodic peripheral vertigo lasting 1-8 hours, horizontal nystagmus, nausea, vomiting.*

DIAGNOSIS: Transtympanic electrocochleography most accurate test during an active episode.   Loss of nystagmus with caloric testing seen with Meniere. Audiometry (loss of low tones especially).

MANAGEMENT:
1. **Symptomatic:** antiemetics: antihistamines (*ex. Meclizine,* Prochlorperazine), *benzodiazepines* (ex. Diazepam), Anticholinergics (ex. Scopolamine). *Decompression if refractory to meds or severe (ex. Tympanostomy tube). Labyrinthectomy.*

2. **Preventative:** *diuretics (ex. Hydrochlorothiazide)* reduces endolymphatic pressure. *Avoidance of salt/caffeine/chocolate/ETOH** (because they increase endolymphatic pressure).

Meniere SYNDROME is due to an identifiable cause. Meniere DISEASE is idiopathic.

ACOUSTIC (VESTIBULAR) CN VIII NEUROMA

- *Cranial Nerve VIII/8 Schwannoma* – benign tumor of Schwann cells, which produce myelin sheath.

CLINICAL MANIFESTATIONS
*Unilateral sensorineural hearing loss is an acoustic neuroma until proven otherwise.** Tinnitus, headache, *facial numbness,* continuous disequilibrium/vertigo (unsteadiness while walking).

DIAGNOSIS: *MRI.* CT scan. Usually unilateral. *If bilateral, suspect Neurofibromatosis type II.*

MANAGEMENT: Surgery or focused radiation therapy (depending on age, tumor location, size etc).

NOSE/SINUS DISORDERS

ACUTE SINUSITIS

• <u>Acute = **1 - 4 weeks.**</u> In order of frequency = maxillary > ethmoid > frontal > sphenoid.

ETIOLOGIES
• *Same organisms associated with acute otitis media* **- S. Pneumo, H. flu, GABHS, M. catarrhalis.**
• *Often occurs with <u>CONCURRENT RHINITIS OR FOLLOWS VIRAL URI,</u>* dental infections.*
• URI leads to edema, which blocks drainage of the sinuses ⇨ fluid buildup ⇨ bacterial colonization.

CLINICAL MANIFESTATIONS
1. ***Sinus pain/pressure: worse with bending down & leaning forward.***
   <u>Maxillary:</u> MC* cheek pain/pressure may radiate to upper incisors.   <u>Frontal:</u> CN VI palsy.
   <u>Ethmoid:</u> tenderness to the high lateral wall of the nose. <u>Sphenoid:</u> mid head pressure.

2. ***Headache,*** malaise, ***purulent sputum or nasal discharge,*** fever, nasal congestion.

PHYSICAL EXAMINATION
Sinus tenderness on palpation, ***opacification with transillumination.***

DIAGNOSIS
1. Clinical diagnosis: primary clinical.   *Symptoms should be present > 1 week.**
2. ***CT scan diagnostic test of choice.**   <u>Sinus radiographs:</u> ***Water's view.****

MANAGEMENT
1. ***<u>Symptomatic therapy:</u>*** decongestants, antihistamines, mucolytics, intranasal corticosteroids, analgesics, nasal lavage. Indicated if symptoms <7 days or used as adjunctive treatment.

2. ***<u>Antibiotics:</u> symptoms should be present for >10-14 days**** or earlier if facial swelling, febrile etc.
   - *<u>AMOXICILLIN DRUG OF CHOICE,</u>** x 10-14 days.
   - 2nd line: ***Doxycycline, Trimethoprim-sulfamethoxazole*** (Bactrim).
   - Fluoroquinolones or Amoxicillin/clavulanic acid used if recent antibiotic use/refractory cases.

CHRONIC SINUSITIS

• <u>Chronic</u> = symptoms ≥ 12 consecutive weeks.   Same symptoms as acute sinusitis.
ETIOLOGIES
• **<u>Bacterial:</u> S. aureus MC bacterial cause,*** Pseudomonas, anaerobes. Other: ***Wegener's (necrotic).***
• **<u>Fungal:</u> Aspergillus MC fungal cause, Mucormycosis** *2nd MC fungal cause.*

MANAGEMENT: depends on the etiology.

MUCORMYCOSIS:
Fungi (Mucor, Rhizopus, Absidia, Cunninghamella) invade the sinuses & may enter the CNS.
   - Often affects the orbits, sinuses, lungs & central nervous system.
   - Seen in ***immunocompromised patients*** (ex. *DM post transplant, chemotherapy, HIV*).

CLINICAL MANIFESTATIONS
Acute sinusitis symptoms. Mucormycosis may be associated with ***black eschar on palate, face.****

MANAGEMENT: ***IV Amphotericin B 1st line.*** Posaconazole. May need surgical debridement.

RHINITIS

3 MAIN TYPES
    ❶ **ALLERGIC:** *MC type overall* - IgE-mediated mast cell histamine release.**

    ❷ **INFECTIOUS:** *Rhinovirus MC infectious cause** (common cold). GABHS & Strep less common.

    ❸ **VASOMOTOR** – nonallergic/noninfectious dilation of the blood vessels (ex. temperature change).

CLINICAL MANIFESTATIONS
1. Sneezing, nasal congestion/itching, ***clear rhinorrhea***. Eyes, ears, nose & throat may be involved.
2. *Allergic associated with **nasal polyps** & tends to be **worse in the morning.***

PHYSICAL EXAMINATION
1. **Allergic:** *PALE/VIOLACEOUS, BOGGY TURBINATES, nasal polyps* with *COBBLESTONE MUCOSA of the conjunctiva.**
2. **Viral:** *ERYTHEMATOUS TURBINATES.*

MANAGEMENT
Avoidance and environmental control, exposure reduction. ***Intranasal corticosteroids if allergic.***

1. ***Oral antihistamines***: decreases itching, sneezing, pruritus & rhinorrhea (little effect on congestion).
    Nonsedating: Cetirizine, Fexofenadine, Loratadine.   Minimally sedating: Desloratadine.
    Sedating: Brompheniramine, Chlorpheniramine, Hydroxyzine, Diphenhydramine.

2. ***Decongestants:*** **MOA:** improve congestion (little effect on rhinorrhea, sneezing, pruritus).
    Intranasal: *Oxymetazoline, Phenylephrine, Naphazoline.*   Oral: *Pseudoephedrine.*
       ***Intranasal decongestants** used >3-5 days may cause* rhinitis medicamentosa* *(rebound congestion).*

3. ***Intranasal steroids:*** *most effective med for allergic rhinitis (especially with* nasal polyps).*

4. Mast cell stabilizers can be used in allergic rhinitis. Anticholinergics may help for rhinorrhea.

NASAL POLYPS

ETIOLOGIES
1. *Allergic rhinitis MC.*   May be seen with Cystic Fibrosis.

2. **Samter's triad:** ❶ *asthma +* ❷ *nasal polyps +* ❸ *Aspirin/NSAID sensitivity/allergy.*

CLINICAL MANIFESTATIONS
Most are incidental findings but if large, they can cause obstruction or anosmia (decreased smell).

DIAGNOSIS
1. Signs of allergic rhinitis: pale/violaceous, boggy turbinates, cobblestone mucosa of the conjunctiva.
2. Nasal polyps (masses) with inspection of the nose.

MANAGEMENT
1. ***Intranasal corticosteroids treatment of choice.****

2. Surgical removal may be needed in some cases only if medical therapy is unsuccessful.

EPISTAXIS

ANTERIOR *MC.* Risk factors: nasal trauma (nose picking, blowing nose forcefully etc.), low humidity in a hot environment (dries nasal mucosa), rhinitis, ETOH, antiplatelet medications.
***Kiesselbach's plexus* MC site of bleeding in _anterior_ epistaxis.**

POSTERIOR: hypertension & atherosclerosis MC risk factors.
***Palatine artery* MC site for _posterior_ (**may cause **bleeding in _both nares_ & posterior pharynx).**

MANAGEMENT
1. ***Direct pressure* 1st line therapy for most cases.*** Pressure applied @ least 10-15 minutes with the patient in the seated position *leaning forward* (to reduce vessel pressure).

2. ***Topical decongestants/vasoconstrictors:*** may be adjunctive therapy with direct pressure.
   Phenylephrine, Oxymetazoline* nasal (Afrin), *Cocaine. Cautious use in patients c HTN.

3. Cauterization: ex. silver nitrate if the above measures failed & the bleeding site can be seen.

4. Nasal packing: if direct pressure & vasoconstrictors are unsuccessful or in severe bleeding.
   May consider antibiotic (Cephalexin or Clindamycin) to prevent toxic shock syndrome if packed.

5. Adjunct therapy: avoid exercise for a few days, avoid spicy foods (they cause vasodilation).
   Bacitracin & humidifiers helpful to moisten the nasal mucosa.

- ***Septal hematoma associated with loss of cartilage if the hematoma is not removed.****

NASAL FOREIGN BODY

- Most commonly seen in children.

CLINICAL MANIFESTATIONS
1. Asymptomatic
2. ***Mucopurulent nasal discharge, foul odor, epistaxis,*** *nasal obstruction (mouth breathing).*

DIAGNOSIS
1. Direct visualization (head light & otoscope). Rigid or flexible fiberoptic endoscopy.

2. Radiographs not usually needed (±helpful if button batteries are suspected & not visualized).

MANAGEMENT
1. Foreign body removal
   - via positive pressure technique: having the patient blow his or her nose while occluding the nostril opposite of the foreign body. Oral positive pressure: parent blows into the mouth while occluding the unaffected nostril (used in smaller children).

   - Instrument removal

MOUTH DISORDERS

ACUTE PHARYNGITIS/TONSILLITIS

- *Viral MC overall cause** -   Adenovirus, Rhinovirus, Enterovirus, Epstein-Barr virus, Respiratory syncytial virus, Influenza A & B, Herpes zoster virus.

- <u>Bacterial:</u> *Group A Beta Hemolytic Streptococcus (GABHS/S. pyogenes) MC bacterial cause.**

CLINICAL MANIFESTATIONS
1. Sore throat, pain or swallowing or with phonation. Other symptoms based on the etiology.

MANAGEMENT
1. <u>**Symptomatic:**</u> fluids, warm saline gargles, topical anesthetics, lozenges, NSAIDs.
2. <u>**Antibiotics if S. pyogenes:**</u> *Penicillin,* Amoxicillin. PCN allergy: Erythromycin or Clindamycin.

STREPTOCOCCAL PHARYNGITIS   ("STREP THROAT")

Group A Beta Hemolytic Streptococcus (GABHS) aka *Streptococcus pyogenes.*

CLINICAL MANIFESTATIONS
1. Sore throat.

	CENTOR CRITERIA INTERPRETATION
❶ *fever* (>38°C/*100.4°F*)	**0-1** ⇨ no antibiotic or throat culture needed (<10% for strep).
	<u>Note</u> if 5-15y, throat cultures should be sent in all cases.
❷ *pharyngotonsillar exudates.*	**2-3** ⇨ throat culture
❸ *tender <u>ANTERIOR</u> cervical lymphadenopathy.*	2 points: 15% chance of strep positivity. 32% if 3 points
❹ *absence of cough.*	**4-5** ⇨ give antibiotics (56% chance).
Each one assigned 1 point	Modified Centor: <15y ⇨ add 1 point
	>44y ⇨ Subtract 1 point

40 - 60% positive predictive value for a culture of the throat to test positive for Group A Streptococcus bacteria. The absence of all four variables indicates a negative predictive value >80%. The high negative predictive value suggests that the **Centor criteria can be more effectively used for ruling out strep throat** than for diagnosing strep throat.

DIAGNOSIS
1. <u>**Rapid antigen detection test:**</u> 95% specific but only 55-90% sensitive (most useful if positive, but ***if negative, throat cultures should be obtained*** *especially in children 5-15y).*

2. <u>**Throat culture:**</u> *definitive diagnosis** (gold standard).

MANAGEMENT
Normal course of illness is 3 -5 days. The course is shortened by 48 hours with treatment, therefore treatment is given mostly to prevent complications (ex rheumatic fever).
   1. *Penicillin G or VK 1st line.**   Amoxicillin, Amoxicillin/clavulanic acid (Augmentin).

   2. *Macrolides if PCN allergic.* Other alternatives include Clindamycin, Cephalosporins.

COMPLICATIONS
1. *Rheumatic fever* (preventable with antibiotics).
2. *Glomerulonephritis* (not preventable with antibiotics).
3. Peritonsillar abscess, cellulitis.

PERITONSILLAR ABSCESS   (QUINSY)

• Tonsillitis ⇨ cellulitis ⇨ abscess formation.

• *MC Strep pyogenes (GABHS), Staph aureus, polymicrobial* (including anaerobes).

CLINICAL MANIFESTATIONS
1. *dysphagia, pharyngitis,* **muffled "HOT POTATO VOICE",*** *difficulty handling oral secretions,* **trismus,** UVULA DEVIATION TO CONTRALATERAL SIDE,* *tonsillitis, anterior cervical lymphadenopathy.*

DIAGNOSIS
CT scan 1st line test to differentiate cellulitis vs. abscess.

MANAGEMENT:
1. *Antibiotics + aspiration or I & D (incision & drainage).*
    - *Ampicillin/Sulbactam* (Unasyn); *Clindamycin; Penicillin G* plus *Metronidazole.*

2. *Tonsillectomy indications: recurrent strep infections, recurrent peritonsillar infections, chronic tonsillitis.*

LARYNGITIS

• Inflammation of the larynx. Infectious MC cause or trauma (vocal abuse – singers, screaming etc.)

ETIOLOGIES
• *Viral infection MC*- Adenovirus, Rhinovirus, Influenza, Respiratory Syncytial virus, Parainfluenza
• Bacterial causes include M. catarrhalis & Mycoplasma pneumoniae.

CLINICAL MANIFESTATIONS
1. *Hoarseness hallmark,* aphonia,* pharyngitis, rhinitis, cough.

MANAGEMENT
1. *Supportive:* vocal rest, warm saline gargles, anesthetics, lozenges, increased fluid intake.

ORAL CANDIDIASIS (THRUSH)

• *Caused by Candida albicans.** Candida is part of the normal flora but can become pathogenic due to local or systemic immunosuppressed states (ex. HIV, chemotherapy, use of steroid inhalers without spacer, antibiotic use, diabetics, denture use, etc).

CLINICAL MANIFESTATIONS
1. *Mouth or throat pain.*

DIAGNOSIS:
1. **Clinical:** *white curd-like plaques (± LEAVE BEHIND ERYTHEMA/BLEEDS IF SCRAPED).**

2. **Potassium Hydroxide (KOH) smear:** *BUDDING YEAST/PSEUDOHYPHAE.**

MANAGEMENT
1. *nystatin liquid tx of choice.**
2. Clotrimazole troches, Oral Fluconazole.

ORAL LEUKOPLAKIA

• Precancerous hyperkeratosis due to chronic irritation (ex. tobacco, cigarette smoking, ETOH, dentures).
• Up to 6% show dysplasia or *squamous cell carcinoma*. Diagnosis of exclusion.

CLINICAL MANIFESTATIONS
Painless white patchy lesion that cannot be scraped off* (in comparison to Candida which is painful & can be scraped off).

MANAGEMENT
Cryotherapy, laser ablation. Biopsy to assess for cancer risk.

ERYTHROPLAKIA

• Precancerous lesions similar to leukoplakia but with an erythematous appearance.

• **90% of erythroplakia is either dysplastic or evident of squamous cell carcinoma.**

ORAL HAIRY LEUKOPLAKIA

• **Caused by Epstein-Barr virus*** (Human herpesvirus-4).
• *MC in immunocompromised* (HIV, post transplant, chronic steroid, chemotherapy).

CLINICAL MANIFESTATIONS
1. **painless, white plaque** along the LATERAL TONGUE BORDERS **or** BUCCAL MUCOSA **±smooth, or irregular "hairy" or "feathery"** lesions with prominent folds or projections* (appearance may change daily). CANNOT be scraped off.

MANAGEMENT
No specific treatment required (may spontaneously resolve). Antiretroviral tx, ablation.

APHTHOUS ULCERS (CANKER SORE, ULCERATIVE STOMATITIS)

• Unknown cause but may be associated with human herpes virus 6.

CLINICAL MANIFESTATIONS
1. Small **round or oval painful ulcers (yellow, white or grey centers) with erythematous halos.** MC on buccal or labial mucosa (nonkeratinized mucosa).

MANAGEMENT
1. **Topical analgesics,** topical oral steroids (ex Triamcinolone in orabase, Fluocinonide), Vitamin B & C.

2. Cimetidine may be used in some patients with recurrent ulcers.

SIALOLITHIASIS (SALIVARY GLAND STONES)

• *MC in Wharton's duct (submandibular gland duct); Stensen's duct* (parotid gland duct).

CLINICAL MANIFESTATIONS
Postprandial salivary gland pain & swelling.

MANAGEMENT
1. **Conservative:** *sialogogues* (ex. ***tart, hard candies, lemon drops,*** Xylitol-containing gum or candy to increase salivary flow), increase fluid intake, gland massage.
   - Avoid anticholinergic drugs if possible (anticholinergics decrease salivation).

2. Extracorporeal lithotripsy, intraoral stone removal if no response to conservative therapy.

ACUTE BACTERIAL SIALADENITIS (SUPPURATIVE SIALADENITIS)

• *Bacterial infection of parotid or submandibular salivary glands.* ± occur with dehydration, chronic illness. *S. aureus MC* or mixed aerobic/anaerobic infections.

CLINICAL MANIFSTATIONS
1. Acute pain, swelling & erythema near the gland especially with meals.

2. Tenderness at the duct opening (±pus if the duct is massaged).

3. Local pain, dysphagia, trismus (reduced opening of the jaw due to spasms of the muscles of mastication). May develop fever & chills if severe.

DIAGNOSIS
1. **CT Scan:** to assess for associated abscess/extent of tissue involvement.

MANAGEMENT
1. **Sialogogues:** ex. tart hard candies or lemon drops used to increase salivary flow.

2. **Antibiotics:** *Antistaphylococcus (Dicloxacillin or Nafcillin)* plus Metronidazole or Clindamycin if severe.

ORAL LICHEN PLANUS

• Idiopathic cell-mediated autoimmune response *(↑ in patients with HCV infection).**

CLINICAL MANIFESTATIONS
*Lacy leukoplakia of the oral mucosa common (Wickham striae).**

MANAGEMENT
Local or systemic corticosteroids.

ACUTE HERPETIC GINGIVOSTOMATITIS

- **Primary manifestation of HSV-1 in children.** MC occurs between 6 months – 5 years.

CLINICAL MANIFESTATIONS
1. sudden onset of fever, anorexia ⇨ **gingivitis (gum swelling, friable/bleeding gums);** vesicles on the oral mucosa, tongue & lips ⇨ *grey/yellow lesions.*

MANAGEMENT
Usually self-limiting. Acyclovir in severe cases.

ACUTE HERPETIC PHARYNGOTONSILLITIS

- **Primary manifestation of HSV-1 in adults.**

CLINICAL MANIFESTATIONS
fever, malaise, headache, sore throat

PHYSICAL EXAM
vesicles that rupture ⇨ **ulcerative lesions with grayish exudates** in the posterior pharyngeal mucosa.

MANAGEMENT:
Oral hygiene - lesions usually resolve within 7-14 days.

LUDWIG'S ANGINA

- Cellulitis of the sublingual & submaxillary spaces in the neck.
- MC secondary to dental infections (anaerobic infections).

CLINICAL MANIFESTATIONS:
Swelling & erythema of the upper neck & chin with PUS ON THE FLOOR OF THE MOUTH.

DIAGNOSIS
CT scan test of choice.

MANAGEMENT
Antibiotics: Ampicillin/sulbactam (Unasyn); Penicillin **plus** Metronidazole or Clindamycin.

SELECTED REFERENCES

Wong TY, Mcintosh R. Hypertensive retinopathy signs as risk indicators of cardiovascular morbidity and mortality. Br Med Bull. 2005;73-74:57-70.

Casson RJ, Chidlow G, Wood JP, Crowston JG, Goldberg I. Definition of glaucoma: clinical and experimental concepts. Clin Experiment Ophthalmol. 2012;40(4):341-9.

Kingman S. Glaucoma is second leading cause of blindness globally. Bull World Health Organ. 2004;82(11):887-8.

Lempert T, Neuhauser H. Epidemiology of vertigo, migraine and vestibular migraine. J Neurol. 2009;256(3):333-8.

Shin JE, Kim CH, Park HJ. Vestibular abnormality in patients with Meniere disease and migrainous vertigo. Acta Otolaryngol. 2013;133(2):154-8.

Walker MF. Treatment of vestibular neuritis. Curr Treat Options Neurol. 2009;11(1):41-5.

Richards A, Guzman-cottrill JA. Conjunctivitis. Pediatr Rev. 2010;31(5):196-208.

Coroneo MT. Pterygium as an early indicator of ultraviolet insolation: a hypothesis. Br J Ophthalmol. 1993;77(11):734-9.

Badano JL, Mitsuma N, Beales PL, Katsanis N. The ciliopathies: an emerging class of human genetic disorders. Annu Rev Genomics Hum Genet. 2006;7:125-48.

Kingman S. Glaucoma is second leading cause of blindness globally. Bull World Health Organ. 2004;82(11):887-8.

Post RE, Dickerson LM. Dizziness: a diagnostic approach. Am Fam Physician. 2010;82(4):361-8, 369.

Gariano RF, Kim CH. Evaluation and management of suspected retinal detachment. Am Fam Physician. 2004;69(7):1691-8.

Pearlman AN, Conley DB. Review of current guidelines related to the diagnosis and treatment of rhinosinusitis. Curr Opin Otolaryngol Head Neck Surg. 2008;16(3):226-30.

Raut VV. Management of peritonsillitis/peritonsillar. Rev Laryngol Otol Rhinol (Bord). 2000;121(2):107-10.

Lempert T, Neuhauser H. Epidemiology of vertigo, migraine and vestibular migraine. J Neurol. 2009;256(3):333-8.

Dykewicz MS, Hamilos DL. Rhinitis and sinusitis. J Allergy Clin Immunol. 2010;125(2 Suppl 2):S103-15.

Martín-navarro CM, Lorenzo-morales J, Cabrera-serra MG, et al. The potential pathogenicity of chlorhexidine-sensitive Acanthamoeba strains isolated from contact lens cases from asymptomatic individuals in Tenerife, Canary Islands, Spain. J Med Microbiol. 2008;57(Pt 11):1399-404.

Lodi G, Sardella A, Bez C, Demarosi F, Carrassi A. Interventions for treating oral leukoplakia. Cochrane Database Syst Rev. 2006;(4):CD001829.

Roden MM, Zaoutis TE, Buchanan WL, et al. Epidemiology and outcome of zygomycosis: a review of 929 reported cases. Clin Infect Dis. 2005;41(5):634-53.

Mcewan J, Giridharan W, Clarke RW, Shears P. Paediatric acute epiglottitis: not a disappearing entity. Int J Pediatr Otorhinolaryngol. 2003;67(4):317-21.

PHOTO CREDITS

CHAPTER 6 – REPRODUCTIVE, OBSTETRICS AND GYNECOLOGY

DIAGNOSTIC TESTS USED IN OB/GYN DISORDERS

PAP SMEAR: screening test for cervical carcinoma, detects early changes that may lead to carcinoma.

COLPOSCOPY: visualization of the cervix & vagina under magnification colposcope (often done with acetic acid to localize any tissue that needs to be biopsied). Office procedure.
> **Ind:** evaluate abnormal cytology results on PAP smear (ex. persistent ASC-US or ASC-US with HPV positivity, HSIL, LSIL), for aid in biopsy to rule out cervical cancer.

ENDOMETRIAL BIOPSY: biopsy of the endometrium via curette or small aspiration tool.
> **Ind:** suspicion of endometrial hyperplasia or carcinoma (follow up of a >4mm endometrial stripe on transvaginal ultrasound).

HYSTEROSCOPY: small fiber optic endoscope used to visualize the uterine cavity or endocervical canal.
> **Ind:** biopsy or excision of myomas, evaluate postmenopausal bleeding, evaluation for possible retained products of conception, endometrial ablation. Office procedure or done in the OR.

LAPAROSCOPY:
Small fiber optic endoscope to visualize the pelvic cavity via umbilical incision.
> **Ind:** for conditions needing laparotomy (ex. unstable ruptured ectopic pregnancy), tubal sterilization, evaluation of the endometrium. Done under general anesthesia.

HYSTEROSALPINGOGRAPHY:
Radiopaque dye is injected via the cervix to visualize the uterine cavity & fallopian tubes.
> **Ind:** used to confirm fallopian tube patency in the evaluation of infertility or to assess tubal rupture.

DILATION & CURETTAGE (D & C):
Dilation of cervix & curettage of the endometrial area with a curette (removes tissue by scraping or scooping) OR "suction curettage" – dilation of cervix with removal of contents by suction vacuum.
> **Ind:** tx of molar pregnancies, termination of pregnancies in the **4-12 weeks of gestation/1st trimester:** (ex. elective, inevitable, incomplete, septic, inevitable abortions), suction curettage may be used to manage postpartum hemorrhage associated with retained products of conception (POC). Also used diagnostically to visualize the uterine cavity to exclude endometrial cancer (used with hysteroscopy to localize area).

DILATION & EVACUATION (D & E):
> **Ind:** tx for molar pregnancies, termination of pregnancies **13-24 weeks gestation** (ex. elective, inevitable, incomplete, septic, inevitable abortions), suction curettage may be used to manage post partum hemorrhage associated with retained products of conception (POC). May be used after a miscarriage to ensure that uterus is completely empty.
> - Suction curettage with manual or electric vacuum aspiration & instruments (ex curette, forceps).

MANUAL VACUUM ASPIRATION: "mini suction".
> **Ind:** a method of abortion as early as 3 weeks gestational age. Does not require dilation.

MEDICAL ABORTION:
> **Mifepristone + Misoprostol** *safe up to 9 weeks gestational age.* Mifepristone given initially with administration of Misoprostol 24-72h afterwards. More effective than Methotrexate. Mifepristone is a progestin antagonist (without progesterone, the endometrium can't maintain the pregnancy & sloughs off). Misoprostol is a prostaglandin analog that causes uterine contraction, facilitating the abortion.
> **Methotrexate + Misoprostol** safe *up to 7 weeks gestational age.* Methotrexate followed by Misoprostol 3-7 days later. Methotrexate is a folic acid antagonist.

BASIC PHYSIOLOGY

MENSTRUAL CYCLE OVERVIEW

Understanding the roles of the hormones in the menstrual cycle are critical to understand this chapter.

Follicular phase: during the 1st 14 days (follicular phase), the endometrium thickens under the influence of **_estrogen_**. In the ovaries, a dominant follicle matures, leading to ovulation.

Luteal phase: after ovulation, the ruptured follicle becomes the corpus luteum, secreting progesterone (& some estrogen). **_Progesterone_** enhances the lining of the uterus to prepare it for implantation. If there is no implantation, the corpus luteum degenerates, leading to a steep decrease in both estrogen & progesterone. The steep drops in both hormones leads to menstruation.

PHASE 1: FOLLICULAR (Proliferative)

Days 1-12

_ESTROGEN PREDOMINATES._*

- **_Pulsatile GnRH_** from the hypothalamus ⇨ ↑FSH & LH from the pituitary gland to stimulate the ovaries.

Ovaries:

- ↑**_FSH_** causes **_follicle & egg maturation in the ovary._**
- ↑**_LH stimulates_** the maturing follicle to **_produce estrogen._**

Endometrium (Uterus)

Estrogen "builds" up the endometrium (proliferative).

Estrogen causes NEGATIVE FEEDBACK in HPO system:

(Hypothalamus-Pituitary-Ovarian)

- The ↑'ing levels of estrogen inhibits hypothalamic GnRH release as well as pituitary release of LH & FSH (so no new follicles start maturing).

OVULATION: Days 12-14

- The ↑estrogen being released from the mature follicle **_switches from NEGATIVE TO POSITIVE FEEDBACK_** on GnRH, causing mutual ↑'**_es in estrogen, FSH & LH._**
- The sudden **_LH surge causes ovulation_** (egg release).

PHASE 2: LUTEAL PHASE (Secretory)

Days 14 - 28

_PROGESTERONE PREDOMINATES._*

- The LH surge also causes the ruptured follicle to become the corpus luteum. The corpus luteum secretes **_progesterone_** & _estrogen_ to maintain the endometrial lining. Estrogen & progesterone switches back to negative feedback.

If pregnancy occurs:

The blastocyst (maturing zygote) keeps the corpus luteum functional (secreting estrogen & progesterone, which keeps the endometrium from sloughing).

MENSTRUAL CYCLE

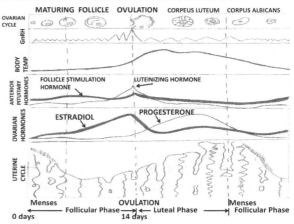

MENSTRUATION (1st days of Follicular)

If the egg is not fertilized, the corpus luteum soon deteriorates (causing a **_fall of progesterone & estrogen levels_**). This has 2 effects:

- The endometrium is no longer maintained & sloughs off, leading to **_menstruation._**

- The negative feedback on GnRH subsides, causing ↑pulsatile GnRH secretion. This leads to ↑FSH & LH, which starts the follicle maturation process all over again.

GnRH pulses >1 an hour favor LH secretion.   Less frequent pulses favor FSH secretion

MENSTRUAL DISORDERS

DYSFUNCTIONAL (ABNORMAL) UTERINE BLEEDING (DUB)

DUB: *abnormal frequency/intensity of menses* due to ***NONORGANIC CAUSES.**** *Diagnosis of exclusion.**

- Normal cycle: 24-38 days with menstruation lasting 4.5-8 days (average loss 30ml -range spotting to 80ml).

Amenorrhea:	absence of menstrual period.
Cryptomenorrhea:	light flow or spotting.
Menorrhagia:	***heavy or prolonged*** bleeding @ normal menstrual intervals.
Metrorrhagia:	irregular bleeding ***between expected menstrual cycles.***
Menometrorrhagia:	irregular, excessive bleeding between expected menstrual cycles.
Oligomenorrhea:	***infrequent menstruation*** (prolonged cycle length >35 days but <6 months).
Polymenorrhagia:	***frequent*** cycle interval (<21 days).

ETIOLOGIES

❶ **CHRONIC ANOVULATION:** *(90%).** Due to disruption of the hypothalamus-pituitary axis.
Seen especially with ***extremes of age*** (teenagers soon after menarche or perimenopausal).
- ***UNOPPOSED ESTROGEN:**** without ovulation, there is no progesterone = unopposed estrogen ⇨↑endometrial overgrowth with ***irregular, unpredictable shedding (bleeding)*** as the endometrium outgrows its own blood supply.

❷ **OVULATORY:** (10%).
- ***Regular cyclical shedding.**** ⊕ ovulation with *prolonged progesterone secretion* (due to ↓ estrogen levels) ⇨ ↑blood loss from endometrial vessel dilation & ***prostaglandins*** ⇨ menorrhagia.

DIAGNOSIS

- ***DIAGNOSIS OF EXCLUSION:**** must exclude organic causes (r/o reproductive, systemic, iatrogenic causes). ***If w/u shows no evidence of organic cause & negative pelvic exam*** ⇨ **DUB is the dx.***
- Workup (w/u) includes: hormone levels, transvaginal US. Endometrial biopsy if endometrial stripe >4mm on transvaginal US or in women >35y (to rule out endometrial hyperplasia or carcinoma).

MANAGEMENT

Goals: control acute bleeding, prevent future bleeding & minimize endometrial cancer risk.
1. **Acute Severe Bleeding:** ***High-dose IV estrogens or high dose OCPs.*** Reduce dose as the bleeding improves. Dilation & curettage (D&C) may be used if IV estrogen fails.

2. **ANOVULATORY: (90%)**
   - ***Oral Contraceptive Pills (OCPs): 1st line**** - *regulates the cycle, thins the endometrial lining & reduces menstrual flow.* ↓'es endometrial cancer risk by reducing unopposed estrogen.
   - **Progesterone:** ***if estrogen is contraindicated.*** ex. Medroxyprogesterone acetate.
   - GnRH agonists: Leuprolide causes temporary amenorrhea (if given in a continuous fashion).

3. **OVULATORY:** (10%)
   - Oral Contraceptive Pills (OCPs): regulate the cycles, thins endometrial lining.
   - Progesterone: orally or IUD (Mirena reduces bleeding in 79-94%).
   - GnRH agonists: Leuprolide with add-back progesterone (to reduce the S/E of Leuprolide).

4. **SURGERY**
   Surgery done if not responsive to medical treatment.
   - ***Hysterectomy: definitive management.***
   - ***Endometrial ablation:*** endometrium destruction in patients who don't want a hysterectomy.

DYSMENORRHEA

- **Dysmenorrhea** = *PAINFUL MENSTRUATION* that affects normal activities

PRIMARY DYSEMONORRHEA: *not due to pelvic pathology. Due to ↑prostaglandins** ⇨ *painful uterine muscle wall activity.* Pain usually starts 1-2 years after onset of menarche in teenagers.

SECONDARY DYSMENORRHEA: *due to pelvic pathology** (ex *endometriosis, adenomyosis, leiomyomas, adhesions, PID).* Increased incidence as women age (especially >25y).

CLINICAL MANIFESTATIONS
- *DIFFUSE PELVIC PAIN RIGHT BEFORE OR WITH THE ONSET OF MENSES** (± lower abdomen, suprapubic or pelvic pain that may radiate to the lower back & legs). May be associated with headache, nausea, vomiting. Cramps usually lasts 1-3 days.

PHYSICAL EXAMINATION: normal (may have uterine tenderness). Findings depend on the cause.

MANAGEMENT
1. *NSAIDs: 1ˢᵗ line.** **MOA:** *inhibits prostaglandin-mediated uterine activity* (best to start before onset of symptoms/menstruation and given for 2-3 days).
   <u>Supportive:</u> local heat & vitamin E started 2 days prior to & for 3 days into menses.

2. *Ovulation suppression: OCPs/Depo-Provera/vaginal ring* significantly reduces symptoms.

3. **Laparoscopy:** if medications fails (done to r/o secondary causes ex. endometriosis or PID). Endometriosis MC secondary cause in younger patients (adenomyosis with increasing age).

PREMENSTRUAL SYNDROME

- *Cluster of physical, behavioral & mood changes* with CYCLICAL OCCURRENCE *during the LUTEAL PHASE* of the menstrual cycle.
- Symptoms seen in 75-85% of patients. Significant disruption only in 5-10%.

Premenstrual Dysphoric Disorder (PMDD): severe PMS with functional impairment.

CLINICAL MANIFESTATIONS
1. **Physical:** bloating, breast swelling/pain, headache, bowel habit changes, fatigue, muscle/joint pain.
2. **Emotional:** depression, hostility, irritability, libido changes, aggressiveness.
3. **Behavioral:** food cravings, poor concentration, noise sensitivity, loss of motor senses.

DIAGNOSIS
- *Symptoms initiate during the luteal phase (1-2 weeks before menses), relieved within 2-3 days of the onset of menses* plus at least *7 symptom-free days during the follicular phase.*

MANAGEMENT
Lifestyle modifications: stress reduction, exercise, caffeine & salt restriction. NSAIDs, Vitamin B6 & E.
1. **SSRIs:** for the emotional symptoms (ex. Fluoxetine, Sertraline, Paroxetine, Citalopram), SNRIs.
2. **OCPs:** induces anovulation. *Drosperinone-containing OCPs for PMDD.*
3. GnRH: continuous dosing with estrogen add-back therapy if no response to SSRIs or OCPs.
4. Bloating: Spironolactone (androgen inhibitor taken during the luteal phase to relieve symptoms of breast tenderness & bloating), calcium carbonate, low salt diet.
5. *Refractory* breast pain: not responding to the above treatments - ± Danazol, Bromocriptine.

AMENORRHEA

Amenorrhea: *absence of menses.* Workup: pregnancy test, serum prolactin, FSH, LH, TSH.

PRIMARY AMENORRHEA: *failure of menarche onset* (menstruation) by age 15y (in the presence of secondary sex characteristics) or 13y (in the absence of 2ry sex characteristics).

ETIOLOGIES OF PRIMARY AMENORRHEA

	UTERUS PRESENT	UTERUS ABSENT
BREAST PRESENT	<u>Outflow obstruction:</u> transverse vaginal septum, imperforate hymen	• Mullerian agenesis (46 XX) • Androgen insensitivity (46 XY)

BREAST ABSENT	• *Elevated:* ↑FSH, ↑LH = Ovarian causes
	   - Premature ovarian failure (46XX)
	   - Gonadal dysgenesis (ex. Turner's 45X<u>O</u>)
	 • *Normal/Low:* ↓FSH, ↓LH
	   - *Hypothalamus-Pituitary Failure*
	   - Puberty delay (ex athletes, illness, anorexia)
		Rare. Usually caused by a defect in testosterone synthesis. Presents like a phenotypic immature girl with primary amenorrhea (will often have intrabdominal testes).

SECONDARY AMENORRHEA: *absence of menses for >3 months in a patient with previously normal menstruation* (or >6 months in a patient who was previously oligomenorrheic).

ETIOLOGIES OF SECONDARY

1. ***PREGNANCY: MC CAUSE OF SECONDARY AMENORRHEA.****
   1st step in amenorrhea workup is to rule out pregnancy (***order β–hCG***).
2. **HYPOTHALAMUS dysfunction:** (35%) disruption of normal pulsatile hypothalamic secretion of GnRH that directly leads to subsequent ↓FSH and/or ↓LH secretion by the pituitary gland.
   ETIOLOGIES: hypothalamic disorders, anorexia (or weight loss 10% below ideal body weight), exercise, stress nutritional deficiencies, systemic disease (ex. Celiac disease).
   DIAGNOSIS: *Normal/↓FSH & LH;* low estradiol, normal prolactin.
   MANAGEMENT: stimulate gonadotropin secretion: ***Clomiphene***, Menotropin (Pergonal).

3. **PITUITARY Dysfunction** (ex. prolactin-secreting pituitary adenoma): 19%
   Dx: *↓FSH, LH, ↑prolactin** (galactorrhea). MRI of pituitary sella. Prolactin inhibits GnRH.
   Management: Transsphenoidal surgery (tumor removal).

4. **OVARIAN Disorders:** 40%. *Polycystic Ovarian Syndrome.* ***Premature Ovarian Failure:*** follicular failure or follicular resistance to LH or FSH. Turner's syndrome.
   CLINICAL: *symptoms of estrogen deficiency* (similar to menopause): hot flashes, sleep & mood disturbances, dyspareunia, dry/thin skin, vaginal dryness/atrophy.
   DIAGNOSIS:
   - ↑FSH &↑LH, ↓estradiol ⇨ *ovarian abnormalities* (primary disorder).
   - Normal/↓FSH, LH ⇨ pituitary or hypothalamus abnormalities (secondary or tertiary).
   PROGESTERONE CHALLENGE TEST: 10mg medroxyprogesterone for 10 days.
   - ⊕ *withdrawal bleeding* ⇨ *ovarian* (patient is anovulatory or oligoovulatory) & there is enough estrogen present (which built up endometrial lining).
   - *No withdrawal bleeding* ⇨ ❶ *hypoestrogenic* ex. hypothalamus-pituitary failure OR ❷ *Uterine:* ex. Asherman's or uterine outflow tract (ex. imperforate hymen).

5. **UTERINE disorder:** *scarring of the uterine cavity (Asherman's syndrome = acquired endometrial scarring* 2ry to postpartum hemorrhage, s/p D&C or endometrial infection.
   Dx: pelvic US: absence of normal uterine stripe. Hysteroscopy: to diagnose & treat.
   Mgmt: Estrogen treatment to stimulate endometrial regeneration of the denuded area.

MENOPAUSE

- *Cessation of menses >1 year due to loss of ovarian function.* Average age in the US is 50-52y.

- Premature menopause = menopause before age 40y. May occur sooner in patients with diabetes mellitus (DM), smokers, vegetarians, malnourished patients.

CLINICAL MANIFESTATIONS
1. **Estrogen deficiency changes**: menstrual cycle alterations, vasomotor instability (including *hot flashes*), mood changes, skin/nail/hair changes, ↑cardiovascular events, hyperlipidemia, osteoporosis, dyspareunia (painful intercourse) due to vaginal atrophy, urinary incontinence. *Atrophic vaginitis: thin, yellow discharge, vaginal pH >5.5, pruritus.*
2. Irregular menstrual cycles but no premenstrual symptoms.

PHYSICAL EXAMINATION
1. ↓bone density, skin: thin/dry, decreased elasticity. Vaginal: atrophy thin mucosa.

DIAGNOSIS
1. **FSH *ASSAY MOST SENSITIVE INITIAL TEST**** (↑*serum FSH* >30 IU/mL)

2. **↑serum FSH, ↑LH, ↓estrogen:*** due to depletion of ovarian follicles. Androstenedione levels don't change. Estrone is the predominant estrogen after menopause.

COMPLICATIONS
1. *Loss of estrogen's protective effects* ⇨ ↑osteoporosis (↑fractures), ↑cardiovascular risk & ↑lipids.

MANAGEMENT
1. ***Vasomotor insufficiency/hot flashes***: **estrogen, progesterone**, Clonidine, SSRIs, Gabapentin.

2. Vaginal atrophy: estrogen (transdermal, intravaginal).

3. Osteoporosis prevention: Calcium + Vitamin D, weight bearing exercise, **bisphosphonates**, calcitonin, estrogen (with or without progesterone), *SERM (ex Raloxifene, Tamoxifen).*

4. ***Hormone Replacement Therapy (HRT):*** risks vs. benefits must be considered.
   a. **Estrogen only:**
      - Benefits: **most effective symptomatic treatment** (ex. mood changes, hot flashes, vaginal atrophy). Transdermal or vaginal preferred vs. PO. No increased risk of breast cancer.

      - Risks: ↑**risk of endometrial cancer** (unopposed estrogen) so **often used in patients with no uterus** *(ex. s/p hysterectomy),* **thromboembolism** (CVA, DVT, PE), liver disease.

   b. ***Estrogen + Progesterone:***
      Continuous: same dose daily doesn't cause menstrual-like bleeding.
      Sequential (cycling): dose changes - can cause menstrual like bleeding but less often than normal cyclical bleeding.
         - Benefits: symptomatic relief, ↓heart & stroke risk, ↓osteoporosis & dementia. ***Protective against endometrial cancer.** *Often used if the patient still has an intact uterus* (progestin protects against unopposed estrogen that may lead to endometrial cancer).

         - Risks: venous thromboembolism. ± slightly ↑risk of breast cancer (controversial).

LEIOMYOMA (UTERINE FIBROIDS)   FIBROMYOMA

- **Leiomyoma:** *benign uterus smooth muscle tumor.* MC benign gynecologic lesion.
- *GROWTH RELATED TO ESTROGEN PRODUCTION:* **regresses after menopause*** (if it grows after menopause, think other causes). ±↑ with pregnancy or change in size with the menstrual cycle.
- MC in 30s (*especially >35y*). *5x MC in African-Americans.*
- Types: Intramural, submucosal, subserosal, parasitic.

CLINICAL MANIFESTATIONS
1. Most are asymptomatic. ***Bleeding MC presentation*** (*menorrhagia*), dysmenorrhea.
2. Abdominal pressure/pain related to size of tumors & location. Bladder: frequency, urgency.

PHYSICAL EXAMINATION
- ***Large, irregular hard palpable mass* in the abdomen or pelvis** during bimanual exam.

DIAGNOSIS: pelvic US: focal heterogenic masses with shadowing. Also used to observe for growth.

MANAGEMENT
1. **Observation:** *majority don't need treatment.* Decision to treat is determined by symptoms, size/rate of tumor growth & the desire for fertility.

2. **Medical:** inhibition of estrogen (↓'es endometrial growth).
   - **Leuprolide:** is a *GnRH agonist* that causes **GnRH inhibition when given continuously** (shrinks the uterus temporarily until natural menopause). **Most effective medical treatment** (can shrink as much as 50% but will return to normal size once therapy is stopped). *Usually used if near menopause or preoperatively (prior to hysterectomy).*
   - Progestins: cause endometrial atrophy ⇨ decreases bleeding. Ex. Medroxyprogesterone.

3. **Surgical:**
   - **Hysterectomy:** *definitive treatment.* **Fibroids are the MC cause for hysterectomy.***
   - **Myomectomy:** used especially **to preserve fertility.**
   - Endometrial ablation, artery embolization. Both may affect the ability to conceive.

ADENOMYOSIS

- *Islands of endometrial tissue within the myometrium* (muscular layer of the uterine wall).
- Ectopic endometrial tissue induces hypertrophy & hyperplasia of the surrounding myometrium ⇨ diffusely enlarged uterus. MC presents later in the reproductive years.

CLINICAL MANIFESTATIONS
- *Menorrhagia* (progressively worsens), *dysmenorrhea*, ±infertility.

PHYSICAL EXAMINATION
- *TENDER, SYMMETRICALLY* (uniformly) enlarged *"BOGGY UTERUS"** "globular" enlargement.

LEIOMYOMA	ADENOMYOSIS
Asymmetric	**Symmetric**
Firm	Soft
Nontender	*Tender*

DIAGNOSIS: diagnosis of exclusion of 2^{ry} amenorrhea (rule out pregnancy first). MRI.
- Post-total abdominal hysterectomy examination of uterus: definitive diagnosis.

MANAGEMENT
1. *Total abdominal hysterectomy: only effective therapy.*
2. Conservative treatment: used to preserve fertility: analgesics, low dose OCPs.

ENDOMETRITIS

- **_Infection of the uterine endometrium._** Chorioamnionitis (fetal membrane infection).
- Usually polymicrobial (often vaginal flora, aerobic & anaerobic bacteria).

RISK FACTORS
- **Postpartum or postabortal uterine infection:** **_C-section biggest risk factor,_**_*_ prolonged rupture of membranes >24 hours, vaginal delivery, dilation & curettage (or evacuation).

DIAGNOSIS
- **_Fever_** (>38°C)/100.4°F), **_tachycardia, abdominal pain & uterine tenderness after C-section,_** _2-3 days postpartum or_ **_postabortal_** (may present later). Mainly a clinical diagnosis.
- May have vaginal bleeding/discharge (may have foul smelling lochia).

MANAGEMENT
1. **Infection post C-section:** **_Clindamycin + Gentamicin._** May add Ampicillin for additional group B Streptococcus coverage. Ampicillin/sulbactam is an alternative.
2. Infection after vaginal delivery or chorioamnionitis: _Ampicillin + Gentamicin._
Prophylaxis with 1st gen cephalosporin x 1 dose during C-section to reduce the incidence.

ENDOMETRIOSIS

- Presence of endometrial tissue (stroma & gland) outside the endometrial (uterine) cavity. The **_ectopic endometrial tissue_** _responds to cyclical hormonal changes._ ~10% incidence.
- **_OVARIES MC SITE,_**_*_ _posterior cul de sac,_ broad & uterosacral ligaments, rectosigmoid colon, bladder.

RISK FACTORS: _nulliparity,_ family history, early menarche. **_Onset usually <35y.*_**

CLINICAL MANIFESTATIONS
1. **Classic triad:** ❶ _cyclic_ **_premenstrual pelvic pain_** ±low back pain ❷ **_Dysmenorrhea_** (painful menstruation) & ❸**_Dyspareunia_** (painful intercourse); **_Dyschezia_** (painful defecation).
2. ±pre-post menstrual spotting. Asymptomatic in $^1/_3$ affected.

3. **_Infertility:_** >25% of all causes of female infertility.

DIAGNOSIS
1. Physical Exam: usually normal. ±fixed tender adnexal masses.
2. **Laparoscopy with biopsy:** **_definitive dx.*_**   Used to visualize structures for presence of tissue.
   - Raised, patches of thickened, discolored scarred or "powder burn" appearing implants of tissue.
   - **Endometrioma:** endometriosis involving the ovaries large enough to be considered a tumor, usually filled with old blood appearing chocolate-colored (_CHOCOLATE CYST_).*

MANAGEMENT
Medical (Conservative) _ovulation suppression:_
1. Premenstrual pain: **_Combined OCPs*_** + _NSAIDs (for pain)._
2. Progesterone: suppresses GnRH, causes endometrial tissue atrophy, suppresses ovulation.
3. Leuprolide: GnRH analog causes pituitary FSH/LH suppression.
4. Danazol: testosterone (induces pseudomenopause - suppresses FSH & LH & mid-cycle surge).

Surgical:
5. **Conservative Laparoscopy with ablation:** used if fertility desired (preserves uterus & ovaries).
6. **Total Abdominal Hysterectomy** with Salpingo-oophorectomy (TAH-BSO): if no desire to conceive.

ENDOMETRIAL HYPERPLASIA

- ***Endometrial gland proliferation*** cytologic atypia (***precursor to endometrial carcinoma****).*
- ***Hyperplasia due to continuous ↑UNOPPOSED ESTROGEN**** (unopposed by progesterone). Ex. ***chronic anovulation***, PCOS, perimenopause, obesity (conversion of androgen ⇨ estrogen in adipose tissue), Hyperplasia often occurs within 3 years of estrogen-only therapy. ***MC postmenopausal.***

CLINICAL MANIFESTATIONS
- ***Bleeding:*** *Menorrhagia, metrorrhagia, postmenopausal bleeding.* ±vaginal discharge.

DIAGNOSIS
1. **Transvaginal Ultrasound (TVUS):** *ENDOMETRIAL STRIPE* **>4 mm*** *(screening test).*
2. **Endometrial Bx:** *definitive diagnosis.**
   Indications: >35y, ↑endometrial stripe seen on TVUS, patients on unopposed estrogen therapy, ***Tamoxifen***, AGS on Pap smear or persistent bleeding c endometrial stripe <4mm.

MANAGEMENT
1. Endometrial hyperplasia **without atypia:**   ***Progestin**** *(PO or IUD-Mirena).*   Repeat endometrial biopsy in 3-6 months.
      MOA: stops estrogen from being unopposed, limiting endometrial growth.

2. Endometrial hyperplasia **with atypia:** ***hysterectomy**** (TAH ±BSO).
   Progestin treatment if not a surgical candidate or if patient wishes to preserve fertility.

ENDOMETRIAL CANCER

- ***MC gynecologic malignancy in the US.**** (2 times more common than cervical cancer).
- *4th MC malignancy incidence in women overall (after breast ⇨ lung ⇨ colorectal).*
- ***MC postmenopausal**** (75%) ***50-60y peak.*** Perimenopausal 25%, premenstrual 5-10%

- ***Estrogen-dependent cancer.***   Associated with antecedent endometrial hyperplasia.
- **Risk Factors:** ***↑estrogen exposure:**** *nulliparity, chronic anovulation, PCOS, obesity, estrogen replacement therapy,* *late menopause, Tamoxifen* (estrogen stimulates endometrial growth)**;** HTN, Diabetes mellitus.

- ***Combination OCPs are protective against both ovarian & endometrial cancers.****

CLINICAL MANIFESTATIONS
1. ***ABNORMAL UTERINE BLEEDING: postmenopausal bleeding**** (causes of 10% postmenopausal bleeding). Pre or perimenopausal ⇨ ***menorrhagia*** or metrorrhagia.

DIAGNOSIS
1. **Endometrial biopsy:** ***Adenocarcinoma MC*** *(>80%),* Sarcoma 5%.
2. **Ultrasound:** Usually ***endometrial stripe >4mm.*** May rule out other causes of bleeding.

MANAGEMENT:
1. **Stage I:** ***Hysterectomy*** (TAH-BSO) ±post-op radiation therapy.
      Most are well differentiated (one of the most curable of the gynecologic cancers).
2. **Stage II, III:** TAH-BSO + lymph node excision ± post-op radiation therapy.
3. Stage IV (advanced): systemic chemotherapy.

POST MENOPAUSAL BLEEDING

ETIOLOGIES:
• *MC benign:* vaginal/endometrial atrophy, cervical polyps, submucosal fibroids; 10% **Endometrial CA.***

DIAGNOSIS
• ANY postmenopausal bleeding in a woman not on HRT (or on HRT with abnormal bleeding) should raise suspicion for endometrial carcinoma, hyperplasia or leiomyosarcoma.
 1. *Transvaginal US*
    - Endometrial stripe <4mm ⇨ repeat US in 4 months. If continued bleeding, ±biopsy.
    - *Stripe >4mm ⇨ endometrial biopsy.*
    - If focal thickening of endometrium ⇨ hysteroscopy.

PELVIC ORGAN PROLAPSE

• **Uterine Prolapse:** uterine herniation into the vagina.
• **Risk factors:** *weakness of pelvic support structures: MC after childbirth (especially traumatic),* ↑pelvic floor pressure: multiple vaginal births, obesity, repeated heavy lifting.

CYSTOCELE: posterior *bladder* herniating into the *anterior vagina.*

ENTEROCELE: pouch of Douglas (*small bowel*) into the *upper vagina.*

RECTOCELE: distal sigmoid colon (rectum) herniates into the *posterior distal vagina.*

GRADES:
I	descent into upper $^2/_3$ of the vagina.
II	cervix approaches introitus.
III	outside introitus.
IV	entire uterus outside of the vagina – complete prolapse.

CLINICAL MANIFESTATIONS
 1. *Pelvic or vaginal fullness, heaviness "falling out" sensation.*
 2. Lower back pain (especially with prolonged standing).
 3. Vaginal bleeding, purulent discharge.
 4. Urinary frequency, urgency, stress incontinence.

PHYSICAL EXAMINATION
• *Bulging mass especially with ↑intrabdominal pressure* (ex. Valsalva).

MANAGEMENT:
 1. **Prophylactic:** *Kegel exercises* (strengthens pelvic floor muscles), weight control.

 2. **Nonsurgical:** pessaries (symptomatic relief), estrogen treatment (improves atrophy).

 3. **Surgical:** Hysterectomy; Uterosacral or sacrospinous ligament fixation.

OVARIAN DISORDERS

FUNCTIONAL OVARIAN CYSTS

- *Follicular cysts* occur when follicles fail to rupture & continue to grow. **Corpus luteal cysts:** fail to degenerate after ovulation. Theca Lutein: excess β-hCG causes hyperplasia of theca interna cells.
- Common in reproductive years (usually unilateral). Most spontaneously resolve within a few weeks.

CLINICAL MANIFESTATIONS
1. *Most are asymptomatic* until they rupture, undergo torsion or become hemorrhagic ⇨ *unilateral RLQ or LLQ pain.* Menstrual changes (abnormal uterine bleeding), dyspareunia.

PHYSICAL EXAMINATION
1. Unilateral pelvic pain/tenderness. May have a mobile palpable cystic adnexal mass.

DIAGNOSIS:
1. **Pelvic US:** Follicular: smooth, thin-walled unilocular. Luteal: complex, thicker-walled with peripheral vascularity. Order β-hCG to rule out pregnancy.

MANAGEMENT:
1. *Supportive: most cysts <8cm are functional* & *usually spontaneously resolve* ⇨ rest, NSAIDs, *repeat ultrasound after 6 weeks.* OCPs ± prevent recurrence but doesn't treat existing ones.
   - If >8 cm/persistent or cysts found postmenopause ⇨ ± laparoscopy or laparotomy.

OVARIAN CANCER

- *2nd MC gynecologic cancer* (after endometrial). *HIGHEST MORTALITY OF ALL GYNECOLOGIC CANCERS.*

RISK FACTORS
⊕ *family hx** ⇨ 7% lifetime risk (Normal 1-2%), *↑# of ovulatory cycles* (infertility, nulliparity, >50y,* late menopause), *BRCA1/BRCA-2* (15-40%), Peutz-Jehgers, Turner's syndrome.

PROTECTIVE FACTORS: *OCPs protective* (↓'es # of ovulatory cycles),* high parity, TAH.

CLINICAL MANIFESTATIONS
Rarely symptomatic until late in disease course (extensive METS). Presents usually 40-60y.
1. Abdominal fullness/distention, back or abdominal pain, early satiety. Urinary frequency.
2. Irregular menses, menorrhagia, postmenopausal bleeding, constipation (intestinal compression).

PHYSICAL EXAMINATION
1. Palpable abdominal or ovarian mass (solid, fixed, irregular), ± *ascites.**
2. Sister Mary Joseph's node: METS to the umbilical lymph nodes.

DIAGNOSIS
1. **Biopsy:** *90% epithelial** (seen especially postmenopausal). Germ cell seen in patients <30y.
2. Transvaginal US useful screening in high-risk patients. Mammography to look for 1ry in breast.

MANAGEMENT
1. **Early stage:** TAH-BSO + selective lymphadenectomy.
2. **Surgery:** tumor debulking. *Serum CA-125 levels used to monitor treatment progress.**
3. **Chemotherapy:** Paclitaxel (Taxol) + Cisplatin or Carboplatin.

BENIGN OVARIAN NEOPLASMS

- In reproductive age, 90% of ovarian neoplasms are benign. Risk of malignancy ↑'es with age. *DERMOID CYSTIC TERATOMAS MC BENIGN OVARIAN NEOPLASM.**

MANAGEMENT: Removal (due to potential risk of torsion or malignant transformation).

POLYCYSTIC OVARIAN SYNDROME (PCOS)

- Endocrine syndrome characterized by triad of ❶*AMENORRHEA* (chronic anovulation)* ❷ *OBESITY** ❸*HIRSUTISM** (androgen excess). PCOS is due to *insulin resistance.** 10% of US population.

PATHOPHYSIOLOGY
- Exact cause unknown but associated with abnormal function of hypothalamus-pituitary-ovarian axis
  ⇨ *↑INSULIN & ↑LH-DRIVEN ↑ IN OVARIAN ANDROGEN PRODUCTION.** Obesity is a risk factor.

CLINICAL MANIFESTATIONS
1. **Menstrual irregularity**: *2ry amenorrhea* (50%), *oligomenorrhea* (70%).
2. **Increased androgen**: *hirsutism** (50%) - coarse hair growth on midline structures (face, neck abdomen), acne, ±male pattern baldness.
3. **Insulin resistance**: *Type II DM, obesity (80%).* Hypertension.

PHYSICAL EXAMINATION
- *Bilateral enlarged, smooth, mobile ovaries* on bimanual examination, *acanthosis nigricans.**
- Cysts are immature follicles with arrested development due to abnormal ovarian function.

DIAGNOSIS
1. Exclude other disorders: thyroid (TSH), pituitary adenoma (prolactin levels), ovarian tumors, Cushing's syndrome (dexamethasone suppression test).
2. **Labs:** *↑testosterone,** ↑DHEA-S (intermediate of testosterone); *LH:FSH ratio ≥3:1** (normal 1.5:1).
3. GnRH agonist stimulation test: rise in serum hydroxyprogesterone.
4. Lipid panel (to check for insulin resistance), glucose tolerance test (for DM).
5. **Pelvic US:** *bilateral enlarged ovaries with peripheral cysts, "string of pearls"** appearance.

MANAGEMENT
1. *Combination OCPs: mainstay of tx.* Normalizes bleeding*, induces regular menses, treats hirsutism *(suppresses androgen)*; ↓LH levels, ↓'es endometrial hyperplasia. Estrogen stimulates hepatic production of sex-hormone binding globulin, reducing androgen levels. Progesterone ↓'es action of testosterone at target organs by receptor antagonism. Avoid androgenic progesterone (avoid Norgestrel or Levonorgestrel).
2. *Anti-androgenic agents for hirsutism*: *Spironolactone** (structurally similar to testosterone but blocks testosterone receptors), *Spironolactone is teratogenic* so must be used with OCPs. May be added if symptoms persist after OCPs. *Leuprolide, Finasteride* are other anti-androgenics.
3. **Infertility:** *Clomiphene* (selective estrogen receptor modulator) gonadotropin reestablishes ovulation in anovulatory women who wish to get pregnant. *Metformin in patients with abnormal LH:FSH ratios may improve menstrual frequency by reducing insulin.*
4. **Lifestyle changes**: diet, exercise, weight loss.
5. **Surgical**: to restore ovulation in patients who desire to have children in whom Clomiphene is ineffective (ex. wedge resection)

COMPLICATIONS:
1. chronic anovulation = ↑ risk for infertility, ↑*endometrial hyperplasia & endometrial carcinoma.** (due to unopposed estrogen); Insulin resistance = ↑risk of atherosclerosis & hypertension.

CERVICAL DISORDERS

PAP SMEAR CERVICAL CYTOLOGY RESULTS

CYTOLOGY (PAP RESULTS)	DESCRIPTION	MANAGEMENT
A) Negative for intraepithelial lesion or malignancy (no neoplasia)	INCLUDES • *Normal Pap smear* • Reactive cellular changes with inflammation, cellular repair, changes associated with IUD, Bacterial Vaginosis, Trichomoniasis	*No HPV ⇨ Follow routine PAP screening:* **If >25y & HPV ⊖ ⇨** 2 options: ❶ cytology & HPV testing in 12 months OR ❷ Genotype for HPV 16,18
B) SQUAMOUS CELL Abnormalities		
ASC-US _Atypical Squamous Cells of Undetermined Significance_	• May be due to multiple reasons. The main goal is to see if HPV related or not. • 70% of ASC-US regresses @ 24 months but HPV+ lesions have higher risk or progression to carcinoma	*If ≥25y 2 possible management options:* HPV testing or repeat PAP: • ❶ *Do HPV testing*.* **HPV Negative ⇨ *repeat PAP & HPV cotesting in 3y;* HPV Positive ⇨ *Colposcopy with biopsy*** • ❷ Repeat PAP in 1y. If negative resume PAP screening colposcopy if positive. 21-24y c ASCUS or LSIL ⇨ repeat PAP in 1y OR HPV testing <21y c ASCUS ⇨ repeat PAP in 1 year
ASC-H _Atypical Squamous Cells can't exclude HSIL (ASC-H)_	• Higher chance of cancer than ASCUS	• *Colposcopy* allows for visualization of cervix using magnification after applying dilute acetic acid for accentuation of lesions.
LSIL: Low grade Squamous Intraepithelial Lesion	• MC associated c cellular changes seen c *transient HPV infection.* • *Includes CIN I* • 50% regress in 24mos May progress to cancer in 7y	• 25-29y ⇨ *Colposcopy with biopsy* **≥30y:** • *HPV Negative ⇨ Repeat cytology in 1 year* • *HPV positive ⇨ Colposcopy with biopsy*
HSIL: High grade Squamous Intraepithelial Lesion	• Include *CIN II, CIN III & Carcinoma in situ*	• *Colposcopy with biopsy in all ages*
C) GLANDULAR CELL Abnormalities		
Atypical Glandular Cells		• Colposcopy for all glandular cells abnormalities. • Glandular abnormalities may be indicative of endometrial neoplasia.
Atypical Glandular Cells favor neoplastic: features suggestive but not sufficient for diagnosis of adenocarcinoma.		
Endocervical Carcinoma in situ, Adenocarcinoma, Endometrial Cells		

CERVICAL BIOPSY HISTOLOGY RESULTS (In follow up of Abnormal Pap Smears)

- *MC associated with HPV.* CIN (Cervical Intraepithelial Neoplasia) is a precursor for cervical carcinoma
- *Transformation zone (squamocolumnar junction) of the cervix highest risk for malignancy (junction of squamous cell of* ectocervix & the glandular columnar cells near of the endocervical canal).

CYTOLOGY (PAP RESULTS)	HISTOLOGY (BX RESULTS)	DESCRIPTION	MANAGEMENT
LSIL: Low grade Squamous **I**ntraepithelial **L**esion (Includes CIN I) Usually results of transient HPV infections (esp in young women). May progress to cancer in 7 years	1. CIN 1	• Cellular changes seen with HPV • **CIN I = MILD dysplasia:** contained to *basal 1/3 of epithelium*	**OPTIONS:** • *Observation:* 75% resolve by immune system within 1y. May be option if <20y • *Excision:* - *LEEP* (Loop Electrical Excision Procedure) - *Cold knife cervical conization* • ± Ablation
HSIL: High grade Squamous **I**ntraepithelial **L**esion: Includes: CIN II, CIN III & Carcinoma in situ HSIL usually from persistent HPV infections. Often p-16 positive.	2. CIN 2	• **CIN II = MODERATE** dysplasia including *2/3 thickness of basal epithelium*	*HSIL lesions (CIN 2 & CIN 3):* excision or ablation mainstay of tx (because of high risk of progression) • *Excision:* - *LEEP (Loop Electrical Excision Procedure)* - *Cold knife cervical conization*
	3. CIN 3	• **SEVERE** dysplasia: *>2/3 – up to full thickness of basal epithelium* • *Full thickness = carcinoma in situ (but has not invaded the basement membrane) – preinvasive cancer*	• *Ablation:* Energy-assisted destruction of lesions via: - *Cryocautery* - *Laser cautery* - *Electrocautery*

CERVICAL CARCINOMA

- *Human papilloma virus associated with 99.7%* especially 16, 18** (70%), *31 & 33,* 45, 52 & 58.

- *3rd MC gynecologic cancer* (#1 = endometrial cancer; #2 = ovarian cancer).

- *45y average age of diagnosis.* MC METS locally: vagina, parametrium, pelvic lymph nodes.

RISK FACTORS:
HPV, early onset of sexual activity, ↑# of partners, smoking, CIN, *DES* exposure (Diethylstilbestrol was a synthetic estrogen used in OCPs), Immunosuppression, STIs.

- **2 TYPES:** *Squamous:* 90%; Adenocarcinoma: 10% *(clear cell carcinoma linked with DES).**

It takes on average 2-10 years for carcinoma to penetrate the basement membrane.

CLINICAL MANIFESTATIONS
- *POST COITAL BLEEDING/SPOTTING* MC SX.* Metrorrhagia. Pelvic pain, ±watery vaginal discharge.

DIAGNOSIS
Colposcopy with biopsy.* Pap smear with cytology used for screening.

MANAGEMENT:

Stage 0	Carcinoma in situ	LOCAL TREATMENT 1. **Excision** (LEEP, Cold knife conization) Excision preferred 2. **Ablation:** (cryotherapy or laser) 3. TAH-BSO
Stage Ia1	Microinvasion	**Surgery:** Conization, TAH-BSO, XRT
Other Stage I, IIA		TAH-BSO; XRT + Chemo tx (Cisplatin)
Stage IIb-Iva	**Locally Advanced:** II: extends locally beyond cervix III: lower $1/3$ of vagina IVa: Local METS (ex bladder, rectum)	Radiation (XRT) + Chemo (Cisplatin ±5FU)
IVb or recurrent	IVb: Distant METS	Palliative radiation therapy, chemotherapy (Surgery is not likely to be curative)

HPV VACCINE & CERVICAL CANCER PREVENTION
Recommendations: *given at age 11 up to 26 years of age.* 2 types.
1. Gardasil: quadrivalent HPV vaccine that targets *HPV 6, 11, 16, 18.*

2. Gardasil 9: targets the same as Gardasil (6, 11, 16, 18) as well as HPV types 31, 33, 45, 52, & 58.

Schedule:
- individual <15y should receive 2 doses of HPV vaccine at least 6 months apart.
- ≥15y should receive *3 doses over a minimum of 6 months.* Classically administered at day 0, at 2 month & at 6 months. Minimum interval between first 2 doses is 4 weeks, minimum interval between the second & 3rd is 12 weeks.

HPV vaccine is contraindicated if immunosuppressed, pregnant or lactating.

CERVICAL CANCER SCREENING GUIDELINES

ORGANIZATION	AGE TO INITIATE	AGE TO DISCONTINUE	Recommended screening test & frequency	
			Age 21 to 29	Age ≥30
ACS/ASCCP/ASCP (2012)	21	65	Pap test every 3years (preferred)	Co-testing (pap test & HPV) q5y (preferred) or Pap every 3years
USPSTF (2012)	21	65	Pap every 3years	Pap every 3years
				Co testing (pap & HPV) every 5 years
ASCCP/SGO (2015)	21	N/A	Can consider primary HPV testing q3y for women ≥25y	Can consider primary HPV testing every 3years
ACP (2015)	21	65	Pap every 3years	Pap every 3years
				Can consider primary HPV testing every 5 years
ACOG (2016)	21	65	Pap every 3years	Co testing (pap & HPV) q5y (preferred).
			Can consider primary HPV testing q3y for women ≥25y	Pap every 3years Can consider primary HPV testing q3y for women ≥25y

ACS=American Cancer Society; ASCCP = American Society for Colposcopy & Cervical pathology; ASCP = American Society for Clinical Pathology; USPSTF = United States Preventive Services Task Force; SGO = Society of Gynecology & Oncology; ACP = American College of Physicians; ACOG: American College of Obstetricians & Gynecologists.

CERVICAL INSUFFICIENCY (INCOMPETENT CERVIX)

- Inability to maintain pregnancy 2ry to **premature cervical dilation (especially in 2nd trimester).**
- **Risk factors:** previous cervical trauma or procedure (ex. treatment for CIN), uterus defects, **DES exposure in utero**, multiple gestations.

CLINICAL MANIFESTATIONS: bleeding, vaginal discharge especially in the 2nd trimester.
PHYSICAL EXAMINATION: *painless dilation & effacement of cervix.*

MANAGEMENT:
1. **Cerclage*** (suturing of cervical os) **and bed rest** especially if prior history. If not performed initially, cerclage can also be performed for women who develop a short cervix (≤25 mm) before 24 weeks as determined by ultrasound surveillance.
2. ± weekly injection of 17 α-hydroxyprogesterone in some women with preterm birth history.

BARTHOLIN CYST/ABSCESS

- Bartholin duct obstruction ⇨ retained secretions ⇨ gland enlargement.
- May be infectious (ex *E. coli, Staphylococcus aureus, Neisseria gonorrhoeae*).

CLINICAL MANIFESTATIONS
- **Infected gland:** *tender,* unilateral vulvar mass, edema/inflammation.
- **Noninfected:** *nontender*, unilateral vulvar mass at Bartholin duct location.

DIAGNOSIS: CBC, cultures.

MANAGEMENT
1. Infected: incision and drainage with antibiotics. No intervention needed for asymptomatic cyst.

VAGINAL AND VULVAR DISORDERS

VAGINAL CANCER

- Rare. 1% of gynecological malignancies (usually secondary to another cancer).
- Peak incidence 60-65y. *Squamous cell 95%.   Clear cell if DES exposure in utero.**

CLINICAL MANIFESTATIONS
- Asymptomatic, changes in menstrual period, abnormal vaginal bleeding, vaginal discharge.
MANAGEMENT:
Radiation therapy

VULVAR CANCER

- *90% Squamous (risks include HPV 16, 18, 31).*   Peak incidence 50y.   Linked to DES exposure.

CLINICAL MANIFESTATIONS
1. *Pruritus MC presentation** (70%), vaginal itching, irritation.
2. Asymptomatic (20%).   Post-coital bleeding, vaginal discharge.

DIAGNOSIS
1. *Red/white ulcerative, crusted lesions.* Biopsy

MANAGEMENT
1. Surgical excision, radiation therapy, chemotherapy (ex 5-fluorouracil).

VAGINITIS

ETIOLOGIES
1. *Infectious:* Bacterial vaginosis, Trichomoniasis, Candida, Cytolytic.
2. *Atrophic:* ex postmenopausal;   Allergic reaction.

CLINICAL MANIFESTATIONS
Vaginal burning, pruritus, pain or discharge. Treatment depends on cause (see page 285).

VULVOVAGINAL ATROPHY

- Seen with ↓estrogen states (ex postmenopausal).
CLINICAL MANIFESTATIONS
Vaginal dryness, dyspareunia, vaginal inflammation, infection & recurrent UTIs with ↑pH (loss of lactobacilli which normally converts glucose to lactic acid).

MANAGEMENT
1. *Vaginal estrogens:* cream, vaginal ring, vaginal troches. MOA: reverses atrophic changes.
   S/E: vaginal bleeding, breast pain, nausea, thromboembolism (CVA, DVT, PE), endometrial cancer.
   Less risk compared to PO estrogen. Estrogen ↑'es hepatic production of coagulation factors.

2. *Ospemifene:* SERM. *Estrogen agonist in the vagina* & bone; Estrogen antagonist in breast, uterus.
3. Vaginal moisturizers: improves symptoms (ex. dyspareunia, dryness) but no effect on atrophy.

MASTITIS & BREAST ABSCESS

Mastitis: inflammation of the breast.
- **Infection**: seen **mostly in lactating women** 2ry to nipple trauma (especially **primagravida**). **S. Aureus MC,*** Strep. ± candida.
- **Congestive:** bilateral breast enlargement 2-3 days postpartum.

CLINICAL MANIFESTATIONS OF MASTITIS
1. **INFECTION**: **unilateral*** breast pain (especially one quadrant) with tenderness, warmth, swelling & nipple discharge.

2. **CONGESTIVE**: **bilateral** breast pain & swelling. May have low grade fever & axillary lymphadenopathy.
3. **BREAST ABSCESS:** induration with fluctuance (due to pus). Rare

MANAGEMENT
1. **Infectious:** **supportive** measures (warm compresses, breast pump) + **Anti-staphylococcal antibiotics:** Dicloxacillin, Nafcillin, Cephalosporin. Fluconazole if fungal.
    - **Mothers may continue to nurse or use breast pump.***

2. **Congestive:** if woman does not want to breastfeed ⇨ ice packs, tight-fitting bras, analgesics, avoid breast stimulation. If breast feeding desired, manually empty breast completely after baby is done breastfeeding, local heat, analgesics, continue nursing.
3. **Breast abscess**: **I & D, discontinue breastfeeding from the affected breast.***

FIBROCYSTIC BREAST DISORDER

Fluid-filled breast cyst due to exaggerated response to hormones. MC breast d/o (esp 30-50y).

CLINICAL MANIFESTATIONS
1. Usually multiple, mobile, well demarcated lumps in breast tissue. Often *TENDER,** bilateral. Usually no axillary involvement nor nipple discharge.
2. **Breast cysts may *INCREASE OR DECREASE IN SIZE WITH MENSTRUAL HORMONAL CHANGES.****

DIAGNOSIS: Ultrasound. Fine needle aspiration (FNA) reveals **straw-colored fluid (no blood).**

MANAGEMENT: Most spontaneously. ±FNA removal of fluid if symptomatic.

FIBROADENOMA OF THE BREAST

2nd MC benign breast disorder. 10-20% of women. MC in late teens to early 20s.
Composed of glandular & fibrous tissue (collagen arranged in "swirls").

CLINICAL MANIFESTATIONS
1. Smooth, well-circumscribed, nontender, freely mobile, rubbery lump in the breast. Gradually grows over time & **DOES NOT USUALLY WAX & WANE WITH MENSTRUATION.*** May enlarge in pregnancy. No axillary involvement nor nipple discharge.

MANAGEMENT
Observation - most small tumors resorb with time. ± Excision (not usually done).

BREAST CANCER

Malignancy primarily of the milk ducts (ductal) or the lobules, which produce the milk.
- MC non-skin malignancy in women. 2nd MC cause of cancer death (after lung).
- 1 in 8 lifetime incidence.

RISK FACTORS: ***BRCA 1 & BRCA 2:*** genetic mutation (associated breast & ovarian CA – lifetime breast cancer 60-85%, ovarian 15-40%), 1st degree relative with breast CA, ***age >65y*** *(>50% occur >65y).* ***Hormonal:*** ↑*# of menstrual* **cycles** (nulliparity, 1st full term pregnancy >35y, early onset of menarche (<12y), late menopause, prolonged unopposed estrogen, never having breast fed. ↑***estrogen:*** postmenopausal HRT & ?OCPs; Obesity, ETOH. ***75% have no risk factors.***

Types:
1. Ductal Carcinoma:
- ***Infiltrative ductal carcinoma MC*** (75%). Associated c lymphatic METS especially axillary.

- Ductal carcinoma in situ (DCIS). Does not penetrate the basement membrane.

2. Lobular Carcinoma: infiltrative lobular carcinoma.
  -lobular carcinoma in situ (may not progress but assoc c ↑risk of invasive breast CA in either breast).

3. Medullary, mucinoid, tubular, papillary, metastatic, mammary Paget's disease of the breast.

CLINICAL MANIFESTATIONS
1. ***Breast mass***: Usually ***painless, hard, fixed (non-mobile) lump*** may be mobile early on. 80% present with mass. 90% found by patient. Pain rare (<10%). ±axillary lymphadenopathy. ***MC in Upper Outer Quadrant*** (65%), areola (18%).

2. ***Unilateral nipple discharge***: ±***bloody,*** purulent or green. METS to lung, liver, bone, brain.

PHYSICAL EXAM:
1. **Skin changes**: *asymmetric* redness, discoloration, ulceration, skin retraction (dimpling if Cooper's ligament involvement), changes in breast size & contour, nipple inversion, skin thickening.

2. **Paget's disease of the nipple**: *chronic **eczematous itchy, scaling rash on the nipples & areola*** (may ooze). <5%. A lump is often present.

3. **Inflammatory breast cancer:** *red, swollen, **warm**, itchy breast*. Often with nipple retraction, peau d'orange. Usually not associated with a lump.
   Peau d'orange = skin changes that looks like the peel of an orange due to ***lymphatic obstruction***. Peau d'orange associated with ***poor prognosis.***

DIAGNOSIS
1. **Mammogram**: ***microcalcifications & spiculated*** masses highly suspicious for malignancy.

2. **Ultrasound:** ***recommended initial modality to evaluate breast masses in women <40y.*** (due to high density of breast tissue). May also be used to guide FNA with biopsy.

3. **Biopsy:** Fine needle with biopsy, large needle core biopsy, open (excisional biopsy).

BREAST CANCER

STAGING: Based on T (size), N = nodes (axillary lymph nodes), M metastasis.
Stage 0: precancerous, DCIS or LCIS
Stage I-III: within breast/regional lymph nodes
Stage IV: metastatic breast cancer

MANAGEMENT
1. **Lumpectomy**: *followed by radiation therapy.* Allows for breast conservation.
2. **Mastectomy**: entire breast removed. Ind: diffuse, large tumor, prior XRT to breast etc.
3. **Removal of regional (axillary) lymph nodes**: to determine if METS present.

Adjunctive:
4. **Radiation Therapy/Chemotherapy:**
   - Radiation Therapy done after lumpectomy & may be done post mastectomy to destroy residual microscopic tumor cells. External beam radiation or brachytherapy (internal).
   - Chemotherapy: used in breast cancers stage II-IV & inoperable disease, especially ER negative disease. Ex: Doxorubicin, Cyclophosphamide, Fluorouracil, Docetaxol.

5. **Neoadjuvant Endocrine Therapy:** (Hormone therapy)
   Breast cancer tumors may be Estrogen receptor (ER) positive, Progesterone receptor (PR) positive as well as HER2 positive.
   - **Anti-estrogen: (*Tamoxifen*):** *Useful in tumors that are ER positive (dependent on estrogen for growth).* MOA: *binds & blocks estrogen receptor in breast tissue.*

   - **Aromatase inhibitors:** useful in postmenopausal ER-positive patients with breast cancer. MOA: reduces the production of estrogen. Ex: *Letrozole, Anastrozole.*

   - **Monoclonal Ab treatment:** *useful in patients with HER2 positivity* (Human Epidermal Growth Factor Receptor). HER2 receptors stimulate cancer growth & are associated with more aggressive tumors. Ex: *Trastuzumab (Herceptin).* S/E: cardiotoxicity.

BREAST CANCER SCREENING
1. **Mammogram**: *best screening test* (detects breast cancer as early as 2 years before a mass can be palpated clinically).
   ACS screening guidelines: annually age 45y-54y & q2y age ≥55y ; ACOG: annually ≥40y
   USPSTF guidelines: baseline mammogram every 2 years 50y-74y. Every 2 years at age 40y if increased risk factors. 10y prior to the age the 1st degree relative was diagnosed.

2. **Clinical Breast Exam:** @ least q3y in women age 20-39y (annually after age 40y).

3. **Breast Self Examination**: monthly ≥20y of age *immediately after menstruation or on days 5-7 of menstrual cycle* - less fluid retention & hormonal influence on breast day 5-7. Not shown to reduce long-term overall mortality.

BREAST CANCER PREVENTION IN HIGH-RISK PATIENTS
SERM: *Tamoxifen or Raloxifene can be used in postmenopausal or women >35y with high risk.*
Treatment usually used for 5 years. Tamoxifen preferred (more effective but increased risk of DVT & endometrial cancer compared to Raloxifene). Aromatase inhibitors are an alternative.

OTHER INFECTIOUS DISORDERS

PELVIC INFLAMMATORY DISEASE

- *Ascending infection of the upper reproductive tract* (may lead to sepsis, ectopic pregnancy or infertility). *Usually mixed: MC N. gonorrhoeae & Chlamydia,* G. vaginalis, anaerobes, H. flu, etc.
- ↑**RISK:** multiple sex partners, unprotected sex, prior PID, age 15-19, nulliparous, IUD placement.

CLINICAL MANIFESTATIONS
Pelvic/lower abdominal pain, dysuria, dyspareunia, vaginal discharge, nausea, vomiting.

PHYSICAL EXAMINATION
1. *Lower abdominal tenderness, fever.   Purulent cervical discharge*, *±bleeding.*
2. ⊕ *CHANDELIER SIGN:* *CERVICAL MOTION TENDERNESS* to palpation & rotation so severe they seem to rise off the bed as if "reaching for the chandelier".

DIAGNOSIS
Primarily a clinical diagnosis. Obtain a β-hCG to rule out ectopic pregnancy.
1. ❶ *abdominal tenderness* (±rebound tenderness if severe) + ❷*cervical motion tenderness* + ❸ *adnexal tenderness* plus ≥1 of the following:
    - ⊕ gram stain, temperature >38° C, WBC >10,000, pus on culdocentesis or laparoscopy, pelvic abnormality on bimanual exam or ultrasound, ↑ESR, CRP.
2. Pelvic ultrasound: may be used if adnexal or abscess suspected.
3. Laparoscopy may be done in uncertain cases, severe disease or if no improvement c antibiotics.

MANAGEMENT
1. **Outpatient:** *Doxycycline* (100mg bid x 14d) + *Ceftriaxone** (250mg IM x1) ±Metronidazole.

2. **Inpatient:** *IV Doxycycline + 2nd generation cephalosporin* (ex. *Cefoxitin or Cefotetan*) OR Clindamycin + Gentamicin.

COMPLICATIONS
1. FITZ-HUGH CURTIS SYNDROME: hepatic fibrosis/scarring & peritoneal involvement. *RUQ pain due to PERIHEPATITIS (liver capsule involvement).* May radiate to the right shoulder. Often have normal LFTs. "Violin-string" adhesions on the anterior liver surface.
2. Infertility, Tubo ovarian abscess, ectopic pregnancy & chronic pelvic pain.

TOXIC SHOCK SYNDROME

- Exotoxins produced by *S. Aureus* - May be seen *c tampon use, diaphragm or sponge esp >24h.*

CLINICAL MANIFESTATIONS
1. *High fever* sudden onset (≥39°C/102.2°F), tachycardia, N/V/diarrhea, pharyngitis.

2. *Skin:* erythroderma = *diffuse erythematous macular rash** (resembles sunburn – includes palms & soles), desquamation. Severe: ulcerations, petechiae, vesicles, bullae.
3. *Hypotension*, abdominal tenderness, headache, myalgias, multisystemic involvement.

DIAGNOSIS: CBC, cultures, clinical. Isolation of organism NOT required.

MANAGEMENT
1. Hospital admission, supportive measures (fluid replacement). Clindamycin + Vancomycin.

	BACTERIAL VAGINOSIS	TRICHOMONIASIS	CANDIDA	CYTOLYTIC VAGINITIS
PATHO PHYSIOLOGY	• Decreased Lactobacilli acidophilus (normally maintains vaginal pH) ⇨ overgrowth of normal flora ex *GARDNERELLA VAGINALIS*, anaerobes (Mobiluncus, Peptostreptococcus)* • *MC cause of vaginitis**	• *TRICHOMONAS VAGINALIS:* pear shaped flagellated protozoa • Sexually transmitted	• *Candida albicans overgrowth* (part of the normal flora due to change in normal vaginal environment (ex. use of abx) • ↑c DM, steroid, pregnancy	• *Overgrowth of LACTOBACILLI*
CLINICAL MANIFESTATIONS	• Vaginal odor worse after sex • ± Pruritus • >50% asymptomatic	• Vulvar pruritus, erythema, dysuria • Dyspareunia	• Vaginal & vulvar erythema, swelling, burning, pruritus • Burning when urine touches skin, Dysuria, Dyspareunia	• Vaginal or vulvar pruritus & burning • Dysuria
VAGINAL DISCHARGE	• Copious discharge • *Thin, homogenous, watery GREY-WHITE "FISH ROTTEN"* smell*	• Copious malodorous discharge • *FROTHY YELLOW GREEN DISCHARGE** worse c menses • *STRAWBERRY CERVIX*: (cervical petechiae)*	• *THICK CURD-LIKE/COTTAGE CHEESE DISCHARGE**	Nonodorous discharge white to opaque
VAGINAL pH	>5	>5	Normal (3.8- 4.2)	Normal (3.8- 4.2)
WHIFF TEST	Positive: *FISHY ODOR** with 10% KOH Prep	May be present	Negative	Copious lactobacilli Large # of epithelial cells
MICROSCOPIC	• *CLUE CELLS:* epithelial cells covered by bacteria. • *Few WBC's,* few lactobacilli	• Mobile protozoa (wet mount) • WBC's	• *HYPHAE, YEAST** & spores on KOH prep	
MANAGEMENT	• *METRONIDAZOLE* (Flagyl) x 7 days - Safe in pregnancy - May use gel or PO • *CLINDAMYCIN* - May use gel or PO	• *METRONIDAZOLE* (Flagyl) - *2g oral x 1 dose* OR - 500mg bid oral x 7days - Safe in pregnancy - *Oral preferred* • *TINIDAZOLE*	• *FLUCONAZOLE* (PO x 1 dose) • *Intravaginal antifungals* - Clotrimazole, Nystatin - Butoconazole - Miconazole	• *Discontinue tampon usage* (to decrease vaginal acidity) • *Sodium Bicarbonate* - Sitz bath with NaHCO3 - Douche with NaHCO3
PREVENTION	• *Avoid douching* - Douching promotes loss of Lactobacilli • *Treating partner unnecessary* - Unclear if sexually transmitted. - But reduced recurrence if male uses condoms	• *Spermicidal agents:* ex. nonoxynol 9 reduces transmission *MUST TREAT PARTNER*	• Keep vagina dry, 100% cotton underwear, avoid tight-fitting clothes, avoid use of feminine deodorants & bubble baths	
COMPLICATIONS	Pregnancy- PROM, preterm labor, chorioamnionitis.	Perinatal complications, ↑HIV transmission		

	CHLAMYDIA	GONORRHEA	CHANCROID	HUMAN PAPILLOMA VIRUS
ETIOLOGY	• *CHLAMYDIA TRACHOMATIS* • *MC cause of cervicitis* • Causes LGV in developing countries (rare in US).	• *NEISSERIA GONORRHOEAE* • IP 3-5d	• *HAEMOPHILUS DUCREYI* – Gram-negative bacillus • Uncommon in US • IP 3-5 days	• ↑*Oncogenic: 16 & 18,* 31, 33, 35 Also causes genital warts • Genital warts: 6, 11 have low oncogenic potential
CLINICAL	• May be asymptomatic • Mucopurulent cervicitis • Increased frequency, dysuria • Abdominal pain PID, post coital bleeding • LGV: *PAINLESS genital ulcer* ⇨ *PAINFUL inguinal LAD**	• May be asymptomatic • Vaginal discharge, cervicitis • Increased frequency, dysuria	• Genital Ulcer: soft, shallow *painful*, may have foul discharge from the ulcer • ±small vesicles or papules • *PAINFUL inguinal LAD** LAD = lymphadenopathy	• May be asymptomatic • *Flat, pedunculated or papular flesh-colored growths* "cauliflower like" lesions ± postcoital bleeding
DIAGNOSIS	• *Nucleic acid amplification* (ex. *PCR test most spp/sensitive).** • Cultures, DNA probe	• *Nucleic acid amplification* (ex. *PCR test most specific/sensitive).** • Cultures, DNA probe	• Clinical Diagnosis • Cultures	• *Whitening with 4% acetic acid application** • Clinical diagnosis • ±Colposcopy, biopsy (look for dysplasia or cancer)
MANAGEMENT	*Azithromycin** 1g PO x 1 dose OR *Doxycycline** 100mg PO bidx10 d 2nd line • Erythromycin, Ofloxacin, levofloxacin • *Co-treat for gonorrhea* (coinfection 30-40%) - *Ceftriaxone 250mg IM x 1*	• *Ceftriaxone 250mg IM x 1* * 2nd line • Cefixime • Azithromycin 2g can also be given as an alternative but associated with GI sx. *Co-treat for chlamydia* (coinfection 30-40%) - *Azithromycin** 1g PO x 1 or - *Doxycycline** x10 days	• *Azithromycin** • Ceftriaxone 250mg IM x 1 dose • Erythromycin • Ciprofloxacin	OFFICE TREATMENT • Trichloroacetic acid • Podophyllin – wash off after 4h to minimize irritation. Not used on bleeding lesions • Cryotherapy • Surgical removal OUTPATIENT • Podofilox • Imiquimod (Aldara)
PREVENTION	Avoid sexual intercourse 7 days after treatment			
COMPLICATIONS	• PID, infertility, ectopic pregnancy, premature labor. • Reactive arthritis	• PID, infertility, ectopic pregnancy • Reactive arthritis	• 2ry infections • Scarring	• Cervical Dysplasia • *Cervical Cancer*

HORMONAL CONTRACEPTION

METHOD	DETAILS	FAILURE RATE (Average)	STI PROTECTION	PROS	CONS
COMBINATION OCP's Estrogen + Progesterone	• Prevents ovulation by inhibiting mid cycle LH surge. • Thickens cervical mucosa • Thins endometrium	• 9% • 0.3 % when used correctly	No	• *Improves dysmenorrhea, controls menstrual cycle* • Protection vs. osteoporosis, ovarian cysts, ovarian cancer & endometrial cancer* • Improves acne • Less PID & ectopic pregnancy	• *Smokers should stop OCPs >35y** • *Gallstones, ↑fluid retention, ↑thromboembolism -DVT/PE* • Estrogen: breast tenderness, headache, hypertension. • **Caution in biliary disease, DM, hyperlipidemia,** *liver disease*
COMBINATION OCP's Estrogen + Progestin *(Drospirenone)*	• *As above* • *Anti-mineralocorticoid*	• Similar to combination OCPs	No	• *APPROVED FOR PMDD** • *Helps with bloating* (H₂O retention) during menses	• *CI in women with liver or kidney or adrenal disease*
Progestin only (No Estrogen)	• *"Mini pill"* • Inhibits ovulation • Changes endometrium • Alters ovum transport • Thickens cervical mucus	• Similar to combination OCPs	No	• *SAFE DURING LACTATION (less CI),* • *No estrogenic S/E (headache, HTN, nausea).* Can be used in women >35 years • ↓ovarian & endometrial CA • Less PID (thick cervical mucus)	• *Menstrual irregularities* • *Slightly less effective than combo OCPs* • Slightly higher risk of ectopic than combined OCPs
LONG ACTING PROGESTINS	• *Implanon* (single rod) implanted *Etonogestrel*	• 0.05%	• No	• *Lasts 3 YEARS* • Same benefits as progestins	• Same S/E as progestin pills *Osteoporosis**
	• *Depo Provera Injectable Medroxyprogesterone*	• 5%	• No	• *Lasts 3 MONTHS*	• Same S/E as progestin pills
ORTHO EVRA	• *Transdermal patch* • Norelgestromin/ethinyl estradiol	• 10%	• No	• *Applied every week x 3weeks ⇨ 1 week off* • Better compliance	• 1 week of withdrawal bleeding • Less effective if patient is underweight
NUVARING	• *Flexible plastic vaginal ring* • *Etonogestrel/estradiol*	• 7%	• No	• *Applied 3 week, 1 week off*	• Must be removed during intercourse (but must be replaced within 3 hours) • Withdrawal bleeding

METHOD	DESCRIPTION	FAILURE RATE (Average)	STI PROTECTION	ADVANTAGES	DISADVANTAGES
NATURAL FAMILY PLANNING	• *Abstain from sex during fertile period* - Body temperature - Cervical mucus - Calendar - Urine progestin test	• Up to 25%	No		
COITUS INTERRUPTUS	• Male withdraws penis from vagina before ejaculation	• 20%	No		• Sperm in pre-ejaculatory fluid can lead to pregnancy.
SPERMICIDE: Nonoxynol-9	• *Destroys sperm*	• 27%	Slight ↑risk of HIV	• *Often used with other forms* ex. condoms	• Slight ↑risk of HIV (causes microabrasions).

BARRIER METHOD CONTRACEPTION

METHOD	DESCRIPTION	FAILURE RATE (Average)	STI PROTECTION	ADVANTAGES	DISADVANTAGES
MALE CONDOMS	• Latex, polyurethane & lambskin	• 20%	Yes		• Decreased sensitivity during intercourse.
FEMALE CONDOMS	• Polyurethane with 2 rings to keep in place	• 21%	Yes		• Decreased sensitivity during intercourse
DIAPHRAGM	• Rubber cuplike device that holds spermicide against cervix	• 15%	±	• No systemic side effects • Protects against pelvic infection & cervical dysplasia	• Must remain in place 6-24h after intercourse. • *Requires Pelvic exam & fitting* • *↑Risk of TSS*, cystitis.
FEM CAP	• Silicone rubber cap with strap - covers cervix	• 14%	±	• *No fitting required by health care professional* • *No additional spermicide needed between intercourse*	• ↑*Risk of TSS* if left too long.
CONTRACEPTIVE SPONGE	• Polyurethane sponge with nonoxynol-9	• Nulliparous 12% • Parous 24%	±	• Insert few hours prior	• Must be left in place @ least 6h but no longer than 24h • *Risk of TSS if left too long*

Barrier methods prevents sperm from entering though the cervix

METHOD	DESCRIPTION	FAILURE RATE (Average)	STI PROTECTION	ADVANTAGES	DISADVANTAGES
EMERGENCY CONTRACEPTION (PLAN B)	• Levonorgestrel - (2) 0.75mg tablets 12 hours apart or - 1.5 mg x 1 dose	• Up to 25%	No	*Beneficial if taken within 72h of unprotected sexual intercourse*	*Seek medical attention of no menses initiated 21d after tx* **Doesn't work if already pregnant**
INTRAUTERINE DEVICE (IUD)	• _Mirena:_ levonorgestrel	• 0.2%	No	• *5 YEARS duration of action* • *IUDs most effective form of contraception (besides sterility & abstinence)**	• Placement/removal by HCP • Similar progestin S/E • ↑Risk of PID
	• _Paragard:_ Copper	• 0.8%	No	• *10 YEARS duration of action*	• ↑Risk of PID
STERILIZATION	• _Tubal ligation_	• 0.5%	No	• Permanent	• Surgery, difficult to reverse • ↑Risk of ectopic pregnancy
	• Essure: chemicals or coils to scar portion of Fallopian tubes	• 0.5%	No	• Can be done as in an office procedure	• Difficult to reverse • ↑Risk of ectopic pregnancy

GYN MEDICATIONS

CLOMIPHENE
- **MOA:** partial estrogen receptor agonist (stimulates ovulation via hypothalamus) ⇨ ↑LH & FSH release.
- **Indications:** *induces ovulation in patients with infertility & Polycystic Ovarian Syndrome.*
- **S/E:** toxicity ⇨ ovarian enlargement, multiple gestation pregnancy, hot flashes, visual changes.

GnRH ANALOG LEUPROLIDE (ex. Lupron Depot)
- **MOA:** GnRH analog.
  - _GnRH agonist:_ if given **pulsatile** (natural way the body releases GnRH): *used in infertility.*
  - _GnRH antagonist:_ if given **continuously:** *uterine fibroids* (↓'es estrogen), *prostate Cancer* (↓testosterone), *DUB, PMS.* Continuous dose interrupts normal pulsatile stimulation ⇨ downregulation of FSH &LH ⇨ ↓testosterone & estrogen.
- **S/E:** *hot flashes, depression, osteopenia if given continuously (because ↓'es estrogen).*

PROGESTIN (Ex. Medroxyprogesterone)
- **MOA:** progesterone receptor agonist ⇨ ↓endometrial proliferation, stabilizes endometrium, thickens cervical mucus.
- **Indications:** *Safe OCP in lactating women, abnormal uterine bleeding* (stabilizes endometrium), *Endometrial hyperplasia* (inhibits hyperplasia), OCPs (added to estrogen to prevent unopposed estrogen action on endometrium). **S/E: bone loss.**

ESTROGEN ONLY
- **MOA:** estrogen receptor agonist. *Not usually used orally in women with intact uterus* (↑*risk of endometrial cancer).**
- **Indication:** hypogonadism/ovarian failure, HRT to treat menopausal sx (vaginal atrophy, hot flashes).

DANAZOL
- **MOA:** *hypoestrogenic & hyperandrogenic* ⇨ endometrial atrophy.
- **S/E:** (due to ↑testosterone) – weight gain, acne, hirsutism, virilization.
- **Indications:** *endometriosis* (suppresses LH/FSH production), fibrocystic breast disease, hereditary angioedema

SELECTIVE ESTROGEN RECEPTOR MODULATORS
Tamoxifen
- **MOA:** *estrogen antagonist in breast;*   *Estrogen agonist in endometrium & bone, liver & coagulation system.*
- **Indication:** breast cancer adjuvant tx. *Breast cancer prevention* in high-risk patients. Postmenopausal osteoporosis prevention.
- **S/E:** ↑*risk of endometrial cancer* (unopposed estrogen), ↑*DVT,* induces menopause (so it can cause hot flashes).

Raloxifene
- **MOA:** *estrogen antagonist in breast AND endometrium; Estrogen agonist in bone.*
- **Indications:** *postmenopausal osteoporosis prevention* (HRT), *breast cancer prevention* (↓'es risk of breast cancer) ↑DVT (DVT risk less than seen with Tamoxifen), can cause hot flashes.
- **S/E:** weight gain, acne, hirsutism, virilization.

UNCOMPLICATED PREGNANCY

UNCOMPLICATED PREGNANCY

DIAGNOSIS
- <u>Serum β-hCG</u>: serum quantitative can detect pregnancy as early as 5 days after conception.
- <u>Urine β-hCG</u>: can detect pregnancy 14 days after conception; ↑Serum progesterone.

PHYSICAL EXAMINATION
- **Uterus changes**
  - ***Ladin's sign:*** uterus softening after 6 weeks.
  - **Hegar's sign**: uterine isthmus softening after 6-8 weeks gestation.
  - **Piskacek's sign**: palpable lateral bulge or softening of uterine cornus 7-8 weeks gestation.
- **Cervix changes**
  - **Goodell's sign:** cervical softening due to increased vascularization ~4-5 weeks gestation.
  - Chadwick's sign: bluish coloration of the cervix & vulva ~8-12 weeks.
- <u>Fetal heart tones</u>: 10-12 weeks (towards the end of the 1st trimester). Normal is 120-160bpm.
- <u>Pelvic ultrasound</u>: detects fetus ~5-6 weeks.
- <u>Fetal movement</u>: 16-20 weeks (quickening).

GPA CLASSIFICATION

- **Gravida:** # of times pregnant (regardless if carried to term).
- **Para:** # of births (>20 weeks) including viable or nonviable births (ex. stillbirth). Multiple gestations (ex twins) count as 1 for notation.
- **Abortus:** # of pregnancies lost for whatever reason (miscarriages, abortions).

<u>Ex:</u> G_3P_3 = 3 pregnancies 3 births. $G_4P_3A_1$ = 4 pregnancies, 3 births, 1 miscarriage (or abortion).

FUNDAL HEIGHT MEASUREMENT

12 weeks	above the pubic symphysis
16 weeks	midway between the pubis & umbilicus
20 weeks	***at the umbilicus***
38 weeks	2-3 cm below the xiphoid process

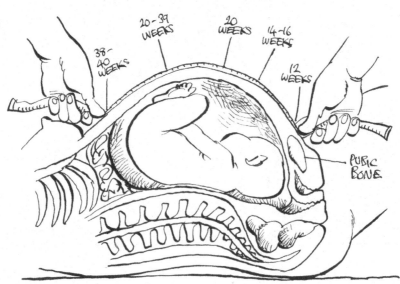

MEASURING FUNDAL HEIGHT

PRENATAL CARE

ESTIMATED DATE OF DELIVERY (EDD) – NAEGELE'S RULE
- *1ST day of last menstrual period plus 7 days subtract 3 months*
  Example: LMP 8/7/16   EDD: 5/14/17

ROUTINE TESTS DURING FIRST PRENATAL VISIT
- Blood pressure, blood type & Rh, CBC, UA (glucose & protein), random glucose, HBsAg, HIV & syphilis, rubella titer, screening for sickle cell & cystic fibrosis. Pap smear.

FIRST TRIMESTER SCREENING/TESTS

Week 1 – 12 of pregnancy
1. **Maternal blood screening tests:**
   - Down syndrome screening may be performed (3 markers):
     Free β-hCG: abnormally high or low may be indicative of abnormalities.
     PAPP-A: usually low with fetal Down syndrome.
     _   PAPP-A = serum pregnancy-associated plasma protein-A.
     Nuchal translucency (ultrasound at 10-13 weeks): ↑thickness is abnormal.
   - **Uterine size & gestation:** if abnormal, chorionic villus sampling (CVS) or amniocentesis can be offered at around 10-13 weeks.

2. **Ultrasound:**
   - Fetal heart tones usually heard around 10-12 weeks by Doppler.
   - Heartbeat at 5-6 weeks via ultrasound of fetus.

3. **Chorionic villus sampling:** may be performed ~10-13 weeks. May be offered to women including those with a prior child with a chromosomal abnormality, maternal age >35y, abnormal 1st or 2nd trimester maternal screening tests, abnormal ultrasound, prior pregnancy losses.
   - Advantage: allows for the option of early termination of the pregnancy if abnormalities are found.
   - Disadvantage: performing it increases the risk of spontaneous abortion.

SECOND TRIMESTER SCREENING/TESTS

Week 13 – 27 of pregnancy
1. *TRIPLE SCREENING*: measured at *15-20 weeks*: ❶α-fetoprotein (α-FP), ❷ β-hCG ❸ estradiol.

α-FP	β-hCG	Estradiol	Diagnosis
Low	*High*	*Low*	*Down Syndrome (Trisomy 21).**
High	N/A	N/A	*Open neural tube defects ex. spina bifida* (or multiple gestation).
Low	Low	Low	Trisomy 18: often born stillborn or die within the 1st year of life.

2. Inhibin-A: high levels may be indicative of chromosomal abnormalities.
3. **Ultrasound:** used to check amniotic fluid level, fetal viability & growth for gestational age.

4. **Amniocentesis:** may be offered to women including those with a prior child with a chromosomal abnormality, maternal age >35y, abnormal 1st or 2nd trimester maternal screening tests, abnormal ultrasound, prior pregnancy losses (same indications as CVS). Usually performed ~15-18 weeks gestation.
5. **Gestational diabetes screening:** *24 – 28 weeks.*

THIRD TRIMESTER SCREENING/TESTS

Week 28 until birth

1. Gestational diabetes screening: 24 – 28 weeks.

2. Repeat antibody titers: in unsensitized Rh negative mothers followed by:
   RhoGAM: @ 28 weeks & within 72 hours after childbirth.*

3. **Group B Streptococcus screening**: at 32-37 weeks (via vaginal-rectal culture).

4. Hemoglobin & Hematocrit: 35 weeks.

5. Biophysical profile: looks at 5 variables including: fetal breathing, fetal tones, amniotic fluid levels, NST & gross fetal movements. 2 points each (maximum score of 10 points).

6. Non Stress Testing
   NON STRESS Testing: baseline fetal heart rate is 120 – 160 bpm.

	DEFINITION	PROGNOSIS	MANAGEMENT
REACTIVE NST	• **≥2 Accelerations in 20 minutes** • **↑Fetal heart rate** ≥15 bpm from baseline lasting ≥15 seconds	• **Fetal well being**	• Repeat weekly or biweekly
NONREACTIVE	• **No fetal heart rate accelerations** **or** ≤15bpm lasting ≤15 seconds	• Sleeping, immature or compromised fetus	• Vibratory stimulation • May try contraction stress

CONTRACTION STRESS TEST: measures fetal response to stress @ times of uterus contraction.

	DEFINITION	PROGNOSIS	MANAGEMENT
NEGATIVE CST	• **No late decelerations** in the presence of 3 contractions in 10 minutes	• **Fetal well being**	• Repeat CST as needed
POSITIVE CST	• **Repetitive late decelerations** in the presence of 3 contractions in 10 minutes	• Worrisome especially if nonreactive NST	• Prompt delivery

INFERTILITY

- **Failure to conceive after 1 year** of regular unprotected sexual intercourse. 60% of couples achieve pregnancy in 1st 3 years in the absence of a cause for infertility.

ETIOLOGIES
Male: 40% of causes (ex abnormal spermatogenesis).
Female: anovulatory cycles or ovarian dysfunction 30%, congenital or acquired disorders.

DIAGNOSIS
- **Hysterosalpingography: helps evaluate tubal patency or abnormalities.**

MANAGEMENT
1. **Clomiphene:* induces ovulation.** Amenorrhea or Oliguria: correct endocrine problems.
2. Intrauterine insemination.
3. In vitro fertilization (especially if fallopian tube defect is present).

COMPLICATIONS OF PREGNANCY

ECTOPIC PREGNANCY

- ***Implantation of fertilized ovum outside of the uterine cavity.***
  Fallopian tube MC* (especially ***ampulla***) 98.3%, abdomen 1.4%, ovarian/cervix 0.15% each
- **RISK FACTORS:**
  High: previous abdominal or tubal surgery (***due to adhesions***), pelvic inflammatory disease, previous ectopic, history of tubal ligation, endometriosis, IUD use, assisted reproduction.
  Intermediate: infertility, history of genital infections, multiple partners.

CLINICAL MANIFESTATIONS
1. **Classic Triad:** ❶ ***unilateral pelvic/abdominal pain*** ❷ ***vaginal bleeding*** & ❸***amenorrhea (pregnancy).*** ***Can also be seen with threatened abortion*** (threatened MC than ectopic).
2. Atypical: vague sx, menstrual irregularities. Severe abdominal/shoulder pain (peritonitis).

3. **Ruptured/Rupturing Ectopic**: severe abdominal pain, dizziness, nausea, vomiting.
   Signs of shock (from hemorrhage): syncope, tachycardia, hypotension.

PHYSICAL EXAMINATION
- ***Cervical motion tenderness, adnexal mass.*** ±Mild uterine enlargement.

DIAGNOSIS
1. **SERIAL quantitative β-hCG**: should double q24-48h. In ectopic, serial β-hCG fails to double (rises <66% expected, decreases or plateaus). If initial value <1,500 ⇨ repeat q2-3 days.

2. **Transvaginal Ultrasound:** presence (or absence) of pregnancy within or outside uterus.
   Absence of gestational sac with β-hCG levels >2,000 strongly suggest ectopic OR nonviable intrauterine pregnancy (IUP).

3. Culdocentesis: nonclotted blood present. Not done often.
4. Laparoscopy: to diagnose (not used often as a diagnostic tool).

MANAGEMENT
1. **UNRUPTURED/STABLE:**
   a. ***Methotrexate:**** MOA: ***destroys trophoblastic tissue*** (disrupts cell multiplication).
      Indications: *hemodynamically stable, early gestation <4cm, β-hCG <5,000, no fetal tones.**
      - Multiple dose: Methotrexate + Leucovorin x 4 doses. β-hCG monitoring day 0 then odd-numbered days. Successful if β-hCG drops ≥ 15% between 2 successive draws.
      - Single dose or Double Dose: monitor β-hCG on days 0,4, 7. Should drop ≥15% by day 4-7.

      Contraindications: *ruptured ectopic, h/o TB*, β-hCG >5,000, ⊕fetal heart tones, noncompliant.

   b. Laparoscopic salpingostomy or salpingectomy if the patient prefers a surgical procedure.
   c. ***RhoGAM*** administration ***if mother is Rh negative.**** Use contraception for at least 2 months.

2. **RUPTURED/UNSTABLE:**
   a. ***Laparoscopic salpingostomy***: ***1st choice**** to remove ectopic gestation (may need reparative procedure to save reproductive organs). Salpingectomy. Laparotomy in severe cases.
   b. RhoGAM administration if mother is Rh negative & unsensitized.

SPONTANEOUS ABORTION

- *Termination of pregnancy BEFORE 20 WEEKS** (MC during 1ST 7 weeks). **Threatened is the only one associated with possible fetal viability.**
- **ETIOLOGIES:** *fetal chromosomal abnormalities MC** (50% of all cases), maternal infection, uterine defects, endocrine abnormalities, malnutrition, immunologic (ex. antiphospholipid syndrome), physical trauma, smoking, drug use etc.

	DEFINITION	PRODUCTS OF CONCEPTION	CERVICAL OS	CLINICAL MANIFESTATION	MANAGEMENT
THREATENED	• *Pregnancy may be viable (progress) or abortion may follow* • MC cause of 1st trimester bleeding	• *No POC expelled from uterus*	• Closed	• **Bloody vaginal discharge** - Spotting ⇔ profuse - ±contractions of uterus. - Uterus size compatible with dates.	• *Supportive:* rest @ home, return to ER if symptoms persist or passage of POC • *Serial β-hCG to see if doubling* • RhoGAM if indicated
INEVITABLE	• Pregnancy not salvageable	• *No POC expelled*	• *Progressive cervix DILATION** >3cm, effaced ± rupture of membranes	• Moderate bleeding >7d • Mod-severe uterus cramping • Uterus size compatible with dates	• **Dilation & Evacuation (D&E)** 2nd trimester • Suction curettage in 1st trimester • RhoGAM if indicated
INCOMPLETE	• Pregnancy not salvageable	• *Some POC expelled some still retained*	• DILATED*	• Heavy **bleeding** • Mod-severe cramping • **Retained tissue** • **Boggy Uterus**	• May be allowed to finish. • **D&E** after 1st. (D&C in 1st) • **Pitocin** • RhoGAM if indicated
COMPLETE	Complete passage of all products	• *All POC expelled from uterus*	• Usually closed	• Pain, cramps & bleeding usually subsides. • Pre pregnancy size of uterus	• RhoGAM if indicated
MISSED	• *Fetal demise but still retained in uterus*	• *No POC expelled*	• Closed	• Loss of pregnancy sx • ±brown discharge	• *D&E.* (D&C if 1st trimester) • *Misoprostol*
SEPTIC	• *The retained POC becomes infected ⇔ infection of uterus & organs*	• *Some POC retained*	• Closed • **Cervical motion tenderness**	• **Foul brownish discharge, fevers, chills** • Uterine tenderness • Spotting ⇔ heavy bleed	• *D&E to remove POC + Broad spectrum Antibiotics* • ±Hysterectomy if refractory

ELECTIVE (INDUCED) ABORTION

MEDICAL: Mifepristone ⇔ Misoprostol 24-72h after (safe up to 9 weeks); Methotrexate ⇔ Misoprostol 3-7d later (safe up to 7 weeks).
- *Mifepristone* (RU-486) is an anti-progestin. *Methotrexate* = antimetabolite (folic antagonist).
- *Misoprostol:* prostaglandin that causes uterine contractions.

SURGICAL: can be performed up to 24 weeks from LMP
- **D & C: *Dilation & Curettage (including suction curettage).*** Used during *4-12 weeks gestation.*
- **D & E: *Dilation & Evacuation: >12 weeks gestation.***

HYPERTENSION DURING PREGNANCY

- *Unknown etiology but all are cause by maternal vasospasm.* Newly elevated BP + protein during pregnancy after 20 weeks.

	TRANSITIONAL (GESTATIONAL) HTN	PREECLAMPSIA	ECLAMPSIA	CHRONIC/PREEXISTING HTN
DEFINITION	• *HTN no proteinuria AFTER 20 WEEKS gestation* - *resolves 12 weeks post partum*	• *HTN + PROTEINURIA* ± edema AFTER 20 WEEKS gestation* - *±earlier in multiple gestation or molar pregnancy*	• *SEIZURES OR COMA* in patients who meet preeclampsia criteria - *Life threatening for mother & fetus*	• *HTN BEFORE 20 weeks gestation or before pregnancy.* - Persists >6w postpartum
CLINICAL MANIFESTATIONS	• *Asymptomatic*	• Sx of HTN: headache, visual symptoms • Fetal growth restriction. Edema caused by proteinuria ⇨ ↓oncotic pressure	• *Abrupt tonic-clonic seizures* 1-2min ⇨ postictal state.* ± headache, visual changes, cardiorespiratory arrest	• Sx of HTN: headache, visual symptoms if severe
DIAGNOSIS	• ↑BP + no proteinuria HTN thought to be due to arteriolar vasoconstriction	**MILD:** BP ≥140/90* - 2 separate occasions @ least 6h apart (but no >1 week apart) - *Proteinuria:* ≥300mg/24h (or >⊕1 on dipstick) **SEVERE:** BP ≥160/110* - *Proteinuria*: ≥5g/24h (>⊕3 on dipstick). - Oliguria: <500ml/24h - *Thrombocytopenia. ± DIC* - *HELLP syndrome*:* Hemolytic Anemia, Elevated Liver enzymes, low Platelets - Sx of HTN: headache, visual sx	• *Same as preeclampsia + seizures* • Hyperreflexia	**MILD:** BP ≥140/90* - 2 separate occasions @ least 6h apart (but no >1 week apart) - *No proteinuria* • Moderate: ≥150/100 • Severe: ≥160/110
MANAGEMENT	• May withhold meds • ±Hydralazine or Labetalol	**MILD** • *DELIVERY at ≥37 weeks* gestation • **Conservative:** if *<34 weeks*: daily weights, BP & dipstick weekly, bedrest. - *Steroids to mature lungs if <34w* & elective delivery is planned. **SEVERE** • *PROMPT DELIVERY ONLY CURE* PLUS • **Hospitalization:** *Magnesium sulfate* (prevent eclampsia/seizures) • BP meds: in acute severe HTN (may be started lower in some cases) –*Hydralazine*, Labetalol, Nifedipine*	• *ABCD's 1st!* • **Magnesium Sulfate:** for seizures. Lorazepam 2nd line (ONLY if refractory to tx) • *Delivery of fetus: once patient is stabilized* • BP meds: Hydralazine, Labetalol	**MILD:** - Monitor q2-4weeks ⇧ weekly @34-36w ⇧ ±delivery @ ≥37 weeks - Weekly NST during 3rd trimester, serial BP and urine protein. • **MODERATE/SEVERE:** Meds if BP ≥150/100 - *Methyldopa tx of choice* - *Labetalol* (β-blocker) - Hydralazine - Nifedipine (CCB) - *Avoid ACEI* & diuretics*

	PLACENTA PREVIA	ABRUPTIO PLACENTAE	VASA PREVIA

DEFINITION	• *Abnormal placenta placement on or close to the cervical os*
	• **Partial:** covering of cervix ahead of fetal presenting part
	• **Complete:** total coverage of the cervical os
	• **Marginal:** within 2-3 cm of the cervical os
		• *Premature separation of placenta from uterine wall* after 20 weeks gestation.
		• *Bloody vaginal discharge*
		  - I: mild, slight bleeding
		  - II: moderate/partial
		  - III: complete (↑risk to fetus & mother)
			• *Fetal vessels traverse the fetal membranes over the cervical os*

CLINICAL MANIFESTATIONS	• *3rd trimester bleeding – sudden onset of PAINLESS* bleeding (bright red) 20-30w. Resolves within 1-2 hours. • *NO ABDOMINAL PAIN; uterine soft NONTENDER*	• *3rd trimester bleeding – continuous often dark red* • *SEVERE ABDOMINAL PAIN* (painful uterine contractions), rigid uterus* ±back, abdominal pain, shock symptoms	• Rupture of membranes ⇨ *PAINLESS vaginal bleed.*
FETAL HEART RATE	• *Normal** (no fetal distress usually).	• *Fetal bradycardia** (fetal distress because interferes with fetal oxygenation)	• *Fetal bradycardia** *(fetal distress)*
DIAGNOSIS	• **Pelvic ultrasound:** to localize placenta (placenta may migrate). *Do not perform pelvic exam!*	• **Pelvic Ultrasound** • *Do not perform pelvic exam!*	• **Pelvic Ultrasound:** vessels crossing the os

MANAGEMENT	• *Hospitalization:* for stabilization. Bed rest
	• *Stabilize fetus:*
	  - *Tocolytics: Magnesium sulfate: inhibits uterine contraction preterm (labor)*
	
	  - *Amniocentesis: to fetal lung maturity. Steroids given between 24-34 weeks to ↑lung maturity*
	
	• *Delivery when stable:* if L:S >2, >36w gestation, blood loss >500ml
	  - *±vaginal:* if partial/marginal
	  - *C-section: if complete when mature.* Complete (↑risk to fetus & mother)
		• *Hospitalization:* for hemodynamic stabilization.
		
		• *IMMEDIATE Delivery:* C-section preferred.
		
		Complications:
		  - *may lead to DIC -* [10%] Disseminated Intravascular Coagulation
			• *Immediate C-section*

RISK FACTORS	• Multiparity, increasing age, smoking	• *Maternal HTN MC cause*,* smoking, ETOH, cocaine, folate deficiency, high parity, increased age, trauma, chorioamnionitis.	

Abruptio placentae & placenta previa 2 MC causes of 3rd trimester bleeding
REMEMBER: Abruptio = **A**bdominal pain; Previa = **P**ainless

ABRUPTIO PLACENTAE	PAINFUL vaginal bleed (often dark red)	⊕ abdominal pain	Tender & rigid uterus	⊕ fetal distress
PLACENTA PREVIA	PAINLESS vaginal bleed (bright red)	No abdominal pain	Soft nontender uterus	Usually no fetal distress

GESTATIONAL DIABETES

- *Glucose intolerance or DM only present during pregnancy.* Usually subsides postpartum.
- **RISK FACTORS:** family or prior history of gestational diabetes, spontaneous abortion, history of infant >4,000g at birth, multiple gestations, obesity, >25y of age, African-American, Hispanic, Asian/Pacific Islander & Native American.

PATHOPHYSIOLOGY

- Caused by placental release of growth hormone, corticotropin releasing hormone & human placental lactogen (HPL) , which antagonizes insulin (works similar to growth hormone as a counterregulatory hormone, increasing glucose availability for the growing fetus).

DIAGNOSIS

1. **Screening: 50g** ORAL GLUCOSE CHALLENGE TEST (nonfasting) *at 24-28 weeks gestation.**
   - *If ≥ 140 mg/dL* after 1 hour ⇨ perform 3 hour oral GTT.

2. **Confirmatory 3-hour** 100g ORAL GLUCOSE TOLERANCE TEST (GTT): *gold standard.**
   Performed in the morning after overnight fast. ⊕ if:
   - fasting >95 mg/dL,   1 hour >180 mg/dL;   2 hour >155 mg/dL;   3 hour >140 mg/dL

MANAGEMENT

Daily fingersticks overnight and after each meal. Diet and exercise recommended.
1. *Insulin: treatment of choice** (doesn't cross placenta). Goal of treatment is fasting glucose <95.
   Indications: fasting blood glucose > 105 or postprandial > 120.
   - NPH/Regular Insulin $^2/_3$ in AM $^1/_3$ in PM.
   - 0.8 IU/kg 1st trimester;   1.0 IU/kg in 2nd trimester;   1.2 IU/kg in 3rd trimester.
2. Glyburide: doesn't cross the placenta (higher risk of eclampsia). Metformin also safe.

3. **Labor induction:** *@38 weeks if uncontrolled/macrosomia.* @ 40 weeks if controlled/no macrosomia. C-section may be delivery method of choice if the child is macrosomic.

Fetal complications: fetal demise, congenital malformation, premature labor, neonate hypoglycemia (from abrupt removal of maternal glucose), hyperglycemia, shoulder dystocia, macrosomia, birth trauma, neonatal hypocalcemia, hyperbilirubinemia.
Maternal complications: preeclampsia, abruptio placentae. >50% chance of developing diabetes mellitus after pregnancy. >50% chance of recurrence with subsequent pregnancies. Mothers should be screened at 6 weeks postpartum for diabetes mellitus and yearly afterwards.

POST PARTUM DEPRESSION

- *Major depression 2 weeks – 12 months postpartum*

	POSTPARTUM BLUES	POSTPARTUM DEPRESSION
ONSET	• 2-4 days postpartum.	• 2 weeks – 2 months postpartum.
DURATION	• Resolves within 10 days.	• 3-14 months.
CLINICAL MANIFESTATIONS	• Mild insomnia, anhedonia, fatigue, depressed mood, irritability. • No thoughts of harming baby.	• Irritability, sleep & mood disturbances, eating changes, anxiety. • *May have thoughts of harming baby.**
MANAGEMENT	• None (self limited).	• May need antidepressants.

GESTATIONAL TROPHOBLASTIC DISEASE (MOLAR PREGNANCY)

Wide array of disorders associated with abnormal placental trophoblastic tissue. 4 types:
❶Molar pregnancy (benign) ❷invasive mole ❸choriocarcinoma & ❹placental site trophoblastic tumor.

HYDATIDIFORM MOLE: *neoplasm due to abnormal placental development with trophoblastic tissue proliferation arising from gestational tissue* (not maternal in origin). MC type. 80% benign.
1. **COMPLETE molar pregnancy:** egg with no DNA fertilized by 1 or 2 sperm. 46XX *all paternal chromosomes*. Associated with higher risk of malignant development into choriocarcinoma (20%).

2. **PARTIAL molar pregnancy:** an egg is fertilized by 2 sperm (or 1 sperm that duplicates its chromosomes). There may be development of the fetus but it is always malformed and never viable. 2 MC Risk factors: prior Molar pregnancy, extremes of maternal age <20y or >35y. Asian.

PATHOPHYSIOLOGY
• Abnormal pregnancy in which a nonviable fertilized egg implants in the uterus with a nonviable pregnancy which will fail to come to term ⇨ *abnormal placental development.*

CLINICAL MANIFESTATIONS
1. *Painless vaginal bleeding* ±begin @ 6 weeks – 4th/5th months MC. ±brownish discharge.
2. *Uterine size/date discrepancies* (ex. larger than expected). Preeclampsia before 20 weeks.
3. **Hyperemesis gravidarum:** due to significant hormonal changes (occurs earlier than usual).
4. Choriocarcinoma: METS to lungs MC, lower genital tract (purple black nodules), pelvic mass.

DIAGNOSIS
1. **β-hCG:** *markedly elevated** (ex >100,000 mIU/mL). Very low maternal serum α-fetoprotein.

2. **Ultrasound:** *"SNOWSTORM"* or *"CLUSTER OF GRAPES"** appearance, absence of fetal parts & heart sounds seen in complete. The cluster of grapes = enlarged cystic chorionic villi.
   - No products of conception seen in complete; Gestational sac may be seen in partial.

MANAGEMENT
1. *Surgical uterine evacuation: suction curettage mainstay** as soon as possible to avoid risk of choriocarcinoma development. Patients are followed weekly until β-hCG levels fall to an undetectable level. Hysterectomy also an option.
   - Rhogam administration to Rh negative mothers. Pregnancy should be avoided 1 year after.

2. *METS: chemotherapy (Methotrexate)** destroys trophoblastic tissue &/or **hysterectomy.** Suspect if β-hCG rises or plateaus after tx, continued hemorrhage after tx, vaginal tumor or pelvic mass.

MULTIPLE GESTATIONS

Dizygotic (fraternal): due to fertilization of 2 ova by two different sperm cells (66%).
Monozygotic (identical): formed from the fertilization of 1 ovum. Increased risk of fetal transfusion syndrome and discordant fetal growth.

MATERNAL COMPLICATIONS: preterm labor, spontaneous abortion, preeclampsia, anemia.

FETAL COMPLICATIONS: intrauterine growth restrictions, placental abnormalities, breech presentation, umbilical cord prolapse, preeclampsia. Multiple gestation considered high risk.

RH ALLOIMMUNIZATION

- Maternal antibodies that bind to fetal RBCs ⇨ neonate hemolytic disease. If the mother of the fetus is Rh negative & father of the fetus is Rh ⊕, there's a 50% chance baby will be positive.

PATHOPHYSIOLOGY

- ***Occurs if Rh negative (Rhesus factor) mother carries an Rh positive fetus*** with exposure to fetal blood mixing (ex during C-section, abruptio placentae, placenta previa, amniocentesis, during vaginal delivery etc). The mixing causes maternal immunization ⇨ maternal anti-Rh IgG antibodies. ***During subsequent pregnancies,*** if she carries ***another Rh positive fetus***, the ***antibodies may cross the placenta & attack the fetal RBCs*** ⇨ ***hemolysis of fetal RBCs.*** <u>At-risk pregnancy</u>: Rh negative mother with Rh+/unknown father.

CLINICAL MANIFESTATIONS

- If subsequent newborn is Rh positive: ***hemolytic anemia, jaundice, kernicterus, hepatosplenomegaly.*** ***<u>Fetal hydrops</u>*** (fluid accumulation in 2 spaces: pericardial effusion, ascites, pleural effusion, subcutaneous edema), congestive heart failure.

DIAGNOSIS

- <u>Pregnant women</u>: ABO blood group, RH-D type. Indirect erythrocyte antibody screen (1:8 – 1:32 is associated with fetal hemolysis). Indirect Coombs.
- <u>Fetus monitoring in 2nd trimester</u>: if present ⇨ amniotic fluid (↑bilirubin). Ultrasound of middle cerebral artery (increased flow 2^{ry} to decreased viscosity of blood in anemia). Percutaneous umbilical blood sampling (decreased hematocrit).

MANAGEMENT

- **Preventative in Mother:** 300 μg ***RhoGAM*** (Rh Immunoglobulin – pooled anti-D IgG binds to fetal RBCs to prevent maternal mixing). ***Given if Rh negative, Ab-negative*** in ***3 indications*** ❶ ***given at 28 weeks gestation*** AND ❷ ***within 72h of delivery*** of an Rh positive baby or ❸ ***after any potential mixing of blood*** (spontaneous abortion, vaginal bleeding, etc.).
- <u>Treatment of Erythoblastosis Fetalis</u>: moderate to severe anemia treated with antigen-negative RBCs through ultrasound-guided umbilical vein transfusion

MORNING SICKNESS & HYPEREMESIS GRAVIDARUM (HEG)

- **MORNING SICKNESS:** nausea &/or vomiting up until 16 weeks.
- **HEG:** ***severe, excessive form of morning sickness*** (nausea, vomiting) associated with weight loss, electrolyte imbalance. Develops during 1st/2nd trimester (persists >16 weeks gestation).

<u>RF</u>: primagravida, previous hyperemesis in past pregnancy, multiple gestations, molar pregnancy.

PATHOPHYSIOLOGY: vomiting center oversensitivity to pregnancy hormones.

CLINICAL MANIFESTATIONS

1. **Hyperemesis gravidarum:** severe nausea/vomiting, weight loss 5% or pre pregnant weight, acidosis (from starvation), metabolic hypochloremic alkalosis (from vomiting).

MANAGEMENT

1. Fluids, electrolyte repletion, multivitamins, early treatment includes high protein foods, small/frequent meals, avoiding spicy/fatty foods. Total parenteral nutrition if severe.
2. **Antiemetics:** ***Pyridoxine (Vit B$_6$) ± Doxylamine 1st line.*** Promethazine, dimenhydrinate.

LABOR & DELIVERY

INTRA PARTUM

- **Braxton-Hicks contractions:** spontaneous uterine contractions late in pregnancy _**not associated with cervical dilation.**_*
- **Lightening:** fetal head descending into the pelvis causing a change in the abdomen's shape and sensation that the baby has "become lighter".
- **Ruptured Membranes:** sudden gush of liquid or constant leakage of fluid.
- **Bloody show:** passage of blood-tinged cervical mucus late in pregnancy. Occurs when the cervix begins thinning (effacement).
- **True labor:** contractions of the uterine fundus with radiation to lower back & abdomen. Regular & painful contractions of the uterus causes cervical dilation & fetus expulsion.

CARDINAL MOVEMENTS OF LABOR

1. **Engagement:** when the fetal presenting part enters the pelvic inlet.
2. **Flexion:** flexion of the head to allow the smallest diameter to present to the pelvis.
3. **Descent:** passage of the head into the pelvis (commonly called "lightening").
4. **Internal Rotation:** fetal vertex moves from occiput transverse position to a position where the sagittal suture is parallel to the anteroposterior diameter of the pelvis.
5. **Extension:** vertex extends as it passes beneath the pubic symphysis.
6. **External rotation:** fetus externally rotates after the head is delivered so that the shoulder can be delivered.

STAGES OF LABOR

3 STAGES OF LABOR.

STAGE I:	Onset of labor (true regular contractions) to _**full dilation of cervix (10 cm).**_* - **Latent phase:** cervix effacement with gradual cervical dilation. - **Active phase:** rapid cervical dilation (usually beginning @ 3-4 cm).
STAGE II:	Time from full cervical dilation until _**delivery of the fetus**_. - **Passive phase:** complete cervical dilation to active maternal expulsive efforts. - **Active phase:** from active maternal expulsive efforts to delivery of the fetus.

STAGE III:	Postpartum until _**delivery of the placenta**_. 0-30 minutes usually (average 5).
	3 signs of placental separation:
	  1. _gush of blood_
	  2. _lengthening of the umbilical cord_
	  3. _anterior-cephalad movement_ of the uterine _fundus (becomes globular and firmer)_ after the placenta detaches.
	Placental expulsion: due to downward pressure of the retroplacental hematoma, uterine contractions

The period 1-2 hours after delivery where the mother is assessed for complications is sometimes called the 4th stage.

APGAR SCORE

Usually done at 1 & 5 minutes after birth.   Repeated at 10 minutes if abnormal.
Score from 1-10: ≥7 = normal;   4-6 fairly low   ≤3 critically low

	0	1	2
Appearance Skin color changes	Blue-gray Pale all over	• *Acrocyanosis: body pink but blue extremities*	• *Pink baby (no cyanosis)*
Pulse	0	• <100	• *≥ 100*
Grimace (Reflex irritability)	No response to stimulation	• Grimaces feebly	• Pulls away, sneezes or coughs
Activity (Muscle tone)	None	• Some flexion	• Flexes arm & legs • Resists extension
Respiration	Absent	• Weak, irregular	• Strong, crying (nml 30-60/min)

POSTPARTUM (PUERPERIUM) 6 week period after delivery

- **Uterus:** at the level of the umbilicus after delivery, involution (shrinks) after 2 days, descends into the pelvic cavity ~2 weeks. Normal size around 6 weeks postpartum.
- **Lochia serosa:** pinkish/brown vaginal bleeding especially postpartum days 4-10 (from the decidual tissue). Usually resolves by 3-4 weeks postpartum.
- **Breasts/menstruation:** breast milk in postpartum days 3-5 bluish-white. If lactating, mothers may remain anovulatory during that time. If not breastfeeding, menses may return 6-8 weeks postpartum.

POSTPARTUM HEMORRHAGE

- Bleeding >500ml if vaginal delivery is performed or >1000ml if C-section is performed.
- Common cause of maternal death within 24 hours of delivery.
- Early: 24 hours postpartum. Delayed > 24 hours up to 8 weeks postpartum.

ETIOLOGIES
1. *Uterine atony*: *MC cause** (uterus unable to contract to stop the bleeding).
2. Uterine rupture, congestion, bleeding disorder, Disseminated Intravascular Coagulation.

Risk Factors: rapid or prolonged labor, overdistended uterus, C-section.

CLINICAL MANIFESTATIONS
1. Hypovolemic shock: hypotension, tachycardia, pale/clammy skin, decreased capillary refill.
2. Uterine atony: *soft boggy uterus* with dilated cervix.

WORKUP
1. CBC to evaluate hemoglobin & hematocrit. Ultrasound may detect the bleeding source.

MANAGEMENT
1. *Bimanual uterine massage.** Treat underlying cause. IV access.

2. **Uterotonic Agents**: *Oxytocin IV, Methylergonovine. Prostaglandin analogs:* IM *Carboprost tromethamine, Misoprostol.* These agents enhance uterine contractions & are only used if the *uterus is soft & boggy.*
3. Suction & curettage may be needed if there are retained products. Antibiotics in some cases.

PREMATURE RUPTURE OF MEMBRANES

- **Risk Factors:** STDs, smoking, prior preterm delivery, multiple gestations.

DIAGNOSIS
1. **Sterile speculum exam**: *visual inspection - pooling of secretions.** Assess for infection.
   - **Nitrazine paper test**: *turns blue if pH >6.5* = PROM is likely.
       Normal amniotic fluid pH (7.0 – 7.3). Vaginal pH usually 3.8 - 4.2.
   - **Fern test**: amniotic fluid - fern pattern (crystallization of estrogen & amniotic fluid).
2. Ultrasound. Avoid digital examination in most cases.

MANAGEMENT
1. Await for spontaneous labor. Monitor for infection (chorioamnionitis or endometritis).

PREMATURE LABOR (PRETERM LABOR) PTL

- **Labor:** *regular uterine contractions* (>4-6/hr) with *progressive cervical changes* (effacement & dilation) *BEFORE 37 WEEKS GESTATION.** *MC cause of perinatal mortality* (70%).

CLINICAL MANIFESTATIONS
1. cramps, uterine contractions, back pain, pelvic pressure, vaginal discharge.

DIAGNOSIS

CERVICAL DILATION	EFFACEMENT	DIAGNOSIS	
≥ 3cm	≥ 80% effacement*	*Premature Labor*	PTL also likely if *>1cm*
2cm-3cm	<80%	PTL is likely	*cervical dilation on*
≤ 2cm	<80%	PTL unlikely	*serial examinations*

1. *Nitrazine pH paper test: turns blue if pH >6.5 (amniotic fluid).* Normal vaginal pH 3.8-4.2
2. *Fern test:* estrogen + amniotic fluid causes delicate crystallization seen with a microscope.
3. *Presence of FETAL FIBRONECTIN** between 20-34 weeks strongly suggests preterm labor.
4. Rule out infections: UTI, Group B strep. *L:S ratio <2:1 = fetal lung immaturity.**

MANAGEMENT: admission to the hospital and observe for signs of infection.
1. *Antenatal steroids*: enhances fetal lung maturity (L:S ratio <2:1, <34 weeks). *Betamethasone.*

2. **TOCOLYTICS**: *suppresses uterine contraction.** *May be given for 48h to delay delivery so steroids can take full effect on the fetus.* Don't delay labor if intrauterine infection is detected.
   - **Indomethacin:** inhibits prostaglandin-mediated uterine contraction. (ex 24-32 weeks).
   - **Nifedipine** (Calcium channel blocker). (ex. 32-34 weeks or 2nd line during 24-32 weeks).
   - **Magnesium Sulfate:** must be admitted if administered. Not used with Nifedipine.
   - **Beta$_2$ agonists:** *Terbutaline* (2nd line 32-34w). S/E: *maternal pulmonary edema.*

3. **Antibiotic prophylaxis:** *includes group B Strep*: ex. Ampicillin followed by PO Amoxicillin and Azithromycin. PCN allergy: Cephazolin followed by PO cephalexin & azithromycin.

DYSTOCIA

- *Abnormal labor progression.* 3 categories: ❶*Power* = uterine contraction ❷*Passenger* = presentation size or position of fetus. Ex *shoulder dystocia*: one or both shoulders lodged at pubic symphysis after delivery of the head. ± lead to Erb's palsy (brachial plexus injury) especially in macrosomic children, multiparity, Gestational DM ❸*Passage* = uterus or soft tissue abnormalities.

MANAGEMENT OF SHOULDER DYSTOCIA
1. **Nonmanipulative:** 1st line: *McRoberts maneuver* (increase pelvic opening with hip hyperflexion).
2. **Manipulative:** *Woods "Corkscrew" maneuver* 180 shoulder rotation.   ± Cesarean section.

INDUCTION OF LABOR

- Stimulation of uterine contractions to initiate labor prior to the onset of spontaneous labor.
- **Indications**: vaginal delivery when prolonged labor may lead to complications for either the mother or the fetus and those risks are greater than continuing the pregnancy.
- **Contraindications:** situations in which the risks of induction of vaginal delivery greater than cesarean delivery: prior uterine rupture, prior C-section, active genital herpes infection, umbilical cord prolapse, placenta previa or vasa previa, transverse fetal lie.

MANAGEMENT

1. **Early induction:** used in women with unfavorable cervices to promote cervical ripening.
   - *Prostaglandin gel* placed directly on the cervix (ex. Cervidil).
   - Balloon catheter or laminaria.

2. **Later induction:** performed when the cervix is dilated <1cm with some effacement
   IV Oxytocin (Pitocin) (uterotonic agent). Monitor uterine activity & fetal heart rate.

3. **Amniotomy** (artificially rupturing the membranes with a small hook) can be done if the cervix is partially dilated and there is effacement of the cervix.

SELECTED REFERENCES

Azziz R, Woods KS, Reyna R, Key TJ, Knochenhauer ES, Yildiz BO. The prevalence and features of the polycystic ovary syndrome in an unselected population. J Clin Endocrinol Metab. 2004;89(6):2745-9.

Master-hunter T, Heiman DL. Amenorrhea: evaluation and treatment. Am Fam Physician. 2006;73(8):1374-82.

Wright TC, Massad LS, Dunton CJ, et al. 2006 consensus guidelines for the management of women with cervical intraepithelial neoplasia or adenocarcinoma in situ. Am J Obstet Gynecol. 2007;197(4):340-5.

Murthy NS, Mathew A. Risk factors for pre-cancerous lesions of the cervix. Eur J Cancer Prev. 2000;9(1):5-14.

Dual protection against unwanted pregnancy and HIV / STDs. Sex Health Exch. 1998;(3):8.

Apgar V. A proposal for a new method of evaluation of the newborn infant. Curr Res Anesth Analg. 1953;32(4):260-7.

Haas DM, Caldwell DM, Kirkpatrick P, Mcintosh JJ, Welton NJ. Tocolytic therapy for preterm delivery: systematic review and network meta-analysis. BMJ. 2012;345:e6226.

Jones RK, Fennell J, Higgins JA, Blanchard K. Better than nothing or savvy risk-reduction practice? The importance of withdrawal. Contraception. 2009;79(6):407-10.

Casey PM, Cerhan JR, Pruthi S. Oral contraceptive use and risk of breast cancer. Mayo Clin Proc. 2008;83(1):86-90.

Oppenheimer LW, Farine D, Ritchie JW, Lewinsky RM, Telford J, Fairbanks LA. What is a low-lying placenta?. Am J Obstet Gynecol. 1991;165(4 Pt 1):1036-8.

Freundl G, Sivin I, Batár I. State-of-the-art of non-hormonal methods of contraception: IV. Natural family planning. Eur J Contracept Reprod Health Care. 2010;15(2):113-23.

Walker CK, Wiesenfeld HC. Antibiotic therapy for acute pelvic inflammatory disease: the 2006 Centers for Disease Control and Prevention sexually transmitted diseases treatment guidelines. Clin Infect Dis. 2007;44 Suppl 3:S111-22.

Shenoy N, Kessel R, Bhagat TD, et al. Alterations in the ribosomal machinery in cancer and hematologic disorders. J Hematol Oncol. 2012;5(1):32.

Bravender T, Emans SJ. Menstrual disorders. Dysfunctional uterine bleeding. Pediatr Clin North Am. 1999;46(3):545-53, viii.

Human papillomavirus vaccine and cervical cancer prevention: Practice and policy implications for pharmacists . Jennifer McIntosh, PharmD, MHS; Deborah A. Sturpe, PharmD, BCPS; Niharika Khanna, MBBS, MD, DGO. *J Am Pharm Assoc (2003)* 2008;48:e1-e17. doi:10.1331/JAPhA.2008.07032

Romond EH, Perez EA, Bryant J, et al. Trastuzumab plus adjuvant chemotherapy for operable HER2-positive breast cancer. N Engl J Med. 2005;353(16):1673-84.

Vaidya JS, Joseph DJ, Tobias JS, et al. Targeted intraoperative radiotherapy versus whole breast radiotherapy for breast cancer (TARGIT-A trial): an international, prospective, randomised, non-inferiority phase 3 trial. Lancet. 2010;376(9735):91-102.

Nelson HD, Tyne K, Naik A, et al. Screening for breast cancer: an update for the U.S. Preventive Services Task Force. Ann Intern Med. 2009;151(10):727-37, W237-42.

Cuschieri KS, Cubie HA, Whitley MW, et al. Persistent high risk HPV infection associated with development of cervical neoplasia in a prospective population study. J Clin Pathol. 2005;58(9):946-50.

Slim R, Mehio A. The genetics of hydatidiform moles: new lights on an ancient disease. Clin Genet. 2007;71(1):25-34.

Kane SC, Dennis A, Da silva costa F, Kornman L, Brennecke S. Contemporary Clinical Management of the Cerebral Complications of Preeclampsia. Obstet Gynecol Int. 2013;2013:985606.

Steer P. The epidemiology of preterm labour. BJOG. 2005;112 Suppl 1:1-3.

Rowan SP, Someshwar J, Murray P. Contraception for primary care providers. Adolesc Med State Art Rev. 2012;23(1):95-110, x-xi.

Legro RS, Kunselman AR, Dodson WC, Dunaif A. Prevalence and predictors of risk for type 2 diabetes mellitus and impaired glucose tolerance in polycystic ovary syndrome: a prospective, controlled study in 254 affected women. J Clin Endocrinol Metab. 1999;84(1):165-9.

PHOTO CREDITS

CHAPTER 7 – ENDOCRINE DISORDERS

HYPOTHALAMIC - PITUITARY AXIS

- The hypothalamus is the command center for the endocrine system. It receives input from the cerebral cortex, the environment (ex. cortisol secretion increases at night) & feedback from the organs it controls.

Hypothalamus – Pituitary - Thyroid Axis in the thyroid gland

Thyroid hormone production is regulated 2 ways:

❶ **TRH-** Thyrotropin-Releasing Hormone is produced by the hypothalamus.
   TRH regulates pituitary TSH secretion.

❷ ***TSH*** – Thyroid Stimulating Hormone (Thyrotropin) is produced by the pituitary gland.
   TSH regulates thyroid gland synthesis/secretion of thyroid hormones (T_3 & T_4).

POSITIVE FEEDBACK MECHANISM:

- Low blood levels of thyroid hormone (T_3/T_4) are sensed by the hypothalamus ⇨ ↑hypothalamic release of TRH ⇨ ↑pituitary release of TSH.

- Increased levels of TSH stimulate the thyroid gland to produce more thyroid hormone, thereby returning the thyroid hormone levels back to normal.

NEGATIVE FEEDBACK MECHANISM:

If thyroid hormone levels become too high, they inhibit the secretion of both hypothalamic TRH secretion & pituitary TSH secretion. This prevents overshoot of the positive feedback mechanism.
   - The pituitary gland & the hypothalamus are regulated by <u>negative feedback</u> of thyroid hormones to keep <u>tight control of hormone levels</u>.

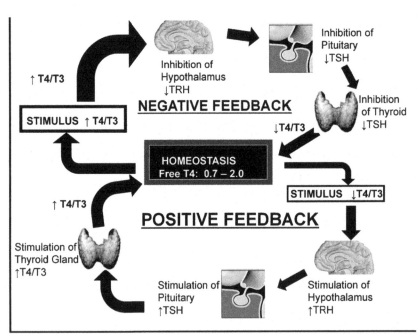

Note: Positive Feedback can also refer to when increased levels of the desired hormone causes further production of that hormone by stimulating the hypothalamus & pituitary gland: 2 important examples are ❶increased cortisol production during times of stress & ❷the positive feedback of estrogen on the hypothalamus & pituitary gland prior to the LH surge that causes ovulation.

THE HYPOTHALAMUS-PITUITARY (HP) AXIS IS SIMILAR FOR:

HYPOTHALAMUS	PITUITARY GLAND	TARGET ORGAN/HORMONE
TRH **T**hyro**t**ropin-**R**eleasing **H**ormone	**TSH** **T**hyroid **S**timulating **H**ormone	**Thyroid Gland:** T3 & T4
CRH **C**orticotropin-**R**eleasing **H**ormone	**ACTH** **A**dreno**C**ortico**T**ropic **H**ormone	**Adrenal Gland:** Cortisol
GnRH **Gon**adotropin-**R**eleasing **H**ormone	**FSH: F**ollicle **S**timulating **H**ormone **LH: L**uteinizing **H**ormone	**Ovaries:** estrogen, progesterone, & small amounts of testosterone. **Testes:** testosterone

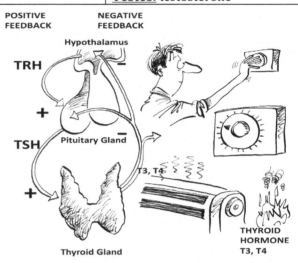

POSITIVE FEEDBACK

The man (hypothalamus) turns on the thermostat (pituitary gland), which turns on the radiator (thyroid gland), which produces the heat (thyroid hormone) to the desired temperature (homeostasis).

NEGATIVE FEEDBACK

When the heat (thyroid hormone) becomes higher than the desired set temperature (homeostasis), this will cause the thermostat (pituitary gland) to shut off so that the radiator (thyroid gland) stops making heat (any new thyroid hormone).

SECONDARY DISORDERS

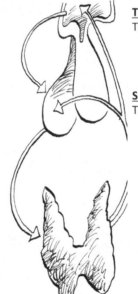

Based on the feedback mechanisms, *secondary (pituitary gland)* & *tertiary (hypothalamic)* disorders have *LABS IN THE SAME DIRECTION.*
- **TSH-secreting PITUITARY adenoma**
  ↑TSH & ↑FreeT$_4$/T$_3$
- **Cushing's disease (PITUITARY adenoma)**
  ↑ACTH & ↑cortisol
- **Hypopituitarism:** low pituitary hormones & low target organ hormones

PRIMARY DISORDERS

Based on the feedback mechanisms, primary disorders have *LABS IN OPPOSITE DIRECTIONS if the problem is the target organ:*

Thyroid gland is the primary problem:
- **Graves, Toxic Goiters, Toxic adenoma**
  ↑FreeT$_4$/T$_3$ & ↓TSH

- **Hashimoto's, Thyroiditis**
  ↓FreeT$_4$/T$_3$ & ↑TSH

Ovaries are the primary problem:
- **Menopause:** ↓estrogen & ↑FSH/LH

Adrenal gland is the primary problem:
- **Addison's disease:** ↓cortisol & ↑ACTH
- **Adrenal adenoma:** ↑cortisol & ↓ACTH

TERTIARY DISORDER
The **hypothalamus** is the problem

SECONDARY DISORDER
The **pituitary gland** is the problem

PRIMARY DISORDER
The **target organ** is the problem

THYROID FUNCTION TESTS

TEST	DESCRIPTION	CLINICAL UTILITY

TSH	Thyroid stimulating hormone	• ***BEST THYROID FUNCTION SCREENING TEST.****
		 • Initial test for suspected thyroid disease.
		 • Used to follow patients on thyroid hormone tx
		   - Low TSH ⇨ decrease dose of levothyroxine
		   - High TSH ⇨ increase dose of levothyroxine
		 • Used with T₄ to manage patients with Grave's.

Free T₄ ***(FT₄)***	***Free thyroxine*** *levels* (metabolically active hormone)	• Ordered when TSH is abnormal to determine thyroid hyperfunction or hypofunction

THYROID ANTIBODIES	• ***Anti-thyroid peroxidase Ab***
	 • ***Anti-Thyroglobulin Ab***
	
	 • ***Thyroid stimulating Ab***
	 (TSH receptor Ab)
		• Used to diagnose ***Hashimoto's*** thyroiditis
		       OR
		   other ***autoimmune*** thyroiditis
		
		 • ***Specific for Graves' disease***

Free T₃	Serum triiodothyronine	• Useful to diagnose hyperthyroidism when TSH is low & T₄ is still normal.
FTI	Free Thyroxine Index	• Used in thyroid disease when the patient has protein abnormalities.

TSH result	Subsequent FT₄ result	Possible Diagnoses
Normal TSH	NO NEED FOR FURTHER TESTING IN MOST PATIENTS	
Elevated TSH *plus* (>5.0 mU/L)	*Low FT₄*	***PRIMARY Hypothyroidism****
	Normal FT₄	***SUBCLINICAL Hypothyroidism****
	High FT₄	***TSH-mediated hyperthyroidism**** ***(2ry or 3ry** – same direction)*
Low TSH *plus* (<0.10 mU/L)	*Low FT₄*	***2ry/3ry hypothyroidism*** (rare) ***If present, usually pituitary.*** May be TSH suppression by drugs: Dobutamine, Octreotide or high-dose Glucocorticoids
	Normal FT₄	Subclinical Hyperthyroidism (Check T4/FT4)
	High FT₄	***PRIMARY hyperthyroidism, thyrotoxicosis*** (May check RAIU to identify cause)

RADIOACTIVE IODINE TEST (RAIU)	POSSIBLE DIAGNOSIS
DIFFUSE uptake	Grave's disease or TSH-secreting pituitary adenoma
Decreased uptake	Thyroiditis (ex. Hashimoto's, postpartum, deQuervain)
Hot Nodule	Toxic Adenoma
Multiple Nodules	Toxic Multinodular goiter
Cold Nodules	Rule out malignancy

SUBCLINICAL HYPOTHYROIDISM

Normal free T4 & T3 levels + ↑TSH. Usually asymptomatic but may develop cardiovascular issues.

MANAGEMENT
1. **Levothyroxine:** *if patient develops hyperlipidemia, TSH >20* mIU/mL *or hypothyroid symptoms.*

CLINICAL MANIFESTATIONS OF THYROID DISORDERS

	HYPOTHYROIDISM	HYPERTHYROIDISM
ETIOLOGIES	<ul><li>Iodine deficiency (dietary)</li><li>Hashimoto's Thyroiditis</li><li>Postpartum Thyroiditis</li><li>Pituitary Hypothyroidism</li><li>Hypothalamic Hypothyroidism</li><li>Cretinism</li><li>Riedel's Thyroiditis</li></ul>	<ul><li>Grave's Disease</li><li>Toxic Multinodular Goiter</li><li>TSH secreting pituitary adenoma</li><li>Excess intake of T3, T4</li><li>Iatrogenic thyrotoxicosis</li></ul>
CLINICAL MANIFESTATIONS		
CALORIGENIC	<ul><li>Decreased Basic Metabolic Rate</li><li>*Cold intolerance* (↓heat production)</li><li>Weight gain (despite ↓appetite)</li></ul>	<ul><li>Increased Basic Metabolic Rate</li><li>*Heat intolerance* (↑heat production)</li><li>Weight loss (despite ↑appetite)</li></ul>
SKIN	<ul><li>Dry, thickened rough skin</li><li>*loss of outer 1/3 of eyebrow*</li><li>Goiter</li><li>Nonpitting edema (myxedema)</li></ul>	<ul><li>Skin warm, moist, soft, fine hair, alopecia, easy bruising</li><li>Goiter</li></ul>
CNS	<ul><li>*Hypoactivity:* Fatigue, sluggishness, memory loss, depression, ↓*DTR*</li><li>Hoarseness of voice</li></ul>	<ul><li>*Hyperactivity:* anxiety, fine tremors, nervousness, fatigue, weakness, tremors, increased sympathetic</li></ul>
GI	<ul><li>Constipation, anorexia</li></ul>	<ul><li>Diarrhea, hyperdefecation</li></ul>
CVS	<ul><li>*Bradycardia, ↓ cardiac output*</li><li>Pericardial effusion</li></ul>	<ul><li>*Tachycardia, palpitations*</li><li>*High-output heart failure*</li></ul>
REPRODUCTIVE	<ul><li>*Menorrhagia*</li></ul>	<ul><li>Scanty periods, gynecomastia</li></ul>
GLUCOSE	<ul><li>Hypoglycemia</li></ul>	<ul><li>Hyperglycemia</li></ul>

CRETINISM

Congenital hypothyroidism due to maternal hypothyroidism or infant hypopituitarism.

CLINICAL MANIFESTATION
1. Macroglossia, hoarse cry, coarse facial features, umbilical hernia, weight gain.
2. Mental development abnormalities may all develop if not corrected.

MANAGEMENT
Thyroid hormone replacement: Levothyroxine.

EUTHYROID SICK SYNDROME

- Abnormal thyroid hormone levels with normal thyroid gland function *seen with nonthyroidal illness* (ex. surgery, malignancies, sepsis, cardiac disease).

DIAGNOSIS
1. ↓*FreeT$_4$/T$_3$* plus ↓*TSH* (often resembles 2ry hypothyroidism lab wise) but TSH may be low, normal or high. *T$_3$ abnormally low.*

2. *Increased reverse T$_3$.**

THYROID STORM (THYROTOXICOSIS CRISIS)

- **_Potentially fatal complication of untreated_** _(or partially treated)_ **_thyrotoxicosis_** usually **_after a precipitating event_** (ex. surgery, trauma, infection, illness, pregnancy).
- **_Rare_** (only occurs in 1-2% of patients with hyperthyroidism). High mortality rate (75%).

CLINICAL MANIFESTATIONS
1. **_Hypermetabolic state: palpitations, tachycardia, atrial fibrillation, high fever, nausea, vomiting, psychosis, tremors_** (which later may progress to coma & hypotension).

DIAGNOSIS
Primary hyperthyroid TFT profile: ↑**_FreeT$_4$/T$_3$_** plus ↓**_TSH_** (TSH may be undetectable).

MANAGEMENT
1. **Anti-thyroid meds**_: IV Propylthiouracil* (PTU) or Methimazole._ In addition to inhibiting thyroid hormone synthesis, PTU also prevents the peripheral conversion of T$_4$ into T$_3$.
2. **_Beta blockers: symptomatic therapy._** Oral/IV sodium iodide: ↓'es thyroid hormone release.
3. Supportive:
    - **_IV glucocorticoids:_** inhibits the peripheral conversion of T$_4$ into T$_3$ & impairs thyroid hormone production. Cardiac monitoring, IV fluids.
    - Antipyretics (**_avoid Aspirin_** because it causes increased T$_3$/T$_4$ release). **_Cooling blankets._**

MYXEDEMA CRISIS

- **_Extreme form of hypothyroidism_** associated with a high mortality rate (60%).
- **_MC seen in elderly women with long standing hypothyroidism in winter (cold weather).*_**

PATHOPHYSIOLOGY
Usually due to an **_acute precipitating factor_** (infection, CVA, CHF, sedative/narcotics) with:
❶ Longstanding, undiagnosed hypothyroidism.
❷ Discontinuation/noncompliance with Levothyroxine therapy.
❸ Failure to start Levothyroxine after radioactive iodine ablation of thyroid in patients c̄ Graves.

CLINICAL MANIFESTATIONS
1. **_Severe signs of hypothyroidism:_** **_bradycardia_**, obtunded (coma), hypothermia, hypoventilation, hypotensive, **_hypoglycemia, hyponatremia_**.

DIAGNOSIS
Serum Studies: primary hypothyroid TFT profile
    1. ↑**_TSH_** (as the pituitary gland tries to increase hormone production of failing thyroid gland).
    2. ↓**FreeT$_4$/T$_3$** _(may be so low that it may be undetectable)._

MANAGEMENT
1. **Thyroid Hormone replacement:** _intravenous Levothyroxine (Synthroid).*_
    - Given while awaiting the results if there is a high suspicion.
2. **Supportive:**
    - ICU admission, antibiotics if an infection is present.
    - **_Passive warming_** (blankets in a warm room). **_Rapid warming contraindicated._**
    - Normal saline.
    - Corticosteroids if adrenal insufficiency is suspected (ex. IV Hydrocortisone).

HYPERTHYROID DISORDERS

TYPE	CAUSE	CLINICAL MANIFESTATIONS	DIAGNOSIS (not all tests need to be done)	MANAGEMENT
GRAVE'S DISEASE	*Autoimmune* MC women 20-40y Circulating *TSH receptor antibodies* cause ↑thyroid hormone synthesis, release & thyroid gland growth *worse with stress (ex. pregnancy, illness)* *Graves MC cause of hyperthyroidism** (90%)	• Clinical Hyperthyroidism • Diffuse, enlarged thyroid. • *THYROID BRUITS** • *OPHTHALMOPATHY*: lid lag, exophthalmos/proptosis (exclusive to Grave)** Hyaluronic acid deposition. *Tx c steroids.* Smoking & iodine may make ophthalmopathy worse. • *PRETIBIAL MYXEDEMA** Nonpitting, edematous, pink to brown plaques/nodules on shin (exclusive to Grave)	• ⊕ *Thyroid- Stimulating Immunoglobulins (Ab)* most spp.* ± Thyroid peroxidase & anti-TG Ab • Hyperthyroid TFTs: ↑FT$_4$/FT$_3$ & ↓TSH (± be subclinical) • RAIU: ↑ *DIFFUSE uptake** Normal Grave's Diffuse uptake seen in TSH-secreting pituitary adenoma also.	• *Radioactive Iodine: MC therapy used.* Destroys thyroid gland. Will need hormone replacement • *Methimazole or PropylThioUracil* • *Beta blockers (ex. Propranolol) for symptomatic relief:* tremors, anxiety, tachycardia, diaphoresis, palpitations, etc • *Thyroidectomy:* if compressive sx, no response to meds, If RAI is contraindicated (ex pregnancy)
TOXIC MULTINODULAR GOITER (TMG) (Plummer's Disease)	Autonomous functioning nodules *MC in elderly*	*BOTH TMG & TA* • Clinical Hyperthyroidism • Diffuse, enlarged thyroid • *No skin/eye changes!* • Palpable nodule(s)	• Hyperthyroid TFTs: ↑ FT$_4$/T$_3$; ↓TSH (± be subclinical) • RAIU: (PATCHY areas of both ↑ & ↓uptake) in TMG TMG	*BOTH TMG & TA* • *Radioactive Iodine: MC therapy* • Surgery (subtotal thyroidectomy) if compressive symptoms present • *Methimazole or PTU:* - *MOA: inhibit hormone synthesis. Methimazole preferred (less S/E)* - *S/E of both: agranulocytosis** (so monitor WBC) & *hepatitis.** • *PTU preferred in pregnancy.* (especially 1st trimester) • *Beta blockers for symptoms of thyrotoxicosis*
TOXIC ADENOMA (TA)	One autonomous functioning nodule	*Compressive sx:* • *Dyspnea, dysphagia, stridor, hoarseness* (laryngeal compression).	• RAIU: ↑LOCAL uptake (hot nodule) in TA TA	
TSH SECERETING PITUITARY ADENOMA	Autonomous TSH secretion by pituitary adenoma	• Clinical Hyperthyroidism • Diffuse, enlarged thyroid • *Bitemporal Hemianopsia** • Mental disturbances	• TFT's:↑FT$_4$/T$_3$; ↑ TSH* (inappropriate TSH elevation in the setting of elevated FT$_4$/T$_3$ (same direction)* • RAIU: DIFFUSE uptake • Pituitary MRI: adenoma	• Transsphenoidal Surgery to remove the pituitary adenoma

HYPOTHYROID DISORDERS

TYPE	CAUSE	CLINICAL MANIFESTATIONS	DIAGNOSIS	DURATION
HASHIMOTO'S thyroiditis (CHRONIC LYMPHOCYTIC) MC cause of hypothyroidism in the US* – 6x MC in women	*Autoimmune* (Anti-thyroid Antibodies) (Ab)	Clinical Hypothyroidism • Painless, enlarged thyroid • May present in euthyroid state (rarely in hyperthyroid state)	• ⊕*Thyroid Ab present: thyroglobulin Ab, antimicrosomial & Thyroid Peroxidase Ab* • *TFTs (usually HypOthyroid)* • ↓Radioactive I- uptake (usually not needed) • Bx: lymphocytes, germinal follicles, Hurtle	• Hypothyroidism usually permanent. • *Levothyroxine therapy** Thyroid hormone replacement
SILENT (LYMPHOCYTIC) THYROIDITIS	*Autoimmune* (Anti-thyroid Ab)	Painless, enlarged thyroid. Thyrotoxicosis ⇔ hypothyroid (depends on when they present)	• ⊕*Thyroid Ab present:* thyroglobulin Ab, antimicrosomial & Thyroid Peroxidase Ab • TFTs: Hyper/Hypothyroid (depends on when they present) • ↓Radioactive Iodine uptake on RAIU scan	• Return to euthyroid state within 12-18 months without treatment. **Aspirin** • *No anti-thyroid meds** • 20% possible permanent hypothyroidism
POSTPARTUM THYROIDITIS	*Autoimmune* (Anti-thyroid Ab)	Painless, enlarged thyroid. Thyrotoxicosis ⇔ hypothyroid (depends on when they present)	• ⊕*Thyroid Ab present:* thyroglobulin Ab, antimicrosomial & Thyroid Peroxidase Ab • TFTs (Hyper/Hypothyroid) (depends on when they present) • ↓Radioactive Iodine uptake on RAIU scan	• Return to euthyroid state in 12-18 months without treatment. **Aspirin**, NSAIDs • *No anti-thyroid meds** • 20% possible permanent hypothyroidism
de QUERVAIN'S THYROIDITIS (GRANULOMATOUS) PAINFUL SUBACUTE	*MC POST VIRAL* * or viral inflammatory reaction. Associated with HLA-B35	*PAINFUL, tender neck/thyroid** *Clinical Hyperthyroidism* (due to neck pain in acute phase) Thyrotoxicosis ⇔ hypothyroid (depend on when they present)	• ↑*ESR (hallmark)** • *NO thyroid Ab** • *TFTs (usually HypERthyroid)* (depends on when they present) • ↓Radioactive Iodine uptake on RAIU scan	• Return to euthyroid state in 12-18 months without treatment. Aspirin (for **pain, inflammation,** ↑'es T4) • *No anti-thyroid meds** • 5% possible permanent hypothyroidism
MEDICATION-INDUCED	*AMIODARONE* (contains iodine), *LITHIUM* Alpha interferon	Painless, enlarged thyroid. Thyrotoxicosis ⇔ hypothyroid (depend on when they present)		Often returns to euthyroid states when med is stopped, Corticosteroids
ACUTE THYROIDITIS (Suppurative)	*S. aureus MC* (any organism may cause it)	May have *PAINFUL fluctuant* thyroid. Usually very ill, *febrile.*	Increased WBC count with left shift. Usually *euthyroid*	Antibiotics Drainage if abscess present
RIEDEL'S THYROIDITIS	*Fibrous* thyroid	Firm hard 'woody' nodule *(similar to anaplastic cancer)**	May develop hypothyroidism	Surgery may be needed

LEVOTHYROXINE: *synthetic T4.* Monitor TSH levels @ 6 week intervals when initiating/changing dose. *Slow, small increases in >50y & patients with cardiovascular disease.* **Monitor elderly, patients with angina, MI, or CHF for adverse reactions** due to increased metabolic rate or withhold until cardiovascular status is stabilized. May need to lower doses of anticoagulants, insulin, and oral antihyperglycemics. Oral cholestyramine may increase T4 requirements. *The MC cause of hypothyroidism in the US is Hashimoto's thyroiditis.* *The MC cause of hypothyroidism worldwide is iodine deficiency.*

THYROID NODULES

Thyroid Nodule: abnormal lump in the thyroid gland.   Prevalence increases with age.

RISK FACTORS: *extremes of age (very young or >60y), history of head/neck irradiation.*
- Most thyroid nodules in women are benign (follicular adenoma or cysts).
- Only 10% are malignant.
- Most thyroid nodules found in men & children are malignant. Papillary cancer MC in women.

CLINICAL MANIFESTATIONS
1. *Most are asymptomatic.*

2. **Compressive sx:** difficulty swallowing or breathing (if large); neck, jaw or ear pain, hoarseness (if it compresses the recurrent laryngeal nerve – rare).

3. Functional nodules: rare. ±Thyrotoxicosis (if active functioning cells are present).

DIAGNOSIS
A. Physical Exam:
   1. **Benign:** *varied:* smooth, firm, irregular, sharply outlined, discrete, painless.

   2. **Malignant:** *rapid growth, fixed in place, no movement with swallowing** (Riedel's thyroiditis/benign fibrotic thyroiditis may also present like this).

B. Thyroid Function Tests: *most patients are euthyroid* (±hyperthyroid or hypothyroid).

C. **Fine Needle Aspiration (FNA) with Biopsy:** *best initial test to evaluate a nodule.**
   1. **Benign nodules:**
      - *Follicular adenoma (colloid) MC type of thyroid nodule** - (50-60%)
      - Adenomas, cyst, localized thyroiditis. *>90% of nodules are benign.*

   2. **Malignant nodules:** (5%). Suspicious (10%) – FNA not as reliable in distinguishing follicular adenoma (benign) from follicular cancer.

D. Radioactive Iodine Uptake Scan:
   1. Indications: usually performed if the FNA is indeterminate.
      - *Cold nodules (no/low iodine uptake) are highly suspicious for malignancy.**
      - Functioning (normal) or hot nodules - lower suspicion.

E. Thyroid Ultrasound
   1. Often used to help obtain a specimen during FNA with biopsy, used to see if nodule is cystic or solid, to monitor a suspicious nodule or to see if a nodule is growing or shrinking. High resolution ultrasound is the most sensitive test in the detection of a thyroid lesion.

MANAGEMENT OF THYROID NODULE
1. **Surgery:** *if thyroid cancer is suspected* or if an *indeterminate FNA with a cold thyroid scan.*
   - Total thyroidectomy vs. subtotal thyroidectomy.

2. *Observation* of suspicious nodules *(usually every 6-12 months)* *often with ultrasound.*

Suppressive therapy with thyroid hormone in an attempt to shrink thyroid nodule in some cases.

THYROID CARCINOMA

- *Roughly 5% of thyroid nodules are malignant.* ↑*suspicion of thyroid nodule in patients <20y of age, cold nodule on RAIU*
- *Most patients with thyroid cancer are euthyroid.* Risks: radiation, oncogenes, tumor suppressor gene disorders.
- *Papillary & Follicular are well differentiated (better prognosis).* Anaplastic poorly differentiated (worst prognosis).

	PAPILLARY	FOLLICULAR	MEDULLARY	ANAPLASTIC
PERCENTAGE	80% (MC type)*	10%	10%	<5%
RISK FACTORS	MC after radiation exposure*	Less often associated with radiation exposure ↑ with iodine deficiency	*Not associated with radiation exposure* MC associated with *MEN 2**	May occur many years after radiation exposure
AGE	*MC in young females*	MC 40-60y		*MC in males >65y*
CHARACTERISTICS	*Least aggressive*	More aggressive than papillary but also slow growing	More aggressive. Arises from parafollicular (C) cells secrete *CALCITONIN**	*Most aggressive* *Rapid growth!* *(often with compressive sx)*
METS	• *Local (cervical)* lymph node *METS common* • *Distant METS uncommon* (when present, usually involves the lung & bone)	• *Local cervical lymph node invasion less common* • *Distant METS common (due to characteristic vascular invasion)* lung, brain, bone, liver, skin.	• *Local cervical lymph node occurs early in disease* • *Distant METS occurs late* (brain, bone, liver, adrenal medulla)	*Local & distant METS* *May invade trachea*
PROGNOSIS	*Excellent (high cure rate)* *Papillary = Popular* (MC type of cancer)	Excellent	Poorer prognosis. These tumors don't take up iodine.	*Poor prognosis** *(only 10% survive 3y after dx)* Most don't live 1y after diagnosis
MANAGEMENT	Controversy exists regarding treatment of well differentiated carcinomas. 2 main surgical options: 1. Total Thyroidectomy 2. Subtotal Thyroidectomy may also be coupled with radioiodine therapy (to destroy residual tumor cells) &/or thyroid/TSH suppression c̄ thyroid hormones (T4) • May monitor thyroglobulin levels 6 months after thyroidectomy to look for residual cells. Done by giving recombinant TSH & then checking thyroglobulin levels.		*Total Thyroidectomy* (including a complete neck dissection of all lymph nodes and surrounding fatty tissues on the ipsilateral side) *Calcitonin levels used to monitor* if residual disease is present after tx or for recurrence.	• *Most are not amenable to surgical resection* • External Beam Radiation • Chemotherapy • *Palliative tracheostomy in* 20% to maintain airway.

- 99% of calcium is in bone. 1% in extracellular fluid. 50% of ECF Ca^{2+} is ionized (active) form.
- Normal calcium levels = 8.5-10 mg/dL. **Vitamin D required for intestinal Ca^{2+} absorption.**
- Ca^{2+} is important for bone, blood clotting, normal cellular function & neuromuscular transmission.
- *Calcium is maintained within a normal range via 3 major hormones:*
  - **Hypocalcemia** stimulates ❶ ↑*parathyroid hormone &* ❷↑**calcitriol (Vitamin D)** secretion: ↑*'es blood* Ca^{2+} via ↑GI/kidney Ca^{2+} absorption & ↑bone Ca^{2+} resorption (via ↑osteoclast activity). Parathyroid hormone also inhibits phosphate reabsorption so phosphate is usually in the opposite direction of the PTH levels in primary parathyroid disorders.
  - **Hypercalcemia** stimulates ❸↑**Calcitonin secretion:** ↓*'es blood* Ca^{2+} (↓Ca^{2+} GI/kidney absorption & ↑bone mineralization.

HYPERPARATHYROIDISM

ETIOLOGIES
- **PRIMARY HYPERPARATHYROIDISM:** *excess* (inappropriate) ↑*PTH production. MC type.**
  - *PARATHYROID ADENOMA MC CAUSE* (80%).
  - *Parathyroid hyperplasia/enlargement* (15-20%).
  - Occurs in 20% of patients taking **Lithium.** MEN I & IIa; Malignant tumor (rare).

MEN 1	Hyperparathyroidism	Pituitary Tumors	Pancreatic Tumors
Men 2A	Hyperparathyroidism	Pheochromocytoma	Medullary Thyroid Carcinoma

- **SECONDARY HYPERPARATHYROIDISM:** ↑*PTH due to hypocalcemia or vitamin D deficiency.* (Parathyroid gland tries to compensate by ↑'ing PTH to increase Ca^{2+} towards normal).
  - **Chronic kidney failure (MC cause of secondary).** Kidneys convert vitamin D to its usable form.
  - Severe calcium deficiency, severe vitamin D deficiency.
- **TERTIARY HYPERPARATHYROIDISM:** prolonged PTH stimulation after 2ry hypoparathyroidism ⇨ autonomous PTH production. Can be seen in post-transplant patients as well.

CLINICAL MANIFESTATIONS OF PRIMARY HYPERPARATHYROIDISM
1. **Signs of hypercalcemia:** *"stones, bones, abdominal groans, psychic moans."* ↓**deep tendon reflexes.**

DIAGNOSIS OF PRIMARY HYPERPARATHYROIDISM
1. **Triad: Hypercalcemia/↑Ca^{2+} + ↑intact PTH + ↓phosphate,*** ↑**24h urine calcium excretion,** ↑vitamin D.
2. Osteopenia on bone scan. Imaging studies to detect parathyroid adenoma.

MANAGEMENT OF PRIMARY HYPERPARATHYROIDISM
1. **Surgery: Parathyroidectomy*** (subtotal/3½ gland) or total (removal of all 4 glands with autotransplantation of parathyroid tissue in the forearm). May be observed in some cases.
2. Vitamin D/ Ca^{2+} supplementation if 2ry. Tx hypercalcemia if symptomatic (ex. IV fluids, Furosemide).

HYPOPARATHYROIDISM

RARE. Either low PTH or insensitivity to its action.
ETIOLOGIES: *2 MC causes are postsurgical or autoimmune.**
1. *accidental damage/removal of the parathyroid glands during neck/thyroid surgery.**
2. *autoimmune destruction of the parathyroid gland.*
3. Radiation therapy, hypomagnesemia (magnesium required for production of PTH), congenital.

CLINICAL MANIFESTATIONS
1. **Signs of hypocalcemia:** *carpopedal spasms, Trousseau's & Chvostek's signs,* ↑**deep tendon reflexes.**

DIAGNOSIS
1. **Triad: Hypocalcemia/↓Ca^{2+} + ↓intact PTH + ↑phosphate.*** Mg^{2+} may be low/normal/high.

MANAGEMENT
Calcium supplementation & Vitamin D *(ex. Ergocalciferol, Calcitriol).* IV calcium gluconate if severe.

	HYPOcalcemia	HYPERcalcemia

ETIOLOGIES	• **HYPOCALCEMIA with ↓PTH:** *Hypoparathyroidism MC overall cause* of ↓Ca⁺² *.*
	 - **Hypoparathyroidism:** parathyroid gland destruction *(autoimmune, post surgical)*
	
	• **HYPOCALCEMIA with ↑PTH:**
	- *Chronic renal dz MC cause if ↑PTH, * Liver dz.*
	- *Vitamin D deficiency* (Osteomalacia & Rickets). ↑PTH in response to hypocalcemia
	- *Hypomagnesemia,* ↑phosphate. *Hypoalbuminemia*
	- High citrate states: ex. blood transfusion
	- Acute pancreatitis, rhabdomyolysis. Meds: PPIs
		• **90% of cases of hypercalcemia are due to: PRIMARY HYPERPARATHYROIDISM OR MALIGNANCY!***
		  • **PTH-mediated:**
		    - *Primary hyperparathyroidism:* MC cause overall
		      Triad: ❶ ↑Ca + ❷ ↑intact PTH + ❸ ↓phosphate*
		      - MEN 1 & 11a, 3ʳʸ hyperparathyroidism
		
		  • **PTH-independent:**
		    - *Malignancy (secretes ↑PTH-related protein), ↓intact PTH*
		    - Vitamin D excess (granulomatous dz, vitamin intoxication)
		    - Vitamin A excess, milk alkali syndrome, *thiazides*, lithium**

CLINICAL MANIFESTATIONS	Hypocalcemia ↓'es excitation threshold for heart, nerves & muscle ⇨ *less stimulus needed for activation/contraction.* • *Neuromuscular:* muscle cramping, bronchospasm, syncope, seizures, *finger/circumoral paresthesias* • *Tetany: Chvostek's sign:* facial spasm with tapping of the facial nerve. *Trousseau's sign:* inflation of BP cuff above systolic BP causes carpal spasms. ↑*DTR* • *Cardio:* CHF, arrhythmias. Skin: dry skin, psoriasis • *GI: diarrhea, abdominal pain/cramps.* • *Skeletal:* abn. dentition, osteomalacia, osteodystrophy	Hypercalcemia ↑'es excitation threshold for heart, nerves & muscle ⇨ *stronger stimulus needed for activation/contraction.* • *Most patients are asymptomatic.* ±Arrhythmias • *Stones: kidney stones* (hypercalciuria ⇨ calcium oxalate & phosphate stones), *Nephrogenic DI: polyuria,* nocturia. • *Bones: painful bones, fractures* (due to ↑bone remodeling). • *Abdominal groans: ileus, constipation,** (decreased contraction of the muscles of the GI tract), nausea, vomiting. • *Psychic moans:* weakness, fatigue, AMS, ↓*DTR,* depression or psychosis may develop. Blurred vision.
LAB FINDINGS	• ↓*ionized Ca²⁺* & total serum Ca²⁺ (<8.5mg/dL) • ±↑Phosphate, ↓Magnesium. Check PTH, BUN/Cr	• ↑*ionized Ca²⁺* (most accurate), ↑Total serum Ca²⁺ (>10mg/dL) • PTH-related protein, 1,25 vitamin D levels, 24h urinary calcium
ECG FINDINGS	• *PROLONGED QT INTERVAL** 	• *SHORTENED QT INTERVAL,* prolonged PR interval, QRS widening.

MANAGEMENT	**Severe/symptomatic:**
	• *Calcium gluconate IV** or IV calcium carbonate
	  - Ca²⁺ carbonate must be given via central line
	
	Mild:
	• *PO Calcium + Vitamin D (Ergocalciferol, Calcitriol)*
	  Calcitriol if renal disease b/c no renal conversion needed
	• *K⁺ & Mg⁺² repletion may be needed in some cases.*
	• Corrected Ca²⁺ in patients with low serum albumin:
	  [0.8 x (nml albumin(4.4) - pts albumin)] + serum Ca²⁺
		Severe/symptomatic:
		• *IV saline** ⇨ *Furosemide* (Lasix) 1ˢᵗ line. Loop diuretics enhance renal Ca²⁺ excretion. *Avoid Hydrochlorothiazide* (causes ↑Ca)*
		• *Calcitonin, Bisphosphonates in severe cases (IV Pamidronate)*
		• Steroids: Vitamin D excess, malignancy (ex. myeloma), granulomas.
		
		Mild:
		• No treatment needed for mild hypocalcemia. Tx underlying cause.

OSTEOPOROSIS

LOSS OF BONE DENSITY over time due to ↑absorption of bone or ↓ decreased formation of new bone.
*Loss of BOTH bone mineral & matrix.** Peak bone mass seen in the 4th decade.

2 TYPES:

1. **PRIMARY:** I: *postmenopausal* & II: *senile.* Osteopenia (↓bone density) = *precursor to osteoporosis.*
   Risk Factors for postmenopausal osteoporosis: Caucasians Asians, thin body habitus, smoking, steroids, kidney disease, ETOH use, low calcium/vitamin D diets, physical inactivity.

2. **SECONDARY:** due to *chronic disease or meds*: hypogonadism, *High cortisol states:* **prolonged high-dose corticosteroid use,** *Cushing's syndrome.* Thyrotoxicosis, hyperparathyroidism, DM, liver disease, low estrogen, malignancy, immobilization, heparin therapy, anticonvulsant treatment.

CLINICAL MANIFESTATIONS

1. Usually asymptomatic. First symptom often due to a pathologic fracture, back pain or deformity.

2. *Pathologic fractures:* MC vertebral, hip & distal radius (Colle's) with or without trauma.
   Postmenopausal: *mostly trabecular bone loss ⇨ ↑vertebral compression & wrist fractures.*
   Senile osteoporosis: *trabecular & cortical bone loss ⇨ ↑hip & pelvic fractures.*

3. *Spine compression: MC upper lumbar & thoracic. Loss of vertebral height* (shortening of stature), kyphosis ("hunchback" bowing forward curvature of spine with forward thrust of head).

4. Back pain: from vertebral spine compression with or without fractures.

DIAGNOSIS

1. **Labs:** *serum calcium, phosphate, PTH & ALP usually normal.** Slight elevations of alkaline phosphatase may occur following acute fractures. ↓Vitamin D; Screen for thyroid, celiac disease.

2. *DEXA scan: best test to show extent of demineralization.** (Dual-energy X-ray Absorptiometry)
   - *Osteoporosis: Bone density T score ≤ -2.5*;* Osteopenia: T score ≤-1.0 to -2.5   Normal = ≥1.0
     T score -1.0 to -1.5 (repeat every 5 years); -1.5 to -2.0 (repeat every 3-5y); < -2.0 (every 1-2y)
3. Radiographs: demineralization. Axial skeleton predominantly affected.

MANAGEMENT

Adequate vitamin D, & exercise (weight lifting, high impact). Periodic height & bone mass measurements.
1. *Bisphosphonates: 1st line tx.** **MOA:** slows down bone loss by inhibiting osteoclast-mediated bone resorption. Take p overnight fast, with water (no food), remain upright for 30 mins, empty stomach - breakfast @ least 30-60mins p. **S/E: pill esophagitis, jaw osteonecrosis, pathological femur fx** (esp IV).
   PO: Alendronate , Risedronate, Ibandronate. IV: Pamidronate & Zoledronic acid (most potent).

2. *Vitamin D: Ergocalciferol associated with ↓progression.* ± add Calcium citrate or carbonate.

3. **Selective Estrogen Receptor Modulator (SERM):** *Raloxifene* used in post menopausal women - reduces progression, protective vs breast cancer, <u>not</u> associated with risk of endometrial cancer.

4. *Estrogen:* in postmenopausal women. Also helps with the symptoms of menopause. **S/E:** ↑risk for endometrial & breast cancer, coronary artery disease, stroke, venous thromboembolism.

5. PTH therapy (Teriparatide). Calcitonin: *last line therapy* (injection or nasal spray).

OSTEOGENESIS IMPERFECTA:

Genetic mutation for type I collagen (necessary for bone integrity). Associated severe osteoporosis, spontaneous fractures in childhood, *blue-tinted sclerae & presenile deafness.**

RENAL OSTEODYSTROPHY

• Bone disorders *(osteitis fibrosis cystica* & *osteomalacia)* associated with *chronic kidney disease.*
PATHOPHYSIOLOGY: failing kidneys do not eliminate phosphate properly & simultaneously poorly synthesize vitamin D ⇨ *hypocalcemia* ⇨ compensatory ↑*PTH* ⇨ osteoids *(↓mineralization).*

CLINICAL MANIFESTATIONS
1. *Bone & proximal muscle pain (in the context of uremia).* ± Pathologic fx, chondrocalcinosis.

DIAGNOSIS
1. *Labs:* ↓*Calcium* & ↑*phosphate,* ↑*PTH (2ʳʸ hyperparathyroidism).* Vitamin D levels vary.
   ↑*PO₄* (inability to excrete PO₄)* + *Hypocalcemia** (due to decreased vitamin D production by the kidney). Hypocalcemia + ↓vitamin D ⇨ ↑PTH (secondary hyperparathyroidism as a response to hypocalcemia attempting to raise the calcium levels towards normal*).*

2. **Radiographs:** *Osteitis Fibrosis Cystica* = periosteal erosions, bony cysts* with thin trabeculum & cortex, *"SALT & PEPPER" APPEARANCE OF THE SKULL** (punctate trabecular bone resorption in the skull). Osteitis Fibrosis Cystica is due to osteoclast activity (↑PTH stimulates osteoclasts to try ↑calcium levels by removing calcium from the bone ⇨ ↑bone resorption – bone cyst formation).

3. *Cystic brown "tumors"* on biopsy* due to appearance (hemosiderin) – not an actual tumor.

MANAGEMENT
1. *Phosphate binders: decreases phosphate: Calcium carbonate, Calcium acetate* (PhosLo). *Sevelamer* (Renagel) used if both calcium & phosphate levels are elevated. Phosphate goal <5.5.

2. *Vitamin D – active forms (ex. Calcitriol)* & calcium.

3. Cinacalcet: MOA: lowers PTH levels by reducing PTH synthesis & secretion by the chief cells of the parathyroid gland. Used in patients with renal osteodystrophy & 2ʳʸ hyperparathyroidism.

OSTEOMALACIA & RICKETS

• Due to *vitamin D deficiency** ⇨ ↓calcium AND phosphate ⇨ *demineralization* ⇨ *"soft bones."*

• In contrast to osteoporosis (where mineral & matrix loss is proportional), *osteomalacia is characterized by decreased mineralization of bone osteoid only – cortical thinning,* layers of demineralized bone.

CLINICAL MANIFESTATIONS
1. **RICKETS (CHILDREN):** *delayed fontanel closure, growth retardation, delayed dentition costal cartilage enlargement* (rachitic rosary), **long bones:** *bowing* + "fuzzy" cortex.

2. **OSTEOMALACIA (ADULTS):** Asymptomatic at 1ˢᵗ. Diffuse *bone pain, muscular weakness* (proximal). Hip pain may cause antalgic gait. *Bowing of long bones.* Hypocalcemia symptoms.

DIAGNOSIS
1. ↓*vitamin D,* ↓*calcium AND* ↓*phosphate,* ↑*alkaline phosphatase.*

2. **Radiographs:** *LOOSER LINES (ZONES):** transverse *"pseudo-fracture" lines* (visible osteoids).

MANAGEMENT: *Vitamin D (Ergocalciferol) first line.** Calcium supplementation in some patients.

	OSTEOPOROSIS	OSTEOMALACIA	RENAL OSTEODYSTROPHY
ETIOLOGIES	• *BONE BREAKDOWN > Bone formation*	• *VITAMIN D DEFICIENCY*	• *Osteomalacia in the setting of CHRONIC KIDNEY DISEASE.*
PATHOPHYSIOLOGY	• Degeneration of already constructed bone ⇨ *↓bone density "BRITTLE BONES"** • Both *demineralization and decreased matrix*	• *Demineralization of bone* during building process ⇨ *"SOFT BONES"**	• Demineralization of bone due to Vitamin D deficiency ⇨ compensatory ↑*PTH** (secondary hyperparathyroidism) • *↓renal phosphate excretion*
CLINICAL SYMPTOMS	• Bone pain, *pathologic fractures more common* • *Loss of vertebral height*	• Bone pain, muscle weakness (proximal) • *Bending (bowing) of bones*	• Symptoms of *osteomalacia*
DIAGNOSIS	• *Normal Ca, Phos, PTH* & ALP • (±↑ ALP if acute fracture) • *DEXA scan**	• *↓Calcium & ↓Phosphate, ↑ ALP* • *LOOSER LINES (ZONES)**	• *↓Calcium & ↑ Phosphate*, ↑ ALP, ↑ PTH • *OSTEITIS FIBROSIS CYSTICA**: *Cystic Brown Tumors*
MANAGEMENT	• *Bisphosphonates** • Vitamin D + Calcium	• *Vitamin D* (Ergocalciferol)* • Calcium	• *Phosphate Binders + Vitamin D (ex. Calcitriol)** - *Calcium carbonate, Calcium acetate* (PhosLo). - *Sevelamer* (Renagel) if patient serum Ca is elevated - Aluminum hydroxide • *Decrease PTH* (via Vit D, phosphate reduction, parathyroidectomy)

ADRENAL DISORDERS

Zona **G**lomerulosa:	**A**ldosterone (Controls Na+ balance)	Outer layer of cortex
Zona **F**asciculata:	**C**ortisol	Middle Layer of cortex
Zona **R**eticularis:	**E**strogens/Androgens	Inner Layer of Cortex

Think "GFR" for the layers of the cortex and "ACE" for the hormones they produce.

CHRONIC ADRENOCORTICAL INSUFFICIENCY

- Disorder where the adrenal gland does not produce enough hormones. *2ry much MC than 1ry.*

PRIMARY (ADDISON'S DISEASE): *adrenal gland destruction (lack of cortisol AND aldosterone).*
1. **AUTOIMMUNE:** *MC cause in industrialized countries** (70-90%). Causes **ADRENAL ATROPHY.***
2. **INFECTION** *(MC worldwide): Tuberculosis,* HIV,* fungal, CMV. Causes **ADRENAL CALCIFICATION.***
3. *Vascular:* thrombosis or *hemorrhage in the adrenal gland (Waterhouse-Friderichsen);* Trauma.
4. Metastatic disease; Medications: **Ketoconazole,** Rifampin, Phenytoin, Barbiturates.

SECONDARY: *pituitary failure of ACTH secretion (lack of cortisol).* Aldosterone intact due to RAAS.
1. ***Exogenous steroid use MC cause of secondary insufficiency as well as OVERALL insufficiency.****
      Especially with abrupt cessation, patients unable to increase cortisol levels during times of 'stress'.
2. Hypopituitarism (rare). Tertiary (hypothalamic disease is very rare).

CLINICAL MANIFESTATIONS
- *2ry or 3ry Adrenal insufficiency usually have normal mineralocorticoid (aldosterone) function.*
   1RY/2RY/3RY: *symptoms due to lack of cortisol =* weakness/muscle ache (99%), myalgias, fatigue.
   Nonspp GI sx: weight/appetite loss (97%) anorexia, nausea, vomiting, abdominal pain (35%),
   diarrhea. Headache, sweating, abnormal menstrual periods, mild hyponatremia, salt craving,
   hypotension (less prominent in 2ry than in 1ry), **hypoglycemia more common in 2ry.**

   1RY ONLY (ADDISON'S DISEASE):
   Symptoms due specifically to *lack of aldosterone, lack of sex hormones & ↑ACTH production:*
   1. **HYPERPIGMENTATION*** (98%) - **↑ACTH stimulation** of melanocyte-stimulating hormone secretion.
   2. ↓ **Aldosterone:** *marked ORTHOSTATIC HYPOTENSION* (syncope, dizziness), **hyponatremia,**
      HYPERKALEMIA* & *non anion gap* **metabolic acidosis,*** (aldosterone normally causes Na+
      retention in exchange for K+ & H+ so deficiency causes the reverse), **hypoglycemia,** low BUN.
   3. **↓Sex hormones in women:** *loss of libido; amenorrhea, loss of axillary & pubic hair.*

DIAGNOSIS
Baseline 8am ACTH, cortisol & renin levels obtained. ↑renin seen especially with primary insufficiency.
1. **HIGH DOSE ACTH (COSYNTROPIN) STIMULATION TEST: *SCREENING test for adrenal insufficiency*** (blood
      or urine cortisol measured before & after IM injection of ACTH. Measured @ 30m & 60m interval).
      - Normal (physiologic) response ⇨ rise in blood/urine cortisol levels after ACTH is given.
      - *Adrenal insufficiency* ⇨ *little or no increase in cortisol levels.* Cortisol < 20 µg/dL.

2. **CRH STIMULATION TEST: *DIFFERENTIATES* between the causes of adrenal insufficiency.***
      - **Primary/Addison (Adrenal)** ⇨ **↑ACTH levels but low cortisol.*** (opposite directions)
      - **Secondary (pituitary)** ⇨ *low ACTH AND low cortisol** (pituitary can't produce enough ACTH).
      - Tertiary (hypothalamus) ⇨delayed, prolonged or exaggerated ACTH response.

MANAGEMENT
Hormone replacement. Glucocorticoids + mineralocorticoids in Addison's; Only glucocorticoids in 2ry*
1. **Synthetic Glucocorticoid:** *Hydrocortisone 1st line,** Prednisone, Dexamethasone. In a patient
      with acute insufficiency, Prednisone & Dexamethasone won't interfere with screening
      (Hydrocortisone will). DHEA may be given in some patients.
2. **Synthetic Mineralocorticoid:** *Fludrocortisone for primary (Addison's disease only).*
      Fludrocortisone not necessary in 2ry because they normally maintain aldosterone secretion.

- Because cortisol is a "stress" hormone, people with chronic adrenal insufficiency must be treated with IV glucocorticoids & IV isotonic fluids before & after surgical procedures (mimicking the body's natural response).
- *During illness/surgery/high fever, oral dosing needs to be adjusted to recreate the normal adrenal gland response to "stress" (ex. triple the normal oral dosing).*
- Everyone should carry a medical alert tag as well as injectable form of cortisol for emergencies.

ADRENAL (ADDISONIAN) CRISIS (ACUTE ADRENOCORTICAL INSUFFICIENCY)

• *Sudden worsening of adrenal insufficiency due to a "stressful" event (surgery, trauma, volume loss, hypothermia, MI, fever, sepsis, hypoglycemia, steroid withdrawal).* Normal response to "stress" is a 3-fold increase in cortisol. These patients are unable to increase cortisol during times of stress to meet the demand.

ETIOLOGIES
1. ***Abrupt withdrawal of glucocorticoids MC cause*** (in patients not gradually tapered off steroids).
2. Previously undiagnosed patients with Addison's disease subjected to "stress".
3. Exacerbation of known Addison's disease (who didn't increase glucocorticoid during stress).
4. Bilateral adrenal infarction (usually due to hemorrhage).

CLINICAL MANIFESTATIONS
Many patients have underlying adrenal insufficiency that manifests during physiologic stress.
1. **Shock*** *primary manifestation* (2ry to mineralocorticoid deficiency ⇨ ↓blood pressure).
   Hypotension, hypovolemia
2. Nonspecific symptoms: abdominal pain, nausea, vomiting, fever, weakness, lethargy, coma.

DIAGNOSIS
1. **Lab Studies:** BMP: ***hyponatremia, hyperkalemia, hypoglycemia***. Cortisol levels, ACTH, CBC.

MANAGEMENT
1. **IV Fluids:** *normal saline* to correct hypotension & hypovolemia (***D5NS if hypoglycemic***).
2. ***Glucocorticoids: IV Hydrocortisone*** (if known Addison's). Dexamethasone (if undiagnosed).
3. Reversal of electrolyte disorders: hyponatremia, hyperkalemia, hypoglycemia, hypercalcemia.
4. ***Fludrocortisone*** (Florinef) – synthetic mineralocorticoid (similar to aldosterone).

ADRENAL INSUFFICIENCY LAB VALUES

	CRH	ACTH	Cortisol	CRH Stimulation Test (ACTH response)	Aldosterone	Renin
Hypothalamus (Tertiary)	Low	low	Low	Exaggerated, prolonged	Low	Normal/low
Pituitary (Secondary)	High	*LOW*	*LOW*	Absent/↓ ACTH	Low	Normal/low
Adrenal (Primary)	High	*HIGH*	*LOW*	↑ACTH	Low	High

Note that primary disorders, ACTH & cortisol go in opposite directions (same direction seen in 2ry/3ry).

CUSHING'S SYNDROME LAB VALUES

	High Dose Suppression Test	ACTH
Cushing's Disease (Pituitary)	***Suppression of cortisol****	Increased
Ectopic ACTH-producing tumor	No suppression	Increased
Adrenal Tumor (cortisol producing)	No suppression	Decreased
Exogenous Steroids	No suppression	Decreased

Note that Cushing's disease is the only one that suppresses during high-dose suppression test.

CUSHING'S SYNDROME (HYPERCORTISOLISM)

Cushing's SYNDROME = *signs & symptoms* related to *cortisol excess.*
Cushing's DISEASE = *Cushing's syndrome caused specifically by* PITUITARY ↑*ACTH secretion.**

CLINICAL MANIFESTATIONS
Symptoms secondary to *excess cortisol & glucocorticoids:*
1. **Redistribution of Fat:**
   - *Central (trunk) obesity, "moon facies", buffalo hump, supraclavicular fat pads.*
2. **Catabolism (breakdown) of protein:**
   - *wasting of extremities* (thin extremities, *proximal muscle weakness*); *skin atrophy* (easy bruising, *striae*); Increased infections (ex. fungal); Hyperpigmentation (especially c ↑ACTH).
3. *Hypertension,** weight gain, osteoporosis, hypokalemia,* acanthosis nigricans.*
4. Mental: depression, mania, psychosis.
5. *Androgen excess*: hirsutism, oily skin, acneiform rash, ↑libido, virilization, amenorrhea.

ETIOLOGIES
Exogenous:
   1. **Iatrogenic:** LONG-TERM HIGH DOSE CORTICOSTEROID THERAPY *(MC CAUSE OVERALL).**
Endogenous:
   2. CUSHING'S DISEASE: (70%) BENIGN PITUITARY ADENOMA* or hyperplasia (secretes ACTH)
   3. **Ectopic ACTH:** (15%) *ACTH-secreting: small cell lung cancer*, medullary thyroid cancer.
   4. **Adrenal tumor:** (15%) *cortisol-secreting adrenal adenoma* (or rarely carcinoma).

DIAGNOSIS
SCREENING Tests for Diagnosing Cushing's Syndrome:
1. *LOW-DOSE DEXAMETHASONE SUPPRESSION TEST:* Dexamethasone is 4x more potent than cortisol. Normal response is cortical suppression. *No suppression = Cushing's syndrome* (Cortisol >5).
2. **24 hour urinary free cortisol levels:** most reliable index of cortisol secretion.
      ↑ urinary cortisol = Cushing's Syndrome.
3. **Salivary Cortisol levels:** ↑cortisol in Cushing's syndrome (usually performed at night).

DIFFERENTIATING tests for causes of Cushing's syndrome:
4. HIGH-DOSE DEXAMETHASONE SUPPRESSION TEST: establishes Cushing's disease from other causes. ACTH production in Cushing's disease is only partially resistant to glucocorticoid negative feedback (adrenal tumors/ACTH producing tumors are independent).
      - *Suppression = Cushing's disease.** The other 3 major causes of Cushing's will not suppress.
      - *No suppression = adrenal or ectopic ACTH-producing tumor.**
5. **ACTH levels**
      - **Decreased ACTH** ⇨ *adrenal tumors* (because adrenal tumors produce high levels of cortisol, suppressing ACTH levels via HPA axis); Decreased ACTH also seen with exogenous steroid use.
      - **Normal/Increased ACTH** ⇨ *Cushing's disease or ectopic ACTH-producing tumor* (because they secrete ACTH independent of the HPA axis).

MANAGEMENT
1. **Cushing's disease (pituitary)** ⇨ *Transsphenoidal surgery.* Radiation therapy if unresectable.

2. **Ectopic ACTH-secreting or adrenal tumors** ⇨ *tumor removal.*
      Ketoconazole or Metyrapone may be used in inoperable patients (↓'es cortisol production).

3. **Iatrogenic steroid therapy** ⇨ *GRADUAL steroid taper* (to prevent Addisonian Crisis).

HYPERALDOSTERONISM

1. **1ry HYPERALDOSTERONISM:** *is RENIN-INDEPENDENT (autonomous).*
   - *Idiopathic or idiopathic bilateral adrenal hyperplasia* (60%). MC in women.
   - *CONN'S SYNDROME: ADRENAL ALDOSTERONOMA** (40%) located in the zona glomerulosa.
   - Unilateral adrenal hyperplasia (rare).
2. **2ry HYPERALDOSTERONISM:** *due to ↑RENIN.* *↑Renin* ⇨ *2ry ↑ in aldosterone via RAAS.*
   - *MC due to renal artery stenosis** or ↓renal perfusion (*CHF*, hypovolemia, nephrotic syndrome).

CLINICAL MANIFESTATIONS
Usually asymptomatic
1. *HYPOKALEMIA:** proximal muscle weakness, **polyuria,*** fatigue, constipation, ↓DTR, hypomagnesemia.

2. *HYPERTENSION:** especially in patients with primary hyperaldosteronism.* HTN may manifest as **headaches,** flushing of the face. Although most of the patients are volume expanded, they are usually **not edematous*** (unless due to underlying disorders in secondary).
   - *Diastolic pressures tend to be more elevated than systolic pressures.**

DIAGNOSIS
1. **Labs:** *HYPOKALEMIA WITH METABOLIC ALKALOSIS** (due to dumping of K⁺ & H⁺ in exchange for Na⁺).
2. Aldosterone: Renin ratio screening: *if hypertensive.* Most sensitive to distinguish 1ry vs. 2ry.
   - *ARR >20 & plasma aldosterone >20 & low plasma renin levels* ⇨ *1ry ↑aldosteronism.**
   - *High plasma renin levels* ⇨ *2ry hyperaldosteronism.*
3. **Definitive tests:** Saline infusion test: no decrease in aldosterone levels if 1ry ↑aldosteronism.
   Sodium loading: high urine aldosterone in 1ry ↑aldosteronism.
4. **CT/MRI:** to look for adrenal or extra-adrenal mass. ECG may show signs of hypokalemia (U wave).

MANAGEMENT
1. **CONN'S SYNDROME:** *excision* of adrenal aldosteronomas + *Spironolactone (blocks aldosterone).*
2. **HYPERPLASIA:** *Spironolactone (blocks aldosterone), ACEI,* CCB. Correct electrolyte abnormalities.
3. **SECONDARY (RENOVASCULAR HTN):** *angioplasty definitive. ACE Inhibitors (blocks aldosterone).*

PHEOCHROMOCYTOMA

- *CATECHOLAMINE-SECRETING ADRENAL TUMOR* (chromaffin cells). *Secretes norepinephrine & epinephrine autonomously & intermittently* (triggers include surgery, exercise, pregnancy, meds: ex TCA, opiates, Metoclopramide, glucagon, histamine). Rare (0.1-0.5% of patients with hypertension).
- *90% benign; 10% malignant. May be associated with MEN syndrome II.*

CLINICAL MANIFESTATIONS
1. *Hypertension: most consistent finding (secondary HTN)** may be temporary or sustained.
2. *"PHE":** Palpitations, Headaches* (paroxysmal), *Excessive sweating.* Chest or abdominal pain, weakness, fatigue, weight loss (despite increased appetite).

DIAGNOSIS
1. *↑24h urinary catecholamines* including metabolites *(↑metanephrine & ↑vanillylmandelic acid).**
2. MRI or CT of abdomen to visualize adrenal tumor. Labs: hyperglycemia, hypokalemia.

MANAGEMENT
1. *Complete adrenalectomy.*

Preoperative nonselective α-blockade: PHENOXYBENZAMINE OR PHENTOLAMINE x7-14d ⇨ *followed by beta blockers* or calcium channel blockers to control HTN. Think "PHE" for symptoms & management.
DO NOT initiate therapy with β-blockade to prevent unopposed α-constriction during catecholamine release triggered by surgery or spontaneously, which could lead to life threatening hypertension.

ANTERIOR HYPOPITUITARISM

- Pituitary destruction or deficient hypothalamic pituitary stimulation. Congenital or acquired ex. tumor, infiltrative disease, *bleeding into pituitary (ex Sheehan's syndrome)*, pituitary infarction, XRT.

CLINICAL MANIFESTATIONS
1. **Growth Hormone deficiency:** children/infancy: growth retardation, **_dwarfism, fasting hypoglycemia_**. Adults: mild-moderate central obesity, increased ↑BP, ↑LDL, ↓CO ↓bone mass, impaired concentration.

2. **TSH deficiency:** *hypothyroidism (cretinism in infancy)* ↓T₃ & T₄ + inappropriately ↓TSH.*

3. **Gonadotropin deficiency:** childhood: delayed puberty, failure of epiphyseal closure ⇨ tall individuals, eunochoid features. In adults: amenorrhea, lack of 2ry sex characteristics, infertility, ↓libido, impotence.

MANAGEMENT
Hormone replacement: If deficient in TSH ⇨ levothyroxine; ACTH ⇨ corticosteroids; GH ⇨ Growth Hormone; FSH/LH/GnRH ⇨ estrogen, progesterone, testosterone.

ANTERIOR PITUITARY TUMORS

- *Most are benign MICROadenomas that are:* ❶ **_functional_** (hypersecretion of pituitary gland hormones), ❷ **_nonfunctional_** ❸ **_compressive:_** *local sx (ex. optic chiasm "mass effect"* ⇨ BITEMPORAL HEMIANOPSIA).*

TYPES OF ANTERIOR TUMORS
1. **PROLACTINOMAS:** **_MC type._*** Prolactin responsible for lactation & suppression of pregnancy during lactation, ↓FSH & gonadotropin-releasing hormone. **_Dopamine inhibits prolactin release._**
   Clinical Manifestations: Women: oligomenorrhea, **_amenorrhea, galactorrhea,_*** infertility. Men: impotence, decreased libido, hypogonadism, infertility.

2. **SOMATOTROPINOMA:** *Growth hormone-secreting* pituitary adenoma ⇨ **_acromegaly/gigantism._**
   Clinical Manifestations: **_acromegaly in adults & gigantism in children._** **_DM & glucose intolerance_** (GH is a counterregulatory hormone that increases glucose). Enlargement of hands, feet, skull & jaw (macrognathia), coarse facial features, ↑spaces between the teeth, headache, deepened voice, thickened moist skin (*doughy*). DM, weight gain, kidney stones.
   Diagnosis of Acromegaly: ⇨ ↑INSULIN-LIKE GROWTH FACTOR (SCREENING TEST).* Confirmatory test = *oral glucose suppression test*: ↑GH levels in acromegaly (normal response is ↓GH).

3. **ADRENOCORTICOTROPINOMAS:** *secretes ACTH*
   Clinical Manifestations: **_Cushing's disease* & hyperpigmentation_** due to ↑ACTH, causing ↑MSH (melanocyte stimulating hormone comes from the same precursor).

4. **TSH-SECRETING ADENOMAS:** *secrete TSH*
   Clinical Manifestations: **_thyrotoxicosis sx._** ↑T₃, T₄ *& inappropriately ↑TSH (same direction).*

DIAGNOSIS
1. *MRI - STUDY OF CHOICE TO LOOK FOR SELLAR LESIONS/PITUITARY TUMORS.*
2. Endocrine studies: prolactin, growth hormone, ACTH, TSH, FSH, LH.

MANAGEMENT
1. *Transsphenoidal surgery (TSS):* *management of choice for removal of ACTIVE or compressive tumors (except prolactinomas).* *Medical treatment is first line for prolactinomas.** Observation if nonfunctional, small microadenomas. Microadenoma = <10mm.
2. **Acromegaly:** *TSS + Bromocriptine* (Dopamine agonist ↓'es GH production). XRT
   Octreotide: Somatostatin analogue that inhibits GH secretion – S/E: diarrhea, cholecystitis. Pegvisomant: growth hormone antagonist. May be added to Octreotide.
3. *Prolactinoma:* *Cabergoline* or Bromocriptine (dopamine agonists inhibit prolactin).* XRT

HYPERPROLACTINEMIA

ETIOLOGIES
1. Pathologic: ***prolactinomas (MC cause),*** hypothyroidism, acromegaly, cirrhosis, renal failure.
2. Pharmacologic: ***dopamine antagonists*** *(Metoclopramide, Promethazine, Prochlorperazine)* because dopamine is an inhibitor of prolactin. SSRIs, TCAs, Cimetidine, estrogen.
3. Physiologic: pregnancy, stress, exercise.

CLINICAL MANIFESTATIONS
Increased prolactin levels inhibits gonadotropin-releasing hormone ⇨ ↓FSH/LH:
  Women: oligomenorrhea, ***amenorrhea, galactorrhea,**** infertility, vaginal dryness.
  Men: impotence, decreased libido, hypogonadism, infertility. Gynecomastia is rare.

WORKUP: includes TSH, BUN, Cr, LFTs, beta hCG, prolactin. Pituitary MRI if adenoma is suspected.

MANAGEMENT
1. Stop offending drugs.
2. **Dopamine agonists:** ***Cabergoline* or Bromocriptine.*** S/E: orthostatic hypotension, dizziness, nausea, fatigue. Cabergoline associated with less S/E than Bromocriptine.
3. Surgical treatment in selected patients. May need follow up radiation therapy.

GYNECOMASTIA

- Benign enlargement of the breast in males due to increased effective estrogen (increased production or reduced degradation) or due to decreased androgens. Seen in 3 main groups:
  1. Infants: due to high maternal estrogen.
  2. during puberty: especially 10 – 14 years (classically may last between 6 months – 2 years).
  3. older males: due to decreased androgen production.

ETIOLOGIES
1. Idiopathic, persistent pubertal gynecomastia.
2. **Medications:** Spironolactone, Ketoconazole, Cimetidine, 5-alpha reductase inhibitors, Digitalis/Digoxin, GnRH agonists (ex. Leuprolide).
3. Others: cirrhosis, testicular tumors (ex. choriocarcinomas), hyperthyroidism, chronic renal disease, Klinefelter syndrome. Alcoholism.

CLINICAL MANIFESTATIONS
1. palpable mass of tissue ≥ 0.5 cm in diameter centrally located (usually underlying the nipple), symmetrical, classically bilateral and often tender to palpation.

DIAGNOSIS
Clinical. Check testosterone levels. Mammogram if breast cancer is suspected.

MANAGEMENT
1. **Supportive:** depends on cause: ex stop offending medications, observation if early in the disease course (most regress spontaneously). Ideal treatment should start within the first 6 months of onset (after 12 months, the tissue may undergo fibrosis).
2. **Medical:**
   - **Selective estrogen modulators (SERM):** ex. ***Tamoxifen***.
   - Aromatase inhibitors blocks estrogen synthesis. Androgens: used in hypogonadism.
3. Surgical: if medications fail, large breasts, cosmetically unappealing, fibrosis etc.

DIABETES MELLITUS

Hyperglycemia due to ❶ *inability to produce insulin* ❷ *insulin resistance* or BOTH.

TYPES OF DIABETES MELLITUS
1. **Type I DM:** *pancreatic beta cell destruction* (patient is **no longer able to produce insulin**).
   - *Most commonly presents in children/young adults (onset usually <30y).*
   - *Type 1A autoimmune beta cell destruction* triggered by 1 or more environmental factors.
   - Type 1B: non-autoimmune beta cell destruction.

2. **Type 2 DM:** combo of ❶*insulin resistance &* ❷*relative impairment of insulin secretion.*
   - Etiology likely due to *genetic & environmental factors:* especially *weight gain & decreased physical activity.* 90% of type 2 diabetics are overweight. *MC >40y.*

   - **Type 2 Risk Factors:** h/o impaired glucose tolerance, family history, 1º relative, Hispanic, African American, Pacific Islander, HTN, hyperlipidemia, delivery of baby >9lbs, syndrome X/insulin resistance: "CHAOS"- Chronic HTN, Atherosclerosis, Obesity (central), Stroke.

3. **GESTATIONAL DIABETES:** during pregnancy.

PRESENTATION OF PATIENTS WITH TYPE I DM:
1. Most are asymptomatic (may be an incidental finding).

2. **Classic sx:** *polyuria, polydipsia, polyphagia, weight loss.* Diabetic ketoacidosis, HHS.

COMPLICATIONS OF DIABETES MELLITUS:
NEUROPATHY:
   - *Sensorimotor:* paresthesias, abnormal gait, ↓proprioception *"stocking glove"* pattern, pain, ↓DTR.
   - *Autonomic: orthostatic hypotension,* gastroparesis: N/V/D, constipation, impotence, incontinence.
   - *Cranial nerve III palsy: pupil size remains normal* unlike other causes of CN III palsy.

RETINOPATHY: painless deterioration of small retinal vessels. ± cause permanent vision loss.
   Dx: funduscopy, angiography.
   - **Nonproliferative (Background):** *microaneurysms earliest change* ⇨ exudative changes leakage of lipoproteins *(hard exudates* – deep yellow with sharp margins, *circinate) or blood (dot or flame-shaped hemorrhages)* ⇨ *cotton wool spots* (aka soft exudates – fluffy gray-white infarction of nerve fiber layer ischemia); closure of retinal capillaries, retinal venous beading (tortuous/dilated veins).

   - **Proliferative:** *neovascularization:* *new, abnormal blood vessel growth, hemorrhage.*

   - **Maculopathy:** *macular edema, blurred vision, central vision loss.* Can occur at any stage.

NEPHROPATHY: progressive kidney deterioration leading to *microalbuminuria (first sign of diabetic nephropathy).* Increased blood pressure accelerates renal deterioration.
   Dx: *ALBUMINURIA,* anemia, acidosis. Kidney bx: *KIMMELSTIEL-WILSON:* nodular glomerulosclerosis
   - *pink hyaline material* around the glomerular capillaries (protein leakage).
   Management: *ACE inhibitors* (reduces protein leakage & slows progression), low Na⁺ diet.
   Diabetes Mellitus is the most common cause of end stage renal disease (HTN 2nd MC).

MACROVASCULAR: atherosclerosis ⇨ coronary artery disease, peripheral vascular disease, stroke.

Increased risk of infections: due to vascular insufficiency & immunosuppression from hyperglycemia.

HYPOGLYCEMIA: a complication of the management of diabetes mellitus. Usually due to too much insulin use, too little food or excess exercise.

1. **CLINICAL MANIFESTATIONS:**
   - **Autonomic:** sweating, tremors, palpitations, nervousness, tachycardia.
   - **CNS:** headache, lightness, confusion, slurred speech, dizziness.

2. **DIAGNOSIS:** random blood sugar 50-60 mg/dL. Sx occur @60. Brain dysfunction begins @50.

3. **MANAGEMENT:**
   - **Mild <60:** ⇨10-15g fast acting carbohydrate, fruit juice, hard candies. Recheck in 15 minutes.
   - **Severe/unconscious <40 mg/dL:** ⇨ *IV bolus of D50 or inject glucagon SQ.*

If unknown cause: order C-peptide, plasma insulin levels & anti-insulin antibodies.

DIAGNOSIS OF DIABETES MELLITUS

Normal fasting blood glucose levels are between 70-100 mg/dL.

GLUCOSE TEST	IMPAIRED TOLERANCE	DIABETES MELLITUS(mg/dL)	COMMENTS
FASTING PLASMA GLUCOSE	110 - 125	≥ 126	- Fasting @ least 8 hours on **2 occasions.** - **GOLD STANDARD.***
2-HOUR GLUCOSE TOLERANCE TEST	≥140-199	≥ 200	- *Oral glucose tolerance test. (GTT).* - *3h GTT* gold standard in gestational diabetes
HEMOGLOBIN A$_{1C}$	5.7 – 6.4 %	≥ 6.5%	*Indicates average blood sugar* ***10-12 weeks prior** to measurement*
RANDOM PLASMA		≥200	in a patient with classic diabetic symptoms or complications.

SCREENING: ADA: all adults ≥45 every 3 years OR any adult with BMI ≥25kg/m^2 & 1 additional risk factor.
USPSTF: (2015) any 40-70 year old that is overweight or obese (every 3 years).

MANAGEMENT & GOALS OF DIABETES MELLITUS

- *Diet, exercise & lifestyle changes: should be tried first in Type II DM!** ⇨oral antihyperglycemic agents.*
   - ± insulin if unable to control glucose with trial of diet, exercise, lifestyle changes & meds.
   - **Diet:** *Carbohydrates 50-60%; Protein 15-20%, 10% unsaturated fats.*

- Insulin therapy initiated in Type I DM. Insulin preferred for glucose control in gestational DM.

- **Glucose control goals:**
   Hgb A$_{1C}$ <7.0% (✓q3 months if not controlled; ✓twice a year if controlled).
   - Pre-prandial blood glucose goal 80 - 130 mg/dL.
   - Post-prandial blood glucose goal <180 mg/dL (1h).

- **Lipid control:** (in mg/dL) LDL <100; HDL ≥ 40; TG <150

- **Neuropathy:** *Gabapentin,* ±Tricyclic antidepressants. Foot care (wide, loose-fitting shoes, nail trimming, podiatrist monitoring at least yearly).

- **Retinopathy:** DM control, laser photocoagulation tx, Bevacizumab (proliferative), Vitrectomy. Yearly eye screening by an ophthalmologist.

- **Nephropathy:** DM control, *ACE Inhibitors if microalbuminuria.** Low sodium diet. Yearly screening for microalbuminemia. Yearly checks of BUN & creatinine.

ANTI-HYPERGLYCEMIC AGENTS

	MECHANISM OF ACTION	SIDE EFFECTS/CAUTION
BIGUANIDES *Metformin* (Glucophage) Phenformin	• Mainly ↓'es *HEPATIC GLUCOSE PRODUCTION,* ↑'es peripheral glucose utilization. • ↓GI intestinal glucose absorption, ↑insulin sensitivity *no effect on pancreatic beta cells* ⇨ *NO HYPOGLYCEMIA, NO WEIGHT GAIN.* • Usually *1st LINE PO MEDICATION** used to control Type II DM. ↓'es triglycerides.	• *Lactic acidosis,* Not given if hepatic or renal impairment* Cr >1.5 • GI complaints common. Metallic taste. • **Macrocytic anemia** (↓B_{12} absorption). • Metformin should be stopped 24h before given iodinated contrast & resumed 48h afterwards with monitoring of creatinine.
SULFONYLUREAS 1st gen: *Tolbutamide, Chlorpropamide* 2nd gen: *Glipizide* (Glucotrol). *Glyburide, Glimepiride*	• Stimulates *PANCREATIC INSULIN RELEASE** *from beta cells (insulin secretagogue –* non glucose dependent) • 2nd generation: less S/E (so preferred), shorter half-lives	• *HYPOGLYCEMIA MC S/E** • GI upset (reduced if taken c food), Dermatitis **Disulfiram reaction***, sulfa allergy • *Cardiac dysrhythmias,* **WEIGHT GAIN** CP450 inducer (drug-drug interactions)
MEGLITINIDES Repaglinide (Prandin), Nateglinide	• Stimulates *pancreatic beta cell insulin release* (insulin secretagogue)*	• *Hypoglycemia* (less than sulfonylureas) because glucose-dependent. Weight gain
α - GLUCOSIDASE INHIBITORS: *Acarbose* (Precose) *Miglitol* (Glyset)	• *DELAYS INTESTINAL GLUCOSE ABSORPTION** (inhibits pancreatic alpha amylase and intestinal α-glucosidase hydrolase). • Does not affect insulin secretion.	• *Hepatitis* (↑LFTs) • GI: flatulence, diarrhea, abdominal pain. • Cautious use in patients with gastroparesis, inflammatory bowel disease, on bile acid resins.
THIAZOLIDINEDIONES Pioglitazone (Actos) Rosiglitazone (Avandia)	• ↑ *INSULIN SENSITIVITY @ PERIPHERAL* *RECEPTOR SITE -ADIPOSE & MUSCLE TISSUES** • *No effect on pancreatic beta cells.*	• *Fluid retention & edema** (CHF), hepatotoxicity, fractures. • *Cardiovascular toxicity c Avandia** (MI) • ↑bladder cancer risk with Pioglitazone
GLUCACON-LIKE PEPTIDE 1 (GLP-1) AGONISTS: *Exenatide* (Byetta), *Liraglutide* (Victoza)	• Mimics *incretin* ⇨ ↑*insulin secretion,* ↓glucagon secretion. Given by injection. • *Delays gastric emptying.** No weight gain.	• Hypoglycemia (less than sulfonylureas - glucose dependent), *pancreatitis.* • *CI if history of gastroparesis,** thyroid CA.
DPP-4 INHIBITOR: Sitagliptin (Januvia) Linagliptin (Tradjenta)	• Dipeptidylpeptase inhibition ⇨inhibition of degradation of GLP-1 ⇨ ↑ GLP-1.	• Pancreatitis, renal failure, GI symptoms.
SGLT-2 INHIBITOR: SGLT = Sodium-Glucose Transport Canagliflozin, Dapagliflozin	• SGLT-2 inhibition lowers renal glucose threshold ⇨ ↑*URINARY GLUCOSE EXCRETION.*	• Thirst, nausea, abdominal pain, UTIs.

INSULIN THERAPY FOR DIABETES

Most type I diabetics need 0.5 - 1.0 units/kg day. Adjust dose as needed.

Insulin Goals:
- Fasting blood glucose 80 - 130 mg/dL
- Postprandial glucose <180 mg/dL

TYPE OF INSULIN	ONSET	PEAK	DURATION	INSULIN COVERAGE
RAPID- ACTING *Lispro* (Humalog) *Aspart* (Novolog) Glulisine	5-15min	1h	3-4h	***Given at the same time of meal.*** Often used with intermediate or long acting insulin.
SHORT- ACTING *Regular (Humulin-R)*	30m – 1h	2-3h	4-6h	***Given 30-60 minutes prior to meal.*** Often used with intermediate or long acting insulin
INTERMEDIATE NPH (Humulin N) (Novolin N)	2-4h	4-12h	16-20h	***Covers insulin for about half day (or overnight).*** Often combined with rapid or short-acting insulin. *NPH often given @ bedtime*
Lente (Humulin L) (Novolin L)				
LONG ACTING *Detemir (Levemir)*	6-8h	12-16h	20-30h	***Covers insulin for 1 full day (basal insulin)*** • *Glargine causes fewer hypoglycemic episodes than NPH.* • *Long acting should not be mixed with other types of insulin* in the same syringe
Glargine (Lantus)	4	No peak	24-36h	

PRE-MIXED: Humulin 70/30 (NPH/reg), Novolin 70/30, Novolog 70/30 (NPH, aspsart), Humulin 50/50

These are generally given twice daily before mealtime. 70/30 (NPH/Regular)

DAWN PHENOMENON:

Normal glucose ***until rise in serum glucose levels between 2am - 8 am.*** Results from decreased insulin sensitivity & ***nightly surge of counter regulatory hormones*** (during nighttime fasting).

MANAGEMENT: ***bedtime injection of NPH*** (to blunt morning hyperglycemia). ***avoiding carbohydrate snack late at night,*** insulin pump usage early in the morning.

SOMOGYI EFFECT: ***nocturnal hypoglycemia followed by rebound hyperglycemia*** (due to surge in growth hormone).

MANAGEMENT: ***prevent hypoglycemia: decreasing*** nighttime NPH dose or give bedtime snack.

INSULIN WANING: progressive rise in glucose from bed to morning (seen when NPH dose evening dose is administered before dinner).

MANAGEMENT: ***move insulin dose to bedtime or increase the evening dose.***

DIABETIC KETOACIDOSIS & HYPEROSMOLAR HYPERGLYCEMIA

- Diabetic ketoacidosis (DKA) & Hyperosmolar Hyperglycemic Syndrome (HHS) are results of *INSULIN DEFICIENCY* & counterregulatory hormonal excess in diabetics as a direct **response to stressful triggers ex:**
  - **Infection (MC),* infarction, noncompliance c insulin**/dosage Δ, undiagnosed diabetics.

- Cortisol is a stress hormone (↑'es glucose). These patients are unable to meet the demand of increased insulin requirements in response to hyperglycemia especially during stress.
- **Differ by the presence of ketoacidosis (DKA) & severity of hyperglycemia (higher in HHS).**
- DKA: younger patients with type I DM;   HHS: usually older with type 2 DM (higher mortality).

PATHOPHYSIOLOGY OF DIABETIC KETOACIDOSIS (DKA)
Insulin deficiency ⇨ ❶ hyperglycemia ❷ dehydration ❸ ketonemia (high anion gap metabolic acidosis) ❹ potassium deficit.   Usually occurs in Type I (may occur in some type II).

PATHOPHYSIOLOGY IN HYPEROSMOLAR HYPERGLYCEMIC SYNDROME (HHS):
Usually occurs in patients with type 2 DM with some illness leading to reduced fluid intake (MC infection). ❶dehydration, increased osmolarity, hyperglycemia ❷ potassium deficit ❸ absence of severe ketosis (Type II diabetics make enough insulin to prevent ketogenesis usually).

CLINICAL MANIFESTATIONS OF DKA AND HHS
1. **Hyperglycemia**: thirst, polyuria, polydipsia, nocturia, weakness, fatigue, confusion, nausea, vomiting, chest pain, **abdominal pain (in DKA). Mental status changes in HHS.**

2. **Physical Exam:** tachycardia, tachypnea, hypotension, (fever if infection), decreased skin turgor. **DKA: KETOTIC BREATH (fruity with acetone smell) & KUSSMAUL'S RESPIRATION*** (deep continuous respirations as lung attempts to blow off excess CO_2 to reduce acidemia).

DIAGNOSIS OF DKA AND HHS:

	HHS	Mild DKA	Moderate DKA	Severe DKA
Plasma Glucose (mg/dL)	**>600**	**>250**	>250	>250
Arterial pH	**>7.30**	**<7.30**	7.0-7.24	<7.0
Serum Bicarbonate (mEq/L)	>15	**15-18**	10 to <15	<10
Ketones (Urine/Serum)	Small	**Positive**	Positive	Positive
Serum Osmolarity	**>320**	Variable	Variable	Variable

Initial management: ABC, mental status, vital signs, volume status, screen for precipitating event.

MANAGEMENT OF DKA/HHS
1. **IV FLUIDS: Critical 1st step***
   - **Isotonic 0.9% NS** until hypotension/orthostasis resolves ⇨ **0.45% NS.** When glucose levels reach 250 ⇨ switch to **D5 0.45 (½) normal saline** to prevent hypoglycemia from the insulin therapy.

2. **INSULIN (REGULAR):** lowers serum glucose & switches body from catabolic to anabolic state ⇨ ↓gluconeogenesis, reduced ketone & fatty acid production.

3. **POTASSIUM:** (1st verify renal output). **Despite serum K levels, patient is always total body potassium deficient***   Correction of DKA invariably will cause hypokalemia. K+ repletion recommended if potassium is low/normal (ex. 20-40mEq/L if K+ <5.5). If potassium is high ⇨ hold repletion & then replete K+ when serum K+ falls into the normal range.

4. Bicarbonate: only in severe acidosis (especially since the acidosis usually resolves with IV fluids & insulin). Associated with many complications (ex. increased rate of cerebral edema).
   Treatment goals: closing of the anion gap in DKA. Normal mental status in HHS.

MULTIPLE ENDOCRINE NEOPLASIA I (MEN 1) Wermer's

- *RARE Inherited* disorder of 1 or more overactive endocrine gland tumors *(3 P's):*
  PARATHYROID: 90%; **PANCREAS:** 60%; **PITUITARY** 55%

- *Most tumors are benign* (especially before 30y). Associated with Menin gene defect.

CLINICAL MANIFESTATIONS
HYPERPARATHYROIDISM: *MC endocrine abnormality (90%)*
1. **CLINICAL MANIFESTATIONS:** *hypercalcemia:* "stones, bones, abdominal groans, psychic moans".
2. **DIAGNOSIS:** *hypercalcemia, ↑intact PTH, ↓phosphate, ↑24h urine Calcium.*
3. **MANAGEMENT:** parathyroidectomy.

PANCREATIC tumors: *2nd MC involvement. These tumors have highest malignant potential!*
- **GASTRINOMAS (ZES):** *MC of all entero-pancreatic tumors.** Tend to be small & multiple.
  Clinical Manifestations: *multiple peptic ulcers,* epigastric pain, reflux, diarrhea, weight loss, GI bleed, GI perforation. Poor prognosis with pancreatic, METS & high gastrin levels.

- **INSULINOMAS:** *2nd MC entero-pancreatic tumor.* Develops from pancreatic beta cells.
  Clinical manifestations: *Whipple's triad:** ❶ fasting or exertional *hypoglycemia* ❷ blood glucose <50 mg/dL during attack ❸ symptom improvement with glucose intake.
  Diagnosis: inappropriately ↑insulin with fasting, ↑*C-peptide** & ↑pro-insulin levels.
  CT/US. 90% solitary & benign (malignancy suspected if >6 cm or liver/nodal METS).
  Management: *surgical removal,* frequent small carbohydrate meals + Octreotide until surgery.

- **GLUCAGONOMAS:** MC @ the head of the pancreas.
  Clinical Manifestations: *necrolytic migratory erythema* 70% (migratory spread of erythematous blisters & swelling across areas with increased friction & pressure),
  Type II DM, muscle wasting (hypo aminoacidemia), cachexia, DVT/PE.
  Management: surgical removal. *Octreotide:* inhibits glucagon release.

- **VIPomas:** Vasoactive Intestinal peptide tumors. Clinical manifestations: *W*atery *d*iarrhea, *h*ypokalemia, *a*chlorhydria (= WDHA), hypovolemia, dehydration (daily loss 5-10 liters stool/day). Management: correct dehydration, surgery (distal pancreatectomy).

- **SOMATOSTATINOMAS:** MC seen in the duodenum & pancreas
  Clinical Manifestations: *triad* ❶steatorrhea ❷cholelithiasis ❸type II DM. Hypochlorhydria
  Management: resect primary tumor & debulk hepatic METS if present.

- **Others:** carcinoid tumors, nonfunctioning polypeptide malignant tumors, lipomas.

PITUITARY ADENOMAS:
- *Prolactinomas 60% : MC type.* amenorrhea, galactorrhea, infertility. Impotence in men.
- Somatotropinomas (20%) - acromegaly (due to excessive growth hormone).
- Corticotropinomas (15%) - *Cushing's disease* (due to excessive ACTH).
  Diagnosis: MRI preferred.
  Management: *Transsphenoidal resection. Cabergoline or Bromocriptine for prolactinoma.*

SCREENING IN PATIENTS WITH MEN I
1. Routine Labs for monitoring patients: *genetic testing for a defect in the menin gene.*
   - *PTH & calcium:* to detect hyperparathyroidism (often the 1st sign of MEN I).
   - *Gastrin:* Gastrinomas MC pancreatic manifestation.
   - *Prolactin:* MC pituitary tumor involved in MEN I.

MULTIPLE ENDOCRINE NEOPLASIA 2 (MEN 2)

- *RARE Inherited autosomal dominant d/o* (RET proto oncogene). *Multiple endocrine gland tumors:*

MEN 2A (90%)	medullary thyroid carcinoma	Pheochromocytoma	Hyperparathyroidism
MEN 2B (5%)	medullary thyroid carcinoma	Pheochromocytoma	Neuromas, Marfanoid
Familial MTC:	medullary thyroid carcinoma		

- **MEN 2B** associated with presence **mucosal neuromas & Marfan-like body habitus.**

- **MEN 2B** have more **aggressive form of medullary thyroid carcinoma (presents in infancy).**

CLINICAL MANIFESTATIONS AND MANAGEMENT OF MEN 2

MEDULLARY THYROID CARCINOMA: *usually first feature.* Medullary thyroid carcinoma originates from parafollicular C cells (they *secrete calcitonin*).* May secrete CEA, ACTH, serotonin, melanin.
- 25% of all medullary thyroid carcinomas are hereditary (occurring in MEN 2).
- **Clinical Manifestations:** palpable neck mass. Compressive sx: hoarseness, dysphagia, dyspnea. Paraneoplastic syndrome: *watery diarrhea & flushing.* Metastatic sx: liver METS common.

- **Management: *total thyroidectomy.*** Parathyroid glands are left behind or transplanted. Prophylactic thyroidectomy within 1st 6 months of life (in 2B), by 5-6y old in 2A.

PHEOCROMOCYTOMA: usually appears between 10-30y, usually occurs after MTC. **Adrenal medullary tumor with intermittent secretion of catecholamines** (norepinephrine & epinephrine).
- **Clinical Manifestations: *P*alpitations, *H*eadache, *E*xcessive sweating** (intermittent)

- **Diagnosis: *24h urinary metanephrines & catecholamines.*** Adrenal CT or MRI.
- **Management:** complete adrenalectomy. Preoperative nonselective α-blockade 2 weeks preop.

HYPERPARATHYROIDISM: *seen only in MEN 2A! (10-35%)* Unlike MEN1, hyperparathyroidism rarely the presenting feature. All known MEN 2A patients screened annually (intact PTH & serum calcium).
- **Clinical Manifestations: *hypercalcemia*** "stones, bones, abdominal groans, psychic moans".

- **Diagnosis: *hypercalcemia,*** ↑intact PTH, ↓phosphate, ↑24h urine calcium excretion.
- **Management:** parathyroidectomy: subtotal (3½ gland removal) or total (4 gland removal with auto transplantation of parathyroid tissue in forearm).

SEEN IN 2B ONLY:
1. **NEUROMAS:** *seen in 2B only!* Mucosal neuromas of the lips, tongue, eyelids, conjunctiva, nasal & laryngeal mucosa.

2. **MARFAN-LIKE BODY HABITUS:** *seen in 2B only!* Includes high arched palate, pectus excavatum, scoliosis.

SCREENING OF MEN 2
1. Genetic testing for RET proto-oncogene and screening:
2. Routine Labs for monitoring patients:
   - **Calcitonin:** basal & stimulated calcitonin levels correlate with tumor burden.
   - **Epinephrine:** produced by pheochromocytoma.
   - **PTH & calcium:** to detect primary hyperparathyroid tumors.

METABOLIC SYNDROME (SYNDROME X, INSULIN RESISTANCE SYNDROME)

- Syndrome of multiple metabolic abnormalities that increase the risk for complications such as diabetes mellitus & cardiovascular disease. This includes:

PATHOPHYSIOLOGY
Key component is **insulin resistance.** Free fatty acids are released, which causes an increase in triglyceride & glucose production as well as reduction in insulin sensitivity, leading to insulin resistance & hyperinsulinemia. The high levels of insulin cause sodium reabsorption, leading to hypertension.

DIAGNOSIS
ATP III criteria: at least 3 of the following 5:
1. ↓HDL: <40 mg/dL in men & < 50 mg/dL in women.
2. ↑Blood pressure: ≥135 systolic or ≥85 mmHg diastolic (or drug tx for HTN).
3. ↑Fasting triglyceride levels: ≥150 mg/dL (or drug tx for high triglycerides).
4. ↑Fasting blood sugar: ≥ 100 mg/dL (or drug treatment for high glucose).
5. ↑Abdominal obesity: waist circumference >40 inches in men & >35 inches in women.

MANAGEMENT
1. Lifestyle: weight reduction, exercise and increased physical activity, diet (rich in fruits, vegetables, lean poultry, fish, whole grains).

2. Weight loss: in addition to behavioral. Medical options includes:
   - short term use of **Phentermine** (3 months only). Sympathomimetic with unknown MOA.
   - **Phentermine/Topiramate** (no restriction on treatment duration).
       S/E: insomnia, constipation, palpitations, headache, paresthesias.

   - **Lorcaserin:** selective serotonin agonist (5-HT2C receptor) that induces satiety.

   - **Orlistat:** inhibits fat absorption.

   - Bariatric surgery may be used in some patients.

3. LDL treatment: diet, statins, Ezetimibe, bile acid sequestrants.

4. Triglyceride treatment: fibrates are usually the drug of choice.
       Other drugs include: statins, Nicotinic acid & high-dose omega 3.

5. Increasing HDL: Nicotinic acid is the most effective drug in increasing HDL levels.
       Other drugs include: statins, fibrates, bile acid sequestrants.

6. Lowering blood pressure: diet, exercise. ACE inhibitors, ARBs

7. Insulin resistance: biguanides (Metformin), thiazolidinediones.

SELECTED REFERENCES

Bennedbaek FN, Perrild H, Hegedüs L. Diagnosis and treatment of the solitary thyroid nodule. Results of a European survey. Clin Endocrinol (Oxf). 1999;50(3):357-63.

Brender E, Lynm C, Glass RM. JAMA patient page. Adrenal insufficiency. JAMA. 2005;294(19):2528.

Ironside JW. Best Practice No 172: pituitary gland pathology. J Clin Pathol. 2003;56(8):561-8.

Sarwar N, Gao P, Seshasai SR, et al. Diabetes mellitus, fasting blood glucose concentration, and risk of vascular disease: a collaborative meta-analysis of 102 prospective studies. Lancet. 2010;375(9733):2215-22.

Carney JA. Familial multiple endocrine neoplasia syndromes: components, classification, and nomenclature. J Intern Med. 1998;243(6):425-32.

Ripsin CM, Kang H, Urban RJ. Management of blood glucose in type 2 diabetes mellitus. Am Fam Physician. 2009;79(1):29-36.

Kitabchi AE, Umpierrez GE, Miles JM, Fisher JN. Hyperglycemic crises in adult patients with diabetes. Diabetes Care. 2009;32(7):1335-43.

Schlumberger M, Carlomagno F, Baudin E, Bidart JM, Santoro M. New therapeutic approaches to treat medullary thyroid carcinoma. Nat Clin Pract Endocrinol Metab. 2008;4(1):22-32.

Utiger RD. Medullary thyroid carcinoma, genes, and the prevention of cancer. N Engl J Med. 1994;331(13):870-1.

Lee NC, Norton JA. Multiple endocrine neoplasia type 2B--genetic basis and clinical expression. Surg Oncol. 2000;9(3):111-8.

Baloch Z, Carayon P, Conte-devolx B, et al. Laboratory medicine practice guidelines. Laboratory support for the diagnosis and monitoring of thyroid disease. Thyroid. 2003;13(1):3-126.

Ziegler R. Hypercalcemic crisis. J Am Soc Nephrol. 2001;12 Suppl 17:S3-9.

Assessment of fracture risk and its application to screening for postmenopausal osteoporosis. Report of a WHO Study Group. World Health Organ Tech Rep Ser. 1994;843:1-129.

Nieman LK, Ilias I. Evaluation and treatment of Cushing's syndrome. Am J Med. 2005;118(12):1340-6.

Sarwar N, Gao P, Seshasai SR, et al. Diabetes mellitus, fasting blood glucose concentration, and risk of vascular disease: a collaborative meta-analysis of 102 prospective studies. Lancet. 2010;375(9733):2215-22.

Saborio P, Tipton GA, Chan JC. Diabetes insipidus. Pediatr Rev. 2000;21(4):122-9.

tandards of medical care in diabetes--2009. Diabetes Care. 2009;32 Suppl 1:S13-61.

Eledrisi MS, Alshanti MS, Shah MF, Brolosy B, Jaha N. Overview of the diagnosis and management of diabetic ketoacidosis. Am J Med Sci. 2006;331(5):243-51.

Berkman J, Rifkin H. Unilateral nodular diabetic glomerulosclerosis (Kimmelstiel-Wilson): report of a case. Metab Clin Exp. 1973;22(5):715-22.

Asa SL, Ezzat S. The cytogenesis and pathogenesis of pituitary adenomas. Endocr Rev. 1998;19(6):798-827.

Standards of medical care in diabetes--2012. Diabetes Care. 2012;35 Suppl 1:S11-63.

PHOTO CREDITS

CHAPTER 8 – NEPHROLOGY & UROLOGY

• The urinary system consists of 2 kidneys connected to the bladder by 2 ureters. The bladder, controlled by a sphincter, contracts to expel urine via the urethra with **parasympathetic (acetylcholine) stimulation** (remember cholinergic "SL<u>U</u>DD-C" with the U for urination).

• **Functions of the Kidney**: the kidneys regulate blood pressure, body volume, excrete waste (ex drugs, toxins, uric acid, urea), regulate solute concentration (ex Na^+, K^+, Ca^+, Mg^+), regulate extracellular pH, assist in the synthesis of red blood cells (via erythropoietin) & synthesize vitamin D.

THE NEPHRON IS THE FUNCTIONAL UNIT OF THE KIDNEY

• **Nephron:** functional unit of the kidney (1,000,000 nephrons). Nephrons are responsible for urine formation via filtration, secretion & reabsorption.

❶ FILTRATION

• **GLOMERULUS:** network of capillaries involved in the 1st step of urine formation by filtering the blood. Blood enters the glomerulus via the **a**fferent (approaching) arteriole & leaves the glomerulus via the **e**fferent (exiting) arteriole. Plasma ultrafiltrate flows from the glomerulus into the Bowman's capsule. The **Bowman's capsule** is a crescent-shaped structure that receives the ultrafiltrate from the glomerulus and is the beginning of the nephron. The Bowman's capsule & the glomerulus = renal corpuscle.

• **Filtration:** the plasma filtrate passes through 3 layers: 1) the capillary endothelium 2) the basement membrane (with a net negative charge) and 3) the podocytes of Bowman's capsule. A molecule's ability to be filtered by the glomerulus is based on the size, charge & shape of the molecule. Smaller molecules such as water, salt ions, glucose, amino acids & urea pass easily. Larger molecules such as blood cells & proteins (especially if negatively charged) do not pass through easily, so **urine does not normally contain cellular elements or proteins.**

• **GLOMERULAR FILTRATION RATE (GFR):** Measures the functional capacity of the kidney to filter blood. Normally the GFR is 125ml/min = 7.2L/h = 180L/day.
   99% of filtered fluid is reabsorbed. GFR depends on age, sex, body size, race.

❷ SECRETION

• **Most active secretion happens in the distal convoluted tubule**: ex organic acids (uric acid), K^+, H^+, drugs, foreign substances, creatinine (from muscle activity), uric acid, bile salts. <u>Secretion</u> = *removal of substances from the blood to be excreted* into the urine.

❸ REABSORPTION

Most reabsorption occurs at the proximal tubule (the rest occurs along the length of the nephron).
Active vs. passive reabsorption:
• **Active transport:** requires energy (ATP) ex. the Na/K pump. 2ry active: symporter (1 substance moving down its concentration gradient facilitates the other molecule to move in the same direction– ex. Na symporter with glucose or amino acids); antiporter (they move in opposite directions – ex. Na antiporter with H^+).
• **Passive transport:** Na^+ symporter (glucose, amino acids), ion channels, osmosis of water (ex in medulla).

Factors affecting reabsorption:
• **Saturation:** a high concentration of a solute can exceed the threshold of the kidney's ability to reabsorb it. Ex. Normally, the kidney reabsorbs nearly all of the glucose. The renal threshold for glucose is a serum level of 180mg/dL. **Clinical correlation:** *if serum glucose rises above 180mg/dL, it reaches saturation & glucose begins to spill into the urine.*
Rate of flow: increased rate of flow decreases reabsorption.

EARLY PROXIMAL CONVOLUTED TUBULE (75% of Na)

- <u>TUBULAR REABSORPTION</u> of vital substances is the primary function of the proximal tubule.
- Isotonic reabsorption of <u>all organic nutrients</u> (ex. all glucose & amino acids), most bicarbonate, sodium, chloride & 75-90% of H_2O.
- Generates & secretes ammonia (buffers pH).
- Angiotensin II acts in the proximal tubule to ↑Na & H_2O reabsorption.
    PTH acts on this segment to ↑phosphate excretion.
- ***Acetazolamide & Mannitol are diuretics that work at the proximal tubule.***

LOOP OF HENLE (25% of Na)

❶ **Thin DESCENDING Limb of Loop of Henle**
- <u>Passively absorbs H_2O</u> (permeable to H_2O) but <u>impermeable to sodium & solutes</u> (based on the hypertonicity of the medulla).

❷ **THICK ASCENDING Limb (TAL) of Loop of Henle**
- ***Impermeable to H_2O*** but ***actively reabsorbs Na^+, K^+, Cl^- via Na/K/2Cl co-transporter.***
- Indirectly aids in the <u>reabsorption of magnesium (Mg^+) & calcium (Ca^+)</u>.
- TAL helps <u>maintain the hyperosmotic medullary gradient needed to produce a concentrated urine</u> (in the presence of ADH).*
- ***Loop diuretics* work at the thick ascending limb of the loop of Henle** ⇨ inhibits the kidney's concentrating ability ⇨ ***production of very dilute urine* ⇨ *strongest class of diuretics.****

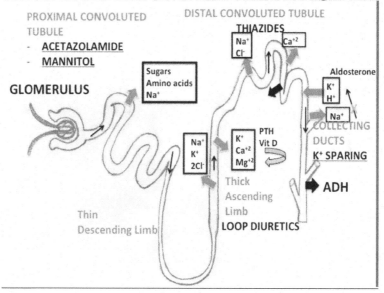

S/E OF LOOP DIURETICS

- **Hypocalcemia, Hypomagnesemia, Hypokalemia:** since loop diuretics affect the thick ascending loop's ability to reabsorb Na^+, K^+, Cl^- & indirectly inhibit Mg^+ & Ca^+ reabsorption, Loop diuretics may cause hypokalemia, hypomagnesemia, hypocalcemia, hypochloremia.

- **Hypochloremic metabolic alkalosis:** since chloride (negatively charged) ions are lost due to the reduced absorption of chloride, the body reabsorbs more bicarbonate (also negatively charged) to maintain electroneutrality, leading to the perpetuation of the metabolic alkalosis.

- **Hyponatremia:** although they promote sodium loss, loop diuretics prevent the concentration of urine, which can lead to hyponatremia (but not as common as thiazide diuretics). Although loops are stronger diuretics, thiazides are more likely to cause hyponatremia.

EARLY DISTAL CONVOLUTED TUBULE (~5% of Na)

- TUBULAR SECRETION main job.   Most active secretion happens at the distal convoluted tubule: ex organic acids, toxins, drugs, K+, H+.
- Dilutes urine by actively reabsorbing Na+ & Cl-, variable H_2O absorption (under control of ADH & aldosterone).
- *Parathyroid hormone acts on the distal tubule to ↑Ca+ reabsorption* (↑Ca+/Na+ exchange)
- *__Thiazide diuretics__ work here, impairing urinary dilution.   May cause __hyponatremia__ in setting of increased free water intake.*   In order to prevent hyponatremia, the kidney must make a dilute urine to excrete free excess water. *Thiazides impair urinary dilution.*

DISTAL COLLECTING TUBULES (1-2% of Na)

- Distal tubule DETERMINES THE FINAL OSMOLARITY OF URINE (via Aldosterone & ADH).

- **ALDOSTERONE:** ↑aldosterone ⇨ ↑Na+ reabsorption (in exchange for ↑secretion of K+ & H+). Although it is only 1-2% of total Na reabsorption, the distal tubule determines how much of excess Na+ intake from the diet is reabsorbed.
- Clinical correlation: this is why *__hyperaldosteronism is associated with hypokalemia & metabolic alkalosis.__* The exact opposite is seen in aldosterone-deficient states.
- *This is the site of action of potassium-sparing diuretics. Aldosterone inhibition by __potassium-sparing diuretics are associated with hyperkalemia & metabolic acidosis.__*

ANTIDIURETIC HORMONE (ADH):

- *__ADH:__* permeable to H_2O only in the presence of ADH.
  Presence of ADH ⇨ concentrated urine.   ADH absence ⇨ dilute urine.
- *↑ADH ⇨ production of a* __concentrated urine during times of hypovolemia, hyperosmolarity & ↑RAAS activation.__

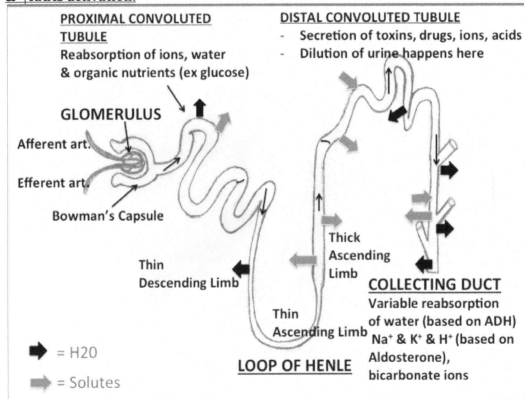

DIURETIC	MECHANISM OF ACTION	INDICATIONS	SIDE EFFECTS & CONTRAINDICATIONS
PROXIMAL TUBE DIURETIC			
MANNITOL	*Osmotic diuretic:* ↑es urine volume by ↑'ing tubular fluid osmolarity (since mannitol is filtered but not easily reabsorbed).	• *Intracranial HTN* (↓'es intracranial CSF pressure) • Oliguria (trauma, shock) • Glaucoma, Acute kidney injury	**S/E:** *PULMONARY EDEMA** (due to ↑fluid shift) **CI:** anuria
ACETAZOLAMIDE	*CARBONIC ANHYDRASE INHIBITOR* in the *proximal tubule* ⇨ *NaHCO₃* diuresis. *Mild diuretic, acidifies the blood* in patients with metabolic alkalosis	• *Glaucoma* (↓'es intraocular pressure), • *Intracranial HTN* (↓'es intracranial CSF pressure) • Urinary alkalinization • Metabolic alkalosis	• *Hyperchloremic metabolic acidosis* (due to loss of bicarbonate). • Hypokalemia, *sulfa allergies* • *Kidney stones* (calcium & phosphate)
LOOP DIURETICS			
FUROSEMIDE (Lasix) **BUMETANIDE** (Bumex)	Inhibits water, *Na⁺-K⁺-Cl⁻* transport across thick ascending *LOOP OF HENLE* ⇨ dilute urine *(strongest class of diuretics)**	• *HTN* • *Edema:* pulmonary edema, CHF, nephrotic syndrome, cirrhosis.	• *Hypokalemia/hypocalcemia/↓ Mg* • *Hyperglycemia & Hyperuricemia (caution in DM, gout).** • *Ototoxicity, Sulfa allergy* • Acute Interstitial Nephritis (all sulfa drugs) • Hypochloremic metabolic alkalosis • NSAIDs decrease its efficacy
TORSEMIDE	↑*PG synthesis* ⇨ ↑*renal blood flow* Lowers urinary Ca⁺² excretion.	• *Hypercalcemia*	
ETHACRYNIC ACID	*Similar action to furosemide (but does not contain sulfonamide)*	• *Diuresis c̄ sulfa allergy* • *Can be used in pts with gout*	• *More ototoxicity compared to Lasix*
THIAZIDE DIURETICS			
HYDROCHLOROTHIAZIDE Chlorthalidone Indapamide Metolazone Chlorothiazide	*Blocks NaCl & water reabsorption* at the early *distal diluting tubule.* ⇨ *diuresis & inability to produce dilute urine** Lowers urinary Ca⁺² excretion.	• *HTN* (if no comorbidities, elderly, African Americans). • Nephrolithiasis • *Nephrogenic DI* HCTZ ↓'es ability to *dilute urine**	• *HypOnatremia,** *HYPERCALCEMIA,** *hypokalemia,* hyperlipidemia. • *Hyperuricemia & hyperglycemia,* therefore *caution in pts c̄ DM, gout.* • *Sulfa allergies,* Metabolic alkalosis. Sexual dysfunction
POTASSIUM SPARING			
SPIRONOLACTONE **EPLERENONE**	*Inhibits aldosterone-mediated Na/H₂O absorption in cortical collecting tubule* while facilitating the reabsorption of K⁺ (potassium-sparing). Weak diuretic	• *CHF (reduces mortality)* • Most useful in combo with loop to minimize K loss. • *Hyperaldosteronism*	• *Hyperkalemia,** *metabolic acidosis* (K⁺ & H⁺ not exchanged for Na⁺). • *Spironolactone causes gynecomastia** *(anti-androgen effects)*
TRIAMTERENE **AMILORIDE**	*Blocks Na⁺ within cortical collecting tubule*	• Lithium-induced nephrogenic DI	• *Hyperkalemia, metabolic acidosis*

NEPHROTIC SYNDROME

- Kidney disease characterized by *PROTEINURIA, HYPOALBUMINEMIA, HYPERLIPIDEMIA & EDEMA.**
- Glomerular damage causes large tubular protein loss into the urine (***proteinuria***) ⇨ urinary loss of albumin cause ***hypoalbuminemia*** ⇨↓plasma oncotic pressure ⇨ ***edema. Hyperlipidemia*** as a result of low protein (albumin) stimulating hepatic protein synthesis (including lipoproteins).

ETIOLOGIES
Primary (Idiopathic): etiologies <u>confined</u> to the kidney.
  1. MINIMAL CHANGE DISEASE: *80% of nephrotic syndrome in children,** 20% adults. **Etiologies:** idiopathic ±associated with viral infections, ***allergies*** (ex insect stings, NSAIDs), Hodgkin dz, SLE.
      Diagnosis: *no visible cellular changes seen on simple light microscopy but **podocyte damage seen on electron microscope (LOSS/FUSION/DIFFUSE EFFACEMENT OF THE FOOT PROCESSES).***
      Loss of the negative charge of the glomerular basement membrane (promotes proteinuria).
      Management: ***Prednisone tx of choice:** >90% of children have remission after 3 months.** (80%) in adults. Cytotoxic therapy with Cyclosporine in refractory cases.

  2. FOCAL SEGMENTAL GLOMERULOSCLEROSIS (FSGS): sclerosis (fibrosis) within the glomerulus. Idiopathic, ***HTN (especially African-Americans),** IV heroin abuse, HIV, reflux nephropathy.

  3. MEMBRANOUS NEPHROPATHY: *THICKENED GLOMERULAR BASEMENT MEMBRANE:** idiopathic, SLE, viral hepatitis, malaria, drugs (Pencillamine), hypocomplementemia. **MC in Caucasian males >40y.**
      Usually present with ***nephritic-nephrotic*** picture. Caused by immune complex deposition.

Secondary causes:
  Systemic disorders extrinsic to kidney that affects <u>other organs in addition to kidney</u> ex. diabetes mellitus (MC overall cause of nephrotic syndrome in adults), systemic lupus erythematosus, amyloidosis, hepatitis, Sjögren syndrome, sarcoidosis, medications, infections, malignancy.

CLINICAL MANIFESTATIONS
  1. *EDEMA: peripheral, periorbital edema (especially in children) usually worse in the morning.* Pitting lower extremity edema, ***scrotal edema***. Edema is the predominant feature due to hypoalbuminemia (↓'es oncotic pressure). Ascites & anasarca may develop once albumin <3g/dL.
  2. *Anemia, **DVT*** (*hypercoagulability* - ↑fibrinogen & clotting factors V, VII, VIII, X as the liver tries to make more proteins to ↑oncotic pressure), frothy urine, pulmonary edema, pleural effusions.

DIAGNOSIS
  1. **24-hour urine protein collection:** *GOLD STANDARD.** >3.5g/day = nephrotic syndrome.*
  2. Urinalysis: ***proteinuria*** (3+ or 4+ on dipstick). ***Oval fat bodies "maltese cross shaped"** seen with polarized light microscopy* (due to filtration of lipoproteins into the urine).
  3. ***Hypoalbuminemia*** (<3.4g/dL), ***hyperlipidemia;*** ±↑BUN/creatinine: varying degrees,
  4. Renal biopsy: may differentiate the types. *Usually not needed* if minimal change is suspected.

MANAGEMENT:
  1. *CORTICOSTEROIDS IN MINIMAL CHANGE DISEASE** & FSGS. **Steroid responsiveness - most important determination of prognosis in nephrotic syndrome.** FSGS not as responsive as minimal change. Cyclophosphamide, Cyclosporine.
  2. **Edema reduction:** *diuretics* (thiazides if mild, loop diuretics if severe - removes excess fluid); 1L fluid & sodium restriction, ↑protein diet (to offset urinary protein loss).

  3. ***Proteinuria reduction: ACEI,** ARBs* reduce intraglomerular pressure, directly decrease urinary protein excretion & dilate the glomerular efferent arterioles ⇨ ↑renal blood flow & ↓GFR.

  4. Hyperlipidemia reduction: diet modifications & medications (ex statins).

ACUTE GLOMERULONEPHRITIS (AGN)

- Immunologic inflammation of the glomeruli causing protein AND RBC leakage into the urine.
- *HTN, HEMATURIA (RBC CASTS), DEPENDENT EDEMA (PROTEINURIA) & AZOTEMIA HALLMARK!!!*

ETIOLOGIES

1. **IgA NEPHROPATHY (BERGER'S DISEASE):** *MC cause of AGN in adults <u>worldwide</u>. Often affects young males within days* (24-48h) *after URI or GI infection** (due to IgA immune complexes). IgA is the 1st line of defense in respiratory & GI secretions so infections may cause IgA overproduction. Henoch-Schönlein purpura is a similar disease (but associated with generalized IgA vasculitis).
   Dx: ⊕ *IgA mesangial deposits* on immunostaining. **Management:** *ACE Inhibitors ± Corticosteroids.*

2. **POST INFECTIOUS:** *MC after <u>GABHS</u>** (±occur after any infection). 10-14d after *skin (ex impetigo)* or pharyngeal infection. <u>Classically:</u> *2-14y boy with facial edema up to 3 weeks after Strep with scanty, cola-colored/dark urine** (hematuria & oliguria). **Dx:** ↑*antistreptolysin* (ASO) *titers, Low serum complement (C3).* <u>Biopsy:</u> hypercellularity, ↑monocytes/lymphocytes, immune humps of IgG, IgM & C3 (seldom done as disease usually resolves without complications). **Mgmt:** *Supportive.* ±Antibiotics.

3. **MEMBRANOPROLIFERATIVE/MESANGIOCAPILLARY:** due to SLE, viral hepatitis (ex. *HCV, HBV*), hypocomplementemia, cryoglobulinemia. Usually present with a *<u>mixed nephritic-nephrotic picture</u>*.

RAPIDLY PROGRESSIVE GLOMERULONEPHRITIS (RPGN): *associated with poor prognosis (rapid progression* to end stage renal disease – weeks/months). *<u>Crescent formation on biopsy</u>** (crescents formed due to fibrin & plasma protein deposition collapsing the crescent shape of Bowman's capsule).
   Management: *Corticosteroids + Cyclophosphamide.*
Any cause of AGN can present with RPGN. The following 2 ONLY PRESENT with RPGN:

4. **GOODPASTURE'S DISEASE:** ⊕*ANTI-GBM ANTIBODIES.* Ab vs. type IV collagen of the glomerular basement membrane in kidney & lung alveoli ⇨ *KIDNEY FAILURE & HEMOPTYSIS.** (not due to immune complex deposition). Often occurs p URI. **DX:** *LINEAR IgG DEPOSITS.** **Management:** high dose *Corticosteroids + Cyclophosphamide* + Plasmapheresis (removes antibodies).

5. **VASCULITIS:** characterized by lack of immune deposits, ⊕ ANCA antibodies.
   - *Microscopic Polyangiitis* (vasculitis of small renal vessels): ⊕ *P-ANCA.**
   - *Granulomatosis with Polyangiitis (Wegener's):* necrotizing vasculitis ⇨ ⊕ *C-ANCA.**

CLINICAL MANIFESTATIONS

1. *HEMATURIA: hallmark.** Microscopic or macroscopic/gross *("cola-colored"/dark urine).*
   The presence of <u>gross</u> hematuria in nephritic distinguishes nephritic from nephrotic.
2. EDEMA (85%): *peripheral, periorbital (esp in children)* due to ↓oncotic pressure & ↑Na retention.
3. HYPERTENSION* (80%): secondary to Na+ & H₂0 retention.
4. *Fever, abdominal pain, flank pain* (due to renal capsule expansion), malaise.
5. Acute Kidney Injury: *OLIGURIA** ↓urine output <200ml (not always present).

DIAGNOSIS

1. **Urinalysis (UA):** *hematuria (RBC casts),** dysmorphic RBCs, proteinuria* (usually <3g/d but may be in the nephrotic range), *high specific gravity > 1.020osm.* ± WBCs.
2. ↑*BUN, ↑Cr: varying degrees.* *Renal biopsy gold standard** (not needed if poststrep suspected).

MANAGEMENT

- Glomerulonephritis is usually self-limited with a good prognosis (except in cases of RPGN).
   1. Berger's disease or proteinuria: ACE inhibitors ± Corticosteroids.
   2. Edema, hypervolemia or hypertension: *Loop diuretics (edema)*; beta-blockers, CCBs (for HTN).
   3. Post streptococcal AGN: Supportive, ± Abx. Lupus nephritis: Steroids or Cyclophosphamide.
   4. *<u>Rapidly progressive AGN or severe disease: Corticosteroids plus Cyclophosphamide.</u>**

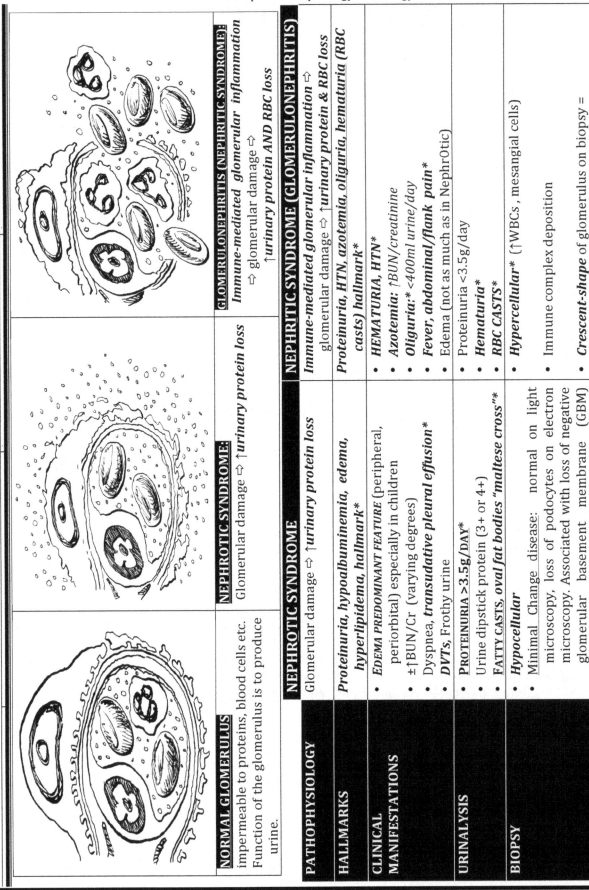

NORMAL GLOMERULUS: impermeable to proteins, blood cells etc. Function of the glomerulus is to produce urine.

NEPHROTIC SYNDROME: Glomerular damage ⇨ *↑urinary protein loss*

GLOMERULONEPHRITIS (NEPHRITIC SYNDROME): *Immune-mediated glomerular inflammation* ⇨ glomerular damage ⇨ *↑urinary protein AND RBC loss*

	NEPHROTIC SYNDROME	NEPHRITIC SYNDROME (GLOMERULONEPHRITIS)
PATHOPHYSIOLOGY	Glomerular damage ⇨ *↑urinary protein loss*	*Immune-mediated glomerular inflammation* ⇨ glomerular damage ⇨ *↑urinary protein & RBC loss*
HALLMARKS	*Proteinuria, hypoalbuminemia, edema, hyperlipidemia, hallmark**	*Proteinuria, HTN, azotemia, oliguria, hematuria (RBC casts) hallmark**
CLINICAL MANIFESTATIONS	• *EDEMA PREDOMINANT FEATURE* (peripheral, periorbital) especially in children • ±↑BUN/Cr (varying degrees) • Dyspnea, *transudative pleural effusion** • *DVTs*, Frothy urine	• *HEMATURIA, HTN** • *Azotemia:* ↑BUN/creatinine • *Oliguria:** <400ml urine/day • *Fever, abdominal/flank pain** • Edema (not as much as in Nephr0tic)
URINALYSIS	• *PROTEINURIA >3.5g/DAY** • Urine dipstick protein (3+ or 4+) • *FATTY CASTS, oval fat bodies "maltese cross"**	• Proteinuria <3.5g/day • *Hematuria** • *RBC CASTS**
BIOPSY	• *Hypocellular* • Minimal Change disease: normal on light microscopy, loss of podocytes on electron microscopy. Associated with loss of negative glomerular basement membrane (GBM) charge which further facilitates albumin loss (albumin has negative charge)	• *Hypercellular** (↑WBCs , mesangial cells) • Immune complex deposition • *Crescent-shape* of glomerulus on biopsy = *rapidly progressing glomerulonephritis**

Mixed Nephrotic/Nephritic picture = hematuria (nephritic) + nephrotic range protein >3.5g/day.

ACUTE KIDNEY INJURY (AKI) ACUTE RENAL FAILURE

- ❶ ↑serum creatinine >50% or ❷ ↑blood urea nitrogen/BUN (azotemia).
- **RIFLE Criteria:** 3 progressive levels of AKI:
  Risk, Injury, Failure with 2 outcome determinants: Loss & End stage renal disease.
- **Phases of AKI:** *oliguric (maintenance) phase* (↓urine output <400mL/d, azotemia, hyperkalemia, metabolic acidosis) ⇨ *diuretic phase* (↑urine output, hypotension, hypokalemia) ⇨ *recovery.*
3 TYPES: ❶ PRErenal ❷ POSTrenal (BOTH rapidly reversible) or ❸ INTRArenal (intrinsic).

PRERENAL

REDUCED RENAL PERFUSION - *hypovolemia.* Nephrons are structurally intact. *MC type of AKI* (40-80%).
Prerenal often leads to intrinsic (ATN) if not corrected. May also be a combined effect of afferent arteriole constriction (ex. *NSAIDs*, IV contrast) plus efferent arteriole dilation (ex. ACEI, ARBs).
Management: *volume repletion* to restore volume & renal perfusion (rapidly responds to treatment).

POSTRENAL:

Obstruction of the passage of urine (ex. BPH). 5-10%. **Management:** removal of the obstruction.

INTRINSIC:

Direct kidney damage: *nephrotoxic, cytotoxic, prolonged ischemic, inflammatory insults to the kidney.*
Structural/functional nephron damage *(CELLULAR CAST FORMATION*) hallmark of intrinsic.*

1. ACUTE TUBULAR NECROSIS (ATN):
Acute destruction/necrosis of the renal tubules of the nephron. Ischemic vs. nephrotoxic.
ISCHEMIC: *prolonged prerenal, hypotension, hypovolemia or post-op.*
NEPHROTOXIC: ❶*exogenous:* **aminoglycosides*** (10-26%), contrast dye, Cyclosporine, medications. ❷ *endogenous:* crystal precipitation (gout), myoglobinuria (rhabdomyolysis), lymphoma & leukemia, Bence-Jones (multiple myeloma). *ATN MC type of intrinsic!* (50%).

  - **UA:** *renal tubular EPITHELIAL CELL CASTS & MUDDY BROWN CASTS** (a variant of epithelial cell casts), waxy/granular casts (formed in damaged tubules); *low specific gravity* (unable to concentrate urine = isosthenuria – due to damage of the tubular cells which normally concentrate urine). Hyperkalemia, ↑Phosphatemia.*
  - **Management:** *remove offending agent(s), IV fluids,* Furosemide (if patient is euvolemic & not urinating). Most patients return to baseline in 7-21 days.

2. ACUTE TUBULOINTERSTITIAL NEPHRITIS (AIN):
Inflammatory or allergic response in interstitium with *sparing of the glomeruli & blood vessels.*
Drug hypersensitivity (70%): *Penicillins, NSAIDs, sulfa drugs,* cephalosporins, Ciprofloxacin, Rifampin, Allopurinol. *Infections* (15%): Strep, Legionella, CMV, EBV, HIV etc.
Autoimmune: 6% SLE, sarcoidosis, cryoglobulinemia; *Idiopathic* 8%.
  - **Clinical Manifestations:** *FEVER, EOSINOPHILIA,* MACULOPAPULAR RASH, arthralgias.*
  - UA: *WBC CASTS ARE PATHOGNOMONIC!* urine eosinophils. ↑Serum IgE.*
  - **Management:** remove the offending agent (most recover kidney function in 1 year).

3. GLOMERULAR (ACUTE GLOMERULONEPHRITIS - AGN) : *hematuria (RBC casts),* HTN, azotemia, proteinuria.* **Management:** high-dose corticosteroids, cytotoxic agents.

4. VASCULAR:
Microvascular: TTP, HELLP syndrome, DIC.
Macrovascular: aortic aneurysm, renal artery dissection, renal artery or vein thrombosis, malignant hypertension, atheroembolic disease (associated with ischemic digits/blue toe syndrome especially post catheterization, CABG, AAA repair).

ACUTE KIDNEY INJURY (AKI) ACUTE RENAL FAILURE

URINALYSIS: *most important noninvasive test regarding the possible etiologies.*

URINARY PATTERN	
RBC CASTS, with hematuria, dysmorphic red cells	*Acute glomerulonephritis (AGN)* or vasculitis.**
MUDDY BROWN (GRANULAR) OR EPITHELIAL CELL CASTS	*ATN (acute tubular necrosis)**
WHITE BLOOD CELL CASTS, pyuria (free WBC cells)	*AIN (acute interstitial nephritis)* or Pyelonephritis** or tubular dz
WAXY CASTS: acellular with sharp edges	Narrow waxy casts: **CHRONIC** ATN/ Glomerulonephritis Broad waxy casts: *end stage renal disease* (tubal dilation).
FATTY CASTS: "maltese crosses", oval fat bodies	*Nephrotic syndrome** (due to hyperlipidemia).
HYALINE CASTS	*Nonspecific (may be seen in normal urine).* Tamm- Horsfall proteins secreted by tubular epithelial cells.
Normal or Near Normal UA: few cells with little or no casts	Acute Kidney injury: *prerenal or postrenal.* Hypercalcemia, multiple myeloma.
Hematuria & pyuria (excluding red cell casts)	*UTI*, acute interstitial nephritis (AIN), glomerular disease, vasculitis.
Hematuria alone	See hematuria section (page 366).
Pyuria alone	*MC due to infection*; sterile pyuria due to tubulointerstitial disease.

	PRERENAL	ATN
Creatinine (Cr)	Increases slower than 0.3mg/dL/day	Increases at 0.3-0.5 mg/dL/day
UNa, FeNa	↓*Urine Na⁺ <20*; *FeNa⁺ <1%**	↑*Urine Na⁺ >40*; FeNa⁺ >2%
URINALYSIS (UA)	*Normal UA* *HIGH SPECIFIC GRAVITY (↑UOsm)*	*EPITHELIAL CELLS, GRANULAR CASTS.** *LOW SPECIFIC GRAVITY**
Response to volume replacement	*Creatinine rapidly improves c̄ IVF*	Creatinine won't improve much
Blood Urea Nitrogen (BUN)/Cr	↑*BUN: Cr >20:1**	10-15:1

$$\text{FENA \%} = \frac{\text{Urinary conc Na}}{\text{Plasma Na}} \times \frac{\text{Plasma creatinine}}{\text{Urine creatinine}} \times 100$$

PRERENAL: ↑*BUN:Cr* 20:1 – in order to conserve H_2O & minimize renal H_2O loss, the kidneys concentrate the urine - a high medullary concentration gradient is needed so that when ADH water pores open, maximum renal H_2O reabsorption will occur. Urea is one of the major solutes responsible for this high medullary gradient so urea reabsorption >> creatinine retention ⇨ ↑*BUN:Cr >20:1. High specific gravity: reflects a concentrated urine = less H_2O in the urine.* **Normal UA:** prerenal is not associated with tubular damage. **Low FeNa:** the kidney holds onto sodium (Na^+) to help replace the volume loss ⇨ less Na^+ is excreted in the urine ⇨↓fraction of excreted Na^+. Because there is no tubular damage, rapid correction of the hypovolemia will cause a faster response to volume replacement in prerenal.

ACUTE TUBULAR NECROSIS: ↑*BUN:Cr* reflects the kidney's failure to excrete both blood urea & creatinine. *Low specific gravity:* reflects renal tubular damage - damage to the cells that normally produce the high medullary concentration gradient means that the medulla is unable to concentrate the urine (isosthenuria). *Cell casts:* cells that make it into the tubules clump together & take the shape of the tubules as they travel through the nephron.

FeNa >2 reflects the fact that the damaged tubules render the kidney unable to reabsorb solutes.

CELLULAR CASTS: cells that make it into the tubules clump together & take the shape of the tubules as they travel through the nephron.

The type of cast is helpful to figure out the possible type of kidney injury:

ACUTE TUBULAR NECROSIS
- **Epithelial cell & muddy brown casts**

ACUTE INTERSTITIAL NEPHRITIS
- **White blood cell casts**

ACUTE GLOMERULONEPHRITIS
- **Red blood cell casts**

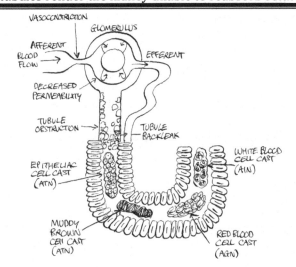

ADULT POLYCYSTIC KIDNEY DISEASE

- *Autosomal <u>dominant</u> disorder* due to mutations of either genes PKD1 (85-90%) or PKD2 (10-15%). 10% of patients with ESRD. Patients usually in 20-40s. Autosomal recessive type seen in children.

- Multisystemic progressive disorder characterized by *formation & enlargement of kidney cysts & cysts in other organs (ex. <u>liver,</u> spleen, pancreas).*
  Vasopressin stimulates cystogenesis ⇨ end stage renal disease (ESRD) over time.

CLINICAL MANIFESTATIONS
1. *<u>Abdominal/flank pain</u>*: may be due to infection, nephrolithiasis or bleeding into the cyst.

2. *<u>Palpable flank mass:</u>* large palpable kidneys on physical examination.

3. *<u>HTN</u>*, hepatomegaly, *hematuria* (may also bleed into the cyst), decreased urine concentrating ability, microalbuminuria.

4. Extrarenal: *cerebral "berry" aneurysms,** *hepatic cysts, <u>mitral valve prolapse,</u>** colonic *diverticula.*

DIAGNOSIS
1. **Renal ultrasound:** *most widely used 1st line diagnostic test.** Genetic testing also done.
2. CT scan/MRI: more sensitive than renal ultrasound.

MANAGEMENT:
1. **Simple cyst:** observation, periodic reevaluation. ACE inhibitors for hypertension.

2. **Multiple cysts:** supportive, ↑*fluid intake* - fluids decreases vasopressin (reducing vasopressin-induced cystogenesis), control HTN. ± Need dialysis or renal transplant.

	HYPOphosphatemia	HYPERphosphatemia
ETIOLOGIES	• **↑Urinary PO₄ excretion:** *1ry Hyperparathyroidism* *Vitamin D deficiency* • **Internal PO₄ redistribution:** respiratory alkalosis, excessive IV Glucose, treatment for DKA, refeeding syndrome in ETOHics (insulin shifts phosphate intracellularly). • **Decreased intestinal absorption:** antacids, phosphate binders	• *Renal failure MC* - ↓Ca^{+2}, ↑*Phosphate*, ↑*iPTH* • *1ry Hypoparathyroidism* - ↓Ca^{+2}, ↑*Phosphate*, ↓*iPTH* • *Vitamin D intoxication* - ↑Ca^{+2}, ↑*Phosphate*, ↓*iPTH* • Iatrogenic • Rhabdomyolysis, Tumor lysis
CLINICAL	• *Diffuse muscle weakness, flaccid* *paralysis (due to ↓ATP)*	• *Soft tissue calcifications* • Most asymptomatic, heart block
MANAGEMENT	Treat the underlying cause. **Phosphate repletion:** if symptomatic or serum PO₄ <2.0mg/dL • potassium phosphate • sodium phosphate	• *Renal failure: phosphate* *binders: Calcium acetate* (PhosLo), *Calcium carbonate,* *Sevelamer* (Renagel) • Decrease dietary phosphate: dairy products, dark colas. • Hydration, Acetazolamide

CHRONIC KIDNEY DISEASE

Chronic kidney disease: progressive functional decline ***≥3 months-years evidence by:***

1. Proteinuria
2. Abnormal urine sediment
3. Abnormal serum/urine chemistries
4. Abnormal imaging studies
5. Inability to buffer pH
6. Inability to make urine
7. Inability to excrete nitrogenous waste
8. ↓ synthesis of Vitamin D/Erythropoietin

CHRONIC KIDNEY DISEASE STAGING

Stage 0: At risk patients: DM, HTN, chronic NSAID use, Africa-American/Hispanic/Asian), age >60, SLE, s/p kidney transplant, family history of kidney disease. ***Normal GFR, normal urine.***

Stage 1: Kidney damage with normal GFR (or >90)
    Kidney damage = proteinuria, Abnormal UA, serum, imaging

Albuminuria
A1 = ACR <30mg/g

Stage 2: GFR 89-60

A2 = ACR 30-300mg/g

Stage 3: GFR 59-30   (3a 59-45) (3b 44-30)

A3 = ACR ≥300mg/g

Stage 4: GFR 29-15

Stage 5: GFR <15   End Stage Renal Disease (ESRD) = uremia requiring dialysis and/or transplant.

Normal Glomerular Filtration Rate (GFR) 120-130

ETIOLOGIES

1. ***Diabetes Mellitus****: MC cause of ESRD** (30%). **Due to diabetic nephropathy.**
2. ***Hypertension: 2nd MC cause of ESRD**** (23%).
3. ***Glomerulonephritis ~10% cases***, Polycystic kidney disease 5%; Rapidly progressive ~2%

PATHOPHYSIOLOGY

1. Nephron destruction (due to various etiologies) ⇨ compensatory hypertrophy of the remaining nephrons ⇨ failure from increased workload leading to fibrosis, sclerosis & tubular dilation.

DIAGNOSIS

1. **PROTEINURIA:** *single best predictor of disease progression.**
   - ***Spot UAlbumin/UCreatinine Ratio (ACR):*** *albuminuria = ACR 30mg/g* especially 1st AM urine.* (>2g glomerular range; less than 2g tubulointerstitial, >3g nephrotic range). ***Preferred over 24h urine collection.*** Spot test estimates grams of protein loss/day.
   - **24-hour urine collection:** alternative to spot ratio but not as good. Total protein, Creatinine Clearance. Normal albumin <30mg/24h; microalbuminemia = 30-300mg/d; macroalbuminemia = >300mg/d; nephrotic range >3g/d. Urine dipstick.
2. **URINALYSIS:** *abnormal sediment*: ***BROAD WAXY CASTS seen in ESRD*** (taking the shape of dilated damaged tubules). ±RBC casts, WBC casts etc.
3. **Estimated GFR:** CKD-Epi most accurate, MDRD.
   Cockcroft used for ***Creatinine clearance*** (ex "renally" dosing medications excreted by the kidney).

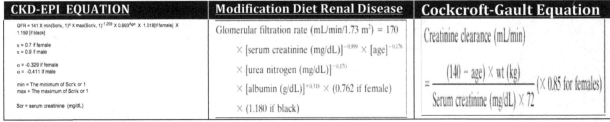

CKD-EPI EQUATION	Modification Diet Renal Disease	Cockcroft-Gault Equation
GFR = 141 X min(Scr/κ, 1)^κ X max(Scr/κ, 1)$^{-1.209}$ X 0.993^{Age} X 1.018[if female] X 1.159 [if black] κ = 0.7 if female κ = 0.9 if male α = -0.329 if female α = -0.411 if male min = The minimum of Scr/κ or 1 max = The maximum of Scr/κ or 1 Scr = serum creatinine (mg/dL)	Glomerular filtration rate (mL/min/1.73 m^2) = 170 X [serum creatinine (mg/dL)]$^{-0.999}$ X [age]$^{-0.176}$ X [urea nitrogen (mg/dL)]$^{-0.170}$ X [albumin (g/dL)]$^{+0.318}$ X (0.762 if female) X (1.180 if black)	Creatinine clearance (mL/min) $$= \frac{(140 - age) \times wt \,(kg)}{Serum\ creatinine\ (mg/dL) \times 72} (\times 0.85\ for\ females)$$

4. ↑***BUN/creatinine***, serum electrolytes, lipid profile. Renal biopsy.
5. **Renal Ultrasound:** ***small kidneys classic*** (large kidneys in diabetic nephropathy, PKD).
6. Miscellaneous: ANA for SLE, depressed serum complement in glomerulonephritis, C-ANCA (Wegener's), P-ANCA (Microscopic polyangiitis), anti-GBM antibodies (Goodpasture's), Hepatitis serologies, HIV, RPR. CBC – normochromic normocytic anemia.

CLINICAL MANIFESTATIONS
Usually not seen until advanced disease:

General: fatigue, malaise, edema, easily bruising, itching, bone pain, anemia of chronic disease, thrombocytopenia.

Cardiac: hypertension, heart failure, uremic pericarditis, coronary artery disease, MI, LVH, arrhythmias.

Pulmonary: dyspnea, pulmonary edema, pleural effusion on CXR, increased risk for pulmonary infections.

GI: anorexia, nausea, vomiting, uremic fetor (urine odor on breath), stomatitis, weight loss, metallic taste..

Neurologic: depression of the CNS, muscle twitching, CVA, uremic encephalopathy.

Metabolic: *metabolic acidosis (decreased by protein restriction).*

Dermatologic: darkening or yellowing of skin, pallor, dry scaly skin, pruritus, *petechiae (platelet dysfunction).*

MANAGEMENT OF COMPLICATIONS OF CHRONIC KIDNEY DISEASE

- **Dietary:** protein, Na^+, water, potassium & phosphate restriction when possible.

PREVENTION OF PROGRESSION (treat modifiable risk factors).
HTN & proteinuria are the 2 most important modifiable risk factors.
1. **HYPERTENSION:**
    - *Blood pressure goal <140/90 – ACEI,* ARBs,* ↓Na/H_2O intake, diuresis.
    - Other cardiovascular complications: CHF, MI, CAD, uremic pericarditis.
2. **PROTEINURIA**
    - *Protein restriction.*
    - *ACEI or ARB for microalbuminuria or proteinuria.* Decreases proteinuria, slows progression.
3. **DIABETES CONTROL**
    - *Hemoglobin A1C <6.5,* hyperlipidemia control (LDL <100 mg/dL, TG <150, HDL >50).

HEMATOLOGIC COMPLICATIONS:
- **ANEMIA:** *anemia of chronic disease (normochromic, normocytic anemia)* due to ↓kidney production of erythropoietin. Anemia of chronic disease: ↑ferritin, ↓ serum Fe, ↓TIBC.
  ± Also have iron deficiency anemia.
    MANAGEMENT: treat with oral FeSO4 (goal ferritin 100-500, goal FeSat 20-50%). *Erythropoietin or Darbepoetin-α if anemia persists after normal iron stores.* Goal is hemoglobin 11-12.

- **COAGULOPATHY:** platelet dysfunction ⇨ petechial, purpura, ↑bleeding times.
    MANAGEMENT: Desmopressin prior to surgical procedures temporarily helps with coagulopathy.

RENAL OSTEODYSTROPHY (BONE DISEASE):
- **Pathophysiology:** Ca^{+2} & phosphate dysregulation ⇨ *bone & proximal muscle pain & pathologic fractures.*

- **DX:** *Osteitis Fibrosis Cystica = periosteal erosions, bony cysts on X ray, "salt & pepper" appearance of the skull on X ray. cystic brown "tumors"* on biopsy (due to appearance – not an actual tumor). Osteitis Fibrosis Cystica is due to osteoclast activity (↑PTH stimulates osteoclasts to try increase calcium levels by removing calcium from the bone ⇨ ↑bone resorption – bone cyst formation). Osteitis Fibrosis Cystica can also be seen in primary hyperparathyroidism.

- **LABS** ↑PO_4* *(inability to excrete PO_4)* + **Hypocalcemia*** (due to decreased vitamin D production by the kidney). *Hypocalcemia + ↓Vitamin D ⇨ ↑PTH (secondary hyperparathyroidism - as a response to hypocalcemia, PTH increases, attempting to raise the calcium levels towards normal).*
    MANAGEMENT: *Vitamin D (Calcitriol) & phosphate binders: Calcium Acetate* (Phoslo); *Sevelamer* (Renagel): *used if both calcium & phosphate levels are elevated.*

Dialysis, renal transplant for end stage disease (stage 5). *Dialysis indicated if GFR ≤ 10mL/min and/or serum creatinine ≥8mg/dL* (In diabetics, GFR ≤ 15ml/min and/or serum creatinine of ≥6).

SYNDROME OF INAPPROPRIATE ADH (SIADH)

- **Non-physiologic excess ↑ADH from pituitary or ectopic source ⇨ ↑FREE WATER RETENTION & impaired water excretion ⇨ HYPONATREMIA & inability of the kidney to dilute the urine** to excrete the excess H_2O.

- The 2 normal stimuli that increases ADH secretion is hypovolemia or hyperosmolarity.
  In SIADH, the patient is both euvolemic & hypoosmolar, so ↑ADH is considered inappropriate.

ETIOLOGIES
Increased ADH secreted from the posterior pituitary gland or an ectopic site:
1. **CNS: MC: stroke (SAH), head trauma, meningitis, CNS tumors, post-op,** hydrocephalus.   HIV.

2. **Pulmonary: small cell lung cancer** (secretes ectopic ADH), infection (ex. Legionella pneumonia).

3. **Meds**: **narcotics, NSAIDs, anticonvulsants, Carbamazepine,** High-dose **IV Cyclophosphamide, antidepressants (TCA/SSRIs), hydrochlorothiazide,** Chlorpropamide, **ecstasy (MDMA).**

4. Endocrine: hypothyroidism, Conn syndrome.

CLINICAL MANIFESTATIONS
Patients usually only become clinically symptomatic with increased oral free H_2O intake.
1. **Symptoms of HYPONATREMIA:*** especially with Na <120 mEq/L.   Neurologic symptoms due to cerebral edema. The cerebral edema is due to relative hypotonicity of the extracellular fluid shifting water into the cells.

DIAGNOSIS
1. **ISOVOLEMIC Hypotonic Hyponatremia:*** **no signs of edema** (but ± have weight gain). Natriuresis prevents edema despite being volume expanded.
   Serum: ↓serum osm* (<280), **↓Na** <135 mg/dL, **hypouricemia & ↓BUN** (all dilutional).

2. **Urine: ↑urine osm*** >300 **= concentrated urine*** despite **↓serum osm** (normally ↓serum osmolarity causes dilute urine to get rid of excess H_2O).
   UNa>20 (since the patient is euvolemic, there is no stimulus to hold onto sodium).

3. Diagnosis may be made in the absence of renal, adrenal, pituitary, thyroid disease or diuretic use.

MANAGEMENT
Treat the underlying cause whenever possible.
1. **H_2O restriction mainstay of treatment*** < 800ml-1 Liter/day.

   Demeclocycline in severe cases (inhibits ADH).

2. **Severe hyponatremia or intracranial bleed ⇨ IV hypertonic saline with furosemide.**
   Hypertonic saline rapidly increases serum sodium levels.   Furosemide ❶limits volume expansion ❷ prevents the kidney from producing a concentrated urine, limiting the hyponatremia.
     - Avoid rapid correction of hyponatremia to prevent central pontine myelinolysis (no faster that 0.5 mEq/L per hour).

DIABETES INSIPIDUS

❶ADH (Vasopressin) deficiency (central DI)   OR
❷ insensitivity to ADH (nephrogenic) ⇨ *inability of the kidney to concentrate urine* ⇨
   production of LARGE AMOUNTS OF DILUTE URINE.

ETIOLOGIES

1. CENTRAL DI: *decreased ADH production:* MC type.* Idiopathic MC, autoimmune destruction
   of the posterior pituitary, *head trauma*, tumor (brain, pituitary), infection, sarcoid granuloma.

2. NEPHROGENIC DI: *partial or complete insensitivity to ADH.**
   - *Drugs: Lithium,* Amphotericin B, Demeclocycline.* **Hypercalcemia & hypokalemia**
     (disrupts kidney's concentrating ability), acute tubular necrosis, hyperparathyroidism.

CLINICAL MANIFESTATIONS

- Patients usually only become *clinically symptomatic with decreased oral free water intake.*
1. *POLYURIA* (up to 20 liters/day) + POLYDIPSIA* (to maintain H_2O balance). *Nocturia** (may
   manifest as enuresis in children).

2. *Hypernatremia (↑serum Osm) if severe or decreased oral H_2O intake.*

3. Dehydration, hypotension, rapid vascular collapse in severe cases.

DIAGNOSIS

1. **FLUID DEPRIVATION TEST**: *establishes the diagnosis of diabetes insipidus.**
   - Normal response ⇨ progressive urine concentration (to conserve H_2O ⇨ ↑'ing Uosm).

   - *DI: continued production of dilute urine* (↓ Uosm <200 & low specific gravity < 1.005).*

2. **DESMOPRESSIN (ADH) STIMULATION TEST**: *differentiates nephrogenic from central DI.**
   Administer Desmopressin (ADH):
   - **Central DI:** ⇨ *reduction in urine output (↑Uosm) indicating a response to ADH.*

   - **Nephrogenic DI:** ⇨ *continued production of dilute urine (no response to ADH).*

MANAGEMENT

1. **Central DI:**
   - *Desmopressin/DDAVP: synthetic ADH.** Intranasal, injection or oral forms.
   - *Carbamazepine* (↑'es ADH). Chlorpropamide.

2. **Nephrogenic DI:** *Na^+/protein restriction* ⇨ *Hydrochlorothiazide,** Indomethacin.
   - *Low solute diet* (Na^+/protein intake & excretion) decreases urine output.
   - *Hydrochlorothiazide* causes a mild hypovolemia (promoting water retention) & inhibition
     of the diluting segment of the distal renal tubule. Amiloride may be used if due to lithium.
   - Indomethacin increases concentration ability & potentiates the effect of ADH.

3. *If symptomatic* ⇨ *hypotonic fluid* (pure water orally is preferred, D5W, ½ normal saline).

SODIUM HOMEOSTASIS

- The kidney has a separate mechanism for adjusting the *total body sodium (Na) levels.*
- The kidney *regulates Na+ via aldosterone. Aldosterone causes Na+ retention.*

↑ Aldosterone is released in response to:
1. *Hypovolemia =* low blood pressure = decreased intravascular volume (↓Na + water).
      Low blood pressure (decreased effective arterial volume) causes juxtaglomerular cells in the kidney to release renin, activating the Renin-Angiotensin-Aldosterone system (RAAS). The increased aldosterone promotes sodium retention.
2. *Hyperkalemia:* aldosterone causes increased potassium excretion in exchange for Na+ reabsorption.

Water homeostasis is determined by ADH. The 2 stimuli that ↑ADH are hypovolemia or hyperosmolarity.

Na+ homeostasis determined by aldosterone. The 2 stimuli that ↑aldosterone are hypovolemia or hyperkalemia.

Note: *since volume is Na+ plus water, hypovolemia stimulates both aldosterone & ADH secretion.*

SODIUM DISORDERS OVERVIEW

- Sodium homeostasis is important to the vital function of all cells.
- Sodium is the dominant extracellular cation & cannot freely cross membranes.
- *Serum Na concentration [Na] is the major determinant of serum osmolality (tonicity):*

$$\textit{Serum osm = 2x [sodium concentration]} + \text{[glucose concentration]}/18 + \text{[BUN]}/2.8$$

For practical purposes, *twice the Na concentration roughly equals serum osmolality* because urea & glucose are responsible for less than 5% of the total osmotic pressure.
Ex: Normal serum osmolality 285-295. Normal Na = 135-145. 2x (135 to 145) = 270 to 290

- *Abnormal Serum [Na] concentration is due to problems with water control* (regulated primarily by ADH). Hydration is the amount of free water (free from Na).
  - Free water exists in the intracellular space.
      *Over*hydration: *Increased free water = decreased serum [Na] = hyponatremia*
      *De*hydration: *decreased free water = increased serum [Na] = hypernatremia*

- *Abnormal extracellular fluid volume size (ECFV) is due to problems with total body Na control* because *Total body Na+ determines ECFV* (since sodium is the dominant extracellular cation and is unable to freely cross membranes. Clinically, ECFV is ❶ interstitial fluid volume and ❷ intravascular space volume. *Extracellular volume is (Na + water).*
      Hypervolemia = ↑Total Body Na+
      Iso/Euvolemia = Normal Total Body Na+
      Hypovolemia = ↓Total Body Na+

HYPERVOLEMIA	HYPOVOLEMIA	ISOVOLEMIA
peripheral and presacral edema	*poor skin turgor*	absence of the
pulmonary edema	*dry mucous membranes*	signs of hyper
jugular venous distension	*flat neck veins*	or hypervolemia
hypertension	*hypotension*	
decreased hematocrit	increased hematocrit	
decreased serum protein	increased serum protein	
decreased BUN: creatinine	*increased BUN: creatinine ratio >20:1*	
	UNa <20 mEq/L	

HYPONATREMIA

- Hyponatremia = ↓Serum [Na] <135 = *INCREASED FREE WATER.**
- Due to ❶*impaired kidney ability to excrete free water (due to ↑ADH secretion)* where the kidney is unable to make a dilute urine in the setting of ❷*increased water intake.*
- *Clinically significant hyponatremia is HYPOTONIC HYPONATREMIA (true hyponatremia).*

ETIOLOGIES OF HYPONATREMIA
❶HYPERTONIC Hyponatremia
- Dilutional drop in serum [Na] due to the presence of osmotically active molecules *(ex glucose in hyperglycemia* or mannitol infusion).* The hyperosmolality causes water to shift from the intracellular to extracellular space. This is not true hyponatremia because it is a state of decreased free water. *True hyponatremia associated with increased free water.*

❷ISOTONIC Hyponatremia
- *Lab artifact/error* due to *hypertriglyceridemia or hyperproteinemia.* It is not true hyponatremia because free water is normal.

❸HYPOTONIC Hyponatremia
- *"TRUE HYPONATREMIA" (clinically significant).* Kidney unable to excrete free water (make dilute urine) to match oral free water intake. *Associated with ↑ free water.*
- Volume status (which reflects Total Body Na⁺) is a clue to the causes:

HYPOVOLEMIC Hyponatremia: ↓volume (Na⁺ +water) AND (↑free water).
> *Impaired free water excretion:* volume depletion ⇨ *extracellular fluid (ECF) volume contraction* ⇨RAAS activation ⇨↑*ADH release* to protect ECF volume leads to impaired free water excretion. *Increased free water intake:* because angiotensin II (from RAAS activation) is a potent thirst stimulator, free water intake in setting of kidney H_2O retention exacerbates the hyponatremia.
>> **Renal volume loss:** *diuretics (Thiazides,* K⁺-sparing diuretics), ACE Inhibitors, aldosterone insufficiency (Na⁺ spills into urine).* **UNa >20** (indicating renal Na⁺ loss).
>> **Extrarenal volume loss:** bleeding, diarrhea/vomiting, pancreatitis, excessive perspiration. **UNa <10** (indicating kidney response to hypovolemia by trying to hold onto Na⁺ to help maintain volume).

ISO/EUVOLEMIC Hyponatremia: normal volume (Na +water) AND (↑free water).
- *Syndrome of Inappropriate ADH secretion (SIADH):* disease where high ADH is not inhibited by decreased osmolarity (decreased serum [Na]). MC CNS/pulmonary.
- *Hypothyroidism, adrenal insufficiency:* unknown mechanism.
- Reset hypothalamic osmostat: hypothalamus sets lowers baseline serum [Na] levels.
- Water intoxication: *1ry polydipsia:* excess water intake > normal kidney water excreting capacity.
- *MDMA (ecstasy):* drug-induced SIADH coupled with marked free water intake
- Tea & Toast syndrome/beer potomania: *decreased solute intake. The kidney needs solutes to aid in H_2O excretion, without it, there is impaired H_2O excretion.*

HYPERVOLEMIC Hyponatremia: ↑volume (Na +water) AND (↑free water).
> Although there is increased volume, the volume is pushed into the interstitium (edema) out of the intravascular space (reducing the effective circulating intravascular volume). This reduces blood flow to the kidney. The kidney is unable to distinguish this from hypovolemia so it stimulates the same processes as outlined in hypovolemia.
>> **Edematous states:** *congestive heart failure, nephrotic syndrome, cirrhosis*

	HYPOnatremia	HYPERnatremia
ETIOLOGY	• Due to ❶ **impaired kidney free water excretion** *(increased ADH secretion)* where the kidney is unable to make dilute urine in the setting of ❷ ↑'ed *water intake*. • Remember Na disorders are a problem with water handling (not total body sodium)!!	• *MC caused by net water loss* (free water loss, hypotonic fluid loss) or hypertonic sodium gain *(iatrogenic)*. • *Sustained hypernatremia seen when appropriate water intake is not possible*/impaired (ex. infants, elderly, debilitated patients) or impaired thirst mechanism.
CLINICAL MANIFESTATIONS	• Symptoms vary with degree & rapidity of hyponatremia. • *CNS dysfunction due to cerebral edema:* hypotonicity shifts water intracellularly ⇨ cerebral edema. — Nonspecific neuro sx: fatigue, headache, nausea, vomiting, muscle cramps, lethargy, AMS, ↓DTR. — Neuro Complications: seizures, coma, permanent brain damage, death, respiratory arrest.	• Symptoms vary with degree and rapidity of hypernatremia. • *CNS dysfunction:* hypertonicity shifts water out of cells ⇨ *shrinkage of brain cells.* — Confusion, lethargy, coma, muscle weakness, lethargy, seizures
LAB FINDINGS	• *Serum Na <135.* May order urine Na & urine osmolality.	• *Serum Na >145.* May order urine Na & urine osmolality.
MANAGEMENT	• **Hypotonic Hyponatremia:** — *ISOvolemic: H₂O restriction.* (<1.5L/d). Tx cause. — *HYPERvolemic: H₂O + Na restriction.* — *HYPOvolemic: normal saline* (volume expansion decreases hypovolemic stimulus for ADH secretion). • **Hypertonic Hyponatremia: normal saline until hemodynamically stable ⇨ switch to ½ normal saline** • **Severe (Iso or Hyper) volemic Hyponatremia:** — *Hypertonic saline + Furosemide*** (rapidly ↑'es Na).	• *HYPOTONIC FLUIDS:* — *Preferred route is oral* (or feeding tube if present). — *Only hypotonic fluids are appropriate:* Ex. pure water orally, D5W, 0.45%NS, 0.2% saline. — except for cases of frank circulatory compromise, 0.9% normal saline is unsuitable for hypernatremia!
CORRECTION	• *Correct ≤0.5mEq/L/h to PREVENT DEMYELINATION.**	• *Correct ≤0.5mEq/L/h to PREVENT CEREBRAL EDEMA.**

HYPONATREMIA

Critical hyponatremia: Tx c̄ hypertonic saline + Loop diuretic

Serum Osm (STEP 1)

Low — HYPOTONIC HYPONATREMIA (TRUE)

Normal — Lab Error (↑Protein, ↑Triglycerides)

High — Hyperglycemia Mannitol

ECF Volume (STEP 2)

Low (HYPOVOLEMIA)

RENAL LOSS (UNa >20)
Diuretics
- *Thiazides*
- K-sparing
- ACE-I ARBs
- IV RTA, Hypoaldosteronism
Mgmt: Normal Saline (correct the volume)

EXTRA-RENAL LOSS (UNa <10), FeNa <1)
- Bleeding
- Burns
- GI (N/V, diarrhea)
- Pancreatitis

Normal (ISOVOLEMIA)
• SIADH, post op
• Hypothyroidism
• Adrenal Insufficiency
• Water Intoxication
• 1° Polydipsia
Mgmt: Water Restriction

High (HYPERVOLEMIA)

Una <20
• CHF, Cirrhosis
• Nephrosis

UNA >20
• Acute/Chronic Renal Failure
Mgmt: H₂O/salt restriction

*Note: all have ↑ADH
• SIADH: inappropriate
• The rest appropriate

REVIEW OF HYPERNATREMIA

ECF Volume

❶ HYPOvolemic

Renal loss: U$_{Na}$ ≥ 20 U$_{osm}$ 300-600
• Severe Hyperglycemia
• Osmotic Diuretics

Extra-renal loss (U$_{Na}$ <10), U$_{osm}$ ≥400)
• Sweating
• Resp Loss
• GI loss (N/V/D)
• Dehydration

❷ ISOvolemic Uosm <250
• Diabetes insipidus
• Reset Osmostat

❸ HYPERvolemic
• Hypertonic Saline
• Mineralocorticoid Excess

HYPONATREMIA

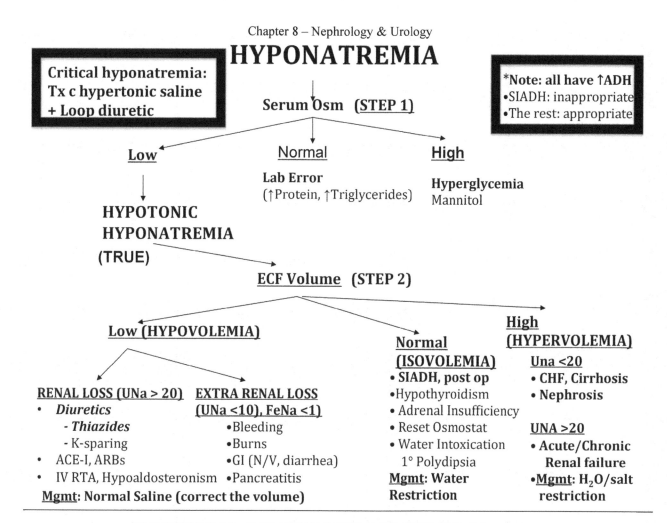

Critical hyponatremia:
Tx c hypertonic saline
+ Loop diuretic

*Note: all have ↑ADH
• SIADH: inappropriate
• The rest: appropriate

Serum Osm (STEP 1)

Low — **Normal** — **High**

Normal: Lab Error (↑Protein, ↑Triglycerides)

High: Hyperglycemia / Mannitol

HYPOTONIC HYPONATREMIA (TRUE)

ECF Volume (STEP 2)

Low (HYPOVOLEMIA)

RENAL LOSS (UNa > 20)
• *Diuretics*
  - *Thiazides*
  - K-sparing
• ACE-I, ARBs
• IV RTA, Hypoaldosteronism

EXTRA RENAL LOSS (UNa <10), FeNa <1)
• Bleeding
• Burns
• GI (N/V, diarrhea)
• Pancreatitis

Mgmt: Normal Saline (correct the volume)

Normal (ISOVOLEMIA)
• SIADH, post op
• Hypothyroidism
• Adrenal Insufficiency
• Reset Osmostat
• Water Intoxication
  1° Polydipsia
Mgmt: Water Restriction

High (HYPERVOLEMIA)
Una <20
• CHF, Cirrhosis
• Nephrosis

UNA >20
• Acute/Chronic Renal failure
• **Mgmt:** H_2O/salt restriction

REVIEW OF HYPERNATREMIA

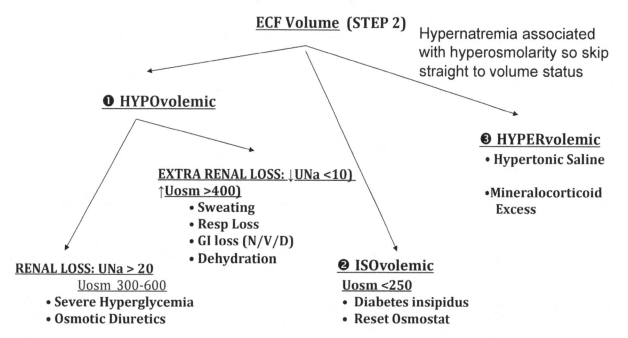

ECF Volume (STEP 2)

Hypernatremia associated with hyperosmolarity so skip straight to volume status

❶ HYPOvolemic

EXTRA RENAL LOSS: ↓UNa <10)
↑Uosm >400)
• Sweating
• Resp Loss
• GI loss (N/V/D)
• Dehydration

RENAL LOSS: UNa > 20
Uosm 300-600
• Severe Hyperglycemia
• Osmotic Diuretics

❷ ISOvolemic
Uosm <250
• Diabetes insipidus
• Reset Osmostat

❸ HYPERvolemic
• Hypertonic Saline

• Mineralocorticoid Excess

	HYPOmagnesemia	HYPERmagnesemia
ETIOLOGIES	• **GI losses:** *Malabsorption: ETOHics,* Celiac disease, small bowel bypass, diarrhea, vomiting, laxatives. • **Renal losses:** - *Diuretics:* thiazides, loop diuretics. - Diabetes mellitus, renal tubular acidosis. - **Meds:** *proton pump inhibitors (omeprazole),* Amphotericin B, Cisplatin, Cyclosporine, Aminoglycosides.	• RARE. 2 MC causes ❶ *renal insufficiency* or ❷ *increased Mg intake* (ex. overcorrection of hypomagnesemia). - *Acute or chronic renal failure:* ↓Mg excretion. - **Iatrogenic:** excess IV Mg administration in the treatment of asthma, eclampsia, torsades de pointes. - Excess ingestion of Magnesium: vitamins, antacids, milk alkali syndrome. - Lithium toxicity, Adrenal sufficiency.
CLINICAL MANIFESTATIONS	• **Neurovascular:** AMS, lethargy, weakness, muscle cramps, vertigo, seizures, *↑DTR, tetany.* • **Hypocalcemia***: Trousseau's & Chvostek's signs are due to impaired PTH secretion/release because magnesium is needed to make parathyroid hormone. • **Cardiovascular:** arrhythmias, palpitations (due to hypomagnesemia & associated hypokalemia).	• Nausea, vomiting, skin flushing, dizziness, muscle weakness, AMS, *↓DTR (hyporeflexive).* • Severe: hypotension, bradyarrhythmias, AV conduction blocks, respiratory depression, tachyarrhythmias.
LAB FINDINGS	• Hypomagnesemia. ± hypokalemia & hypocalcemia	• Hypermagnesemia. ± hyperkalemia & hypercalcemia
ECG FINDINGS	• *Prolonged PR & QT interval,* wide QRS, A-fib, V-fib, Ventricular tachycardia (R on T), *Torsades* R ON T PHENOMENON TORSADES DE POINTES	• Similar to hypomagnesemia Prolonged PR & QT interval, wide QRS • May show ECG signs of hyperkalemia • Arrhythmias
MANAGEMENT	**MILD** • Oral Magnesium: ex. Magnesium oxide. **SEVERE** • *IV Magnesium Sulfate. Also used in Torsades de pointes* • Hypocalcemia & hypokalemia associated with hypomagnesemia are often refractory to treatment until magnesium is repleted.*	**MILD TO MODERATE:** • *IV fluids + Furosemide* (Lasix): enhances renal magnesium excretion. Also used if severe **SEVERE** • *Calcium Gluconate:* antagonizes the toxic effects of magnesium & stabilizes the cardiac membrane. • Dialysis in severe cases.

	HYPOkalemia	HYPERkalemia
ETIOLOGIES	• Increased urinary/GI losses: *MC causes - diuretic therapy,* *vomiting, diarrhea.* RTA: classic distal (Type I), proximal (II) • Increased intracellular shifts: *metabolic alkalosis,* *β-2 agonists, hypothermia,* Chloroquine use, vitamin B12 tx, insulin. • Hypomagnesemia. • Decreased potassium intake: very rare unless superimposed with another cause.	• ↓Renal excretion: *acute or chronic renal failure* (especially if on dialysis & coupled with increased K⁺ intake (ex bananas)). <u>↓aldosterone:</u> hypoaldosteronism, adrenal insufficiency. • *Meds: K⁺ supplements, K⁺-sparing diuretics, ACEI/ARB's, digoxin,* *β-blockers, NSAIDs,* Cyclosporine. • *Cell lysis:* rhabdomyolysis, burns, hypovolemia, thrombocytosis, tumor lysis syndrome, leukocytosis (intracellular release of K⁺ from cell lysis). • K⁺ redistribution: *metabolic acidosis** (DKA), catabolic states • *Pseudohyperkalemia: venipuncture MC,* lab error.
CLINICAL MANIFESTATIONS	• **Neuromuscular:** severe muscle weakness (including respiratory), rhabdomyolysis, *nephrogenic DI: POLYURIA** (affects renal concentrating ability), myoglobinuria, cramps, nausea/vomiting, ileus, ↓DTR. • **Cardiovascular:** palpitations, arrhythmias.	Serum levels & symptoms not consistent. Rapidity in serum K⁺ change influences symptoms more than levels. • **Neuromuscular:** weakness (progressive ascending), fatigue, paresthesias, flaccid paralysis. • **Cardiovascular:** palpitations, cardiac arrhythmias. • **GI:** abdominal distention, diarrhea.
LAB FINDINGS	• BMP: potassium < 3.5 mEq/L. Magnesium, glucose, bicarbonate ordered in the workup.	• *Potassium >5.0* mEq/L. Glucose, bicarbonate part of the workup. • ±CBC (hemolysis), ±CK (rhabdomyolysis).
ECG FINDINGS	• *T wave flattening (earliest change)* ⇨ *prominent U wave** ±Hypomagnesemia changes Prominent U wave	• *Tall peaked T waves** ⇨ *QR interval shortening, wide QRS,* prolonged PRI ⇨ *P wave flattening* ⇨sine wave ⇨ arrhythmias. Peaked T waves
MANAGEMENT	• *Potassium replacement:* KCl oral if possible IV KCl given for rapid treatment/severe sx. • High dose KCl given in central line. *Hypokalemia associated with ↑risk of digoxin toxicity.** • Potassium sparing diuretics: *Spironolactone, Amiloride* • *If hypomagnesemia present, it may be hard to replenish potassium (so tx hypomagnesemia)* • Use nondextrose IV solutions (because dextrose induced insulin release will shift K⁺ into cells).	Repeat blood draw to verify not from hemolysis during blood draw (since venipuncture may cause cell lysis). • *IV Calcium gluconate:** *stabilizes the cardiac membrane* used for *severe symptoms, K⁺ > 6.5,* ⊕ *significant ECG findings.* Given over 30-60min. Given simultaneously with other tx for hyperkalemia. • *Insulin (with glucose): insulin shifts K⁺ intracellularly* glucose given to prevent hypoglycemia from insulin. • Sodium polystyrene sulfonate (*Kayexalate*): *enhances GI potassium excretion. Lowers total body K⁺* • *Beta₂ agonists:* 4-8 times dosing use for asthma. 12-20mg via nebulizer. • Bicarbonate: not usually given unless metabolic acidosis also present • Loop diuretics, Fludrocortisone (synthetic mineralocorticoid). • Dialysis if severe.

EPIDIDYMITIS & ORCHITIS

- Epididymal pain & swelling thought to be secondary to retrograde infection or reflux of urine. *Epididymitis usually bacterial. Orchitis usually viral.*

- **ACUTE EPIDIDYMITIS-ORCHITIS:**
    - **Men <35y:** *Chlamydia MC,* * Neisseria gonorrhoeae*, Ureoplasma, E. coli, Treponema, Trichomonas & Gardnerella.   ± *Viral in children (Mumps MC cause).* *

    - **Men >35y & children:** *Enteric organisms MC:* * E coli, Klebsiella,* Pseudomonas, Proteus.

- **CHRONIC EPIDIDYMITIS:** >6 weeks 2^{ry} to inadequate treatment of acute cases, chronic disease, Mycobacterium tuberculosis.

- **ACUTE ORCHITIS:** *Viral: Mumps,* * Coxsackie, Rubella, Echovirus, Parvovirus. *$1/3$ of postpubertal men with mumps have concomitant orchitis.* * Mumps parotitis precedes the onset of orchitis by 3-10 days. Bacterial/pyogenic infections (unusual), trauma, idiopathic.

CLINICAL MANIFESTATIONS

1. *gradual (over a few days) onset of scrotal pain, erythema & swelling* MC unilateral. ± Groin or abdominal pain. ± associated with *fever* & chills, irritative sx (dysuria, urgency, frequency). Symptoms may follow acute strain (sex, lifting a heavy object, exercise).

2. **Physical Examination:** epididymal tenderness & induration.
    - *POSITIVE PREHN's sign:* * relief of pain with elevation of the affected scrotum.*

    - *Positive (normal) cremasteric reflex:* * elevation of the testicle after stroking the inner thigh.

    - Scrotal erythema may be present. Testicles usually in normal (vertical) position.

DIAGNOSIS

1. **Scrotal ultrasound:** *enlarged epididymis,* INCREASED TESTICULAR BLOOD FLOW* ± reactive hydrocele. Radiologic studies usually not needed for mumps orchitis.

2. **UA:** *pyuria (↑WBC)/bacteriuria.* ⊕WBCs & no visible organisms in smear ⇨ chlamydia, gonorrhea.

3. CBC: leukocytosis; urine culture, STD testing: gonorrhea, chlamydia, RPR & HIV.

MANAGEMENT

1. **Symptomatic treatment:** *bed rest, scrotal elevation, cool compresses & analgesics* (NSAIDs).

2. **Acute epididymitis:**
    - *Gonorrhea & chlamydia, <35y: Doxycycline* (100mg bid x 10d) *plus Ceftriaxone (250mg IMx1).* Azithromycin is an alternative to Doxycycline.

    - *Enteric organisms, >35y: fluoroquinolones* * (ex. Ofloxacin, Levofloxacin)
        Children: *Cephalexin or Amoxicillin.*

3. Chronic epididymitis: 4-6 week trial of antibiotics.

TESTICULAR TORSION

- ***Spermatic cord twists & cuts off testicular blood supply*** due to congenital malformation ("bell clapper" deformity of the process vaginalis), which allows the testicle to be free floating in the tunica vaginalis (90%) causing it to twist on itself. ***True urologic emergency!***

- ***65% occur in teenagers* (10-20y).*** Incidence decreases with age (rare before 10 years).

CLINICAL MANIFESTATIONS:

1. *ABRUPT **onset of scrotal, inguinal or lower abdominal pain (usually <6 hours), ± nausea & vomiting.**** If nausea/vomiting presents, suspect torsion (usually absent in epididymitis).

2. Physical Examination:
   - *Swollen, tender, retracted (high-riding) testicle ± horizontal lie.*
   - NEGATIVE PREHN'S SIGN*: **no pain relief with scrotal elevation.****
   - *NEGATIVE (ABSENT) CREMASTERIC REFLEX:** no elevation of the testicle after stroking the inner thigh.
   - *"Blue dot sign" at the upper pole = torsion of appendix of testis.**

DIAGNOSIS

1. **Testicular Doppler Ultrasound:** *best initial test* - avascular testicle (↓blood flow).**

2. Emergency surgical exploration is required if ultrasound is unable to exclude torsion.
3. Radionuclide scan (not used as frequently).

MANAGEMENT

1. ***Detorsion & orchiopexy within 6 hours & in obvious cases.***
   Orchiopexy = testicle fixation in the scrotum
2. Orchiectomy if the testicle is not salvageable.

CRYPTORCHIDISM

- ***Undescended testicle.*** ↑**risk:** ***premature infants*** (30% of premature vs. 5% in full term infants), ***low birth weight.*** Most descend spontaneously (~70%). MC right-sided.

CLINICAL MANIFESTATIONS

1. Empty, small scrotum, ±inguinal fullness (MC located in inguinal canal). 10% bilateral.

COMPLICATIONS

Testicular cancer (in both the affected & unaffected testicle), subfertility (body temperature ↓'es sperm formation, scrotum ~9 degrees cooler than core body temperature), testicular torsion & inguinal hernia. Early diagnosis & treatment prevents some of the complications.

MANAGEMENT

1. ***Orchiopexy:*** recommended as ***early as 6 months of age (ideally performed before 1 years old).***

2. **Observation** *can be done only if <6 months of age.* Most descend by 3 months of age (rarely spontaneously descend after 6 months of age). Orchiopexy = testicle fixation in scrotum.

3. hCG or gonadotropin releasing hormone: human chorionic gonadotropin stimulates testosterone & hormonal testicular descension. May be used prior to orchiopexy (not used often).

4. Orchiectomy recommended if detected at puberty to reduce testicular cancer risk.

TESTICULAR CANCER

- MC solid tumor in young men **_15-40y (average 32y)._**
- 5 year survival 90% with treatment (associated with good prognosis – very curable)

RISK FACTORS:
1. **_Cryptorchidism:*_** in both the undescended & normal testicle. Cryptorchidism is associated with a 40-fold ↑risk. **_MC right-sided_** (because cryptorchidism occurs MC on the right side).
2. MC in Caucasians. Klinefelter's syndrome.

GERMINAL CELL TUMORS (97%): *usually malignant*
- **SEMINOMA (SGCT)**: *MC type in men 30s-40s.* The 4 S's of Seminoma
     Seminomas are **_Simple (lack tumor markers_** = normal serum α-fetoprotein & β-hCG), **_Sensitive (sensitive to radiation), Slower growing_** & associated with **_Stepwise spread._**

- **NONSEMINOMATOUS (NSGCT)**:
     Embryonal cell carcinoma, teratoma, yolk sac (MC in young boys ≤10y), choriocarcinoma (worst prognosis). Mixed tumors (seminomatous + nonseminomatous components). Mixed tumors are treated like nonseminomas.
     Nonseminomas associated with ↑serum α-fetoprotein, ↑β–hCG & radioresistance.*

NONGERMINAL CELL TUMORS (3%):
Nongerminal cell tumors can spread hematogenously & cause pulmonary symptoms.
- Leydig cell tumors: may be benign. May secrete hormones (ex. androgens or estrogens), which may lead precocious puberty in children or gynecomastia/loss of libido in adults.
- Sertoli cell tumors: often benign. May secrete hormones (ex. estrogens, androgens).
- Gonadoblastoma, Testicular lymphoma.

CLINICAL MANIFESTATIONS:
1. **_painless testicular nodule, solid mass or enlargement*_** unable to be separated from testicle. May have dull pain or testicular heaviness. Any hematoma or hydrocele 2^{ry} to minor scrotal trauma should raise suspicion for testicular cancer.   ⊕ **_Hydrocele present_** *in 10%.*

2. *Gynecomastia in <10%* (seen especially with Leydig or Sertoli tumors that secrete estrogen). Rarely, tumors present with signs of METS: hemoptysis (pulmonary), supraclavicular lymph node neck mass, abdominal mass (retroperitoneal).   Seminomas may spread to the bone.

DIAGNOSIS
1. **Scrotal ultrasound**: seminomas (hypoechoic mass); non = cystic, inhomogenous masses.

2. **Alpha-fetoprotein, β-hCG, LDH**.
    - β-hCG often elevated in nonseminomatous (especially choriocarcinoma).
    - α-fetoprotein ↑'ed in many NSCGT. Not usually elevated in seminoma & choriocarcinoma.

MANAGEMENT
1. **Low-grade (Stage I) Nonseminoma (limited to testes):**
     orchiectomy with retroperitoneal lymph node dissection.*

2. **Low-grade Seminoma:** *orchiectomy* ⇨ *radiation.*

3. **High-grade Seminoma:** **_debulking chemotherapy_** ⇨ **_orchiectomy & radiation._**

HYDROCELE

- **Cystic testicular fluid collection** ⇨ testicular mass. **MC cause of painless scrotal swelling.**

Communicating: peritoneal/abdominal fluid enters the scrotum via a patent processus vaginalis that failed to close.

Noncommunicating: derived from fluid from the mesothelial lining of the tunica vaginalis (no connection to the peritoneum).

Infants: **congenital** (due to incomplete obliteration of the processus vaginalis). Congenital defects usually close within the 1st year of life & may not require treatment.

Adults: **usually acquired:** injury, infection or inflammatory etiologies.

CLINICAL MANIFESTATIONS
1. **painless scrotal swelling** (may increase throughout the day). ±dull ache or heavy sensation. **Communicating: swelling worse with Valsalva.**
2. ⊕**transillumination** on physical examination. Must rule out testicular tumor (also painless).

MANAGEMENT
1. Usually no treatment needed (most resolve by the child's first birthday).
2. Surgical repair may be needed if it persists beyond 1 year of age, older patients with communicating hydroceles (elective) or hydroceles associated with complications.

VARICOCELE

- **Cystic testicular mass of <u>varicose veins:</u>** pampiniform venous plexus & internal spermatic vein. Asymptomatic varicoceles may be seen in up to 10% of population.

- **<u>MC occurs on left side</u>*** (85-95%) because left spermatic vein enters the left renal vein at a 90 degree angle. **<u>MC surgically correctable cause of male infertility</u>** (seen in ~30% of infertile men because the increased temperature from the increased venous blood flow inhibits spermatogenesis).

CLINICAL MANIFESTATIONS
"bag of worms"* superior to the testicle. Usually painless but ±cause a dull ache or heavy sensation.
- Dilation usually decreases when patient is supine or with testicular elevation.
- **Dilation worsens when patient is upright or with Valsalva.**

MANAGEMENT: Observation in most. Surgery in some cases (spermatic vein ligation, varicocelectomy).

Sudden onset of **left-sided varicocele in older man** ⇨ possible **renal cell carcinoma.**
Right-sided varicocele in children <10y ⇨ possible **retroperitoneal malignancy.**

SPERMATOCELE (EPIDIDYMAL CYST)

- Epididymal cystic (scrotal mass) that contains sperm.

CLINICAL MANIFESTATIONS
1. painless, cystic mass in the head of the epididymis *superior, posterior* & **separate from the testicle.**

PHYSICAL EXAMINATION:
Freely movable mass above the testicle that **transilluminates easily.**

MANAGEMENT: no treatment usually necessary unless the mass is bothersome.

Hydrocele, varicocele & spermatocele can be confirmed on testicular ultrasound.

CYSTITIS & PYELONEPHRITIS

RISK FACTORS
A. **Women:** sexual intercourse "honeymoon cystitis", spermicidal use (especially with diaphragm).
   pregnancy: progesterone & estrogen ⇨ ureter dilation, inhibition bladder peristalsis.
   postmenopausal: ↓bladder tone, estrogen deficiency alters normal vaginal flora.
B. **Males** *rare for males to have UTI (males should receive workup to r/o GU abnormalities).*
   >50y (BPH, Prostate cancer) ↑risk with insertive anal intercourse, uncircumcised.
C. **Children/Neonates:** vesicourethral reflux, newborns c FUO. Other: diabetes mellitus, catheter.

ETIOLOGIES
- ***E. COLI* (80%) MC organism in complicated/uncomplicated cases.**** Other gram-negative uropathogens: *Proteus, Enterobacter, Klebsiella, Pseudomonas.* Usually ascending infection.
- ***Staph. saprophyticus: especially sexually active women.**** *Enterococci* with indwelling catheters.

CLINICAL MANIFESTATIONS
1. **ACUTE CYSTITIS:** dysuria (burning), ↑frequency, urgency, hematuria, suprapubic discomfort.
2. **PYELONEPHRITIS:** *fever & tachycardia, back/flank pain, ⊕ CVA tenderness, nausea/vomiting.**

DIAGNOSIS
1. **Urinalysis (UA):**
   - ***Pyuria:**** [>5 WBC/hpf (esp >10)], ⊕ leukocyte esterase; ***If WBC casts ⇨ pyelonephritis.**
   - ⊕ nitrites (90% bacteria causing UTIs), **hematuria,** ± cloudy urine, bacteriuria, ↑pH c Proteus.
2. **Dipstick:** ⊕ leukocyte esterase, nitrites, hematuria. Cystitis associated c WBCs but not WBC casts.

3. **Urine culture:** *definitive diagnosis.** Indications: complicated UTI, infants/children, elderly, males, urologic abnormalities, refractory to treatment, catheterized patients.
   Women: ≥ 10^5 (100,000) - clean catch specimen.* Epithelial (squamous cells) = contamination.
   Men: ≥10^2 – 10^4 + symptoms = acute urethral syndrome.

DIFFERENTIAL DIAGNOSIS
1. Vaginitis: vaginal discharge, odor, itching, dyspareunia, dysuria.
2. Urethritis: sexual intercourse with new partner, dysuria (usually develop gradually over weeks).

MANAGEMENT OF CYSTITIS
➢ ↑fluid intake, void after intercourse. **Phenazopyridine** (Pyridium) bladder analgesic (turns urine orange). *Not used more than 48h due to ↑S/E: methemoglobinuria, hemolytic anemia.*
Uncomplicated Cystitis: options include:
   ❶ *Nitrofurantoin* (Macrobid) 100 bid x 5-7d. Not used if pyelonephritis is suspected.
   ❷ *Fluoroquinolones* ex. Ciprofloxacin 250mg bid x 3d.
   ❸ *Trimethoprim-sulfamethoxazole* double strength (Bactrim-DS) bid x3d. Increased resistance.
   Fosfomycin, Cefpodoxime. Post coital ⇨ single dose (ex. Trimethoprim-sulfamethoxazole).

Complicated Cystitis:
   Complicated = *underlying condition with risk of therapeutic failure:* symptoms >7 days, pregnancy, diabetics, immunosuppression, indwelling catheter, anatomic abnormality, elderly, males.
   Fluoroquinolone PO or IV, Aminoglycosides x 7-10 (or 14) days (depending on severity).

Pregnant: tx for 7-14 days ⇨ **Amoxicillin,*** Amoxicillin/clavulanate, Cephalexin, Cefpodoxime, **Nitrofurantoin,** Fosfomycin. Sulfisoxazole is safe except in last days of pregnancy ⇨ ↑kernicterus.

Pyelonephritis:
   Fluoroquinolone PO or IV, *Aminoglycoside* ***x14d*** (7 days may be used in healthy, young women).

PARAPHIMOSIS

• **_FORESKIN BECOMES TRAPPED BEHIND THE CORONA OF GLANS_ & forms tight band, constricting penile tissues.** _Foreskin cannot be pulled forward._ The ring of tissue impairs blood & lymphatic flow ⇨ gangrene & auto-amputation (days to weeks). **_Urologic emergency!_**

CLINICAL MANIFESTATIONS
• Enlarged, painful glans with constricting band of foreskin behind the glans.

DIFFERENTIAL DIAGNOSIS
• **Phimosis** (inability to retract foreskin over the glans). Not emergent. Management is circumcision.

MANAGEMENT
1. **_Manual reduction:_** restore original position of the foreskin. Reduce edema with cool compresses or pressure dressing then gentle pressure to restore the foreskin to its normal position.
2. **_Pharmacologic therapy:_** granulated sugar, injection of hyaluronidase. Incision (ex. dorsal slit).

PROSTATITIS

• _Prostate gland inflammation 2ry to an **ascending infection.**_

ACUTE PROSTATITIS:
• **>35y:** _gram-negatives:_ **_E coli MC,_**_*_ _Pseudomonas, Klebsiella,_ Proteus, Serratia, Enterobacter.

• **<35y:** **_Chlamydia & Gonorrhea MC,_**_*_ E. coli, Treponema, Trichomonas, Gardnerella.
• Viral may be seen in children (Mumps MC cause in children).

CHRONIC PROSTATITIS:
E coli 75-80%, enterococci, Trichomonas, HIV, inflammatory. Structural or functional abnormality, recurrent UTIs. Acute prostatitis may progress to chronic.

CLINICAL MANIFESTATIONS
• **_fever/chills in acute_** (fever not common in chronic), malaise, arthralgias.
• **Irritative sx:** frequency, urgency, dysuria
• **Obstructive sx:** hesitancy, poor or interrupted stream, straining to void, incomplete emptying.
• _Lower back/abdominal pain, **perineal pain in acute prostatitis.**_ Sx usually milder in chronic.
• Chronic prostatitis usually presents as recurrent UTIs/intermittent dysfunction.

PHYSICAL EXAMINATION
1. **Acute Prostatitis:** **_exquisitely TENDER, normal or hot, boggy prostate._**_*_ Boggy = prostatitis.
2. **Chronic Prostatitis:** **_usually NONtender, boggy prostate._**_*_

DIAGNOSIS
1. **Urinalysis & urine culture**: positive in acute prostatitis. UA/culture often negative in chronic.
2. **_Avoid prostatic massage in ACUTE prostatitis_**_*_ (may cause bacteremia).
   Prostatic massage often done in chronic prostatitis to increase bacterial yield on UA/culture.
3. **Transrectal ultrasound:** may be _helpful for suspected prostatic abscess or calculi._

MANAGEMENT
1. Acute Prostatitis:
>35y: **_fluoroquinolones or Trimethoprim-sulfamethoxazole_** x ~4-6 weeks (outpatient).
If hospitalized: IV fluoroquinolones ± Aminoglycoside OR Ampicillin ± Gentamicin.
<35y: tx for gonorrhea & chlamydia: **_Ceftriaxone plus Doxycycline_** (or Azithromycin).

2. **Chronic Prostatitis:** fluoroquinolones, Trimethoprim-sulfamethoxazole x 6-12 weeks.
   _Transurethral resection of the prostate (TURP) for refractory chronic prostatitis.__*_

BENIGN PROSTATIC HYPERTROPHY (BPH)

- ***Prostate hyperplasia** (periurethral/transitional zone)* ⇨ ***bladder outlet obstruction.*** Common in older men (discrete nodules in the periurethral zone). Hyperplasia is part of the normal aging process & is hormonally dependent on ↑***dihydrotestosterone production.***

CLINICAL MANIFESTATIONS: <u>Irritative symptoms:</u> frequency, urgency, nocturia.
   <u>Obstructive symptoms:</u> hesitancy, weak/intermittent stream force, incomplete emptying.

DIAGNOSIS
1. **Digital Rectal Exam (DRE):** *uniformly enlarged, firm, rubbery prostate.**
2. ↑<u>Prostate Specific Antigen (PSA):</u> correlated with risk of sx progression. Normal <4ng/mL.
3. <u>Urine cytology:</u> if ↑risk of bladder cancer (h/o tobacco use, irritative bladder sx or hematuria).

MANAGEMENT
1. ***Observation:*** mild symptoms (monitored annually). Avoid antihistamines & anticholinergics.

2. **5-A REDUCTASE INHIBITORS:** **Finasteride** (Proscar) & **Dutasteride** (Avodart)
   MOA: *androgen inhibitor - inhibits the conversion of testosterone* to dihydrotestosterone ***suppressing prostate growth, reduces bladder outlet obstruction.*** Doesn't provide immediate relief but ***has positive effect on clinical course of BPH* (size reduction & ↓need for surgery)*** unlike α-1 blockers.
   S/E: sexual or ejaculatory dysfunction, decreased libido, breast tenderness/enlargement.

3. ***α-1 BLOCKERS:*** ***Tamsulosin most uroselective*** (Flomax), Alfu<u>zosin</u>, Doxa<u>zosin</u>, Tera<u>zosin</u>.
   Ind: ***provides rapid symptom relief but no effect on the clinical course of BPH.****
   MOA: ***smooth muscle relaxation of prostate & bladder neck*** ⇨ ***↓urethral resistance/↓obstruction*** ⇨ ***increased urinary outflow.*** α-1a activation in the prostate & urethra normally cause contraction/decreased flow.
   S/E: ***nonselective - dizziness & orthostatic ↓BP*** (due to α-1b blockage), retrograde ejaculation.

4. <u>**Surgical:**</u> ***transurethral resection of prostate (TURP)*** – removes excess prostate tissue, relieving the obstruction. <u>S/E</u> sexual dysfunction, urinary incontinence. Laser prostatectomy.

PROSTATE CANCER

- *Slow growing tumor usually* (most patients die with prostate cancer rather than from it).
Risk Factors: ***Genetics; Diet:*** ***high fat intake,**** *obesity, African-American.* ***Adenocarcinoma*** (>95%).
CLINICAL MANIFESTATIONS
1. Often asymptomatic until invasion of bladder, urethral obstruction or bone involvement.
2. **Urethral obstruction:** ↑urinary frequency, urgency, urinary retention, ↓urinary stream.
3. **Back pain/bone pain:** ↑ *incidence of METS to bone,** weight loss.

DIAGNOSIS
1. ↑**Prostate Specific Antigen (PSA):** PSA >10ng/mL ↑*likelihood for prostate cancer & METS.*
2. **Digital rectal exam (DRE):** *hard, nodular, enlarged asymmetrical prostate.**
3. **Ultrasound with needle biopsy:** if PSA >4ng/mL. If >10 ⇨ bone scan to rule out METS.

MANAGEMENT
1. **Local disease:** ±active surveillance/observation if low grade.
   radical prostatectomy. <u>S/E or prostatectomy:</u> incontinence & impotence.
2. **Advance disease:** ***External beam radiation therapy, androgen deprivation*** (orchiectomy + GnRH agonists). Chemotherapy. If bone pain/METS ⇨ ±localized radiation, cryotherapy.

Screening is controversial. DRE & PSA done if ≥50y; African-Americans or family history ⇨ ≥ 40y.

BLADDER CANCER

- *TRANSITIONAL CELL (TCC) MC** (90%); 10% (squamous cell, adenocarcinoma, sarcoma, small cell).

RISK FACTORS: *SMOKING MC** >60%, *occupational exposure: dyes, rubber, leather* (beauticians, auto workers), *age >40y, white males 3x MC,* schistosomiasis, chronic bladder infection; *Cyclophosphamide** (Cyclophosphamide also causes hemorrhagic cystitis), *Pioglitazone.*

CLINICAL MANIFESTATIONS: *PAINLESS GROSS or microscopic HEMATURIA** (80-90%), irritative sx.

DIAGNOSIS: *cystoscopy with biopsy** (can be diagnostic or curative – ± be able to do excision). IVP.

MANAGEMENT
- *Most present early & respond well to treatment* but has the highest rate of recurrence of all cancers.
  1. **Localized or superficial:** *transurethral resection (electrocautery)* & follow-up every 3 months.
  2. **Invasive disease (advanced or involving muscular layer):** *radical cystectomy,* Chemotx, XRT.
  3. **Recurrent Bladder CA:** *BCG* (Bacillus Calmette-Guérin) *vaccine intravesicular** if electrocautery unsuccessful - immune reaction stimulates cross reaction with tumor antigens. Do not use BCG if immunosuppressed or if gross hematuria is present (may cause BCG-related sepsis).

RENAL CELL CARCINOMA

- *95% of tumors originating in the kidney.* Tumor of the proximal convoluted renal tubule cells (they are very metabolically active cells so they are the most prone to dysplasia).
- Characterized by lack of warning signs, variable presentations & resistance to chemo/XRT

RISK FACTORS: *smoking, dialysis, HTN, obesity, men,* cadmium/industrial exposure.

CLINICAL MANIFESTATIONS:
Classic triad: ❶*hematuria* (90%) ❷*flank/abdominal pain* ❸*palpable mass;* Malaise, weight loss.
- *L-sided varicocele** (blocks left testicular vain drainage).
- *HTN & hypercalcemia common* (↑PTH-related proteins leads to hypercalcemia).

DIAGNOSIS: *CT scan usually the first test.* Renal ultrasound, MRI.

MANAGEMENT:
  1. **Stage I-III** ⇨ *radical nephrectomy;** Immune therapy (ex *interleukin-2,* molecular-targeted tx). Renal cell cancer is usually resistant to chemotherapy & radiation therapy.
  2. Bilateral involvement or patient with solitary kidney ⇨ partial nephrectomy.

WILMS TUMOR (NEPHROBLASTOMA)

- *Nephroblastoma MC in CHILDREN within the 1st 5y of life.* MC abdominal malignancy in children.
- May be associated with other GU abnormalities (ex. cryptorchidism, hypospadias, horseshoe kidney).

CLINICAL MANIFESTATIONS:
*Painless, palpable abdominal mass MC manifestation** (doesn't cross midline), *hematuria, ±HTN (due to ↑renin secreted by tumor), anemia,* ±abdominal pain, nausea, vomiting, anorexia, fever.

DIAGNOSIS: *abdominal ultrasound: best initial test.* **CT with contrast or MRI:** more accurate test.
MANAGEMENT
  1. *Nephrectomy followed by chemotherapy. 80-90% cure rate!* Lung common site for METS.
  2. Post surgery radiation therapy if it extends beyond renal capsule, pulmonary METS or large tumor.

NEPHROLITHIASIS

RISK FACTORS
Decreased fluid intake (MC), males, medications (loop diuretics, antacids, chemotherapeutic drugs), gout (uric acid stones), hypercalcemia, polycystic kidney disease, UTIs (ex. urea-splitting organisms).

4 TYPES:
1. *Calcium oxalate MC** & phosphate* (80%) - ↑protein & salt intake inhibit Ca^{+2} reabsorption.

2. *Uric acid:* 5-8%. High protein foods ⇨ ↑purine ⇨ uric acid. Acidic urine promotes formation.

3. *Struvite stones (Mg ammonium phosphate)* may form *staghorn calculi** in the renal pelvis due to urea-splitting organisms *(ex. Proteus,* Klebsiella, Pseudomonas, Serratia, Enterobacter).*

4. Cystine 1-3% (genetic disorder).

CLINICAL MANIFESTATIONS
1. *RENAL COLIC: sudden, CONSTANT upper/lateral back/flank pain* over the costovertebral angle *radiating to the groin/anteriorly,** nausea/vomiting. ± Unable to find a comfortable position.

2. ⊕ *Costovertebral angle tenderness (CVAT).* Usually afebrile. ± *Hematuria,* frequency, urgency.

3. **Proximal ureter** ⇨ *flank, CVAT.* Midureter ⇨ *midabdominal;* **Distal ureter (VUJ)** ⇨ *groin pain.*

DIAGNOSIS
1. **UA:** *microscopic or gross hematuria** (85%), nitrites (if infectious). Obtain culture if infectious.

Urinary pH	STONE TYPE MOST LIKELY
5.5 – 6.8	Calcium (oxalate & phosphate)
<5.0 (acidic)	Uric acid, Cystine
>7.2 (alkaline)	*associated with struvite stones**

Examine urinary sediment for crystals. Patients often given a strainer to take home for later stone analysis

2. *Noncontrast CT Abdomen/pelvis** MC initial diagnostic test ordered.*
3. Renal ultrasound: detects stones or complications (ex. hydronephrosis). Used if CT contraindicated.
4. KUB radiographs: *only calcium & struvite stones are radiopaque* (visible on radiographs).
5. Intravenous pyelography (gold standard). Determines extent of obstruction & severity.

MANAGEMENT
STONES < 5-mm IN DIAMETER
80% chance of spontaneous passage.
1. *IV fluids, analgesic, antiemetics.** Tamsulosin* (alpha-blocker that may facilitate passage).

2. Stones at the *ureterovesicular junction (narrowest point of the urinary tract)** & ureteropelvic junction may make passage of small stones difficult.

STONES > 7-mm IN DIAMETER
20% chance of spontaneous passage. Alkalinize the urine to a pH >6.5 to dissolve uric acid stones.

1. *Extracorporeal shock wave lithotripsy:* may be used to break up larger stones that are less likely to pass spontaneously. May need multiple treatments to reduce the size of the stones.

2. *Uretoscopy ± stent: used to provide immediate relief to an obstructed or at-risk kidney.**

3. *Percutaneous nephrolithotomy:* most invasive ⇨ used for *large stones (>10mm), struvite*, or if other less invasive modalities fail. Incision made in the back & the stone is removed via a tube.
Prevention: increase fluid intake, decrease protein intake.

NORMAL ERECTION PHYSIOLOGY

ERECTIONS are caused by ❶ *INCREASED PENILE ARTERIAL INFLOW* & ❷ *DECREASED PENILE VENOUS OUTFLOW*.

- *Parasympathetic stimulation* ⇨ ↑nitric oxide ⇨ ↑cyclic GMP ⇨ penile artery dilation (increased arterial inflow) & corpus cavernosal smooth muscle relaxation (allowing it to fill with blood). Prostaglandins also play a role. Indirect venous constriction (by the enlarged sinusoids) reduces venous outflow, maintaining erectile rigidity.

FLACCID *state is achieved by sympathetic stimulation** ⇨ norepinephrine ⇨ penile arterial vasoconstriction (reduced inflow) & venous dilation (increased outflow). *cGMP-specific phosphodiesterase* breaks down cyclic GMP ⇨ reduces arterial vasodilation ⇨ flaccid state.

ERECTILE DYSFUNCTION

- Consistent inability to generate or maintain an erection.

PATHOPHYSIOLOGY

- Neurologic (ex. DM), psychogenic, vascular (atherosclerosis), prolactinoma, trauma, surgery, medications: ex beta-blockers, hydrochlorothiazide, calcium channel blockers, SSRIs, TCAs.
- Abrupt onset most likely psychological, gradual worsening indicates systemic causes.

DIAGNOSIS: history & physical exam, testosterone level, other hormone testing. Nocturnal penile tumescence used to evaluate sleep erections. Duplex ultrasound to evaluate penile blood flow.

MANAGEMENT

1. *Phosphodiesterase-5 inhibitors: Sildenafil* (Viagra), *Tadalafil* (Cialis), *Vardenafil* (Levitra). **MOA:** phosphodiesterase-5 inhibition ⇨ ↑*nitric oxide levels &* ↑cyclic GMP ⇨ ability to achieve & maintain erection. **S/E:** headache, flushing, hearing loss. **CI:** *not used with nitrates or patients with cardiovascular disease** (may cause severe hypotension – synergistic nitric oxide).
2. Intracavernosal injection therapy: prostaglandin E_1 (Alpradostil), Papaverine or combination of Papaverine plus Phentolamine (causes vasodilation – increased arterial inflow).
3. Other: vacuum pumps, penile revascularization, penile prosthesis.
4. Testosterone: hormone replacement if testosterone is low (ex. androgen deficiency).

PRIAPISM

- Prolonged, painful erections without sexual stimulation. Infection & impotence common complications.
- **Ischemic (low-flow):** *decreased venous outflow* may lead to a compartment syndrome. *MC type.*
- **Nonischemic (high-flow):** due to *increased arterial inflow.* Commonly related to perineal or penile trauma.

ETIOLOGIES

1. *Idiopathic MC* (50%), *sickle cell disease* (10%), injection of erectile agent for erectile dysfunction, drugs (ex cocaine, marijuana), alcohol. Trauma (high flow) may cause rupture of the cavernosal artery.
2. Meds: PDE-5 inhibitors, antidepressants (esp Trazodone), antipsychotics, anticonvulsants, alpha blockers.
3. Neurologic: head trauma, meningitis, subarachnoid hemorrhage, postoperative.

DIAGNOSIS: primarily based on history and physical examination. Blood gas may be performed in erection >4h.
1. Cavernosal blood gas: high-flow results similar to ABG, low-flow shows hypoxemia, hypercarbia & acidemia.
2. Doppler ultrasound: Normal or high blood flow in nonischemic, minimal or absent blood flow in ischemic.

MANAGEMENT OF LOW-FLOW
1. *Phenylephrine* (intracavernous injection). *1st line medication.** **MOA:** alpha-agonists cause contraction of the cavernous smooth muscle which ↑'es venous outflow. **CI:** cardiac or cerebrovascular history
2. **Terbutaline:** orally or SQ (constricts cavernosal artery, reducing arterial inflow) may be used if <4 hours.
3. **Needle aspiration** of corpora to remove blood especially if >4 hours duration ±Phenylephrine. Ice packs.
4. Shunt surgery may performed if not responsive to medical & aspiration therapy.

MANAGEMENT OF HIGH-FLOW
1. *Observation* (since it is not ischemic). ±nonpermanent arterial embolization or surgical ligation if refractory.

HEMATURIA

Terminal hematuria ⇨ *bladder or prostate. Throughout* ⇨ *bladder, ureter, kidneys. Initial* ⇨ *urethra.*

ETIOLOGIES
1. *<40y: GU infection MC,* nephrolithiasis. >40y: urinary tract cancer,* prostatic disease.*
2. Upper GU tract: nephrolithiasis, kidney disease, renal cell CA, trauma, DM, sickle cell trait or sickle cell disease.
3. Lower GU tract: BPH (MC cause of microscopic hematuria), urothelial cell cancer (in the absence of infection).
4. Pseudo hematuria: Rhabdomyolysis, beets, rhubarb, myoglobinuria (contains heme), hemoglobinuria.
5. Meds: Ibuprofen, Phenazopyridine, Rifampin. Cyclophosphamide causes hemorrhagic cystitis.

DIAGNOSIS
UA/urine culture usually done 1st* to rule out benign causes - UTI, pyelonephritis, trauma, viral illness, sexual activity, exercise. CT angiography, MRI, US.
Cystoscopy, IVP & urine cytology is part of the workup in patients >40y.
1. **Cystoscopy:** *best test to evaluate for bladder or urethral cancer* (ex. hematuria without infection)
2. Intravenous pyelogram: useful to evaluate the kidney, ureters etc. but uses contrast dye.
3. Ultrasound: to evaluate the kidney & to rule out kidney stones.
4. Cytology: may be used to rule out bladder cancer.

URETHRITIS

CLINICAL MANIFESTATIONS
Urethral discharge or pruritus. Dysuria seen in both gonococcal & nongonococcal urethritis.
1. **Gonococcal Urethritis:** abrupt onset of symptoms (especially within 3-4 days). Opaque, yellow, white or clear thick discharge, pruritus. Up to 20% of patients are asymptomatic.

2. **Non-Gonococcal (NGU):** *Chlamydia MC cause of nongonococcal urethritis.* 5-8 days ⇨ purulent or mucopurulent discharge, Pruritus. Hematuria, pain with intercourse. Up to 40% asymptomatic. Others include: Ureaplasma urealyticum, Trichomonas vaginalis.

COMPLICATIONS
1. **Men:** epididymitis, prostatitis, infertility, reactive arthritis (urethritis, conjunctivitis & arthritis), septic arthritis.
2. **Women:** pelvic inflammatory disease, infertility, ectopic pregnancy, premature delivery, septic arthritis.

3. **Children/Infants:** neonatal pneumonia & **Neonatal Conjunctivitis (Ophthalmia neonatorium):** Neonatal eye infection during passage through an infected birth canal.
   -Day 2-5 ⇨ Gonococcal. Erythromycin ophthalmic ointment used as prophylaxis against gonococcal infection (otherwise child may be at increased risk of blindness).
   -Day 5-7 ⇨ Chlamydia.

DIAGNOSIS: *Nucleic acid amplification** most sensitive & specific for both chlamydia & gonorrhea.

MANAGEMENT
25-30% of patients have co-infection of both gonorrhea & chlamydia so treatment of both is recommended:
1. **Gonococcal: *Ceftriaxone 250mg IM x 1 dose.*** Azithromycin 2g orally x 1 dose can be given if true allergy to cephalosporin (but it is not ideal & eradication must be documented). Cefixime.

2. **Nongonococcal: *Azithromycin*** 1g orally x 1 dose or ***Doxycycline*** 100mg orally bid x 10 days.
Recurrent NGU: 1 time dose of Metronidazole + Erythromycin x 7 days. Treat other causes as needed.

RENOVASCULAR HYPERTENSION (RENAL ARTERY STENOSIS)

- *HTN due to <u>renal artery stenosis</u> 1 or both kidneys ⇨ perceived hypotension by kidney ⇨ ↑RAAS.*

- *MC CAUSE OF SECONDARY HTN!* - HTN due to ↑RAAS activation.*

- *Suspect if HTN onset <20y or >50y, severe HTN, HTN resistant to ≥3 drugs, ⊕abdominal bruit or if patient develops <u>acute kidney injury after the initiation of ACE Inhibitor therapy.</u>* *

ETIOLOGIES: ❶ *Atherosclerosis MC in elderly** ❷ *<u>Fibromuscular dysplasia MC cause in women <50y.</u>* *

CLINICAL MANIFESTATIONS: *severe/refractory HTN; <u>abdominal (renal) bruit,</u>* headache.*

DIAGNOSIS
1. <u>Noninvasive:</u> options include CT or MR angiography (MRA safe if poor renal function) & ultrasound. <u>Captopril renography:</u> ↑plasma renin activity 1 hour after Captopril administration (ACEI reduce GFR & renal blood flow causing a reactive ↑ in plasma renin). Used to determine kidney function.

2. *<u>Renal arteriography: most definitive (gold standard).</u>* * Do not use if renal failure is present.

MANAGEMENT
1. **Surgical:** revascularization
   - *Angioplasty with stent – definitive.** Done if ↑Cr > 4, ↑Cr with ACEI tx, >80% stenosis.
   - Bypass may be performed if angioplasty with stent is unsuccessful.

2. **ACE inhibitors***/ARBs (inhibits aldosterone & angiotensin II-mediated vasoconstriction. *However, ACEI/ARB contraindicated if bilateral stenosis or solitary kidney** because ACEI markedly reduces renal blood flow & GFR in these patients* ⇨ acute kidney injury!* Diuretics.

ENURESIS

<u>Primary monosymptomatic enuresis (bedwetting)</u> distinct episodes of urinary incontinence while sleeping in children ≥5 years in the absence of symptoms of infection.
Enuresis spontaneously resolves in most cases.

MANAGEMENT
1. **Behavioral:** motivational therapy (especially in children 5-7y), education & reassurance. Use of washable products, room deodorizers. Bladder training: regular voiding schedule, deliberate voiding prior to sleeping, waking the child up to urinate intermittently. Avoidance of caffeine-based & drinks with high sugar content. Fluid restriction.

2. **Enuresis alarm:** usually *used if children fail to respond to behavioral therapy.* Often attempted before medical therapy. A sensor is placed on a bed pad or in the undergarments and goes off when wet. Most effective long-term therapy. Usually continued until there is a minimum of 2 weeks of consecutive dry nights.

3. *<u>Desmopressin</u>** (DDAVP): used in nocturnal polyuria with normal bladder function capacity. Better for short-term use. <u>MOA:</u> *synthetic antidiuretic hormone (ADH),* which reduces urination. May cause hyponatremia so patients may use liberal amounts of salt to reduce the incidence.

4. **Tricyclic antidepressants:** may be used if they fail the above treatments. <u>MOA:</u> stimulates ADH secretion, detrusor muscle relaxation & decreases time spent in REM sleep. Ex. *Imipramine.*

- **Incontinence: *involuntary loss of urine.*** Normally, sympathetic tone closes the bladder neck & increases pelvic floor tone. During micturition, parasympathetic tone increases, allowing bladder neck relaxation. Functional incontinence: a problem that keeps the patient from quickly getting to bathroom.
- Mixed: combination of stress & urge in 40-60%. Detrusor overactivity & impaired urethral function: bladder training & pelvic exercises + medications for urge.

	STRESS INCONTINENCE	URGE INCONTINENCE	OVERFLOW INCONTINENCE
DEFINITION	• urine leakage due to ↑ *intraabdominal pressure.* Rare in men.	• urine leakage *accompanied by or preceded by urge.**	• *Urinary retention (incomplete bladder emptying)*
PATHOPHYSIOLOGY	• ↑ *intrabdominal pressure > urethral resistance to urine flow.** - *Laxity of the pelvic floor muscles:* childbirth, surgery, postmenopausal estrogen loss, post prostatectomy.	• *Detrusor muscle overactivity"* involuntary detrusor muscle contraction. **"OVERACTIVE BLADDER"** - Detrusor muscle stimulated by muscarinic acetylcholine receptors	• ↓ *detrusor muscle activity (atony)* **"UNDERACTIVE BLADDER"** - DM, multiple sclerosis, autonomic dysfunction, spinal injury. - *Bladder outlet obstruction: BPH*
CLINICAL MANIFESTATIONS	• ↑ *intraabdominal pressure from sneezing, coughing, laughing ⇨ urine leakage.* • Worse when upright.	• *Urgency, frequency, small volume voids, nocturia*	• Small volume voids, frequency, dribbling. • ↑*post void residual >200ml.*
MANAGEMENT	• *PELVIC FLOOR EXERCISES**: 87% improvement - Kegel exercises, biofeedback. • *ALPHA AGONISTS* (19-74% improvement). - *Midodrine, Pseudoephedrine.* - MOA: ↑'es urethral sphincter tone & ↑'es urethral urine flow resistance. • Surgery: {88% improvement} - Increases urethral outlet resistance (including artificial sphincter). • Anti-incontinent devices: vaginal cones help to strengthen the pelvic floor muscles. • Estrogen: cream or estradiol-impregnated vaginal ring.	• *BLADDER TRAINING* (75% improvement). Timed frequent voiding, ↓fluid intake • *ANTICHOLINERGICS: 1st line meds in urge* - Oxybutynin (Ditropan XL) *antispasmodic & anticholinergic.* - *Tolterodine* (Detrol) - **MOA: *Blocks cholinergic receptors in the bladder* ⇨ ↑'ing bladder capacity,** ↑'es the volume threshold for initiating an involuntary contraction ⇨ ↓*involuntary contraction strength* - *S/E: dry mouth, constipation, dry eyes, blurred vision, increased heart rate.* • Tricyclic antidepressant: *Imipramine* - **MOA: *central & peripheral anticholinergic effect & alpha-adrenergic agonist*** (bladder muscle relaxation, ↑'es bladder outlet resistance, antispasmodic effect on detrusor muscle & ↑'ed urethral sphincter tone). • *Mirabegron:* β-3agonist ⇨ bladder relaxant • Surgical: increases bladder compliance: injection of Botox, bladder augmentation. • Diet: avoidance of spicy foods, citrus fruit, chocolate, caffeine.	• **BLADDER ATONY** • *Intermittent or indwelling catheterization 1st line treatment** • *Cholinergics: Bethanacol* - ↑'es detrusor muscle activity. **BPH** • *α-1 blockers: Tamsulosin* - <u>MOA</u>: smooth muscle relaxation of the prostate & bladder neck, decreases urethral resistance & obstruction.

SELECTED REFERENCES

Crumley SM, Divatia M, Truong L, Shen S, Ayala AG, Ro JY. Renal cell carcinoma: Evolving and emerging subtypes. World J Clin Cases. 2013;1(9):262-275.

Trojian TH, Lishnak TS, Heiman D. Epididymitis and orchitis: an overview. Am Fam Physician. 2009;79(7):583-7.

Chou R, Croswell JM, Dana T, et al. Screening for prostate cancer: a review of the evidence for the U.S. Preventive Services Task Force. Ann Intern Med. 2011;155(11):762-71.

Calle EE, Rodriguez C, Walker-thurmond K, Thun MJ. Overweight, obesity, and mortality from cancer in a prospectively studied cohort of U.S. adults. N Engl J Med. 2003;348(17):1625-38.

Tan N, Margolis DJ, Mcclure TD, et al. Radical prostatectomy: value of prostate MRI in surgical planning. Abdom Imaging. 2012;37(4):664-74.

Ringdahl E, Teague L. Testicular torsion. Am Fam Physician. 2006;74(10):1739-43.

Hayes-lattin B, Nichols CR. Testicular cancer: a prototypic tumor of young adults. Semin Oncol. 2009;36(5):432-8.

Shaw J. Diagnosis and treatment of testicular cancer. Am Fam Physician. 2008;77(4):469-74.

Lane DR, Takhar SS. Diagnosis and management of urinary tract infection and pyelonephritis. Emerg Med Clin North Am. 2011;29(3):539-52.

Mehta RL, Kellum JA, Shah SV, et al. Acute Kidney Injury Network: report of an initiative to improve outcomes in acute kidney injury. Crit Care. 2007;11(2):R31.

Qaseem A, Hopkins RH, Sweet DE, Starkey M, Shekelle P. Screening, monitoring, and treatment of stage 1 to 3 chronic kidney disease: A clinical practice guideline from the American College of Physicians. Ann Intern Med. 2013;159(12):835-47.

Macdonald R, Wilt TJ. Alfuzosin for treatment of lower urinary tract symptoms compatible with benign prostatic hyperplasia: a systematic review of efficacy and adverse effects. Urology. 2005;66(4):780-8.

UA guideline on management of benign prostatic hyperplasia (2003). Chapter 1: Diagnosis and treatment recommendations. J Urol. 2003;170(2 Pt 1):530-47.

Zeegers MP, Tan FE, Dorant E, Van den brandt PA. The impact of characteristics of cigarette smoking on urinary tract cancer risk: a meta-analysis of epidemiologic studies. Cancer. 2000;89(3):630-9.

Neoadjuvant chemotherapy in invasive bladder cancer: update of a systematic review and meta-analysis of individual patient data advanced bladder cancer (ABC) meta-analysis collaboration. Eur Urol. 2005;48(2):202-5.

Baltimore RS. Re-evaluation of antibiotic treatment of streptococcal pharyngitis. Curr Opin Pediatr. 2010;22(1):77-82.

Salama AD, Levy JB, Lightstone L, Pusey CD. Goodpasture's disease. Lancet. 2001;358(9285):917-20.

Cohen HT, Mcgovern FJ. Renal-cell carcinoma. N Engl J Med. 2005;353(23):2477-90.

Tournade MF, Com-nougué C, De kraker J, et al. Optimal duration of preoperative therapy in unilateral and nonmetastatic Wilms' tumor in children older than 6 months: results of the Ninth International Society of Pediatric Oncology Wilms' Tumor Trial and Study. J Clin Oncol. 2001;19(2):488-500.

Hodson EM, Willis NS, Craig JC. Corticosteroid therapy for nephrotic syndrome in children. Cochrane Database Syst Rev. 2007;(4):CD001533.

Nickel JC. Prostatitis. Can Urol Assoc J. 2011;5(5):306-15.

Bellomo R, Ronco C, Kellum JA, Mehta RL, Palevsky P. Acute renal failure - definition, outcome measures, animal models, fluid therapy and information technology needs: the Second International Consensus Conference of the Acute Dialysis Quality Initiative (ADQI) Group. Crit Care. 2004;8(4):R204-12.

Mehta RL, Kellum JA, Shah SV, et al. Acute Kidney Injury Network: report of an initiative to improve outcomes in acute kidney injury. Crit Care. 2007;11(2):R31.

Qaseem A, Hopkins RH, Sweet DE, Starkey M, Shekelle P. Screening, monitoring, and treatment of stage 1 to 3 chronic kidney disease: A clinical practice guideline from the American College of Physicians. Ann Intern Med. 2013;159(12):835-47.

Hodson EM, Willis NS, Craig JC. Corticosteroid therapy for nephrotic syndrome in children. Cochrane Database Syst Rev. 2007;(4):CD001533.

Levey AS, Bosch JP, Lewis JB, Greene T, Rogers N, Roth D. A more accurate method to estimate glomerular filtration rate from serum creatinine: a new prediction equation. Modification of Diet in Renal Disease Study Group. Ann Intern Med. 1999;130(6):461-70.

Levey AS, Stevens LA, Schmid CH, et al. A new equation to estimate glomerular filtration rate. Ann Intern Med. 2009;150(9):604-12.

Eubanks PJ, Stabile BE. Osteitis fibrosa cystica with renal parathyroid hormone resistance: a review of pseudohypoparathyroidism with insight into calcium homeostasis. Arch Surg. 1998;133(6):673-6.

Cockcroft DW, Gault MH. Prediction of creatinine clearance from serum creatinine. Nephron. 1976;16(1):31-41.

Locatelli F, Aljama P, Canaud B, et al. Target haemoglobin to aim for with erythropoiesis-stimulating agents: a position statement by ERBP following publication of the Trial to reduce cardiovascular events with Aranesp therapy (TREAT) study. Nephrol Dial Transplant. 2010;25(9):2846-50.

Zietse R, Van der lubbe N, Hoorn EJ. Current and future treatment options in SIADH. NDT Plus. 2009;2(Suppl_3):iii12-iii19.

Adrogué HJ, Madias NE. Hyponatremia. N Engl J Med. 2000;342(21):1581-9.

Elliott MJ, Ronksley PE, Clase CM, Ahmed SB, Hemmelgarn BR. Management of patients with acute hyperkalemia. CMAJ. 2010;182(15):1631-5.

Halperin ML, Kamel KS. Potassium. Lancet. 1998;352(9122):135-40.

Al-ghamdi SM, Cameron EC, Sutton RA. Magnesium deficiency: pathophysiologic and clinical overview. Am J Kidney Dis. 1994;24(5):737-52.

PHOTO CREDITS

CHAPTER 9 – NEUROLOGY

Central Nervous System: consists of the brain & spinal cord.
Peripheral Nervous System: consists mainly of the peripheral nerves

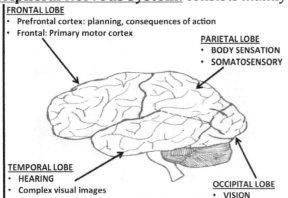

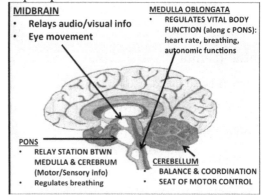

I. CEREBRUM

1. ***Cortex: functions in higher brain processes such as thought & action. Controls all voluntary activity (with the help of the cerebellum).*** 2 hemispheres. The right side may be more associated with creativity, left side with logic. The corpus callosum is a bundle of axons that connects the 2 hemispheres. The cerebral cortex is divided into 4 lobes:
    - Frontal Lobe: reasoning, problem solving, parts of speech, movement & emotion.
    - Parietal Lobe: perception/recognition of stimuli, orientation & movement.
    - Temporal Lobe: memory, perception/recognition of auditory stimuli & speech.
    - Occipital Lobe: visual processing.

2. Basal ganglia: voluntary motor movement, coordination, cognition & emotion.

3. Limbic system: includes the thalamus, hypothalamus, amygdala & hippocampus.
    - Amygdala: located in the temporal lobe. Involved in memory, emotion and fear.

    - Hippocampus: learning, memory. Converts short-term memory into long-term memory.

II. DIENCEPHALON

THALAMUS: located deep in the forebrain.
- Processes nearly all sensory & motor information. Relays info to & from the overlying cortex - last relay site to all sensory input (except olfaction) before the information about sensory input reaches the cortex.

HYPOTHALAMUS
- Located below & ventral to the thalamus. ***Controls homeostasis.***

III. BRAINSTEM: controls vital life functions (including breathing, heart rate & blood pressure).
- **Midbrain:** controls eye movement, relays visual & auditory information.
- **Pons:** *regulates breathing, serves as a relay station between the cerebral hemisphere & the medulla.* Involved in motor control & sensory input.
- **Medulla oblongata:** extension of spinal cord (located between the pons & spinal cord). Regulates vital body functions (along with the pons) such as heart rate, breathing, autonomic centers, swallowing & coughing.

IV CEREBELLUM
- Located posterior to the medulla. Maintains posture & balance, coordinates voluntary movement & controls certain head & eye movements.

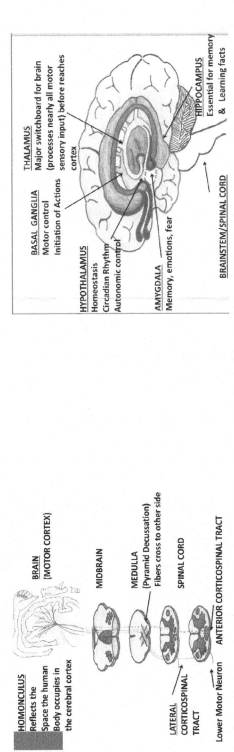

BASAL GANGLIA DISORDERS: since the basal ganglia is involved in coordinated movement, emotion & cognition, problems can lead to movement disorders (*dyskinesias, dystonias, Parkinsonism, Huntington's disease*) or *behavior control* (*Tourette's, obsessive compulsive*).

	"EXTRAPYRAMIDAL SYMPTOMS"
DYSKINESIA	*Involuntary spasms, repetitive motions or abnormal voluntary movement.*
DYSTONIA	*Sustained contraction* (muscle spasm) especially of antagonistic muscles (ex simultaneous biceps & triceps contraction) ⇨ *twisting of the body, abnormal posturing* (ex: torticollis, writer's cramp).
MYOCLONUS	Sudden, *brief, sporadic involuntary jerking/twitching* of 1 muscle or muscle group (not suppressible).
TICS	Sudden, *repetitive nonrhythmic movements or vocals* using specific muscle groups. Tics are **suppressible** (unlike myoclonus which is not suppressible). Ex. Tourette syndrome.
CHOREA	*Rapid involuntary jerky, uncontrolled, purposeless movements.* Ex. **Huntington chorea** (due to caudate nucleus atrophy in the basal ganglia), Sydenham's chorea (rheumatic fever)
MUSCLE SPASMS	Muscle contractions. **Tonic:** *prolonged sustained contraction/rigidity;* **Clonic:** *repetitive rapid movements*
TREMORS	Rhythmic movement of a body part. – **Resting tremor:** tremor at rest (ex Parkinson disease) – **Postural tremor:** tremor occurs while holding position against gravity. – **Intentional tremor:** tremor occurs during movement or when approaching nearer to a target.

PARKINSONISM: disorders associated with tremor, bradykinesia, rigidity, and postural instability. Includes:

❶ *Parkinson disease:* loss of the dopamine producing cells of the substantia nigra (in the basal ganglia).

❷ *Dopamine antagonists: medications that block dopamine include the typical antipsychotics (Haloperidol, Droperidol, Fluphenazine, Chlorpromazine) > atypical antipsychotics (ex. Olanzapine, Clozapine, Risperidone).* Antiemetics: *Prochlorperazine, Promethazine, Metoclopramide.*

❸ *Lewy body disease:* loss of dopaminergic neurons leads to motor features similar to Parkinson disease. Loss of anticholinergic neurons lead to dementia (similar to Alzheimer's), visuospatial dysfunction & recurrent visual hallucinations.

❹ Other: head trauma, HIV, carbon monoxide or mercury poisoning, CNS dysfunction (ex stroke, meningitis).

HUNTINGTON DISEASE

- **_Autosomal dominant_** neurodegenerative disorder. Mutation on chromosome 4.
- Huntingtin gene ⇨ neurotoxicity as well as cerebral, putamen & caudate nucleus atrophy.

CLINICAL MANIFESTATIONS
Symptoms usually appear 30-50y of age. Initial ❶ behavioral ⇨ ❷ chorea* & ❸ dementia.
1. **Behavioral changes:** personality, cognitive, intellectual & psychiatric including irritability.

2. **Chorea**: rapid, involuntary or arrhythmic movement of the face, neck, trunk & limbs initially. Chorea worsened with voluntary movements & stress (usually disappears with sleep).

3. **Dementia**: most develop dementia before 50y (primarily executive dysfunction).
4. Gait abnormalities/ataxia (often irregular & unsteady). Incontinence, facial grimacing.

PHYSICAL EXAM
1. Restlessness, fragility. Quick, involuntary hand movements. Brisk deep tendon reflexes.

DIAGNOSIS
1. **CT scan:** _CEREBRAL & CAUDATE NUCLEUS ATROPHY._* MRI shows similar findings. Genetic testing.

2. PET scan: decreased glucose metabolism in the caudate nucleus & putamen.

MANAGEMENT
1. No cure. **_Usually fatal within 15-20 years_** after presentation (due to disease progression).

2. **Chorea management:** antidopaminergics: typical & atypical antipsychotics, Tetrabenzine. Benzodiazepines may help with chorea & sleep. No medication stops disease progression.

ESSENTIAL FAMILIAL TREMOR (BENIGN)

- Autosomal dominant _inherited disorder_ of unknown etiology.
- Onset of age is usually in the 60s but may occur at any age.

CLINICAL MANIFESTATIONS
1. _INTENTIONAL TREMOR - **postural, bilateral** ACTION **tremor of the hands, forearms, head, neck or voice.**_* MC in the _upper extremities & head (titubation)_ - usually spares the legs.
   - **worsened with emotional stress & intentional movement.** On finger to nose testing, _tremor increases as the target is approached._*
   - **_Tremor shortly relieved with ETOH ingestion._***

2. No abnormal physical exam findings, **no other significant neurologic findings** besides the tremor (patient ± cogwheel phenomenon).

MANAGEMENT
Treatment not usually needed.
1. **_Propranolol may help if severe or situational._***

2. Primidone (barbiturate) if no relief with Propranolol, instead of Propranolol or with it.

3. Alprazolam (benzodiazepine) 3rd line.

PARKINSON DISEASE

- ***Idiopathic dopamine depletion**** ⇨ failure to inhibit acetylcholine in the ***basal ganglia*** (Ach is an excitatory CNS neurotransmitter, *dopamine is inhibitory*).   Onset of symptoms 45-65y MC.
- Cytoplasmic inclusions ***(Lewy bodies), loss of pigment cells seen in the substantia nigra.****

CLINICAL MANIFESTATIONS
1. **Tremor:** often 1st symptom.   ***RESTING* tremor MC sign*** *(ex. "pill rolling").*
   - worse at rest & with emotional stress.
   - ***lessened with voluntary activity, intentional movement*** & sleep.
   - *Usually confined to one limb or one side* for years before it becomes generalized.

2. **Bradykinesia:** ***slowness of voluntary movement & ↓automatic movements***
   ex. lack of swinging of the arms while walking & shuffling gait.

3. **Rigidity:** increased resistance to passive movement ***(cogwheel,*** flexed posture).   Festination = increasing speed while walking.   Normal deep tendon reflexes.   Usually no muscle weakness.

4. **Face involvement:** relatively immobile face ***(fixed facial expressions),*** widened palpebral fissure, ***Myerson's sign:*** *tapping the bridge of nose repetitively causes a sustained blink.* Decreased blinking. Seborrhea of the skin common.

5. **Instability**: ***postural instability*** usually a late finding ("pull test" – stand behind patient & pull shoulders ⇨ patient falls or takes steps backwards). Dementia in 50% (usually a late finding).

MANAGEMENT
Drug treatment not used early in the course of the illness if symptoms are mild.
1. **Levodopa/Carbidopa** (Sinemet): ***most effective treatment.**** *Levodopa is converted to dopamine* (Carbidopa reduces amount of Levodopa needed, reducing S/E of Levodopa).
   S/E: nausea, vomiting, hypotension, somnolence, dyskinesia & "wearing off bradykinesia" associated with long-term use.

2. **Dopamine agonists: Bromocriptine, Pramipexole, Ropinirole.**
   MOA: directly stimulates dopamine receptors. Less S/E than Levodopa. Sometimes ***used in young patients to delay the use of Levodopa.*** If patient is not sensitive to Levodopa, they may develop an insensitivity to dopamine agonists.
   S/E: orthostatic hypotension, nausea, headache, dizziness, sleep disturbances, anorexia.

3. **Anticholinergics: Trihexyphenidyl, Benztropine** (Cogentin).
   MOA: ***blocks excitatory cholinergic effects.***
   Ind: ***<70y with tremor predominance**** *(doesn't improve bradykinesia).*
   S/E: constipation, dry mouth, blurred vision, tachycardia, urinary retention. **CI: *BPH, glaucoma.***

4. **Amantadine**: (↑'es presynaptic dopamine release) & improves long-term levodopa induced dyskinesias.   May help early on with mild symptoms.

5. **MAO-B Inhibitors** ex. **Selegiline, Rasagiline**
   MOA: *increases dopamine* in the striatum (MAO-B normally breaks down dopamine).

6. Catechol-O-Methyltransferase (COMT) inhibitors: **Entacapone, Tolcapone.** Adjunctive tx.
   MOA: prevents dopamine breakdown. Ex. S/E: GI sx, brown discoloration of urine.

TOURETTE SYNDROME

- Onset usually in childhood (2-5y) MC in boys. ± associated with obsessions-compulsions.

CLINICAL MANIFESTATIONS:

1. **Motor tics:** *of the face, head & neck* (blinking, shrugging, head thrusting, sniffling).

2. **Verbal or phonetic tics:** ex. grunts, throat clearing, obscene words (coprolalia), repetitive phrases, repeating the phrases of others (echolalia).
3. Self-mutilating tics: hair pulling, nail biting, biting of the lips etc.

MANAGEMENT:

1. *Habit reversal therapy.* 50% have symptom resolution by 18y.
2. Dopamine blocking agents: ex. *Haloperidol, Risperidone, Fluphenazine, Pimozide.* Tetrabenzine.
3. Alpha-adrenergics: ex. Clonidine, Guanfacine. Clonazepam may also be used as adjunct.

AMYOTROPHIC LATERAL SCLEROSIS (ALS)   LOU GEHRIG'S DISEASE

- Necrosis of BOTH upper & lower motor neurons ⇨ *progressive MOTOR degeneration.*

CLINICAL MANIFESTATIONS

1. Muscle weakness, *loss of ability to initiate & control motor movements.*

2. *MIXED UPPER MOTOR & LOWER MOTOR NEURON SIGNS:* *
    - Upper motor neuron sx: spasticity, stiffness, hyperreflexia.
    - Lower motor neuron sx: progressive bilateral fasciculations, muscle atrophy, hyporeflexia, muscle weakness.
3. Bulbar symptoms: dysphagia, dysarthria, speech problems. Eventual respiratory dysfunction.

4. *Sensation, urinary sphincter & voluntary eye movements are spared.* *

MANAGEMENT

1. *Riluzole* reduces progression for up to 6 months. Usually fatal within 3-5 years after onset.

CEREBRAL PALSY

- CNS disorder associated with muscle tone & postural abnormalities due to brain injury during perinatal or prenatal period.

CLINICAL MANIFESTATIONS

1. *Spasticity: hallmark.* *Varying degrees of motor deficits.* Often associated with intellectual/learning disabilities & development abnormalities. May develop seizures.

PHYSICAL EXAMINATION

1. Hyperreflexia, limb-length discrepancies, congenital defects.

MANAGEMENT

1. Multidisciplinary approach.
2. Improving spasticity: Baclofen, Diazepam. Antiepileptics for seizures.

RESTLESS LEGS SYNDROME (Willis-Ekbom disease)

- Sleep-related movement disorder. Usually primary but may occur secondary to CNS iron deficiency, pregnancy, peripheral neuropathy etc.

DIAGNOSIS
1. An uncomfortable or unpleasant sensation (itching, burning, paresthesias, etc) in the leg that creates an urge to move the legs. Symptoms:
   - worsen at night & tend to occur with prolonged periods of rest or inactivity. During sleep, periodic limb movements may disturb sleep or cause the patient to awake from sleep.
   - improve with movement.

MANAGEMENT
1. **Dopamine agonists**: *tx of choice.** ex. ***Pramipexole, Ropinirole.***
2. Alpha-2-delta calcium channel ligands: ex. ***Gabapentin,*** Pregabalin.
3. Benzodiazepines: may be used as adjunctive treatment. Ex. Clonazepam.
4. Opioids may be used in disease resistant to the aforementioned medications.

Iron supplementation recommended in patients with a serum ferritin levels lower than 75 mcg/L because of the association with iron deficiency in the central nervous system.

GUILLAIN BARRÉ SYNDROME

- Acute/subacute acquired inflammatory ***demyelinating polyradiculopathy*** of the ***peripheral nerves***.

- ↑ ***Incidence with CAMPYLOBACTER JEJUNI*** *(MC)* or other ***antecedent respiratory or GI infections***, CMV, EBV, HIV, mycoplasma. Immunizations, postsurgical.

PATHOPHYSIOLOGY
- Immune-mediated demyelination & axonal degeneration slows nerve impulses ⇨ symmetric weakness & paresthesias. Post-infection immune response cross-reacts with peripheral nerve components (molecular mimicry).

CLINICAL MANIFESTATIONS
1. ***Ascending weakness & paresthesias (usually symmetric).*** ↓*DTR (LMN lesion).* May involve the muscles of respiration or the bulbar muscles (swallowing abnormalities). CN VII palsy.
2. ***Autonomic dysfunction***: *tachycardia, hypotension or hypertension,* ***breathing difficulties.***

DIAGNOSIS
1. **CSF: *high protein with a normal WBC (cell count).**** This is known as *albuminocytological dissociation.* May be due to altered neuronal capillary-CSF barrier defect.
   - the high protein (>400mg/L) usually seen after 1-3 weeks of symptom onset.
2. Electrophysiologic studies: decreased motor nerve conduction velocities & amplitude.

MANAGEMENT
1. **PLASMAPHERESIS** best if done early. MOA: removes harmful circulating auto-antibodies that cause demyelination. Equally as effective as IVIG. Patients are usually hospitalized.

2. **INTRAVENOUS IMMUNE GLOBULIN (IVIG):** suppresses harmful inflammation/Auto-antibodies & induces remyelination. Most recover within months.
3. Mechanical ventilation if respiratory failure develops. ***Prednisone contraindicated.***

PROGNOSIS: 60% full recovery in 1 year (10-20% left with permanent disability).

MYASTHENIA GRAVIS

- *Autoimmune* peripheral nerve disorder. *MC in young women.** Associated HLA-DR3.
- *75% have **thymic abnormality (hyperplasia or thymoma)*** or other autoimmune disorders. May occur postpartum.

PATHOPHYSIOLOGY

- Inefficient skeletal muscle neuromuscular transmission due to *autoimmune antibodies against acetylcholine (nicotinic) postsynaptic receptor** at the *neuromuscular junction* (↓ACh receptors) ⇨ progressive weakness with repeated muscle use & recovery after periods of rest.

CLINICAL MANIFESTATIONS

- 2 categories: ❶ *ocular* (usually 1ˢᵗ presenting symptom & more severe) & ❷ *generalized.*
  1. ***OCULAR weakness:*** extraocular involvement ⇨ ***diplopia,*** eyelid weakness/***ptosis*** (more prominent with upward gaze). Weakness worsened with repeated use. Pupils are spared.

  2. ***GENERALIZED muscle weakness***: least in the morning ***worsened with repeated muscle use throughout the day (relieved with rest).*** Normal sensation/ deep tendon reflexes.
     - **Bulbar** (oropharyngeal) **weakness** - with prolonged chewing, dysphagia.
     - **Respiratory muscle weakness**: may lead to ***respiratory failure = myasthenic crisis.***

DIAGNOSIS

1. ⊕ ***Acetylcholine receptor antibodies.***   ⊕ MuSK (muscle-specific tyrosine kinase) antibodies.
2. **Edrophonium (Tensilon) test: *rapid response to short-acting IV Edrophonium*** in limb MG.
3. CT scan or MRI of the chest may show thymoma or thymus gland abnormality.
4. Ice pack test: place ice on eyelid for 10 minutes ⇨ improvement of ptosis in ocular MG.

MANAGEMENT

1. ACETYLCHOLINESTERASE INHIBITORS:
   Pyridostigmine* or *Neostigmine* 1ˢᵗ *line management.
   Short acting Edrophonium only used for diagnostic purposes.
   MOA: *increases acetylcholine* (by decreasing acetylcholine breakdown). Normally acetylcholinesterase breaks down acetylcholine in the synapse.
   S/E: abdominal cramps/diarrhea, ***cholinergic crisis.***
   cholinergic crisis: *excess acetylcholine* due to Ach-esterase inhibition ⇨ *weakness, nausea, vomiting, pallor, sweating, salivation, diarrhea, miosis, bradycardia, respiratory failure.* In myasthenia gravis, it can be difficult to determine if the weakness & respiratory failure is from *myasthenic crisis (severe manifestation of myasthenia gravis)* or cholinergic crisis (result of too much acetylcholine from acetylcholinesterase inhibitors). ***If flaccid paralysis improves with Tensilon ⇨ myasthenic crisis. If flaccid paralysis worsens with Tensilon ⇨ cholinergic crisis.***

2. IMMUNOSUPPRESSION: *Plasmapheresis or IVIG used in myasthenic crisis for rapid response.*
   Chronic: Corticosteroids. Azathioprine or Cyclosporine are steroid alternatives.

3. **Thymectomy** if thymoma. ± helpful if not due to thymoma (thymus is the source of antibody).
4. *Avoid fluoroquinolones & aminoglycosides (may exacerbate myasthenia).*

Ddx: MYASTHENIC SYNDROME (LAMBERT-EATON): MC associated with small cell lung cancer.
Antibodies against presynaptic voltage-gated calcium channels prevents acetylcholine release.
Unlike Myasthenia Gravis, ***weakness improves with repeated use in Lambert-Eaton.***

MULTIPLE SCLEROSIS

- *Autoimmune, inflammatory demyelinating disease* of the CNS of idiopathic origin. Associated with axon degeneration of *white matter* of the brain, optic nerve & spinal cord.
- MC in *women & young adults 20-40y.* Associated with CNS IgG production & T-cell reaction.

❶ *Relapsing-remitting disease MC:** episodic exacerbations.
❷ Progressive disease: progressive decline without acute exacerbations.
❸ Secondary progressive: relapsing-remitting pattern that becomes progressive.

CLINICAL MANIFESTATIONS
1. **Sensory deficits**:
   - *Pain, fatigue (75%), numbness, paresthesias in the limbs,* muscle cramping.
   - *Trigeminal Neuralgia (suspect MS in young patients with trigeminal neuralgia).*

   - **Uhthoff's phenomenon:** *worsening of symptoms with heat (ex. exercise, fever, hot tubs).*

   - **Lhermitte's sign:** *neck flexion causes lightning-shock type pain radiating from the spine down the leg.*

2. *Optic neuritis* (retrobulbar):* *unilateral eye pain worse with eye movements, diplopia, central scotomas, vision loss (especially color).*

   - **Marcus-Gunn pupil:** during swinging-flashlight test *from the unaffected eye into the affected eye, the pupils appear to dilate* (due to less than normal pupillary constriction). This response is due to the brain perceiving the delayed conduction of affected optic nerve as if light was reduced.

3. **Motor:** *upper motor neuron* involvement *= spasticity & positive (upwards) Babinski.**
4. Spinal cord symptoms: bladder, bowel or sexual dysfunction.
5. CHARCOT'S NEUROLOGIC TRIAD: ❶nystagmus ❷staccato speech & ❸ intentional tremor.

DIAGNOSIS
MS is mainly a clinical diagnosis – at least 2 discrete episodes of exacerbations.
1. **MRI with gadolinium:** *MRI test of choice in helping to confirm MS.**
   WHITE MATTER PLAQUES (hyperdensities) with high intensity is hallmark finding. There should be proof at least 2 areas of white matter involvement before the diagnosis is made.

2. **Lumbar Puncture:** *↑IgG (oligoclonal bands) in CSF:** small discrete bands in the gamma globulin region seen on electrophoresis, which reflects inflammatory cells penetrating the blood brain barrier.

MANAGEMENT
1. **ACUTE EXACERBATIONS**
   - *IV Corticosteroids* (high-dose)*1ˢᵗ line.* Immunomodulators: ex. Cyclophosphamide.
   - *Plasmapheresis if not responsive to Corticosteroids.*

2. **RELAPSE-REMITTING/PROGRESSIVE DISEASE**
   - *β-interferon* or *Glatiramer acetate* (Copaxone) decrease #/severity of relapses.

*Amantadine is helpful for the fatigue in MS.** Baclofen & Diazepam for spasticity.

BELL PALSY

Idiopathic, unilateral CN VII (7)/facial nerve palsy ⇨ hemifacial weakness/paralysis* due to inflammation or compression.   Lower motor neuron lesion.
***Strong association with Herpes simplex virus reactivation.**   MC on the right side (60%).

RISK FACTORS
- Diabetes mellitus, pregnancy (esp 3rd trimester), *post URI,* dental nerve block.

CLINICAL MANIFESTATIONS
1. <u>Sudden</u> onset of *ipsilateral hyperacusis (ear pain)* 24-48 hours ⇨ ***UNILATERAL facial paralysis:** <u>unable to lift affected eyebrow,</u>** wrinkle forehead, smile on affected side, loss of the nasolabial fold, drooping of the corner of mouth, *taste disturbance (anterior ²/₃),* biting inner cheek, eye irritation (due to decreased lacrimation & inability to fully close eyelid).   Bell phenomenon: eye on the affected side moves laterally & superiorly when eye closure is attempted. ***Weakness/paralysis ONLY affects the face*** (not extremities).

DIFFERENTIAL DIAGNOSIS: upper motor lesions (ex. CVA).
- ***If upper face is OK (able to wrinkle both sides of the forehead) it is NOT Bell palsy.****

DIAGNOSIS: Diagnosis of exclusion.   Incomplete palsies have a better prognosis.

MANAGEMENT: No treatment is required (most cases resolve within 1 month).
1. *Prednisone (especially if started within 1st 72h of sx onset).** Decreases nerve inflammation.
2. *Artificial tears* (replaces lacrimation, reduces vision problems). ± Eye patch to sleep if severe.
3. ± Acyclovir in severe cases have been shown to improve symptoms/timing of recovery.

PROGNOSIS
- Function often begins to return within 2 weeks with significant improvements within 4 months with or without treatment.
- Restoration of taste usually precedes motor recovery.

HEADACHES

- **PRIMARY** (90%): *migraine, tension, cluster or rebound.*
    - Primary = idiopathic in nature.   Tension & migraine MC in women.
- **SECONDARY** (4%): meningitis, subarachnoid hemorrhage, intracranial hypertension, hypertensive crisis, acute glaucoma. Suspect 2ry if abrupt or progression of severity.

TENSION HEADACHE

- MC overall type of headache. Mean age of onset ~30y. Thought to be due to mental stress.

CLINICAL MANIFESTATIONS
1. *Bilateral,* tight, band-like, vise-like** constant daily headache. Worsened with stress, fatigue, noise or glare (not worsened with activity like with migraines).   Usually not pulsatile.
2. ***No nausea, vomiting or focal neurologic symptoms**** (ex. no photophobia nor phonophobia).

MANAGEMENT
- Treated like migraines – 1st line: NSAIDs, aspirin, acetaminophen.   Anti-migraine medications.
- TCAs (ex. Amitriptyline) in severe or recurrent cases, prophylaxis. Beta-blockers. Psychotherapy.

MIGRAINE HEADACHE

- MC in women. *2 types: __migraine without aura (common)__* & rarer *__migraine c aura (classic).__* MC cause of morning headache. Family history (80%).
- Thought to be caused by vasodilation of the blood vessels innervated by the trigeminal nerve. Neurological findings thought to be due to internal carotid artery constriction.

CLINICAL MANIFESTATIONS
1. *__LATERALIZED, pulsatile/throbbing headache__ associated with nausea/vomiting, photophobia & phonophobia* usually 4-72 hours in duration. May be bilateral.
   - *Worse with physical activity*, stress, lack/excessive sleep, ETOH, specific foods (ex. chocolate, red wine), OCPs/menstruation.

2. *__Auras: visual changes MC__** ex. light flashes (photopsia), zig zag lines of light (teichopsia), scotomas (blind spots that may scintillate), aphasia (impairment of language), weakness, numbness. Auras usually last <60 minutes (5-20 minutes common) ⇨ headache onset.

MANAGEMENT:
1. SYMPTOMATIC (ABORTIVE):
   - *__Triptans or Ergotamines__. MOA: serotonin 5HT-1 agonists* ⇨ vasoconstriction.
     S/E: *chest tightness from constriction*, nausea, vomiting, abdominal cramps
     CI: *coronary artery or peripheral vascular disease, uncontrolled HTN (due to vasoconstriction)*; hepatic or renal disease. Pregnancy.

   - *__Dopamine blockers:__ IV Phenothiazines: __Metoclopramide__, Promethazine, Prochlorperazine.*
     Ind: antiemetics for nausea & vomiting. *Given with Diphenhydramine* (Benadryl) *to prevent EPS, dystonic reactions* & parkinsonism symptoms due to decreased dopamine.

   - IV fluids & placing the patient in a dark, quiet room helps most suffering an acute attack.
   - Mild symptoms: *NSAIDs/acetaminophen 1st line.* Codeine or barbiturates may be used. Some migraine medications have caffeine added to it to improve symptoms.

2. PROPHYLACTIC:
   - *Anti-HTN meds: (ß-blockers, calcium channel blockers)*; tricyclic antidepressants (TCAs), *anticonvulsants* (Valproate, Topiramate), NSAIDs.

TRIGEMINAL NEURALGIA (TGN) (TIC DOULOUREUX)

PATHOPHYSIOLOGY: compression of the trigeminal nerve root (by superior cerebellar artery or vein) 90%. Idiopathic 10%. MC in mid-aged women.

CLINICAL MANIFESTATIONS
1. *__Brief, episodic, stabbing/lancinating pain__** in the 2nd/3rd division of Trigeminal nerve (CN V) lasting seconds-minutes *__worse with touch, eating, drafts of wind__* & movements (often __unilateral__).* Pain starts near mouth & shoots to the eye, ear & nostril on the ipsilateral side.

MANAGEMENT
1. *__Carbamazepine__ (Tegretol) 1st line.** Oxcarbazepine.
   MOA: unknown in TGN. S/E: drowsiness, nausea, vomiting, leukopenia.
2. *Gabapentin* (Neurontin), Baclofen. *Suspect Multiple Sclerosis in younger patients with TGN.*
3. Surgical decompression may be used in severe or recalcitrant cases.

CLUSTER HEADACHE

- Predominantly *young & middle-aged* **males.**

CLINICAL MANIFESTATIONS
- **Severe UNILATERAL periorbital/temporal pain (sharp, lancinating).* Bouts lasting <2 hours with** spontaneous remission. Bouts occur several times a day over 6-8 weeks (clusters). **Triggers: worse at night,* ETOH, stress or ingestion of specific foods.**

PHYSICAL EXAM
   IPSILATERAL **Horner's syndrome*** *(ptosis, miosis, anhydrosis),* **nasal congestion/rhinorrhea, conjunctivitis & lacrimation.**

MANAGEMENT
   1. **100% Oxygen 1st line*** (6-10L).
   2. **Anti-migraine meds** help during attack: **SQ Sumatriptan** or Ergotamines (vasoconstriction).

PROPHYLAXIS
   - **Verapamil (1st line),*** Corticosteroids, Ergotamines, Valproic acid, Lithium, Cyproheptadine.

IDIOPATHIC INTRACRANIAL HTN (PSEUDOTUMOR CEREBRI)

- **Idiopathic increased intracranial (CSF) pressure** & no other cause of intracranial HTN evident on CT or MRI imaging.
- MC in obese women of childbearing age. Meds: *corticosteroid withdrawal*, growth hormone, thyroid replacement, OCPs. Systemic diseases may also be causative in susceptible patients.

CLINICAL MANIFESTATIONS
   1. Signs/symptoms of ↑intracranial pressure: **headache (worse with straining)**, retrobulbar pain, nausea, vomiting, tinnitus, **visual changes** *(may lead to blindness if not treated)*.

DIAGNOSIS
   1. Ocular exam:
      - Funduscopic exam: **papilledema.*** May have visual field loss.
      - ±CN 6 (abducens) palsy = lateral rectus muscle weakness ⇨ limitation of abduction (induces esotropia/turning inward towards the nose) especially looking in the distance.

   2. **CT scan: 1st to rule out CNS mass** ⇨ lumbar puncture: **increased CSF pressure* (otherwise normal CSF).** MRI is an alternative to exclude 2ry causes of ↑CSF pressure.

MANAGEMENT:
   1. **Acetazolamide** (reduces CSF pressure/production) ± Furosemide. ±short-course of steroids.
   2. Optic nerve sheath fenestration or CSF shunting allows evacuation of CSF, improving vision.

CLASSIC CSF FINDINGS

1. MULTIPLE SCLEROSIS	High IgG (oligoclonal bands)
2. GUILLAIN BARRÉ SYNDROME	High protein with normal WBC/cell count
3. BACTERIAL MENINGITIS	High protein with increased WBC (primarily polymorphonuclear neutrophils), decreased glucose
4. VIRAL (ASEPTIC) MENINGITIS	Normal glucose, increased WBCs (lymphocytes)
5. FUNGAL or TB MENGITIS	Decreased glucose, increased WBCs (lymphocytes)
6. IDIOPATHIC INTRACRANIAL HTN	Increased CSF pressure otherwise normal
7. SUBARACHNOID HEMORRHAGE	Xanthocromia, blood in the CSF

NORMAL PRESSURE HYDROCEPHALUS

- Dilation of the cerebral ventricles with normal opening pressures on lumbar puncture.
- Unknown but thought to be due to impaired CSF absorption after a CNS injury (ex. subarachnoid hemorrhage, tumors, CNS infection, inflammatory disease, head injury etc.).

CLINICAL MANIFESTATIONS
Classic triad: ❶ *dementia* ❷ *gait disturbance* & ❸ *urinary incontinence.*
1. **Gait disturbances:** *wide-based, shuffling gait* – described as gait apraxia or *"magnetic"* gait (as if the feet are stuck to the floor). May be associated with postural instability.
2. **Dementia:** includes impaired executive function, psychomotor depression, apathy.
3. **Urinary incontinence.** May present as urinary urgency early in the disease.
4. Other: weakness, lethargy, malaise, rigidity, hyperreflexia & spasticity.

DIAGNOSIS
1. **MRI** or CT scan: *enlarged ventricles* in the absence of or out of proportion to sulcal dilation. MRI is superior to CT scan.

2. **Lumbar puncture:** CSF pressure is usually normal.
   Lumbar tap test = removal of up to 50cc of CSF leads to improvement of symptoms 30-60 minutes after the procedure.

MANAGEMENT
1. ***Ventriculoperitoneal shunt tx of choice.*** Gait abnormalities usually the most improved.

CONCUSSION SYNDROME

- ***Mild traumatic brain injury*** ⇨ ***alteration in mental status*** with or without loss of consciousness.

CLINICAL MANIFESTATIONS
1. ***Confusion:*** confused or blank expression, blunted affect.

2. ***Amnesia:*** pretraumatic (retrograde) or posttraumatic (antegrade) amnesia.
   The duration of retrograde amnesia is usually brief.
3. Headache, dizziness, visual disturbances: blurred or double vision.
4. Delayed responses & emotional changes: emotional instability.
5. Signs of ↑intracranial pressure: persistent vomiting, worsening headache, increasing disorientation, changing levels of consciousness.

DIAGNOSIS
1. ***CT scan: study of choice for evaluating acute head injuries.****
2. **MRI:** study of choice if prolonged symptoms >7-14 days or with worsening of symptoms not explained by concussion syndrome.
3. PET scan may be done to look at glucose uptake (not done often).

MANAGEMENT
1. ***Cognitive & physical rest is the main management of patients with concussion.****
   Patients may resume strenuous activity after resolution of symptoms & recovery of memory & cognitive functions.

DELIRIUM

- **_Acute, abrupt TRANSIENT confused state_** due to an **_identifiable cause (ex medications, infections etc.)._** Rapid onset associated with fluctuating mental status changes & marked deficit in short-term memory. Usually associated with full recovery within 1 week in most cases.

DEMENTIA

- **_Progressive, chronic intellectual deterioration_** of selective functions: **_MEMORY LOSS_** AND loss of impulse control, motor & cognitive functions. Includes language dysfunction, disorientation, inability to perform complex motor activities & inappropriate social interaction. NOT due to delirium, medications or psychiatric illness. Risk factors: age (especially >60y) & vascular disease.
- Includes: Alzheimer's disease, Vascular, Frontotemporal, Diffuse Lewy Body, Creutzfeldt-Jakob.

ALZHEIMER DISEASE

- **_MC type of dementia.*_** Loss of brain cells, **_amyloid deposition (senile plaques)_** in the brain, **_neurofibrillary tangles (tau protein)_**.
- **_Cholinergic deficiency_** ⇨ memory, language, visuospatial changes. Normal reflexes.

CLINICAL MANIFESTATIONS: short-term memory loss (1st symptom). Progresses to long-term memory loss, disorientation, behavioral & personality changes. Usually gradual in nature.

DIAGNOSIS
1. **CT scan:** **_cerebral cortex atrophy on CT scan_**. May be used to rule out other causes as well.

MANAGEMENT
1. **_Ach-esterase inhibitors: Donepezil_** (Aricept), **_Tacrine, Rivastigmine, Galantamine_**.
   MOA: reverses cholinergic deficiency & symptom relief (does not slow down disease progression).

2. **NMDA antagonist:** **_Memantine_** **MOA:** _Blocks NMDA_ receptor, slowing calcium influx & nerve damage. Glutamate is an excitatory neurotransmitter of the NDMA receptor. Excitotoxicity causes cell death. **_NMDA antagonists reduce glutamate excitotoxicity_**. May be adjunctive.

VASCULAR DEMENTIA

- **_2nd MC type._** Brain disease due to chronic ischemia & multiple infarctions **_(ex. lacunar infarcts).*_**
- **_Hypertension_** most important risk factor. HTN control may slow disease progression.

CLINICAL MANIFESTATIONS
1. Cortical: forgetfulness, confusion, amnesia, executive difficulties, speech abnormalities.
2. Subcortical: motor deficits, gait abnormalities, urinary difficulties, personality changes.

FRONTOTEMPORAL DEMENTIA (PICK'S DISEASE)

- Rare type. **_Localized brain degeneration of the frontotemporal lobes.*_** May progress globally.
- **_Marked personality changes*_** (**_preserved visuospatial_**), aphasia. Behavioral symptoms: apathy, disinhibition. ⊕Palmomental & palmar grasp reflexes. Usually no amnesia present. ⊕Pick bodies.

DIFFUSE LEWY BODY DISEASE

- Lewy bodies: abnormal neuronal protein deposits. Diffuse in comparison to (Parkinson disease - localized).
- **_Visual hallucinations,* delusions_**, episodic delirium, Parkinsonism. Dementia occurs later in the disease.

	UPPER MOTOR NEURON (UMN) LESIONS	LOWER MOTOR NEURON (LMN) LESIONS
ANATOMY	• UMN connects cortex to the LMN (in spinal cord) • Neurotransmitter glutamate transmits nerve impulses from upper motor to lower motor neurons (via glutamate receptors on the receiving lower motor neuron).	• LMN are located in the spinal cord & links the UMN to the muscles. • LMN stimulated by glutamate release from UMN causing depolarization of LMN. The LMN terminates at the effector (muscle) at the neuromuscular joint. *Acetylcholine release by the LMN stimulates muscle contraction at the neuromuscular joint.*
ETIOLOGIES	• Stroke (CVA) • Multiple sclerosis • Cerebral palsy • Brain or spinal cord damage (ex traumatic brain injury)	• Guillain-Barré Syndrome • Botulism • Poliomyelitis • Cauda Equina Syndrome • Bell palsy
PARALYSIS	• *SPASTIC PARALYSIS* *(hypertonia)* with ↑*DTR** (due to removal of inhibitory influence of the cortex). • Weakness	• *FLACCID PARALYSIS* *(loss of muscle tone/hypotonia),* ↓*DTR.** • Weakness
FASCICULATIONS	• No fasciculations	• *FASCICULATIONS** (end stage muscle denervation).
BABINSKI	• *UPWARD* *BABINSKI REFLEX* (extension of the great toe & fanning outward of the other toes). This response is only considered normal in an infant & up to 2y old. Considered abnormal in adult or >2y.	• *DOWNWARD BABINSKI REFLEX.**
MUSCLE ATROPHY	• Little or no muscle atrophy	• *MUSCLE ATROPHY.** (neurogenic degeneration)

GLASGOW COMA SCALE (GCS)

	SCORE
Eye opening	
Spontaneous	4
Response to verbal commands	3
Response to pain	2
No eye opening	1
Best Verbal Response	
Oriented	5
Confused	4
Inappropriate words	3
No verbal response	1
Best Motor Response	
Obeys commands	6
Localizing response to pain	5
Withdrawal response to pain	4
Flexion to pain	3
Extension to pain	2
No motor response	1

Score between 3 and 15.

Mild brain injury ≥13   9-12 moderate   ≤8 severe brain injury.

ASTROCYTOMA

- Derived from astrocytes (astrocytes are star-shaped glial cells of the brain & spinal cord that support the endothelial cells of the blood-brain barrier, provide nutrients for cells, maintain extracellular ion balance and also repair the brain after injury).
- Can appear in any part of the brain. *Most often infratentorial in children (supratentorial in adults).*

TYPES OF ASTROCYTOMAS

- **PILOCYTIC ASTROCYTOMA (GRADE I):** (Juvenile Astrocytoma) - typically localized. Considered the ***"most benign"*** (noncancerous) of all the astrocytomas. ***MC in children & young adults.*** Other grade I astrocytomas include cerebellar astrocytoma & desmoplastic infantile.

- **DIFFUSE ASTROCYTOMA** (**Grade II** or **Low-grade**) Types: Fibrillary, Gemistocytic & Protoplasmic. They tend to invade surrounding tissues but grow at a relatively slow pace.

- **ANAPLASTIC ASTROCYTOMA: (Grade III).** Rare but aggressive.

- **GRADE IV ASTROCYTOMA:** *(GLIOBLASTOMA "Multiforme").* ***MC primary CNS tumors in adults.****

- Subependymal Giant Cell Astrocytoma - ventricular tumors associated with tuberculous sclerosis.

CLINICAL MANIFESTATIONS

1. Focal deficits: MC. Depends on the location of the lesion. MC in frontal & temporal areas of the cerebral hemisphere.
   - General sx: headaches (may be worse in the morning, ***may wake patients up at night***, may be positional), cranial nerve deficits, altered mental status changes, neurological deficits, ataxia, vision changes, weakness.
2. Increased intracranial pressure: *due to mass effect* ⇨ *headache, nausea, vomiting, papilledema, ataxia,* drowsiness, stupor.

DIAGNOSIS

1. CT scan or MRI with contrast: Grade I & II non-enhancing. Grade III & IV are enhancing.
2. Brain biopsy: usually guided by imaging studies. Histologic appearance includes:
   - **Pilocytic Astrocytomas (Grade I)** generally form sacs of fluid (***cystic***), or may be enclosed within a cyst. Although they are usually slow-growing, these tumors can become very large. ***Rosenthal fibers*** (eosinophilic corkscrew fibers).

   - **Diffuse Astrocytomas** tend to contain microcysts and mucus-like fluid. They are grouped by the appearance and behavior of the cells for which they are named.

   - **Anaplastic Astrocytomas** tend to have tentacle-like projections that grow into surrounding tissue, making them difficult to completely remove during surgery.

   - ***Astrocytoma Grade IV (glioblastoma)*** may contain cystic material, calcium deposits, blood vessels, and/or a mixed grade of cells.

MANAGEMENT

1. Pilocytic Astrocytoma: Surgical excision. In adults and older children, radiation may follow surgery if the tumor cannot be completely removed.
2. Diffuse Astrocytoma: Surgery if the tumor is accessible & can be completely removed. Radiation may be adjunctive to surgery or for unresectable tumors.
3. Anaplastic Astrocytoma: Surgery ⇨ XRT. ± Chemotherapy after radiation or for tumor recurrence.
4. Astrocytoma Grade IV: Surgery ⇨ XRT (radiation therapy) + Chemotherapy.

GLIOBLASTOMA (GLIOBLASTOMA MUTLIFORME)

- ***MC & MOST AGGRESSIVE OF ALL THE PRIMARY CNS TUMOR IN ADULTS.**** (>50%).
- ***Glioblastoma = Grade IV Astrocytoma:*** heterogenous mixture of poorly differentiated astrocytes.

<u>PRIMARY</u>: *MC* (60%). ***Seen in adults >50y.*** Arises de novo (new). MC type & most aggressive.

<u>SECONDARY</u>: (40%). *MC* <45y. Due to malignant progression from a low-grade astrocytoma (grade II) or anaplastic astrocytoma (grade III). May transform as early as 1 year or >10y.

RISK FACTORS
1. Males, >50y, HHV-6 & cytomegalovirus infections, ionizing radiation.

TYPES
- "Classic": 97%. Presence of extra copies of the epidermal growth factor receptor gene (EGFR). TP53 rarely mutated in this type (note that the others are associated with TP53 mutation).
- Mesenchymal: high rates of mutations & alterations including the gene encoding for neurofibromatosis type I. TP53 often mutated. An alteration of MGMT (a DNA repair enzyme)

CLINICAL MANIFESTATIONS
1. <u>Focal deficits</u>: MC. Depends on the location of the tumor. MC in frontal & temporal areas of the cerebral hemisphere.
   - <u>General</u>: headaches (may be worse in the morning, may wake patients up at night, may be positional), cranial nerve deficits (ex fixed, dilated pupil from a CN III palsy), altered mental status, neurological deficits, ataxia, vision changes, weakness.
   - <u>Frontal Lobe</u>: dementia, personality changes, gait abnormalities, expressive aphasia, seizures.
   - <u>Temporal Lobe</u>: partial complex & generalized seizures.
   - <u>Parietal Lobe</u>: receptive aphasia, contralateral sensory loss, hemianopia, spatial disorientation.
   - <u>Occipital Lobe</u>: contralateral homonymous hemianopia.
   - <u>Thalamus</u>: contralateral sensory loss.
   - <u>Brainstem</u>: papillary changes, nystagmus, hemiparesis.

2. <u>Increased intracranial pressure</u>: *due to mass effect* ⇨ <u>*headache, nausea, vomiting, papilledema, ataxia,*</u> drowsiness, stupor.
   Cushing's reflex: in severe cases: triad ❶***irregular respirations*** ❷ ***hypertension*** & ❸***bradycardia.***

DIAGNOSIS
1. <u>CT scan or MRI with contrast</u>: tumor has a variety of appearances on imaging (depending on the amount of hemorrhage, necrosis or its age). MC seen in the subcortical white matter of the cerebral hemispheres.
   - nonhomogenous mass with a hypodense center and a ***<u>variable ring of enhancement surrounded by edema.</u>**** Mass effect may cause hydrocephalus.
   - May ***cross the corpus callosum (butterfly glioma).***

2. <u>Brain biopsy</u>: usually guided by imaging studies.
   - **Histologic appearance:** presence of small areas of ***<u>necrotizing tissue</u>***(from myelin breakdown) surrounded by anaplastic cells + hyperplastic blood vessels with areas of ***<u>hemorrhage</u>***. Cells may have stem-cell like properties. ***Pseudopalisading:*** tumor cells lining the area of necrosis.

MANAGEMENT
1. Surgical excision, radiotherapy & adjuvant chemotherapy with Temozolomide (alkylating agent). Poor prognosis (often <1 year survival).

MENINGIOMAS

- **Meningiomas:** *usually benign tumors* arising from meningiothelial arachnoid cells of the meninges (covering the brain & spinal cord). Normally, these cells provide a barrier function of the CNS system as part of the meninges, help to clear waste products from the CSF and helps to maintain optic nerve microenvironment). 2nd MC primary CNS neoplasm (after Glioblastoma).
- MC in women (estrogen receptors on tumor cells). *Associated with neurofibromatosis (esp NF-2).*
- *MC arise from dura or sites of dural reflection* (ex. venous sinuses, falx cerebri).

CLINICAL MANIFESTATIONS
1. Most are asymptomatic. Often found incidentally on imaging for other reasons.
2. Focal deficits: includes seizures, progressive spasticity, weakness or other motor/sensory symptoms. Symptoms due to increased intracranial pressure not as common.

DIAGNOSIS
1. CT scan or MRI with contrast: *intensely enhancing, well-defined lesion OFTEN ATTACHED TO THE DURA.** MC sites: parasagittal region, convexities of the hemispheres, sphenoid, & olfactory groove. Calcification of the tumor & increased calcification may be seen on CT scan.

2. Brain biopsy: usually guided by imaging studies.
   - Histologic appearance: *spindle-cells* concentrically arranged in a *whorled pattern.*
     PSAMMOMA BODIES: concentric round calcifications.

MANAGEMENT
1. Asymptomatic: observation if small/asymptomatic.
2. Symptomatic: surgical removal (transarterial embolization may be performed prior to surgery). Radiation therapy may be used if not a surgical candidate or as adjuvant treatment.

CNS LYMPHOMA

- **PRIMARY:** seen without evidence of systemic disease. *Variant of extranodal NHL.* 2ry more common.
- **SECONDARY:** METS from another site (ex NHL in the neck, chest, groin, abdomen) *especially diffuse large B cell lymphoma (90%),** *Burkitt's lymphoma* (10%).

RISK FACTORS
- Immunosuppression (ex. AIDS, post transplant, receiving immunosuppresant treatment).
  Epstein-Barr virus ⊕ in 90% of these patients.

CLINICAL MANIFESTATIONS
1. Focal deficits: MC. Depends on the location of the lesion.
2. Ocular symptoms: visual changes, steroid-refractory posterior uveitis.

DIAGNOSIS
1. CT scan or MRI with contrast: hypointense *RING-ENHANCING LESION** in deep white matter on CT.
2. Biopsy: usually guided by imaging study.
3. Workup includes CT of abdomen/pelvis, PET scan, bone marrow biopsy, slit lamp examination.

MANAGEMENT
1. **Chemotherapy:** *Methotrexate most effective chemotherapy** (given with folinic acid/leucovorin). Chemotherapy not usually given at the same time as radiation therapy (due to increased risk of leukoencephalopathy).
2. **Radiation therapy, Corticosteroids:** partial response.
3. Surgical resection usually ineffective.

OLIGODENDROGLIOMA

- <u>Oligodendrocyte</u> – a type of cell that makes up the supportive (glial) tissue of the brain. These tumors can be found anywhere within the cerebral hemispheres (especially the frontal & temporal lobes).

CLINICAL MANIFESTATIONS
1. May be asymptomatic. May be incidental finding (tumor grows slowly).
2. <u>Focal deficits:</u> includes seizures, headaches & personality changes depends on the tumor location.

DIAGNOSIS
1. CT scan or MRI with contrast.
2. <u>Brain biopsy:</u> usually guided by imaging studies.
   <u>Histologic appearance:</u> soft, grayish-pink *calcified* tumors, areas of hemorrhage &/or cystic. *Chicken-wire capillary pattern* with *"fried-egg shaped"* tumor cells seen with microsope.

MANAGEMENT: surgical resection standard tx. ± Radiation and/or chemotherapy (ex. anaplastic).

EPENDYMOMA

- <u>Ependymal cells</u> line the ventricles & parts of the spinal column. ***MC in children.***
- ***MC seen in 4th ventricle*** (±cause hydrocephalus). ±medulla, ***spinal cord.**** Cauda equina in adults.

CLINICAL MANIFESTATIONS
1. <u>Infants:</u> increased in head size, irritability, sleeplessness & vomiting.
2. <u>Older children/adults:</u> nausea, vomiting, headache.

DIAGNOSIS
1. <u>CT scan or MRI with contrast:</u> hypointense T1, hyperintense T2. Enhances with gadolinium.
2. <u>Brain biopsy:</u> ***perivascular pseudorosettes*** (tumor cells surrounding a blood vessel).

MANAGEMENT: surgical resection ⇨ adjuvant radiation therapy. Chemotx not as helpful usually.

HEMANGIOMAS

- ***Hemangioma:*** abnormal buildup of blood vessels in the skin or internal organs. 2% of all 1ry brain tumors. 10% have von Hippel-Lindau syndrome (hemangiomas, tumors of the liver, pancreas & kidney).
- **Hemangioblastoma**: arises from the blood vessel lining. Benign, slow growing well-defined tumors. MC found in the posterior fossa (***brainstem & cerebellum***). Often >40y. May occur in the cerebral hemispheres or spinal cord. ***Retinal hemangiomas associated with von Hippel-Lindau syndrome.***

- <u>Hemangiopericytoma:</u> originate from the cells surrounding the blood vessels & the meninges. May spread to the lung & liver.

CLINICAL MANIFESTATIONS
1. <u>Hemangioblastoma:</u> headache, nausea, vomiting, gait abnormalities, poor coordination of the limbs. May produce erythropoietin (secondary polycythemia).
2. <u>Hemaniopericytoma:</u> depends on the tumor location.

DIAGNOSIS: CT scan or MRI.
   Biopsy: well-defined borders, usually does not invade surrounding healthy tissue.
   Foam cells with high vascularity.

MANAGEMENT: Surgical resection. Radiation may be used in tumors attached to the brainstem.

ATLAS C1 BURST (JEFFERSON) FRACTURE

- **Bilateral fractures of the anterior & posterior arches of C1** (disruption of the transverse ligament may lead to instability if it occurs with the fracture). ± C1/C2 dislocation.

<u>MOI:</u> vertical compression force through the occipital condyles to the lateral masses of the atlas.

<u>DIAGNOSIS:</u> <u>Lateral radiographs:</u> *increase in the predental space between C1 & the odontoid (dens).* >3mm in adults & >5mm in children.
<u>Open-mouth (odontoid) view:</u> may also show step-off of the lateral masses of the atlas.

MANAGEMENT
1. <u>Nonoperative:</u> hard cervical orthosis vs. halo immobilization for 6-12 weeks.
2. <u>Operative:</u> posterior C1-C2 fusion vs. occipitocervical fusion if unstable (controversial).

HANGMAN'S (C2/AXIS PEDICLE) FRACTURE

- **Traumatic bilateral fractures (spondylolysis) of the pedicles or pars interarticularis of the AXIS vertebra (C2).** May lead to **spondylolisthesis between C2 & C3.**
- **Unstable fracture.** 30% are associated with cervical spinal fractures. Usually no cord injury.

MECHANISM OF INJURY
Extreme hyperextension injuries of the skull, atlas & axis (especially in an already extended neck) & secondary flexion with subsequent subluxation (due to tearing of the posterior longitudinal ligament).

CLINICAL MANIFESTATIONS
1. Neck pain. Neurologic exam is usually intact because the cervical canal is widest at C2 area.

DIAGNOSIS
1. <u>Cervical X rays:</u> subluxation.
2. <u>CT scan:</u> **study of choice.** MRI if vertebral artery injury is suspected.

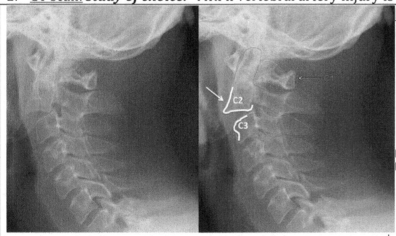

Hangman Fracture
Note slipping of C2 forward compared to C3 (white arrow).

Hangman Fracture
By Lucien Monfils (Own work) [GFDL (http://www.gnu.org/copyleft/fdl.html) or CC BY-SA 3.0 (http://creativecommons.org/licenses/by-sa/3.0)], via Wikimedia Commons

MANAGEMENT
1. <u>Nonoperative:</u> Type I (<3mm horizontal displacement) rigid cervical collar 4-6 weeks. Type II (3-5 mm displacement) closed reduction followed by halo immobilization 8-12 weeks.
2. <u>Operative:</u> Type II (>5mm displacement with severe angulation), Type III facet dislocations.

ODONTOID FRACTURES

Fracture of the dens (odontoid process) of the axis (C2). **MOI:** head placed in forced flexion or extension in an anterior-posterior orientation (ex. forward fall onto the forehead).

TYPES
- Type I: oblique fracture at the tip of odontoid.
- **Type II:** fracture at the base of the odontoid process (dens) where it attaches to C2. *Most common type. Unstable.* High association with nonunion.
- Type III: extends into C2.

DIAGNOSIS: best seen on AP odontoid (open mouth) view.

MANAGEMENT
1. Os odontoideum (aplasia or hypoplasia of the odontoid) ⇨ observation. Type I ⇨ cervical orthosis.
2. Type II in young ⇨ halo immobilization. Surgery if risk factors for nonunion.
   II in elderly ⇨ surgery preferred. Cervical orthosis if not surgical candidates.
3. Type III ⇨ cervical orthosis.

ATLAS FRACTURE & TRANSVERSE LIGAMENTAL INSTABILITY

MECHANISM OF INJURY
Hyperextension & compression injuries.
Low risk of neurologic complications. May be associated with axis fracture.

ATLANTO-OCCIPITAL DISLOCATION

- Extreme flexion injury involving the atlas (C1) & axis (C2). ± associated with odontoid fractures.

ATLANTO-AXIAL JOINT INSTABILITY

- Instability between the atlas (C1) and axis (C2).

MECHANISM OF INJURY
- Traumatic: due to extreme flexion-rotation injuries.
- Non traumatic: degenerative changes: ex Down syndrome, Rheumatoid arthritis, Os odontoideum.

CLINICAL MANIFESTATIONS
Neck pain, neurologic symptoms/deficits. Myelopathic symptoms: muscle weakness, hyperreflexia, wide gait, bladder dysfunction.
RADIOGRAPHS: open-mouth (odontoid) view: may see increase in the atlanto-dens interval.

MANAGEMENT: depends on the cause.

CLAY-SHOVELER'S FRACTURE

- *Spinous process avulsion fracture MC @ the lower cervical (C6 or C7)* or upper thoracic vertebrae.

Mechanism: forced neck flexion with the muscle pulling off a piece of the spinous process, especially after sudden deceleration injuries (ex. MVA). Usually a stable injury (no deficits usually).

MANAGEMENT
1. **Nonoperative:** NSAIDs, rest, immobilization in hard collar for comfort.
2. Surgical excision only used if non union or persistent pain.

FLEXION TEARDROP FRACTURES

- *Anterior displacement of a wedge-shaped fracture fragment* (the so-called teardrop shape of the *anterio-inferior portion* of the superior vertebra). Often associated with loss of vertebral height. **MOI** severe flexion & compression causes the vertebral body to collide with an inferior vertebral body.

- Most commonly occurs in the lower cervical spine. Often associated with loss of vertebral height.

- *Highly unstable* (because of disruption of the posterior longitudinal ligament).
  May cause anterior cervical cord syndrome.

MANAGEMENT
Surgery
 (due to its highly unstable nature)

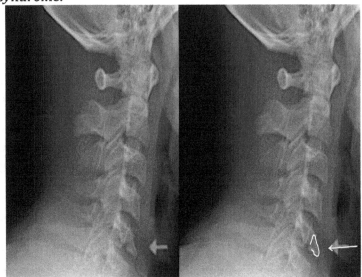

EXTENSION TEARDROP FRACTURES

- Triangular-shaped avulsion fracture of the *antero-inferior* corner of the vertebral body as a result of rupture of the anterior longitudinal ligament. **MOI:** abrupt neck extension.

- *MC seen at C2*. May be seen at C5 – C7 and associated with a *central cord syndrome.* No loss of vertebral height. Unstable.

MANAGEMENT: cervical collar

BURST FRACTURES

- Burst fracture due to nucleus pulposus of the intervertebral disc being forced into the vertebral body, causing it to shatter or 'burst' outwards. Usually as a result of a vertical compression injury.
- **MOI:** axial loading injury causing vertebral compression injuries of the cervical & lumbar spine.

1. Stable: all the ligaments are intact and usually no posterior displacement of the fracture segment.
2. Unstable: >50% compression of the spinal cord, >50% loss of vertebral height, >20 degrees of spinal angulation or associated neurologic deficits. May cause incomplete or complete spinal cord injury (ex. anterior cord syndrome).

- **Radiographs:** comminuted vertebral body and loss of vertebral height (depicted as a vertical fracture on the AP view).

MANAGEMENT
1. Unstable - needs surgical correction.

SUBCLAVIAN STEAL SYNDROME

- Signs & symptoms from reversed (retrograde) blood flow down the ipsilateral vertebral artery to supply the affected arm due to occlusion or stenosis of the subclavian artery. The blood flow to the arm is at the expense of the vertebrobasilar circulation. Left arm MC affected.

ETIOLOGIES: *atherosclerosis (MC)*, Takayasu arteritis, Thoracic outlet syndrome.

CLINICAL MANIFESTATIONS
Most patients are asymptomatic
1. **Symptoms of arm arterial insufficiency:** arm claudication, paresthesias.
    Physical examination: ***blood pressure difference between the arms*** (reduction of blood pressure in the affected arm ***> 15mmHg*** compared to the unaffected arm).

2. **Symptoms of vertebrobasilar insufficiency:** presyncope or syncope, dizziness, neurologic deficits, vertigo, diplopia, nystagmus, weakness, drop attacks, gait abnormalities.

DIAGNOSIS
Continuous wave Doppler, Duplex US, Transcranial Doppler, CT angiography, angiogram.

MANAGEMENT
1. Revascularization or percutaneous transluminal angioplasty in severe cases.

SPINAL CORD SYNDROME - MNEMONICS

ANTERIOR CORD SYNDROME
Because ANT couldn't walk to the bathroom in the TeePee, he peed his pants when his bladder busted into flecks.

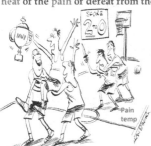

ANT = Anterior Cord Syndrome
- **Couldn't walk:** lower extremity motor deficit

- **TeePee** = loss of <u>T</u>emperature & <u>P</u>ain sensation

- **Peed his pants** = bladder dysfunction, lower extremity involvement

- **Flex** = flexion compression injuries common mechanism

CENTRAL CORD SYNDROME
Because Maleficent developed frostbite when she extended her hand to touch the cold window pane, she couldn't put on her shawl with her weak hands.

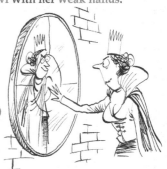

Extension injuries

loss of pain & temperature sensation

upper extremity > lower extremity (especially hands)

Shawl = shawl distribution

BROWN SEQUARD SYNDROME
The MVP on the winning side was oblivious 2(to) the stabbing heat of the pain of defeat from the losing side.

Ipsilateral deficits
- **MVP** = **M**otor, **V**ibratory and **P**roprioception deficits

Contralateral deficits
- pain & temperature deficits occurring usually 2 levels below the level of injury.

Mechanism
Stabbing: penetration injuries

MVP

ANTERIOR CORD SYNDROME
Motor & Sensory deficits in lower extremities

CENTRAL CORD SYNDROME
Motor & Sensory deficits in upper extremities in a "shawl" distribution

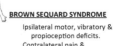

BROWN SEQUARD SYNDROME
Ipsilateral motor, vibratory & propioception deficits.
Contralateral pain & temperature deficits

DEFICITS
MOTOR
SENSORY
VIBRATORY PROPRIOCEPTION

	ANTERIOR CORD	CENTRAL CORD	POSTERIOR CORD	BROWN SÉQUARD
MECHANISM OF INJURY	• MC after blowout vertebral body burst fractures (flexion). • Anterior spinal artery injury or occlusion. • Direct anterior cord compression. • Aortic dissection, SLE, AIDS.	• Hyperextension injuries (ex 50% occur c̄ MVA), falls in elderly, gun shot wounds, tumors, cervical spinal stenosis, syringomyelia. • MC incomplete cord syndrome. • It affects primarily the central gray matter (including the spinothalamic tracts).	• Rare • Damage to posterior cord or posterior spinal stenosis.	• Unilateral hemisection of the spinal cord • MC after *penetrating trauma* (tumors may cause it) • Rare injury.
DEFICITS	**Motor deficit:** • *lower extremity > upper** (corticospinal) **Sensory deficit:** • pain, temperature (spinothalamic tract) • light touch • May develop *bladder dysfunction* (retention, incontinence)	**Motor deficit:** • *upper extremity > lower**. The distal portion of the upper extremity more severe involvement (ex. hands) from corticospinal involvement. **Sensory deficit:** • pain, temperature (spinothalamic tract) deficit greater in the upper extremity > lower extremity. Sometimes described as a *"shawl" distribution.*	• *Loss of proprioception & vibratory sense only**	**Ipsilateral deficits:** - *Motor* (lateral corticospinal tract) - *Vibration & proprioception* (dorsal column) **Contralateral deficits:** - *pain & temperature* (lateral spinothalamic tract) usually 2 levels below the injury (where the spinothalamic tract crosses at the spinal cord level)
PRESERVATION	**Preserved:** • Proprioception, vibration, pressure (dorsal column spared) • Light touch preservation.	**Preserved:** • Proprioception, vibration, pressure (dorsal column spared)	**Preserved:** • Pain & light touch. • No motor deficits	
	Anterior Cord Syndrome	**Central Cord Syndrome**	**Posterior Cord Syndrome**	**BROWN SÉQUARD**

ANTERIOR CIRCULATION ISCHEMIC STROKE LESIONS

NON DOMINANT SIDE LESIONS (usually RIGHT HEMISPHERE) Right side: behavior, learning process, short term memory	DOMINANT SIDE LESIONS (usually LEFT HEMISPHERE) Left side: speech language
• Left hemiparesis • Left sensory loss, L-sided neglect, *anosognosia* • Left homonymous hemianopsia, *apraxia* • Dysarthria, *spatial/time deficits** • *Flat affect, impaired judgment, impulsivity**	• Right hemiparesis • Right sensory loss • Right homonymous hemianopsia • Dysarthria • *Aphasia*, agraphia, decreased math comprehension*

Hemiparesis = weakness **Hemiplegia** = paralysis **Dysarthria** = inability to articulate words. **Apraxia:** loss of ability to execute purposeful movements. **Ataxia** = loss of coordinated movements. **Aphasia** = difficulty remembering words, speaking, writing. **Broca's aphasia:** frontal lobe nonfluency, sparse output *(comprehension relatively preserved).** **Wernicke's aphasia:** fluent aphasia (voluminous, meaningless) with *markedly impaired comprehension**

TRANSIENT ISCHEMIC ATTACK (TIA)

• *TRANSIENT episode of neurological deficits* caused by focal brain, spinal cord, or retinal ischemia *WITHOUT ACUTE INFARCTION. Often lasting <24h* – most resolve in 30-60 minutes. *MC due to embolus* (ex. heart, carotid, vertebrobasilar) or transient hypotension.

• 50% of patients with TIA will have a CVA within 1st 24-48h afterwards (esp if DM, HTN). 10-20% will experience CVA within 90 days.

CLINICAL MANIFESTATIONS

1. Internal Carotid Artery: AMAUROSIS FUGAX* *(monoocular vision loss – temporary "lamp shade down on one eye"), weakness contralateral hand.*

   ICA/MCA/ACA: cerebral hemisphere dysfunction. Other sx: sudden headache, speech changes, confusion. PCA: somatosensory deficits.

2. **Vertebrobasilar: *brainstem/cerebellar symptoms*** (ex. gait & proprioception, dizziness, vertigo).

DIAGNOSIS

1. **CT scan of head: initial test of choice*** to rule out intracranial hemorrhage.
2. **Carotid Doppler: *carotid endarterectomy recommended if patient has internal or common carotid artery stenosis ≥70%**
   (associated with 80% reduction in mortality).
3. **CT angiography, MR angiography,** Transcranial Doppler - images cerebral vasculature for stenosis or occlusion.
4. Blood glucose to rule out hypoglycemia, rule out electrolyte abnormalities, coagulation studies, CBC.
5. **Echocardiogram:** TTE or TEE: to look for cardioembolic sources.
6. ECG: to look for atrial fibrillation (A-fib can cause emboli).
7. ABCD² score: to assess CVA risk: (**A**ge, **B**lood pressure, **C**linical features, **D**uration of sx/**D**iabetes Mellitus).

MANAGEMENT

1. *Aspirin ± Dipyridamole or Clopidogrel (Plavix).* Aspirin/Dipyridamole (Aggrenox). *Thrombolytics contraindicated!*
2. Place in supine position to increase cerebral perfusion. Avoid lowering blood pressure (unless >220/120).
3. Reduce modifiable risk factors: ❶ DM (glucose control), ❷ HTN (BP control) ❸ A fib (Warfarin).

STROKE TYPE	CLINICAL MANIFESTATIONS	DIAGNOSIS	MANAGEMENT
ISCHEMIC STROKE	*MC type (80%). Due to* ❶ *thrombotic MC* (49%)* ❷ *emboli (31%)* ❸ *cerebrovascular occlusion.*		
LACUNAR INFARCT	*Small vessel disease (penetrating branches* of cerebral arteries in pons, basal ganglia. ❶ **Pure motor MC** (hemiparesis, hemiplegia) ❷ **ATAXIC HEMIPARESIS** & clumsiness leg >arm ❸ **DYSARTHRIA (CLUMSY HAND SYNDROME)** ❹ *pure* sensory loss (numbness, paresthesias). *History of HTN 80%**	**CT scan:** *small punched out hypodense areas.* Lesions usually central & in noncortical areas: ex basal ganglia	Aspirin. Control risk factors (<u>HTN</u> & <u>DM</u>). Good prognosis: partial or complete deficit resolution ranging from hours up to 6 weeks.
ANTERIOR CIRCULATION **Middle Cerebral Artery** *MC type** (70%)	• Contralateral sensory/motor loss/hemiparesis: *GREATER IN FACE, ARM** > *leg/foot*. • Visual: contralateral homonymous hemianopsia, *gaze preference towards side of lesion* (x1 – 2 days). • **Dominant** (usually L-side): *aphasia: Broca (expressive), Wernicke (sensory).* math comprehension, *agraphia.* • **Nondominant** (usually R-side): *spatial deficits, dysarthria, left-side neglect, anosognosia, apraxia*	**ISCHEMIC STROKE DIAGNOSIS** *Noncontrast CT scan to rule out hemorrhage in suspected stroke.* CT scan may be normal during 1st 6-24 hours.	**ISCHEMIC STROKE MANAGEMENT** •*Thrombolytics within 3 hours* of onset (4.5 hours in some cases). •Tissue plasminogen activator (rTPA) *Alteplase** given if no evidence of hemorrhage. *Alteplase only rTPA effective in ischemic stroke.** CI: BP ≥185/110, recent bleed/trauma, bleeding d/o.
Anterior Cerebral Artery 2%	• Contralateral sensory/motor loss/hemiparesis: *GREATER IN LEG/FOOT** > *upper extremity* ⇨ abnormal gait. • **Face spared:*** speech preservation. Slow responses • Frontal lobe & mental status impairment: *impaired judgment, confusion. Personality changes* (flat affect)* • *URINARY INCONTINENCE*.* Upper motor neuron weakness. • Gaze preference towards side of the lesion (early on).		•Antiplatelet therapy: Aspirin, Clopidogrel, Dipyridamole. Aspirin used in the acute setting if after 3 hours & thrombolytics aren't given or at least 24h after thrombolytics. •±Anticoagulation tx if cardioembolic
POSTERIOR CIRCULATION **Posterior Cerebral Artery**	• *Visual hallucinations, contralateral homonymous hemianopsia.* "*crossed sx*"** (ipsilateral cranial nerve deficits + contralateral muscle weakness), coma, drop attacks.		•Only lower BP if ≥185/110 for thrombolytics or ≥220/120 if no thrombolytic use or if MAP >130
Basilar Artery **Vertebral Artery**	• Cerebellar dysfunction, CN palsies, ↓vision, ↓bilateral sensory • *Vertigo, nystagmus, N/V, diplopia,* ipsilateral ataxia.		•**Note: strokes with facial involvement involves the lower half of face*** (patient will still be able to raise both eyebrows)!
HEMORRHAGIC STROKE	*20% of strokes. Headache, vomiting favors ICH or SAH*. Impaired consciousness without focal symptoms favors SAH. ↑mortality*		
Spontaneous ICH	*Commonly caused by HTN** especially in **basal ganglia.** LOC, N/V, hemiplegia, hemiparalysis. Sx usually mins-hrs gradually increasing in intensity.	Noncontrast CT (*Do not perform LP if ICH is suspected*).* Mass effect ± cause herniation if LP done).	Supportive vs. hematoma evacuation If↑ intracranial pressure ⇨ Head elevation, ± IV Mannitol, hyperventilation
Subarachnoid Hemorrhage (SAH)	*Sudden "worst h/a of my life"** ⇨ *brief LOC, N/V, meningeal irritation** signs (nuchal rigidity), seizures. MC 2ry to rupture of berry aneurysm* or AVM. No focal neurologic symptoms*	1. CT scan. 2. If CT negative & high suspicion ⇨ Lumbar puncture: xanthochromia (<u>RBC's</u>)* esp if >12h & ↑CSF pressure*	Bedrest, no exertion/straining, anti-anxiety meds, stool softeners; ± cautious lowering of BP (only if >220/120 or MAP >130)
"Berry" Aneurysm	*MC circle of Willis (asymptomatic until SAH)*	*Angiography gold standard*	±Aneurysm clipping or coiling.

4 TYPES OF INTRACRANIAL HEMORRHAGE

EPIDURAL HEMATOMA (HEMORRHAGE)	SUBDURAL HEMATOMA (HEMORRHAGE)	SUBARACHNOID HEMORRHAGE (SAH)	INTRACEREBRAL HEMORRHAGE (ICH)
LOCATION • *Arterial bleed MC* between skull & dura.*	**LOCATION** • *Venous bleed MC*. Between dura & arachnoid due to tearing of cortical bridging veins*. MC in elderly.*	**LOCATION** • *Arterial bleed* between arachnoid & pia*	**LOCATION** • *Intraparenchymal*
MECHANISM • *MC after Temporal bone fracture* ⇨ middle meningeal artery* disruption.*	**MECHANISM** • *MC blunt trauma* often causes bleeding on other side of injury "contre-coup". Venous bleed.*	**MECHANISM** • *MC Berry aneurysm rupture, AVM*	**MECHANISM** • HTN, AVM, trauma, amyloid ArterioVenous Malformation
CLINICAL MANIFESTATIONS • Varies. brief LOC ⇨ lucid interval ⇨ coma; headache, N/V, focal neuro sx, rhinorrhea (CSF fluid). CN III palsy if tentorial herniation.	**CLINICAL MANIFESTATIONS** • Varies. May have focal neuro sx.	**CLINICAL MANIFESTATIONS** • *Thunderclap sudden headache "worse h/a of my life"* ±unilateral, occipital area. ± LOC. N/V, Meningeal sx: stiff neck, photophobia, delirium*.* • *No focal neurologic deficits* usually. • Terson syndrome: retinal hemorrhages.	**CLINICAL MANIFESTATIONS** • *Headache, N/V,* ± LOC, hemiplegia, hemiparesis. Not associated with lucid intervals
DIAGNOSIS • *CT: convex (lens – shaped)* bleed* • *Does NOT cross suture lines. Usually in temporal area**	**DIAGNOSIS** • *CT: concave (crescent-shaped) bleed*.* • *Bleeding can cross suture lines**	**DIAGNOSIS** • *CT scan performed first.* If CT negative ⇨ LP: xanthochromia (RBC's), ↑CSF (ICP) pressure.* • *4-vessel angiography* after confirmed SAH.	**DIAGNOSIS** • CT: intraparenchymal bleed. • *Do NOT perform LP if suspected because it may cause brain herniation!*
MANAGEMENT • ± herniate if not evacuated early. Observation if small. If ↑ICP: Mannitol, hyperventilation, head elevation, ± shunt	**MANAGEMENT** • Hematoma evacuation vs. supportive Evacuation if massive or ≥ 5mm midline shift.	**MANAGEMENT** • Supportive: bed rest, stool softeners, lower ICP. Surgical coiling or clipping. • ± lower BP gradually (ex. *Nicardipine*, *Nimodipine*, Labetalol).	**MANAGEMENT** Supportive: gradual BP reduction. ± IV Mannitol if ↑ICP ±Hematoma evacuation if mass effect

EPIDURAL

SUBDURAL

SUBARACHNOID

INTRACEREBRAL.

TYPES OF MENINGITIS:

❶ BACTERIAL MENINGITIS: bacterial infection of the meninges.
❷ ASEPTIC MENINGITIS: NOT caused by pyogenic bacteria. *Includes viral,* fungal & tuberculosis (viral is often referred to as aseptic).

ACUTE BACTERIAL MENINGITIS

May have a history of sinusitis or pneumonia prior to the development of meningitis.

CLINICAL MANIFESTATIONS

- ❶ *Fevers/chills (95%)* ❷ *meningeal sx:* headache/nuchal rigidity (stiff neck), photosensitivity, nausea/vomiting ⇨ *AMS, seizures*
- ⊕*Kernig's sign*: inability to straighten knee with hip flexion;   ⊕*Brudzinski's sign*: neck flexion produces knee/hip flexion.

DIAGNOSIS

1. Lumbar Puncture (LP): *CSF examination definitive dx*: ↑*100-10,000 PMN (neutrophils),* ↓ *glucose <45,* ↑*total protein,* ↑*CSF pressure.*
   DO NOT wait for lumbar puncture to start empiric antibiotics. Early antibiotic therapy has been shown to increase survival rates.

2. Head CT scan: *done to r/o mass effect BEFORE LP if high risk (>60y, immunocompromised, h/o CNS dz, AMS, focal neuro findings, papilledema).*

AGE	PATHOGENS	EMPIRIC MANAGEMENT
<1 month	*Group B Strep (Streptococcus agalactiae) MC* (70%), *L. monocytogenes, E. coli, S. pneumoniae*	Ampicillin + Cefotaxime or Aminoglycoside [*Ampicillin covers Listeria)* This regimen also used if 1 - 3 months old
1mos – 18 y	*N. meningitidis MC (associated with petechial rash),* *S. pneumo,* H. Influenzae	*Ceftriaxone (or Cefotaxime) + Vancomycin*
18y – 50y	*S. pneumo (50%) MC, N meningitidis (±accompanying petechial rash);* H. influenzae, Listeria monocytogenes, Gram negative rods	
>50y	*S. pneumo, Listeria monocytogenes,* Gram negative rods	Ampicillin + Ceftriaxone (or Cefotaxime) ±Vancomycin

Dexamethasone is recommended if known or suspected Streptococcus pneumoniae also in children if due to H. influenzae-B (reduces hearing loss).*
POST-EXPOSURE PROPHYLAXIS: *Ciprofloxacin* 500mg PO x 1 dose.   Alternative *Rifampin* 600mg PO q12h x 2days.

	NORMAL	BACTERIAL MENIGITIS	VIRAL MENINGITIS	FUNGAL & TUBERCULOSIS
Opening pressure (cm H₂0)	5-20 cm	Increased	Normal or mildly increased	Variable (normal or mildly ↑)
Appearance	Normal	Turbid	Clear	Fibrin webs
Protein (mg/L)	18 – 58	↑*high* >200	<100 (normal or mildly increased)	Increased
Glucose (mg/100mL)	50-80	*Markedly decreased* (<40)	*Normal*	Decreased
WBC Count Pleocytosis = ↑ WBC count	0-5 WBCs (no RBCs)	↑*100-100,000* (pleocytosis) >80% *Neutrophils (PMN's)*	↑ (10-300) *Lymphocytes*	↑ (10-200) *Lymphocytes*
Gram Stain	Negative	Positive (60-90%)	Negative	Negative

If glucose is normal, then viral meningitis is most likely.   If WBC is predominantly neutrophils, then bacterial is more likely.

	VIRAL (ASEPTIC) MENINGITIS	ENCEPHALITIS
DEFINITION	• *Viral infection of the MENINGES*	• *Viral infection of the BRAIN PARENCHYMA*
ETIOLOGIES	• *Enterovirus family MC cause of viral meningitis* (ex. Echovirus, Coxsackie)* especially summer & fall. • *Arboviruses (Arthropod Borne viruses transmitted by insects esp mosquitoes:* St. Louis virus (associated with dysuria & pyuria), West Nile Virus (severe lethargy), Colorado Tick Fever. • Mumps, HSV 1 & 2, HIV	• *HSV-1 MC cause of encephalitis** • Enteroviruses (ex Echovirus, Coxsackie) • Arboviruses: ex. West Nile Virus • Varicella Zoster, Rubeola • Toxoplasmosis, CMV, Rabies (Rhabdovirus)
CLINICAL MANIFESTATIONS	• Headache, fever, mild confusion. • ⊕ **Meningeal sx:** nuchal rigidity, ⊕ Brudzinski & Kernig, photophobia, phonophobia, lethargy. Meningeal symptoms not as intense as seen in bacterial meningitis. • *Associated with NORMAL CEREBRAL FUNCTION:** Not commonly associated with focal neurological deficits nor seizures.	• Headache, fever. **Profound lethargy, AMS** • *Associated with ABNORMAL CEREBRAL FUNCTION.** Since brain parenchyma is affected, encephalitis associated with *focal neurologic deficits: ex. cranial nerve deficits* (esp CN II, IV, VI, VII), sensory & motor deficits, personality, movement, speech & behavioral disorders, *seizures.*
DIAGNOSIS	• **CSF analysis: *most important test to differentiate.*** CT scan done 1st to rule out intracranial mass. - *lymphocytosis, normal glucose,** mildly increased protein. • **MRI:** diffuse enhancement of the meninges. Frontal & temporal enhancement seen with HSV-1 • Serologies, viral cultures.	• CSF analysis same as viral (aseptic) meningitis. - *lymphocytosis, normal glucose,** increased protein. • Brain imaging: temporal lobe MC involved (may show mass effect).
MANAGEMENT	• **Supportive care:** antipyretics, IV fluids, antiemetics.	• **Supportive care:** antipyretics, IV fluids, control cerebral edema, seizure prophylaxis if needed, protect the airway if needed. • *Valacyclovir* if HSV or no identifiable cause of meningitis (HSV associated with poor prognosis). • ± Immunoglobulin if immunocompromised.
PROGNOSIS	• Good prognosis. Usually self-limited (lasting on average 7-10 days). • Increased fatality seen in neonates.	• Associated with higher morbidity & mortality than viral meningitis. • HSV encephalitis associated with up to 70% mortality if not treated

ENCEPHALITIS VS. MENINGITIS:
- *Encephalitis associated with abnormal cerebral function** (sensory/motor deficits, speech/movement disorders). HSV-1 MC cause.
- Meningitis not usually associated with abnormal cerebral function. Echovirus family MC cause.
- Meningoencephalitis: a combination of both meningitis & encephalitis.
- Encephalomyelitis: combination of encephalitis & spinal cord involvement.

SEIZURE CLASSIFICATION	MANIFESTATIONS	MISCELLANEOUS
PARTIAL (FOCAL) SEIZURES	*Confined to small area of brain (focal part of one hemisphere).*	May become generalized.
SIMPLE PARTIAL	*CONSCIOUSNESS FULLY MAINTAINED.* EEG: focal discharge at the onset of the seizures.	May have focal sensory, autonomic, motor sx^ May be followed by transient neurologic deficit (Todd's paralysis) lasting up to 24 hours.
COMPLEX PARTIAL (TEMPORAL LOBE)	*CONSCIOUSNESS IMPAIRED.* Starts focally. EEG: interictal spikes with slow waves in the temporal area. Aura (seconds – minutes) ⇨ impaired consciousness.	*AURAS:* sensory/autonomic/motor symptoms of which the patient is aware of. May precede/accompany or follow. Complex partial includes: *AUTOMATISMS: ex: lip smacking, manual picking, patting, coordinated motor movement* (ex. walking).
GENERALIZED SEIZURES	*Diffuse brain involvement (both hemispheres)*	
❶ ABSENCE (PETIT MAL) Nonconvulsive	*Brief lapse of consciousness;* patient usually unaware of attacks. *Brief staring episodes, eyelid twitching.* NO post-ictal phase.	May be clonic (jerking), tonic (stiffness) or atonic (loss of postural tone). *MC in childhood* ⇨ usually ceases by 20y EEG: bilateral symmetric 3Hz spike & wave action or may be normal.
❷ TONIC-CLONIC (GRAND MAL)	Tonic Phase: *loss of consciousness ⇨ rigidity,* sudden arrest of respiration (usually <60sec) ⇨ clonic phase. Clonic Phase: *repetitive, rhythmic jerking* (lasts <2-3 minutes) ⇨ postictal phase. Postictal phase: *flaccid coma/sleep: variable duration.*	May be accompanied by incontinence, tongue biting or aspiration with postictal confusion. *Auras are prewarnings to seizures* EEG: generalize high-amplitude rapid spiking. May be normal in between seizures.
❸ Myoclonus	*Sudden, brief, sporadic involuntary twitching* No LOC	*May be 1 muscle or groups of muscles*
❹ Atonic	*"Drop attacks" – sudden loss of postural tone*	
Status Epilepticus	Repeated, generalized seizures without recovery >30mins	

^motor: jerky, rhythmic, movements one area (focal) or spread to other parts of the affected limb or body (spread = "Jacksonian March"). Tonic or clonic.
^sensory: paresthesias, numbness, pain, heat, cold, sensation of movement, olfactory, flashing lights (photopsia).
^autonomic: abdominal (nausea, vomiting, pain, hunger); cardiovascular (sinus tachycardia).

MANAGEMENT OF SEIZURES
1. **Absence (Petit Mal):** *Ethosuximide 1st line* (only works for absence); *Valproic acid* 2nd line (S/E: hepatitis, pancreatitis); Lamotrigine.
2. **Grand Mal:** *Valproic acid, Phenytoin, Carbamazepine, Lamotrigine,* Topiramate, Primidone, Levetiracetam, Gabapentin, Phenobarbital, Midazolam
3. **Status Epilepticus:** *Lorazepam or Diazepam ⇨ Phenytoin ⇨ Phenobarbital.* Thiamine + Ampule of D50. Place in lateral decubitus position with all possible harmful objects cleared away from the area. Febrile: Phenobarbital.
4. **Myoclonus:** Valproic acid, Clonazepam.

Benzodiazepines (Lorazepam, Diazepam): increases GABA (GABA is an inhibitory neurotransmitter in the CNS).
Phenytoin: blocks Na+ channels in the CNS (takes longer to work).   **S/E:** *gingival hyperplasia, Steven Johnson Syndrome, hirsutism*
Barbiturates: (Phenobarbital): binds to GABA receptors to ↑GABA-mediated CNS inhibition.
- *Prolactin levels are increased in seizures* (helps to differentiate it from pseudoseizures).
- *EEG helps to establish the diagnosis & localize the lesions.*

ANTICONVULSANT MEDICATIONS

SEIZURE MEDICATION	MECHANISM OF ACTION	INDICATIONS	SIDE EFFECTS
ETHOSUXIMIDE (Zarontin)	Blocks Ca^{+2} channels ⇨ motor cortex depression (elevates stimulation threshold, decreases neuronal firing).	Ind: *drug of choice for absence* (only used in absence)*	S/E: drowsiness, ataxia, dizziness, headache, rash, GI upset (diarrhea), weight gain. Caution: patient with renal or hepatic failure. Monitoring: CBC, UA, ↑LFTs
VALPROIC ACID (Depakene) DIVALPROEX SODIUM (Depakote)	Multiple mechanisms of action: - ↑'es GABA's effects (↑CNS inhibition) - inhibits glutamate/NMDA receptor-mediated neuronal excitation.	Ind: absence sz, complex-partial sz, epileptic seizures (Grand Mal). Acute mania in bipolar disorders.	S/E: *pancreatitis, hepatotoxicity*,* GI problems, thrombocytopenia, monitor levels CI/Cautions: hepatic disorders
LAMOTRIGINE (Lamictal)	Blocks Na & Ca channels, decreasing presynaptic glutamate & aspartate release. Also inhibits glutamate's effects on NMDA receptor ⇨ decreased neuronal activity.	Ind: absence, grand mal & partial complex seizures.	*Rash, Steven Johnson Syndrome (SJS),* headache, diplopia
PHENYTOIN (Dilantin)	MOA: stabilizes neuronal membranes (limits firing of action potentials by blocking Na-dependent channels) – related to barbiturates. *Does not cause CNS depression*	Ind: generalized tonic-clonic seizures, complex partial seizures, *seizure prophylaxis*,* - status epilepticus: started after benzodiazepine.	Monitoring: *drug levels,* CBC, UA, significant drug-drug interactions. S/E: *rash (erythema multiforme/SJS), gingival hyperplasia*,* nystagmus, slurred speech, hematologic cx, *hirsutism,* dizziness, teratogenic, *hypotension, arrhythmias (esp with rapid administration >50mcg/min).*
CARBAMAZEPINE (Tegretol)	Blocks Na+ channels, decreases seizure spread. Exact mechanism in trigeminal neuralgia & bipolar disorder is unknown.	Ind: *seizure disorders, bipolar d/o. trigeminal neuralgia (drug of choice),* central diabetes insipidus.*	S/E: *Hyponatremia (causes SIADH)*, SJS* dizziness, drowsiness, N/V, ↑LFT's, arrhythmias *blood dyscrasias (rare).*
TOPIRAMATE (Topamax)	Blocks Na channels, ↑'es GABA activity, glutamate receptor antagonist.	Grand Mal, partial seizures	Weight loss, nephrolithiasis, paresthesias, headache, hyperthermia
BENZODIAZEPINES LORAZEPAM (Ativan) DIAZEPAM (Valium)	MOA: *potentiates GABA-mediated CNS inhibition* *Lorazepam most effective* (has shorter ½ life than diazepam).*	Generalized sz, absence sz, anxiety, chemo-related N/V, sedation, muscle spasms. Status epilepticus, *benzodiazepine 1st line for status epilepticus** (usually followed by phenytoin "loading" to prevent seizure recurrence).	S/E: sedation, ataxia, paradoxical reaction. *Flumazenil reverses sedation.** CI/Cautions: Suicide risk, *monitor BP after dose.*
PHENOBARBITAL	Barbiturate: binds to GABA receptor potentiating GABA-mediated CNS inhibition	*Status epilepticus after phenytoin if status epilepticus persistent* Febrile seizures in children	S/E: permanent neurologic deficit if injected into or near peripheral nerves. *Depression, osteoporosis, irritability.*

CRANIAL NERVE (CN)		PHYSICAL EXAMINATION	ABNORMALITIES
I. OLFACTORY	S	Smell	
II. OPTIC	S	Visual acuity, visual fields, pupillary light reflex (swinging light test)	Optic neuritis, Marcus Gunn
III. OCULOMOTOR	M	Inferior rectus, ciliary body	Oculomotor, Dilated pupil
IV. TROCHLEAR	M	Superior oblique rectus	
V. TRIGEMINAL	B	Motor: muscles of mastication, closing jaw, moves chin side to side. Sensory: light touch (with cotton wisp) to test the 3 divisions of the nerve (ophthalmic, maxillary & mandibular branches)	Trigeminal Neuralgia
VI. ABDUCENS	M	Lateral rectus (lateral gaze). III, IV & VI help with extraocular movements.	
VII. FACIAL	B	Motor: Muscles of facial expression (including blinking of the eyelid, raising eyebrows, frown smile, close eyes tightly, puff cheeks), tear glands. Sensory: taste (anterior 2/3 of tongue). Somatic fibers to external ear.	Bell's Palsy, CN 7 Palsy, Ramsay Hunt syndrome
VIII. ACOUSTIC (Vestibulocochlear)	S	Hearing: speech, Weber & Rinne test. Vestibular Function: balance & proprioception	Acoustic neuroma
IX. GLOSSOPHARYNGEAL	B	Motor: Swallow, gag reflex. Sensory: taste (posterior 1/3 of tongue)	
X. VAGUS	B	Motor: Voice, soft palate, gag reflex. Sensory: relays to the brain sensory information about organs (ex GI, pulmonary heart)	
XI. ACCESSORY	M	Shoulder shrug, turning head from side to side	
XII. HYPOGLOSSAL	M	Tongue: inspect for fasciculations & asymmetry	

M = Motor, S = Sensory, B = both sensory & motor.   "Some Say Money Matters But My Brother Says Big Bucks Matters More"

	MOTOR	MUSCLES	SENSORY	REFLEXES
C5	Shoulder abduction, Elbow Flexion (palm up)	Deltoid, Biceps	Lateral arm (below deltoid & above elbow), Axillary nerve	Loss of bicep jerk reflex
C6	Elbow flexion (thumb up), Wrist extension	Brachioradialis, Extensor carpi radialis	Thumb, Radial side of the hand	Brachioradialis
C7	Elbow extension, Wrist Flexion	Triceps, Flexor carpi radialis	Radial side of the fingers, Fingers 2, 3, 4	Triceps jerk reflex
C8	Finger flexion	Flexor digitorum superficialis	Median nerve, ±Horner's syndrome	
T1	Finger abduction	Interossei	Medial elbow, Ulnar nerve	

S1-S2 Loss of Ankle Jerk   L3-L4 Loss of Knee Jerk   C5-C6 Loss of Biceps Jerk   C7-C8 Loss of Triceps Jerk.
PERONEAL NERVE: innervates the peroneus longus, peroneus brevis, and the short head of the biceps femoris muscles. Injuries lead to a FOOT DROP*

	NEUROLEPTIC MALIGNANT SYNDROME	SEROTONIN SYNDROME
ETIOLOGIES	↓Dopamine activity (esp D₂). - **Dopamine antagonists:** ex Typical > atypical antipsychotics (Haldol, Chlorpromazine Clozapine, Risperidone). NMS usually *slow in onset* occurs 1-2 weeks after initiation or increasing dose. - Abrupt discontinuation of dopamine agonist medications	↑Serotonin (5-HT$_{1A}$) activity due to ↑dose of serotonergic drugs or potentiation between 2 serotonergic drugs. Usually occurs within 24 hours of the interaction - SSRI's + MAO Inhibitors - SNRI or SSRI + St John's Wort - SSRI + Promethazine
CLINICAL MANIFESTATIONS	4 main sx: (can also be seen with SS but usually more severe in NMS) - **AMS:** delirium, coma - **Autonomic instability:** tachycardia, blood pressure fluctuations, may have respiratory distress, **hyper salivation, incontinence*** - **Hyperthermia:** fever due to muscle rigidity. T >100.4° F, diaphoresis - **Muscle rigidity:** extrapyramidal sx. **bradykinesia, "lead pipe" rigidity** HYPOreflexia	Main sx: - AMS: mood changes, "foggy feeling", **agitation.*** - Autonomic instability: tachycardia, blood pressure fluctuations. - Hyperthermia: fever (from muscle contractions), Diaphoresis - Neurologic changes: tremor, **HYPERreflexia,* myoclonus*** (brief, involuntary twitching of muscle or muscle groups)
DISTINGUISHING FEATURES	- ↑creatinine kinase, LDH, LFTs (Rhabdomyolysis due to muscle tremors & rigidity). ↑WBC count. Normal pupils in NMS - **Hyperthermia:** more severe in NMS - Diarrhea & Mydriasis not associated with NMS	- **Mydriasis (dilated pupils).*** - **Hyperactive GI tract: hyperactive bowel sounds, diarrhea.*** (due to serotonin's effect on enterochromaffin cells of GI tract), **abdominal cramps.** - **Agitation***
MANAGEMENT	- **Prompt discontinuation of drug most important tx.*** Symptoms usually resolve 1-2 weeks after drug is discontinued. - **Supportive care:** cooling blankets for fever, ventilator support if needed, IV fluids. - **Dopamine agonists:** ex. Bromocriptine or Amantadine - **Dantrolene: skeletal muscle relaxer for muscle rigidity, fever**	- **Prompt discontinuation of drug most important tx.*** symptoms usually fully resolve in 1 week. - **Supportive care:** IV fluids, cardiac monitoring, oxygen. - **Benzodiazepines for hyperthermia** (↓muscle contraction) or agitation. - **Serotonin antagonists (ex. Cyproheptadine)** if the above treatments are unsuccessful in stabilizing the patient.

Clinical correlation: Carcinoid syndrome: Besides serotonin being a CNS neurotransmitter. Serotonin is also produced by enterchromaffin cells of the GI tract and regulates GI motility. **Carcinoid syndrome associated with sudden increases of serotonin, causing diarrhea. The flushing is caused by Kallikrein (a precursor to bradykinin). Bradykinin is a very powerful vasodilator.

		INCREASED	DECREASED
GLUTAMATE	*Most abundant excitatory neurotransmitter in CNS.* Released by upper motor neurons (UMN) in the synapse to activate lower motor neurons (LMN). • Also activates NMDA receptor. • Involved in normal brain function, memory, cognition & learning.	• **Alzheimer**-associated excess glutamate causes excitotoxicity & cell death . **NMDA antagonists (ex. Memantine) is sometimes used in Alzheimer disease.** • Glutamate is essential but also toxic at high or low doses.	• Phenylketonuria
GABA Gamma-Aminobutyric Acid	*Most abundant inhibitory neurotransmitter in CNS.* • Regulates muscle tone, protects against overexcitation (ex. seizures).	• ETOH mimics GABA at receptor sites	• **Upper Motor Neuron lesions develop hypertonia (spastic)** muscles no longer able respond to GABA. • **Anxiety, Huntington's disease** • Meds that increase GABA can be used for anxiety & seizures (ex. benzodiazepines).
ACETYLCHOLINE	*Activates the muscle at the neuromuscular junction from the LMN to the effector cell (ex. muscle) regulating movement.*	• *Parkinson Disease* (relative increase of acetylcholine due to depletion of dopamine). • Black widow spider venom, mushroom toxicity, *organophosphate poisoning – pesticides & Sarin gas*	• Alzheimer, Huntington, Major Depression. • Botulism toxin (blocks Acetylcholine release leading to paralysis).
DOPAMINE	*Inhibitory CNS neurotransmitter, which allows for coordinated movement.* Without dopamine, movements will be jerky & rigid instead of fluid-like. • *Motivated behaviors (ex drug addiction)* • Endocrine control • Sexual behavior	• *Schizophrenia* (Dopamine antagonists are used to treat Schizophrenia).	• *Parkinson disease:* Dopamine agonists such as Levodopa-Carbidopa 1st line treatment • Depression • *Neuroleptic Malignant syndrome* treated with Bromocriptine (a dopamine agonist). • Bromocriptine also used to treat prolactinemia & acromegaly (inhibits anterior pituitary prolactin secretion).
NOREPINEPHRINE	• *Excitatory CNS neurotransmitter*	• Anxiety, arousal, selective attention	• ADHD
SEROTONIN	• Involved in regulation of mood, pain, higher cognition, emotion	• *Serotonin syndrome*	• Depression

SELECTED REFERENCES

Jankovic J. Parkinson's disease: clinical features and diagnosis. J Neurol Neurosurg Psychiatr. 2008;79(4):368-76.

Zochodne DW. Autonomic involvement in Guillain-Barré syndrome: a review. Muscle Nerve. 1994;17(10):1145-55.

Conti-fine BM, Milani M, Kaminski HJ. Myasthenia gravis: past, present, and future. J Clin Invest. 2006;116(11):2843-54.

Saidha S, Eckstein C, Calabresi PA. New and emerging disease modifying therapies for multiple sclerosis. Ann N Y Acad Sci. 2012;1247:117-37.

Mackenzie C. Dysarthria in stroke: a narrative review of its description and the outcome of intervention. Int J Speech Lang Pathol. 2011;13(2):125-36.

Abboud H, Ahmed A, Fernandez HH. Essential tremor: choosing the right management plan for your patient. Cleve Clin J Med. 2011;78(12):821-8.

Jankovic J. Parkinson's disease: clinical features and diagnosis. J Neurol Neurosurg Psychiatr. 2008;79(4):368-76.

Walker FO. Huntington's disease. Lancet. 2007;369(9557):218-28.

Hughes RA, Wijdicks EF, Barohn R, et al. Practice parameter: immunotherapy for Guillain-Barré syndrome: report of the Quality Standards Subcommittee of the American Academy of Neurology. Neurology. 2003;61(6):736-40.

Maddison P, Newsom-davis J. Treatment for Lambert-Eaton myasthenic syndrome. Cochrane Database Syst Rev. 2005;(2):CD003279.

Nakahara J, Maeda M, Aiso S, Suzuki N. Current concepts in multiple sclerosis: autoimmunity versus oligodendrogliopathy. Clin Rev Allergy Immunol. 2012;42(1):26-34.

Maher AR, Maglione M, Bagley S, et al. Efficacy and comparative effectiveness of atypical antipsychotic medications for off-label uses in adults: a systematic review and meta-analysis. JAMA. 2011;306(12):1359-69.

Cruccu G, Biasiotta A, Di rezze S, et al. Trigeminal neuralgia and pain related to multiple sclerosis. Pain. 2009;143(3):186-91.

Easton JD, Saver JL, Albers GW, et al. Definition and evaluation of transient ischemic attack: a scientific statement for healthcare professionals from the American Heart Association/American Stroke Association Stroke Council; Council on Cardiovascular Surgery and Anesthesia; Council on Cardiovascular Radiology and Intervention; Council on Cardiovascular Nursing; and the Interdisciplinary Council on Peripheral Vascular Disease. The American Academy of Neurology affirms the value of this statement as an educational tool for neurologists. Stroke. 2009;40(6):2276-93.

Zink BJ. Traumatic brain injury outcome: concepts for emergency care. Ann Emerg Med. 2001;37(3):318-32.

Pelonero AL, Levenson JL, Pandurangi AK. Neuroleptic malignant syndrome: a review. Psychiatr Serv. 1998;49(9):1163-72.

Tyler KL. Herpes simplex virus infections of the central nervous system: encephalitis and meningitis, including Mollaret's. Herpes. 2004;11 Suppl 2:57A-64A.

Rozenberg F, Deback C, Agut H. Herpes simplex encephalitis : from virus to therapy. Infect Disord Drug Targets. 2011;11(3):235-50.

The International Classification of Headache Disorders: 2nd edition. Cephalalgia. 2004;24 Suppl 1:9-160.

Bonte FJ, Harris TS, Hynan LS, Bigio EH, White CL. Tc-99m HMPAO SPECT in the differential diagnosis of the dementias with histopathologic confirmation. Clin Nucl Med. 2006;31(7):376-8.

Singer HS. Tourette syndrome and other tic disorders. Handb Clin Neurol. 2011;100:641-57.

CHAPTER 10 – PSYCHIATRY & BEHAVIORAL SCIENCE

PSYCHOSES

DELUSIONAL DISORDER

- ≥1 ***delusion*** lasting ≥1 month ***WITHOUT other psychotic symptoms.*** ± Nonbizarre = possible but highly unlikely (ex. being poisoned). Apart from the delusion, behavior is not obviously odd or bizarre & there is no significant impairment of function. Not explained by another disorder.

SCHIZOPHRENIA

- **BRIEF PYSCHOTIC DISORDER:** ≥1 psychotic symptom(s) with onset & remission ***<1 month.****
- **SCHIZOPHRENIFORM DISORDER:** meets criteria for schizophrenia but ***<6 months duration.****
- **SCHIZOAFFECTIVE DISORDER:** ***schizophrenia + mood disturbance*** (major depressive or manic episode).

SCHIZOPHRENIA: ***≥6 MONTHS DURATION*** of illness with 1 month of acute symptoms along with ***FUNCTIONAL DECLINE.****

CRITERIA: At least 1 must be hallucination, delusion, or disorganized speech. ***≥2 of the following:***

POSITIVE SYMPTOMS	Thought to be caused by ***excess dopamine receptors*** in mesolimbic pathway
	Hallucinations, delusions, disorganized speech & thinking, abnormal behavior.
HALLUCINATIONS	**Sensory perception without a physical stimuli**
Auditory (MC type)	Sound or a voice. Voice often in "3rd person" or can be command hallucinations.
Visual	Simple (flashing light) or complex (ex. seeing faces).
Olfactory	Stench or foul smells common.
Tactile	Insects on skin or being touched.
Somatic	Sensation arising from within the body.
Gustatory	Can be a part of persecutory delusions (tasting poison in food).
DELUSIONS	**A fixed belief held with strong conviction despite evidence to the contrary**
Persecutory	Person or force is interfering with them, observing them or wishes harm to the patient
Reference	Random events take on a personal significance (directed at them).
Control	Some agency takes control of patient's thoughts, feelings & behaviors.
Grandiose	Unrealistic beliefs in one's powers & abilities.
Nihilism	Exaggerated belief in the futility of everything & catastrophic events.
Erotomanic	Believes another person is in love with them.
Jealousy	Somebody is suspected of being unfaithful.
Doubles	Believes a family member or close person has been replaced by an identical double.

Catatonia may be a specifier of other psych disorders besides schizophrenia.

NEGATIVE SYMPTOMS	Thought to be caused by ***dopamine dysfunction*** in the mesocortical pathway. Serotonin may also play a role.

Flat emotional affect, social withdrawal; Lack of emotional expression, ***avolition*** (lack of self-motivation). Lack of communication & reactivity; Silent patients. Poor eye contact.

- 1% of population. MC in males. Onset often in early 20s for men & late 20s for women.
- **Risk Factors:** ***family history*** (10% incidence in patients with schizophrenic 1st degree relative).
- Patients with schizophrenia have ↓CNS gray matter, ↑size of ventricles, ↑CNS dopamine receptors.

MANAGEMENT
Hospitalization for acute psychotic episodes.
1. **Antipsychotics: *dopamine receptor antagonists.***
   - ***2nd generation: 1st line treatment for schizophrenia.**** *Ex. Risperidone, Olanzapine, Quetiapine.*
      MOA: dopamine & serotonin antagonists. Clozapine may be used in refractory cases (ex. no significant improvement after 2-6 weeks of pharmacological therapy).
   - 1st generation: ex. Haloperidol & Chlorpromazine are better at treating the positive symptoms but are associated with increased extrapyramidal symptoms.

ANTIPSYCHOTIC AGENTS (NEUROLEPTICS)

"TYPICAL" 1ST Generation
 	
BUTYROPHENONES
Haloperidol (Haldol)
 	
Droperidol
 	
PHENOTHIAZINES
Fluphenazine
(Prolixin)
 	
Perphenazine
 	
Chlorpromazine
(Thorazine)
 	
Thioridazine
 	
Chlorpromazine & Thioridazine less associated with EPS but associated with more anticholinergic side effects.
	MOA: blocks CNS dopamine (D_2) receptors ***(dopamine antagonists).****
	Ind: *psychosis, schizophrenia (especially positive symptoms).*
	S/E: due to ↓dopamine activity:
	EXTRAPYRAMIDAL Sx (EPS):* *rigidity, bradykinesia, tremor, akathisia* (restlessness).
	*High incidence seen with Typical Antipsychotics.** 3 followings EPS syndromes include:
	  1. DYSTONIC REACTIONS (Dyskinesia): reversible EPS *hours-days after initiation of typical antipsychotic* due to disruption of Dop-Ach balance (decreased dopamine leads to excess acetylcholine-mediated activation) ⇨ intermittent, spasms, sustained involuntary muscle contractions *(trismus, protrusions of tongue, facial grimacing, torticollis, difficulty speaking).**
	    Management: *Diphenhydramine IV* (has anticholinergic properties) or add an *anticholinergic agent* (ex *Benztropine*). Symptoms usually resolve within 10 minutes of IV administration. Benzodiazepines may be used (normal Dopamine-Acetylcholine balance mediated by GABA-containing neurons).
	  2. TARDIVE DYSKINESIA: *repetitive involuntary movements mostly involving extremities & face – lip smacking, teeth grinding, rolling of tongue.** Seen with *long-term use.**
	  3 PARKINSONISM: (due to ↓dopamine in nigrostriatal pathways) ⇨ rigidity, tremor.
	
	OTHER S/E:
	- NEUROLEPTIC MALIGNANT SYNDROME (NMS): *life threatening disorder due to D_2 inhibition* in basal ganglia ⇨ *mental status changes, extreme muscle rigidity, tremor, autonomic instability (tachycardia, tachypnea, hyperthermia/fever,** profuse diaphoresis, incontinence, blood pressure changes) & leukocytosis. NMS occurs MC in young adults & often occurs within 90 days of initiation/dose increase.
	    Management: *stop offending agent.* Tx hyperthermia with cooling blankets & ice to axilla/groin), ventilatory support. *Dopamine agonists:* ex. *Bromocriptine,* Amantadine, Levodopa/Carbidopa.
	- QT prolongation, cardiac arrhythmias, sedation, anticholinergic side effects, dermatitis, blood dyscrasias, ↑*prolactin** (more than 2nd generation), *weight gain.**
	CI/caution for Haldol: Parkinson disease, anticoagulant use, severe cardiac disorder.

"ATYPICAL" 2nd Generation
Quetiapine (Seroquel)
Olanzapine (Zyprexa)
Clozapine (Clozaril)
Loxapine (Loxatane)
	MOA: *CNS dopamine D_4 receptor & serotonin ($5HT_2$) antagonists.**
	Ind: *1st line for psychotic disorders. Clozapine useful for patients who develop resistance to other antipsychotics** (persistent sx 2-6 weeks on meds).
	S/E:
	  *Extrapyramidal sx: less incidence of EPS compared to 1st generation (especially less with Clozapine & Quetiapine)** because they weakly bind to D_2 receptors.
	  Increased prolactin levels, hyperglycemia, hyperlipidemia, weight gain, NMS.
	CI/cautions: *Clozapine causes agranulocytosis** (monitor CBC weekly) & *myocarditis;** Seizures, *QT prolongation. Marked weight gain & diabetes mellitus with Olanzapine**

BENZISOXAZOLES *Risperidone* (Risperdal) *Ziprasidone* (Geodon)	**MOA:** partial dopamine (D_2) receptor & serotonin $5\text{-}HT_{1A}$ receptor antagonist. serotonin $5\text{-}HT_2$ receptor antagonist. **Ind:** schizophrenia, bipolar, psychosis. Risperdal may be used for Tourette's. **S/E:** EPS, *increased prolactin,** sedation, weight gain, hypotension, prolonged QT.
QUINOLINONES *Aripiprazole* (Abilify)	**MOA:** dopamine (D_2) receptor & serotonin ($5\text{-}HT_2$ & $5\text{-}HT_1$) receptor antagonist. **Ind:** psychotic disorders. Sometimes called a 3rd generation antipsychotic.
LITHIUM	**MOA:** increases norepinephrine & serotonin receptor sensitivity. **Ind:** bipolar disorders: acute mania (mood stabilizer). **S/E:** Endocrine: *hypothyroidism,** sodium depletion, *increased urination & thirst** (must drink 8-12 glasses of H_2O/day),* diabetes insipidus, hyperparathyroidism/*hypercalcemia.* Neuro: *seizures* (monitor EEG changes), tremor, headache, sedation. Cardio: *arrhythmias.* GI: nausea, vomiting, diarrhea, weight gain. CI: pregnancy, severe renal disease, cardiac disease. *Narrow therapeutic index** ⇨ monitor plasma levels every 4 – 8 weeks.
VALPROATE, CARBAMAZEPINE	Anticonvulsants may help suppress impulsive & aggressive behavior

MOOD (AFFECTIVE) DISORDERS

MAJOR DEPRESSIVE DISORDER (MDD)/UNIPOLAR DEPRESSION

- <u>Risk factors:</u> family history, female: male (2:1). Highest incidence 20s-40s.
- <u>MDD</u>: ***Depressed mood or anhedonia (loss of pleasure)*** or loss of interest in activities ***with ≥5 associated symptoms*** *almost every day for most of the days for* <u>***at least 2 weeks***</u>:
  - Fatigue almost all day, insomnia or hypersomnia, feelings of guilt or worthlessness, recurring thoughts of death or suicide, psychomotor agitation, significant weight change (gain or loss), decreased or increased appetite, decreased concentration/indecisiveness.
  - The symptoms are not due to substance use, bereavement or medical conditions.
  - <u>Somatic:</u> constipation, headache, skin changes, chest or abdominal pain, cough, dyspnea.

- ***Symptoms cause clinical distress or impairment*** in social, occupational or other important areas of functioning. ***Absence of mania or hypomania.***

SUBTYPES "COURSE SPECIFIERS" OF MDD

1. SEASONAL AFFECTIVE DISORDER/SEASONAL PATTERN: the presence of depressive symptoms at the same time each year (ex. most common in the winter – "winter blues" – due to reduction of sunlight & cold weather). **Management:** SSRIs, light therapy, Bupropion.
2. ATYPICAL DEPRESSION: shares many of the typical symptoms of major depression but patients experience ***mood reactivity (improved mood in response to positive events).*** Symptoms include significant weight gain/appetite increase, hypersomnia, heavy/leaden feelings in arms or legs & oversensitivity to interpersonal rejection. **Management:** *MAO inhibitors.*
3. MELANCHOLIA: characterized by anhedonia (inability to find pleasure in things), lack of mood reactivity, depression, severe weight loss/loss of appetite, excessive guilt, psychomotor agitation or retardation & sleep disturbance (increased REM time & reduced sleep). Sleep disturbances may lead to early morning awakening or mood that is worse in the morning.
4. CATATONIC DEPRESSION: motor immobility, stupor & extreme withdrawal.

PATHOPHYSIOLOGY

- <u>Alteration in neurotransmitters:</u> serotonin, epinephrine, norepinephrine, dopamine, acetylcholine & histamine. Genetic factors
- <u>Neuroendocrine dysregulation:</u> adrenal, thyroid or growth hormone dysregulation.
- 15% of patients commit suicide (especially men 25-30y & women 40-50y). Higher suicide rates in patients with a detailed suicide plan, white males >45y & concurrent substance abuse.
- Patient Health Questionnaire (PHQ)-2 form for initial screen. If positive, may use PHQ-9 form.

MANAGEMENT

1. ***Psychotherapy: principle therapy in mild - moderate depression.*** Cognitive behavioral therapy: exposure/response prevention, psychoeducation, support groups. Particularly beneficial when combined with medical therapy.

2. **Medications:** *SSRIs often first line medications in mild to moderate;** SNRIs. Bupropion & Mirtazapine 2nd line. TCAs and MAO inhibitors usually 3rd line. ***Antidepressants should be continued for a*** <u>***minimum of 3-6 weeks***</u> ***to determine efficacy.****

3. **Electroconvulsive therapy (ECT)**: *patients who fail to respond to medical therapy, positive previous response to ECT or for rapid response in patients with severe symptoms.* ECT is safe in pregnancy and in the elderly.

PSYCHOTHERAPEUTIC AGENTS

SELECTIVE SEROTONIN REUPTAKE INHIBITORS (SSRIs) *Citalopram* (Celexa) *Escitalopram* (Lexapro) *Paroxetine* (Paxil) *Fluoxetine* (Prozac) *Sertraline* (Zoloft) *Fluvoxamine* (Zyvox)	**MOA:** selectively inhibits CNS uptake of serotonin ⇨ ↑*serotonin* CNS activity **Ind:** *1st line therapy for depression* & anxiety disorder. *Preferred over the other classes in children.* SSRIs *have the advantage of easy dosing, __less side effects__ & __low toxicity in cases of overdose__* (because they don't affect norepinephrine, acetylcholine, histamine or dopamine). **S/E:** common S/E: *GI upset, sexual dysfunction, headache,* changes in energy level (fatigue, restlessness); Anxiety, insomnia, weight changes, SIADH. *Avoid Citalopram in patients with long QT syndrome.* **SEROTONIN SYNDROME*** *(especially if used c MAOI)* ⇨ <u>neuro</u>: *acute AMS seizures,* coma & death; <u>autonomic</u>: *restlessness, diaphoresis, tremor, hyperthermia, nausea, vomiting, abdominal pain, mydriasis, tachycardia*
SEROTONIN & NOREPINEPHRINE REUPTAKE INHIBITORS (SNRI's) *Venlafaxine* (Effexor) *Desvenlafaxine* (Pristiq) *Duloxetine* (Cymbalta)	**MOA:** Inhibits neuronal *__serotonin, norepinephrine, & dopamine__* reuptake. **Ind:** may be used as first line agents, *particularly in patients with significant __fatigue or pain syndromes in association with depression__.* 2nd line agents in patients with no response to SSRIs. Safety, tolerability & side effect profile similar to those of SSRIs including hyponatremia & noradrenergic sx. Other S/E: *__hypertension__,* dizziness. **CI/Cautions:** MAOI use, renal/hepatic impairment, seizures. Avoid abrupt discontinuation. Use with caution in patients with hypertension. *↑Serotonin Syndrome if SNRIs used with St John's Wort.**
TRICYCLIC ANTIDEPRESSANTS (TCA) *Amitriptyline* (Elavil) *Clomipramine* (Anafranil) *Desipramine* (Norpramin) *Doxepin* (Sinequan) *Imipramine* (Tofranil) *Nortriptyline* (Pamelor)	**MOA:** Inhibits reuptake of *__Serotonin & Norepinephrine.__* **Ind:** depression, insomnia, diabetic neuropathic pain, post-herpetic neuralgia, migraine, urge incontinence. *Used less often because of their side effect profile & __severe toxicity with overdose.__** Nondepressed patients experience sleepiness. Depressed patients feel elevated mood. **S/E:** *anticholinergic effects,** sedation, weight gain, *prolonged QT interval* (best indicator of overdose). **Overdose:** *Na channel blocker effects** ⇨ sinus or *__wide complex tachycardia,__** neurologic symptoms, ARDS, SIADH. Sodium bicarbonate may be used for cardiotoxicity. **CI/Caution:** use of MAO Inhibitors, recent MI, seizure history.
TETRACYCLIC COMPOUNDS *Mirtazapine* (Remeron)	**MOA:** enhances central noradrenergic & serotonergic activity **Ind:** depression. Less sexual dysfunction S/E. May be used with Trazodone **S/E:** *sedation,* dry mouth, constipation, weight gain, agranulocytosis. **CI:** use with MAO inhibitors.
BUPROPION HYDROCHLORIDE *Bupropion* (Wellbutrin) (Zyban)	**MOA:** inhibits the neuronal uptake of *dopamine & norepinephrine.* **Ind:** Wellbutrin for depression; Zyban marketed for smoking cessation. **S/E:** seizures, agitation, anxiety, restlessness, weight loss, HTN, headache. *__Less GI distress & sexual dysfunction compared to SSRIs,__** dry mouth. **CI/Cautions:** *seizure disorder,** *eating disorders* (ex. bulimia, anorexia), MAOI use, patients undergoing drug/ETOH detox. Avoid abrupt withdrawal.
MAO INHIBITORS <u>Nonselective (MAO A & B)</u> *Phenelzine* (Nardil) *Tranylcypromine* (Parnate) *Isocarboxazid* (Marplan) <u>Selective MAO B</u> *Selegiline* (Eldepryl) **Less chance of HTN Crisis induced by tyramine c MAO B**	**MOA:** blocks breakdown of neurotransmitters (dopamine, serotonin, epinephrine, norepinephrine) by inhibiting monoamine oxidase. **Ind:** refractory depression; Many types of anxiety & affective disorders. **S/E:** insomnia, anxiety, orthostatic hypotension, weight gain, sexual dysfunction. *Hypertensive crisis** (must avoid tyramine-containing foods -* aged or fermented cheese, wine, beer, aged foods, smoked meats, chocolates, coffee, tea – MAOI prevents breakdown of tyramine, leading to hypertension); **CI:** *MAOI + SSRI may cause <u>Serotonin syndrome:</u>* ⇨ acute AMS, restlessness, diaphoresis, tremor, hyperthermia, seizures occasionally coma & death. *MAOI + TCA may cause delirium & hypertension.*

Trazodone: serotonin antagonist & reuptake inhibitor. *Antidepressant, anti-anxiety & hypnotic effects.*
S/E: sedation, cardiac arrhythmias. Priapism is a rare side effect.

BIPOLAR I DISORDER

- ≥1 MANIC OR MIXED EPISODE* which often cycles with OCCASIONAL DEPRESSIVE EPISODES* (but major depressive episodes are not required for the diagnosis).
- 1% of population. Men = women. *Family history (1st degree relatives) strongest risk factor.*
- Average age of onset is 20s - 30s. New onset rare after 50y. The earlier the onset, the greater likelihood of psychotic features & the poorer the prognosis.

- MANIA: *abnormal & persistently elevated, expansive or irritable mood at least 1 week* (or less if hospitalization is required) c *marked impairment of social/occupational function* ≥3:
   - MOOD: euphoria, irritable, labile or dysphoric.

   - THINKING: racing, flight of ideas, disorganized, easily distracted, expansive or grandiose thoughts (highly inflated self esteem). Judgment is impaired (ex. *spending sprees*)

   - BEHAVIOR: physical hyperactivity, pressured speech, decreased need for sleep (may go days without sleep), increased impulsivity & excessive involvement in pleasurable activities including risk-taking & hypersexuality. Disinhibition, increased goal directed activity. *Psychotic symptoms (paranoia, delusions, hallucinations) may be seen in these patients.*

MANAGEMENT
1. *Mood Stabilizers:*
   - *Lithium 1st line.** *Valproic acid, Carbamazepine*
   - *2nd generation antipsychotics (ex. Olanzapine).* *Haloperidol* (1st generation antipsychotic) or *Benzodiazepines* may be added *if psychosis or agitation develops.*
   - Other treatment may include: electroconvulsive therapy, MAOIs, SSRIs & TCAs (however *antidepressant medications may precipitate mania*).
2. Therapy: cognitive, behavioral & interpersonal. Good sleep hygiene recommended.

BIPOLAR II DISORDER

- ≥1 HYPOMANIC episode + ≥1 MAJOR DEPRESSIVE EPISODE.* Mania or mixed episodes are absent.

- HYPOMANIA: *symptoms similar to manic symptoms* - period of elevated, expansive or irritably mood @ least 4 days that is clearly different from the usual nondepressed mood but *does NOT cause MARKED impairment, no psychotic features & does not require hospitalization usually.* Does not include racing thoughts or excessive psychomotor agitation.

MANAGEMENT: similar to bipolar I (antipsychotics, mood stabilizers & benzodiazepines).
1. Acute Mania: mood stabilizers (ex. *Lithium**), Valproate, 2nd generation antipsychotics
2. Depression: *Lithium*, Valproate, Carbamazepine, 2nd generation antipsychotics
3. Mixed: atypical antipsychotics, Valproate

	MANIA/MIXED	MAJOR DEPRESSION
BIPOLAR I	*Yes*	*Typical but not required.*
BIPOLAR II	*HYPOmania only (no mania)*	*Yes*
CYCLOTHYMIA	No (but may have periods of mood elevation)	No. Associated with relatively mild depressive episodes.
MAJOR DEPRESSIVE DISORDER	No	*Yes*
PERSISTENT DEPRESSIVE DISORDER (DYSTHYMIA)	No	Usually mild but can meet criteria for major in some cases.

"Mixed" symptoms = simultaneous occurrence of ≥3 manic (or hypomanic) symptoms + depression.

PERSISTENT DEPRESSIVE DISORDER   (DYSTHYMIA)

- *Chronic depressed mood >2 years in adults* (>1 year in children/adolescents). *Usually milder than major depression* but can include symptoms of chronic major depression (DSM V consolidated dysthymia & chronic major depressive disorder into persistent depressive disorder).

- There are no symptoms of hypomania, mania or psychotic features.

- *Patients are usually able to function* (may experience mild decreased productivity).

- MC in women. Begins MC in late teens, early adulthood.

- May progress over time to develop into major depressive disorder or bipolar disorder.

CLINICAL MANIFESTATIONS
1. Generalized loss of interest, social withdrawal, *pessimism,* decreased productivity.

2. *Chronic depressed mood >2 years in adults* (>1 year in children/adolescents) for most of the day, more days than not. In that 2 year period, the patient is not symptom free for >2 months at a time.   May say things like *"I've always been this way".*

3. At least 2 of the following conditions must be present: insomnia or hypersomnia, fatigue, low self-esteem, decreased appetite or overeating, hopelessness, poor concentration, indecisiveness.

MANAGEMENT
Similar to depression: psychotherapy principal treatment, *SSRIs first line medical treatment.* Second line treatments include: SNRIs, Bupropion, TCAs and in some cases MAO Inhibitors.

CYCLOTHYMIC DISORDER

- *Similar to bipolar disorder II but LESS SEVERE.** Prolonged period of *milder elevations & depressions in mood.* ~15% may eventually develop bipolar disorder.
- Men = women.

CLINICAL MANIFESTATIONS
1. Recurrent episodes of *hypomanic symptoms* that don't meet criteria for hypomania *"cycling" with relatively mild depressive episodes* (that don't meet the criteria for major depressive disorder) for *at least a 2-year period* in adults (1 year in children). These patients may have symptom free periods, however those symptom-free periods don't last longer than 2 months at any time.

2. Manic or mixed episodes do not occur.

MANAGEMENT: similar to bipolar I: mood stabilizers & neuroleptics.

ANXIETY DISORDERS

PANIC ATTACKS

• Panic attacks are feature of many different anxiety disorders but not a disorder in & of itself.

• **Panic Attack:** episode of intense fear or discomfort that develops abruptly, *usually peaks within 10 minutes & usually lasts <60 minutes.* ≥4 of the following symptoms:

PANIC ATTACK SYMPTOMS: sympathetic overdrive

1. Dizziness	6. Shortness of breath	11. Palpitations, increased heart rate
2. Trembling	7. Chest pain/discomfort	12. Nausea or abdominal distress
3. Choking feeling	8. Chills or hot flashes	13. Depersonalization (being detached from
4. Paresthesias	9. Fear of losing control	oneself) or derealization (feelings of unreality)
5. Sweating	10. Fear of dying	

MANAGEMENT of ACUTE ATTACK

1. **_Benzodiazepines:_** ex. *Lorazepam, Alprazolam* **1ˢᵗ *line*.*** Watch for dependence or abuse.

PANIC DISORDER

• 2-3 times more common in women. Symptom onset usually occurs before 30 years of age.

CRITERIA:

• **_Recurrent, unexpected panic attacks*_** (at least 2 attacks) may or may not be related to a trigger. Usually sudden in onset, peaks within 10 minutes & usually lasts <60 minutes.

• At least one of the following must occur for at least 1 month: ❶ *panic attacks often followed by concern about future attacks,* ❷worry about the implication of the attacks (ex. losing control) or ❸ significant change in behavior related to the attacks.

• Must exhibit *at least 4* of 13 typical symptoms of panic (see panic attack chart above).

• Symptoms are not due to substance use, medical condition or other mental disorder.

• **_± Agoraphobia: anxiety about being in places or situations from which escape may be difficult_** (ex. *open spaces, enclosed spaces, crowds, public transportation or outside of the home alone*). Agoraphobia now seen as a separate entity from panic disorders & can occur with other psychiatric disorders.

MANAGEMENT

LONG TERM Management

1. **_SSRIs 1ˢᵗ line medical treatment:*_** ex. *Paroxetine, Sertraline, Fluoxetine.* SSRI = selective serotonin reuptake inhibitors. Serotonin Norepinephrine reuptake inhibitors (SNRIs) also used (ex. *Venlafaxine).*

2. **Cognitive Behavioral Therapy (CBT):** treatment that focuses on thinking & behavior (ex. relaxation, desensitization, examining behavior consequences etc.). Psychotherapy may be used in mild cases as initial therapy.

ACUTE ATTACK Management

1. **_Benzodiazepines:_** ex. *Alprazolam, Clonazepam.* Watch for dependence or abuse.

GENERALIZED ANXIETY DISORDER

- **GAD:** *excessive anxiety or worry a majority of days* ≥6 *month period* *about various aspects of life.* It is not episodic (as seen in panic disorders), situational (as seen in phobias) nor focal.

- Associated with ≥3 of the following symptoms: fatigue, restlessness, difficulty concentrating, muscle tension, sleep disturbance, irritability, shakiness & headaches. Not due to medical illness.

- More common in females. Onset of symptoms usually occur in early 20s.

MANAGEMENT:
1. *Antidepressants: SSRIs* (ex. *Paroxetine, Escitalopram*); SNRIs (ex. *Venlafaxine*).

2. *Buspirone (Buspar):* stimulates serotonin receptors & blocks dopamine receptors. May take several weeks before clinical improvement. *Buspirone does not cause sedation.* *
   S/E: nausea, restless leg syndrome, extrapyramidal symptoms, dizziness.

3. Benzodiazepines (short term use only); ß-blockers; TCAs (Tricyclic antidepressants).
4. *Psychotherapy:* includes cognitive behavioral therapy.

SOCIAL ANXIETY DISORDER   (Formerly Social Phobia)

- *Persistent (> 6 months),* INTENSE FEAR OF SOCIAL OR PERFORMANCE SITUATIONS *in which the person is exposed to the scrutiny of others* *for fear of embarrassment* (ex. public speaking, meeting new people, eating/drinking in front of people). Exposure to social situations almost always provoke anxiety & cause *expected* panic attacks.
- May realize feelings are excessive & unreasonable. May avoid those situations.

MANAGEMENT
1. *Antidepressants: SSRIs* (ex. *Paroxetine, Fluoxetine, Escitalopram*) or SNRIs (*Venlafaxine*).
2. Beta-blockers: may be used for performance anxiety (ex. Propranolol, Atenolol).
3. Benzodiazepines: if treatment is needed infrequently.
4. **Psychotherapy:** ex. cognitive behavior therapy, insight-oriented therapy

SPECIFIC PHOBIAS

- *Persistent (> 6 months), intense fear/anxiety of a specific situation* (ex. heights, flying), *object* (ex. pigeons, snakes, blood) or *place* (ex. hospital).
- The fear is out of proportion to any real danger.

- The phobic object or situation is actively avoided or endured with intense fear or anxiety.

- *Everyday activities must be impaired by distress or avoidance* of the situation or object.

MANAGEMENT
1. **Exposure/desensitization therapy:** *treatment of choice.* Childhood phobias may disappear or lessen with age.
2. Short-term benzodiazepines & ß-blockers can be used in some patients.

TRAUMA & STRESSOR-RELATED DISORDERS

POSTTRAUMATIC STRESS DISORDER (PTSD)

• *MC seen in young adults*: trauma for men includes combat experience & urban violence; Trauma for women includes rape or assault. Also common in adult survivors of sexual abuse.

CRITERIA:

A. ***Exposure*** to actual or threatened death, serious injury or sexual violence via:
   ❶ direct experience of the traumatic event
   ❷ witnessing the event in person
   ❸ learning the event happened to someone close (family member or friend)
   ❹ experiencing extreme or repeated exposure to aversive details of the traumatic event (ex. first responders collecting human remains during 9/11).

B. ***Presence of ≥1 of the following intrusion symptoms*** after the event that may lead to significant distress or impairment in function (ex. occupational, social or other areas):

   1. ***Re-experiencing: >1 MONTH**** as ***repetitive recollections*** (ex. distressing dreams) & ***dissociative reactions*** (ex. flashbacks in which the person feels/acts as if the event is recurring), leading to physiologic distress &/or physiologic reactions.

   2. ***Avoidance*** of stimuli associated with the traumatic event (reminders of the events).

   3. ***Negative alterations in cognition & mood***: inability to remember an important aspect of the event, persistent exaggerated beliefs (ex. "the world is unsafe"). Horror guilt, anger or shame. May include disinterest in activities.

   4. ***Arousal & reactivity:*** angry outbursts, irritable behavior, reckless or self destructive behaviors, hypervigilance, sleep disturbances, concentration issues, exaggerated startle response.

MANAGEMENT

1. ***Antidepressants: SSRIs 1st line medical treatment:**** ex. *Paroxetine, Sertraline, Fluoxetine.* Tricyclic antidepressants (ex. *Imipramine*). MAO inhibitors. ***Trazodone may be helpful for insomnia.***

2. **Cognitive behavioral therapy:** psychotherapy including individual or group counseling.

ACUTE STRESS DISORDER

• *Similar to PTSD* but *symptoms last <1 MONTH** & symptom onset occurs within 1 month of event.

MANAGEMENT:

1. Counseling/psychotherapy. If persistent ⇨ treat as PTSD.

ADJUSTMENT DISORDERS

• *An EMOTIONAL OR BEHAVIORAL REACTION TO AN IDENTIFIABLE STRESSOR* (ex. job loss, physical illness, leaving home, divorce etc.) or an event *THAT CAUSES A DISPROPORTIONATE RESPONSE* that would normally be expected *within 3 months of the stressor* (does not include bereavement) & resolves usually *within 6 months* of the stressor.

CLINICAL MANIFESTATIONS
Symptoms include one or both of the following:
   ❶ marked distress out of proportion to the severity of stressor.
   ❷ significant impairment in areas of functioning (ex. occupational, social, etc.).

MANAGEMENT:
1. **Psychotherapy** including individual or group therapy is *first line therapy.**
2. Medications may be used in selected cases but they are not the preferred treatment.
3. Patients may self-medicate with alcohol or other drugs.

DISSOCIATIVE DISORDERS

Dissociation: loss or impaired sense of "self". Temporary alteration in consciousness, memory, personality, behavior or motor function. Causes impairment of functioning.

DISSOCIATIVE IDENTITY DISORDER
• *Presence of ≥2 DISTINCT IDENTITIES OR STATES OF PERSONALITIES* that take control of behavior (formerly known as multiple personality disorder). The symptoms of the disruption of the identity may be self-reported and/or observed by others.
• Gaps in the recall of events may occur for everyday and not just for traumatic events.

• MC in women. May be associated with history of *sexual abuse,** PTSD, substance use etc.

DEPERSONALIZATION/DEREALIZATION DISORDER
• *Persistent feelings of detachment or estrangement* from:
   - oneself (depersonalization) ex. "feel out of body" and/or
   - surrounding environment (derealization)
During these experiences, reality testing is intact & the symptoms cause distress.

DISSOCIATIVE AMNESIA
• *Inability to recall personal/autobiographical information.* Often secondary to sexual abuse, stress or trauma. It causes significant impairment in functioning.

• *Dissociative fugue: abrupt change in geographic location** with loss of identity or inability to recall the past.

• Before determining this diagnosis, neurologic testing must be done to rule out seizures or brain tumor as the cause.

Management of dissociative disorders: psychotherapy.

OBSESSIVE-COMPULSIVE & RELATED DISORDERS

Includes: obsessive-compulsive disorder, body dysmorphic disorder, hoarding disorder, trichotillomania (hair-pulling disorder) & excoriation (skin-picking) disorder.

OBSESSIVE-COMPULSIVE DISORDER (OCD)

• <u>OCD</u>: anxiety disorder characterized by a combination of ***thoughts (obsessions) + behaviors (compulsions).*** Men = women but men often present earlier in their teens.

• Mean age of onset 20y (onset rare after 50y).

• <u>OBSESSIONS:</u> ***recurrent or persistent thoughts/images.*** These thoughts are inappropriate, intrusive & unwanted. The patient tries to ignore or suppress the obsessions.

    Specifiers:
- <u>Good/fair insight:</u> recognizes OCD beliefs are not true or may not be true.
- <u>Poor insight:</u> thinks the OCD beliefs are probably true.
- <u>Absent insight/delusional beliefs:</u> completely convinced that the OCD beliefs are true.

• <u>COMPULSIONS:</u> ***repetitive behaviors the person feels driven to perform*** to reduce/prevent stress from the obsession. These compulsions often interfere with their lifestyle/time consuming.

CLINICAL MANIFESTATIONS
1. <u>4 Major patterns:</u> ❶**contamination** (compulsion may include cleaning or hand washing), ❷**pathologic doubt** (ex. forgetting to unplug iron), ❸ **symmetry/precision** (must arrange objects with precision) & ❹ **intrusive obsessive thoughts** without compulsion.

MANAGEMENT:
1. **Antidepressants:** *SSRIs* (Selective Serotonin Reuptake Inhibitors such as *Fluoxetine, Sertraline, Paroxetine*); TCAs (Tricyclic antidepressants); SNRIs (ex. *Venlafaxine*).

2. **Cognitive behavioral therapy:** exposure & response prevention, psychoeducation.

BODY DYSMORPHIC DISORDER

• Excessive <u>PREOCCUPATION THAT ≥1 BODY PART IS DEFORMED OR AN OVEREXAGGERATION OF A MINOR FLAW,</u> which often causes them to be ashamed or feel self-conscious & causes functional impairment.

• May *commit repetitive acts in response to this preoccupation* of physical flaw/defect (mirror checking, skin picking, seeking reassurance) or mental acts (comparison to others).

• MC in females. Often begins in teenage years.
• Patients may also have anxiety disorder or depression.

MANAGEMENT
1. Antidepressants: SSRIs (ex. *Fluoxetine*), TCAs (ex. *Clomipramine*).
2. Psychotherapy

SOMATIC SYMPTOM & RELATED DISORDERS

SOMATIC SYMPTOM DISORDER   (Formerly Somatization Disorder)

- Chronic condition in which the patient has _**PHYSICAL SYMPTOMS INVOLVING ≥1 PART OF THE BODY**_ BUT _**NO PHYSICAL CAUSE**_ CAN BE FOUND.
- MC in women. Onset usually before 30 years of age.
- Many patients previously diagnosed with hypochondriasis are now classified as having somatic symptom disorder.

CRITERIA

- One or more vague somatic symptoms that are distressing or result in significant disruption of daily life. These symptoms cannot be explained by a physical or medical cause.
  - ≥ 2 or more means a high likelihood of somatization disorder:

MNEMONIC	SYMPTOM	SYSTEM
Symptoms	Shortness of breath	Respiratory
Described as	Dysmenorrhea	Reproductive
Body	Burning in sexual organ	Psychosexual
Laments &	Lump in throat (dysphagia)	Pseudo neurological
Ailments	Amnesia	Pseudo neurological
Void a	Vomiting	GI
Physical cause	Painful extremities	Skeletal muscle

- Excessive thoughts, feelings, or behaviors related to the somatic symptoms:
  - disproportionate & persistent thoughts about the seriousness of the symptoms.
  - persistently high level of anxiety about symptoms or health.
  - excessive time & energy devoted to the symptoms & health concerns.

- Although any one of the somatic symptoms may not be continuously present, the state of being symptomatic is persistent (usually > 6 months).
- May or may not be associated with other medical conditions.

- Specifiers: _**with predominant pain**_ (previously pain disorder in DSM IV).

MANAGEMENT
1. _**Regularly scheduled visits to a healthcare provider.**_
   Patients are usually reticent to seek mental health counseling.

ILLNESS ANXIETY DISORDER   (Formerly HYPOCHONDRIASIS)

CRITERIA
- _**PREOCCUPATION WITH THE FEAR OR BELIEF ONE HAS OR WILL CONTRACT A SERIOUS, UNDIAGNOSED DISEASE**_ (despite reassurance and medical workups showing no disease). Symptoms last ≥6 months.
- Somatic symptoms are usually not present. If they are present, they are mild in intensity.
- Age 20-30y. Care seeking type: frequently get tested, "doctor shop". Care avoidance may be seen.

MANAGEMENT
1. _**Regularly scheduled appointments with their medical provider**_ for continued reassurance.

FUNCTIONAL NEUROLOGICAL SYMPTOM DISORDER (CONVERSION DISORDER)

- **_NEUROLOGIC DYSFUNCTION_** suggestive of a physical disorder **_THAT CANNOT BE EXPLAINED CLINICALLY_** (or by neurological pathophysiology). The symptoms cause significant distress or impairment.

- The **SYMPTOMS ARE NOT INTENTIONALLY PRODUCED OR FEIGNED*** (NOT due to malingering).
- Patients often have depression, anxiety, schizophrenia or personality disorders.

CLINICAL MANIFESTATIONS
Symptoms tend to be episodic and may recur during times of stress. MC in females and onset is usually in adolescence or young adulthood.
1. **Motor dysfunction: *paralysis***, aphonia, ***mutism,*** seizures, gait abnormalities, involuntary movements, tics, weakness, swallowing.
2. **Sensory dysfunction: *blindness,*** anesthesia, paresthesias, visual changes, deafness.
3. Patients often have depression, anxiety, schizophrenia or personality disorders.

MANAGEMENT
1. **Psychotherapy:** ex. behavioral therapy is ***treatment of choice.***

FACTITIOUS DISORDER

- **INTENTIONAL FALSIFICATION OR EXAGGERATION OF SIGNS & SYMPTOMS** *of medical or psychiatric illness* for "primary gain" (motivation of their actions is **ASSUMING THE SICK ROLE** TO **GET SYMPATHY).**

- Patients with factitious disorder have an ***inner need to be seen as ill or injured***, but ***NOT for concrete personal gain*** (as seen in malingering). The main difference between factitious and somatic symptom disorder is that patients with factitious deliberately fake their symptoms.
- May suffer from other mental disorders (ex. personality disorders).

TYPES:
1. ***Factitious disorder imposed on self –*** presents themselves as injured, impaired or ill.
2. ***Factitious disorder imposed on another*** *(by proxy)* ex. presents another as injured, impaired or ill (ex. child, elder or mentally disabled family member). It is considered a form of premeditated child or elder abuse.

CLINICAL MANIFESTATIONS
1. **Creation or exaggeration of symptoms of illness**: ex. may hurt themselves to bring on symptoms, alter diagnostic tests, lie or mimic symptoms. May inject themselves with substances to make themselves sick, etc. Medical history may be dramatic but inconsistent.

2. May be ***willing or eager to undergo surgery repeatedly or painful tests*** in order to obtain sympathy. They may "hospital jump", use other aliases or go to different cities to access care. They often have extensive knowledge about medial terminology, hospitals or great detail about their "illness" (may even work in healthcare).

MANAGEMENT: Nonspecific treatment.

Munchausen syndrome is an old term that referred to a severe form of factitious disorder characterized by the predominance of physical symptoms, use of aliases, habitual lying.

MALINGERING

- **INTENTIONAL FALSIFICATION OR EXAGGERATION OF SIGNS & SYMPTOMS** *of medical or psychiatric illness.*

- The primary motivation of their actions is **SECONDARY GAIN*:** financial gain (ex insurance money, lawsuits), food, shelter, avoidance of prison/school/work/military services, to obtain drugs (ex. narcotics). Malingering is not a mental illness.

- Both factitious disorder and malingering are associated with intentionally faking signs and symptoms. The difference is that in malingering, they feign illness for secondary gain whereas in factitious disorder the primary motive is to 'assume the sick role' & get sympathy.

CHILD ABUSE/NEGLECT

CHILD ABUSE & NEGLECT

- **SEXUAL ABUSE**
  - Abuser often male and often known to the victim (has accessibility).
  - Signs may include genital/anal trauma, sexually transmitted diseases, UTIs.

- **PHYSICAL ABUSE**
  - Abuser often female and usually the primary caregiver
  - Signs may include cigarette burns, burns in a stocking glove pattern, lacerations, healed fractures on radiographs, subdural hematoma, multiple bruises or retinal hemorrhages.
  - Hyphema or retinal hemorrhages seen in shaken baby syndrome

- **CHILD NEGLECT**
  - Failure to provide the basic needs of a child (ex. supervision, food, shelter, affection, education) etc.
  - Signs include: malnutrition, withdrawal, poor hygiene and failure to thrive.

EATING DISORDERS

OBESITY

- Obesity associated with ↑risk for coronary disease, diabetes mellitus, breast & colon cancers.

DIAGNOSIS
1. *Body mass index (BMI) > 30 kg/m² or body weight ≥20% over their ideal weight.*
2. **Binge eating (~50%):** recurrent episodes characterized by eating within a discrete time (ex. 2 hour period) more than people would in a similar period with lack of control during an eating episode. Binge eating occurs *at least weekly for 3 months.* ≥ 3 of the following:
   - eating until uncomfortably full, faster than normal, large amounts when not physically hungry, feeling disgusted/depressed/guilty afterwards, eating alone due to embarrassment. Binge eating disorder is a separate diagnosis from obesity.

MANAGEMENT
1. Behavior modification: exercise & dietary changes, group therapy.
2. Medical therapy: antidepressants if there is underlying depression. Treat any complications.
3. **Anti-obesity meds:** *Orlistat* (decreases GI fat digestion); *Lorcaserin* (serotonin agonist)
4. Surgical options: include gastric bypass, gastric sleeve, gastric banding, bariatric surgery.

ANOREXIA NERVOSA

- **REFUSAL TO MAINTAIN A MINIMALLY NORMAL BODY WEIGHT** fueling a relentless desire for thinness with a ***morbid fear of fatness or gaining weight*** (even though they are underweight).
  - Mid teens MC age of onset. 90% are ***women*** (60% are girls age 15-24y). Frequently seen in athletes, dancers (or other conditions requiring thinness). 60% incidence of depression.

CLINICAL MANIFESTATIONS
1. ***Exhibits behaviors targeted at maintaining a low weight*** or certain body image: ex. excess water intake, food-related obsessions (hoarding, collecting).
   - <u>Restrictive type</u>: reduced calorie intake, dieting, fasting excessive exercise, diet pills.
   - <u>Purging type</u>: primarily engages in self-induced vomiting, diuretic/laxative/enema abuse

DIAGNOSIS
1. Body mass index ***(BMI) ≤17.5 kg/m² or body weight <85% of ideal weight.***

2. **Physical examination:** emaciation, hypotension, bradycardia, skin/hair changes (ex. ***lanugo***), dry skin, salivary gland hypertrophy, amenorrhea, arrhythmias, osteoporosis.
3. **Labs:** leukocytosis, leukopenia, anemia; hypokalemia, ↑BUN (dehydration), hypothyroidism.

MANAGEMENT:
1. <u>Medical stabilization:</u> hospitalization for <75% expected body weight or patients who have medical complications. Electrolyte imbalances may lead to cardiac abnormalities.
2. <u>Psychotherapy:</u> cognitive behavioral therapy, supervised meals, weight monitoring.
3. <u>Pharmacotherapy:</u> if depressed ex: SSRIs; atypical antipsychotics (± also help c weight gain).

BULIMIA NERVOSA

- ***Major difference from anorexia*** is patients with ***bulimia have normal weight or ± overweight.***
- More common in females. Average onset of age in the late teens. Concerned about body image.

CLINICAL MANIFESTATIONS
1. ***Binge eating:*** recurrent episodes characterized by eating within a 2 hour period more than people would in a similar period with lack of control during an eating episode. ***Occurs at least weekly for 3 months***. May be triggered by stress/mood changes.

2. ***Compensatory behavior:***
   - ***Purging type:*** primarily engages in self-induced vomiting, diuretic/laxative/enema abuse.
   - <u>Non-purging type</u>: reduced calorie intake, dieting, fasting, excessive exercise, diet pills.

PHYSICAL AND LABORATORY FINDINGS
1. ***Teeth pitting or enamel erosion (from vomiting),*** Russell's sign (calluses on the dorsum of the hand from induced vomiting), parotid gland hypertrophy. Metabolic alkalosis from vomiting.
2. <u>Labs:</u> ± hypokalemia, hypomagnesemia. Electrolyte imbalance may lead to cardiac arrhythmias.

MANAGEMENT
1. <u>Psychotherapy:</u> cognitive behavioral therapy.

2. <u>Pharmacotherapy:</u> Fluoxetine has been shown to reduce the binge-purge cycle (but may have cardiovascular side effects especially if electrolyte abnormalities are present).

PERSONALITY DISORDERS

- 10-15% of population. Pervasive inflexible personality trait causing impaired function or distress.

CLUSTER A DISORDERS

- **_Cluster A:_** SOCIAL DETACHMENT with unusual behaviors: WEIRD, ODD, ECCENTRIC BEHAVIOR.

SCHIZOID PERSONALITY DISORDER

- Long pattern of <u>VOLUNTARY SOCIAL WITHDRAWAL **&** ANHEDONIC INTROVERSION</u> (constricted affect).
  - Usually early childhood onset. _LONER **"hermit-like behavior"**_ (reclusive). **_MC in males._**

CLINICAL MANIFESTATIONS
1. Inability to form relationships. Lifelong pattern of social withdrawal.
2. **_Anhedonic:_** appears indifferent to others, lacks response to praise or criticism or feelings expressed by others. **_Prefers to be alone (little enjoyment in close relationships, sex)._**
3. Appears eccentric, isolated or lonely, _<u>"COLD" FLATTENED AFFECT,</u>_ quiet & usually not sociable.

MANAGEMENT:
1. <u>**Psychotherapy:**</u> including individual or group therapy **_first line management._**
2. <u>Pharmacologic:</u> ± short-term low dose antipsychotics, antidepressants or psychostimulants.

SCHIZOTYPAL PERSONALITY DISORDER

- <u>ODD, ECCENTRIC BEHAVIOR **&** PECULIAR THOUGHT PATTERNS</u>* suggestive of schizophrenia but **_<u>without psychosis (delusions).</u>_** Usually early adulthood onset.

CLINICAL MANIFESTATIONS:
1. **_"odd" in behavior or appearance, inappropriate affect or speech, <u>"MAGICAL THINKING"</u>_*** _(believes in clairvoyance, telepathy, superstition, bizarre fantasies etc.)._ May talk to self in public.
2. _Pervasive discomfort with close relationships._ ± Restricted affect.

MANAGEMENT:
1. <u>**Psychotherapy:**</u> cognitive behavioral, individual or group therapy - **_treatment of choice._**
2. <u>Pharmacologic:</u> ± short term low-dose antipsychotics, antidepressants or benzodiazepines.

PARANOID PERSONALITY DISORDER

- <u>PERVASIVE PATTERN OF DISTRUST **&** SUSPICIOUSNESS OF OTHERS.</u>
- Begins in early adulthood. MC in males.

CLINICAL MANIFESTATIONS:
1. **_<u>Distrust & suspiciousness:</u> misinterprets the actions of others_** as malevolent, sees hidden messages, easily insulted, appears cold & serious, lack of interest in social relationships, bears grudges, doesn't forgive, blames their problems on others. **_Preoccupation with doubt regarding the loyalty of others._**

MANAGEMENT:
1. <u>**Psychotherapy:**</u> cognitive behavioral, individual or group therapy **_treatment of choice._**
2. <u>Pharmacologic:</u> <u>short-term</u> low doses of antipsychotics if severe (ex. Haloperidol) or Benzodiazepines (for anxiety or agitation) if necessary.

CLUSTER B DISORDERS

- **_Cluster B:_** "DRAMATIC, WILD, ERRATIC, IMPULSIVE & EMOTIONAL"

ANTISOCIAL PERSONALITY DISORDER

- Behaviors DEVIATING SHARPLY FROM THE NORMS, VALUES & LAWS OF SOCIETY (harmful or hostile to society). **_May commit criminal acts_** with disregard to violation of laws.
  - **_May begin in childhood as conduct disorders_** but **_must be ≥18y to dx.*_** 3x MC in males.

CLINICAL MANIFESTATIONS
1. **_Inability to conform to social norms_** with _DISREGARD & VIOLATION OF THE RIGHTS OF OTHERS,_ lack of empathy, _pattern of criminal behavior,_ shows little anxiety. Extremely manipulative, deceitful, impulsive, promiscuous, spouse/child abuse, lacks remorse, lies frequently, endangers others (ex. **_drunk-driving common)._**

MANAGEMENT
1. **_Psychotherapy_**: establishing limits.
2. Pharmacologic: not helpful.

BORDERLINE PERSONALITY DISORDER

- **_Unstable, unpredictable mood & affect._** UNSTABLE SELF IMAGE & RELATIONSHIPS. MC seen in women.

CLINICAL MANIFESTATIONS
1. Extreme pattern of instability in relationships but cannot tolerate "being alone." Often have **_'MOOD SWINGS'.*_** Marked sensitivity to criticism & rejection (fear of abandonment).
2. **_'BLACK & WHITE THINKING':_** thinks in extremes "all good" or "all bad" with no middle ground.
3. **_Impulsivity in self-damaging behaviors:_** _suicide threats, self-mutilation, substance abuse, reckless driving, binge eating, spending._

MANAGEMENT
1. **Psychotherapy:** **_treatment of choice._** _Dialectical,_ cognitive behavior & group therapy
2. Pharmacologic: ± short-term low doses antipsychotics, antidepressants or benzodiazepines.

HISTRIONIC PERSONALITY DISORDER

- OVERLY EMOTIONAL, DRAMATIC, SEDUCTIVE.* "ATTENTION-SEEKING".*

CLINICAL MANIFESTATIONS
1. **_Self-absorbed, 'temper tantrums",_** efforts to draw attention to themselves with need to be the **_center of attention._** Often **_inappropriate, sexually provocative, seductive_** with shallow or exaggerated emotions. Seeks reassurance & praise often. May believe their relationships are more intimate than they are in actuality. Can be suggestible (easily influenced by others or circumstances).

MANAGEMENT:
1. **Psychotherapy:** **_treatment of choice.*_** Cognitive behavioral, individual or group therapy.

NARCISSISTIC PERSONALITY DISORDER

• _**Grandiose often excessive sense of SELF-IMPORTANCE* but needs praise & admiration.**_ MC in males.

CLINICAL MANIFESTATIONS:
1. _**Inflated self-image: considers themselves special, entitled, requires extra special attention BUT**_ they have _**fragile self-esteem**_ (occupied with fantasies, jealousy of others, believes others are envious of them & has difficulty with the aging process). Reacts to rejection/criticism with rage. Often becomes depressed. Lacks empathy for others.

MANAGEMENT:
1. **Psychotherapy:** _**treatment of choice.**_ Includes individual or group therapy.

CLUSTER C DISORDERS

• _**Cluster C:**_ ANXIOUS, WORRIED & FEARFUL.

AVOIDANT PERSONALITY DISORDER

• _**Desires relationships but**_ AVOIDS RELATIONSHIPS DUE TO "INFERIORITY COMPLEX"* (intense feelings of inadequacy, sensitive to criticism, fears rejection & humiliation). Timid, shy & lacks confidence.

MANAGEMENT:
1. Psychotherapy: ex. social training, cognitive behavioral or group therapy.
2. Pharmacologic: ± Beta blockers for anxiety or SSRIs for depression.

DEPENDENT PERSONALITY DISORDER

• DEPENDENT, SUBMISSIVE BEHAVIOR (very 'needy' & 'clingy').

CLINICAL MANIFESTATIONS:
1. _**Constantly needs to be reassured, relies on others**_ for decision-making & emotional support, _**will not initiate things,**_ intense discomfort when alone. May volunteer for unpleasant tasks.

MANAGEMENT
1. **Psychotherapy:** including behavioral & group therapy.
2. Anxiolytics or antidepressants may be used in some cases for symptomatic control.

OBSESSIVE-COMPULSIVE PERSONALITY DISORDER

• _**PERFECTIONISTS who require a great deal of ORDER & CONTROL:**_ rigid adherence to routine (rules, lists, details, inflexible, stubborn, lacks spontaneity). Any change in their routine may lead to extreme anxiety. Often makes moral judgment on others.
• _**Preoccupied with minute details**_ (may find it difficult to finish projects, hesitates to delegate work to others, devotes themselves to their work). May avoid intimacy.

MANAGEMENT:
1. Psychotherapy
2. Pharmacologic: ± Beta blockers for anxiety or SSRI's for depression.

CHILDHOOD DISORDERS

AUTISM SPECTRUM DISORDER

- Spectrum of developmental disorders probably linked to a combination of prenatal viral exposure, immune system abnormalities and/or genetic factors. Male: female 4:1.

CLINICAL MANIFESTATIONS
1. **Primary signs:**
   - *__social interaction difficulties:__* significant emotional discomfort or detachment (ex avoiding eye contact, no response to cuddling or affection).
   - *__impaired communication:__* either inability to communicate or has the ability to communicate but chooses not to in social settings. Difficulties in understanding what is not explicitly stated (ex. metaphors, humor in jokes etc.).
   - *__restricted, repetitive, stereotyped behaviors__* & patterns of activities.

2. **Other signs**
   - persistent failure to develop social relationships, failure to show preference to parents over other adults; unusual sensitivity to visual, auditory or olfactory stimuli; unusual attachments to ordinary objects. Savantism (unusual talents).

MANAGEMENT
1. Referral for neuropsychologic testing, behavioral modification strategies, medications.

OPPOSITIONAL DEFIANT DISORDER

- Persistent pattern of negative, hostile & DEFIANT BEHAVIOR TOWARDS ADULTS.

- At least 6 months of the following 3 components: ❶ *angry/irritable mood* (ex. often blames others for their misbehaviors, has negative attitudes & has anger/resentment ❷ *argumentative/defiant behavior* ❸ *vindictiveness.*

MANAGEMENT
1. Psychotherapy: behavioral therapy. No association with psychosis. May progress to conduct disorder.

CONDUCT DISORDER

- Persistent pattern of behaviors that DEVIATE SHARPLY FROM THE AGE-APPROPRIATE NORMS & VIOLATE THE RIGHTS OF OTHERS.

- *Social & academic difficulty.*

- 4 main areas: ❶ *serious violations of laws.* Includes defying authority & sexual disinhibition ❷ *aggressive/cruel to animals* (ex. causes fights, throws tantrums, tortures animals). ❸ *deceitfulness:* includes stealing, lying, lacking guilt/remorse ❹*destruction of property* (ex. *sets fires*).

- Poor prognosis....*__40% develop antisocial personality disorder.__* *MC in boys.*

ATTENTION-DEFICIT DISORDER (ADD) & ATTENTION-DEFICIT HYPERACTIVITY DISORDER (ADHD)

• Neurodevelopmental disorder characterized by problems paying attention, difficulty controlling behaviors & hyperactivity that is not age-appropriate.

DIAGNOSIS

1. Symptoms of hyperactivity/impulsivity or inattentiveness leading to impairment. These symptoms must have on onset **before 12y of age** and must be present for at least 6 months.

2. Symptoms **_must occur in at least 2 settings_** (ex school, home, recreational activities). At least 6 of the following symptoms:

INATTENTIVENESS
1. Easily distracted: misses details, frequently switches from one activity to another, forget things, easily distracted when multiple things are happening simultaneously.
2. Has difficulty maintaining focus on one task or learning something new.
3. Misses details and may make careless mistakes.
4. Forgets things or loses things (ex. pencils) needed to complete activities and tasks.
5. Difficulty in completing assignments.
6. Becomes bored with a task after a few minutes, unless doing something enjoyable.

HYPERACTIVITY/IMPULSIVITY
1. Fidgets and squirms in their seat.
2. Constantly in motion (may often leave their seat).
3. Talks nonstop or excessively.
4. Impatience.
5. Dashes around, touching or playing with everything in sight.
6. Has trouble sitting for long periods (ex doing homework, dinner or school).
7. Difficulty doing quiet tasks.
8. Restlessness.
9. Blurts out appropriate or inappropriate comments, shows unrestrained emotions.
10. Interrupts the conversation or the activities of others.

MANAGEMENT

Multimodal approach:

1. Behavior modification
2. **Sympathomimetic medications (stimulants)**: **_pharmacologic treatment of choice._**
   Methylphenidate *(Ritalin)*, **_Amphetamine/dextroamphetamine_** *(Adderall),*
   Dexmethylphenidate *(Focalin)*
   - **MOA:** blocks norepinephrine & dopamine reuptake. Increases release of norepinephrine & dopamine in the extraneuronal space.
   - **Ind:** ADD, ADHD, narcolepsy, excessive daytime sleepiness.
   - **S/E:** anxiety, hypertension, tachycardia, weight loss, growth delays, addiction.

3. **Nonstimulants:**
   - **_Atomoxetine_** (Strattera).
     MOA: selective norepinephrine reuptake inhibitor. Similar efficacy and side effect profile as stimulants (but side effects occur less often & less addictive ability).

   - Adjunctive medications: Bupropion, Venlafaxine, Guanfacine, Clonidine.

DRUG ABUSE/DEPENDENCE

TOBACCO USE/DEPENDENCE

• Tobacco is a major cause of pulmonary, cardiac and cancer deaths (most modifiable risk factor).

CLINICAL MANIFESTATIONS OF NICOTINE WITHDRAWAL

• Includes restlessness, anxiety, irritability, sleep abnormalities, depression, nicotine craving.

MANAGEMENT

Includes counseling and support therapy, cognitive behavioral therapy.
1. **Nicotine tapering therapy:** gum, nasal sprays, transdermal patches, inhaler, lozenges.

2. **Bupropion:** (Zyban) - antidepressant drug often used in combination with nicotine tapering therapy.

3. **Varenicline:** (Chantix) blocks the nicotine receptors, reducing nicotine activity.

OPIOID USE/DEPENDENCE

• Includes heroin, Oxycodone, Morphine, Meperidine & Codeine.

CLINICAL MANIFESTATIONS

1. Opioid intoxication:
- **Euphoria & sedation:** drowsiness, impaired social functioning, impaired memory, slow or slurred speech. May develop nausea, vomiting. Seizures. Coma.

- **Physical examination findings:** *pupillary constriction** (narcotics are miotics), **respiratory depression.** * May also develop *Biot's breathing* (groups of quick, shallow inspirations followed by regular or irregular periods of apnea), **bradycardia, hypotension,** nausea, vomiting, flushing. Patients on long-term narcotics may develop constipation (opioid receptors in the GI tract reduce GI motility), hypothermia.

2. Opioid Withdrawal:
- Lacrimation, hypertension, pruritus, tachycardia, nausea/vomiting, abdominal cramps, diarrhea, sweating, yawning, **piloerections** * (goose bumps), **pupil dilation (mydriasis),** * **flu-like symptoms: rhinorrhea,** joint pains, myalgias.

MANAGEMENT

1. **Acute intoxication:** *Naloxone** (Narcan):* used in acute intoxication or overdose to acutely reverse the effects of opioids. Onset of action ~2 minutes IV (~5 minutes IM). ~30-60 minute duration of action. Most commonly used in patients with *respiratory depression.*

2. **Withdrawal**
   - Symptomatic control: Clonidine (decreases sympathetic symptoms), Loperamide for diarrhea, NSAIDs for joint pains & muscle cramps. Buprenorphine + Naloxone.
   - Methadone tapering. Benzodiazepines may be helpful in some cases of mild withdrawal.

3. **Long term management of dependence or detoxification:**
   - Methadone maintenance program. Suboxone (Buprenorphine + Naloxone).

	INTOXICATION		WITHDRAWAL	
	BEHAVIORAL/MOOD EFFECTS	PSYCHOLOGICAL EFFECTS	ONSET	SYMPTOMS
ETHANOL BENZODIAZEPINES	Disinhibition **Depression:** slurred speech, impaired judgment & somnolence. Ataxia. Labile Mood: erratic behavior, aggression *Flumazenil used to treat benzodiazepine intoxication**	Prolonged reaction time, muscular incoordination, facial flushing **Chronic:** - **Wernicke's encephalopathy:** triad of ataxia, confusion & oculomotor palsy (due to thiamine/B1 deficiency). - **Korsakoff syndrome** amnesia (both retrograde & antegrade) - Hepatomegaly, palmar erythema, cirrhosis, Dupuytrens contractures, gynecomastia, testicular atrophy. - Increased mean corpuscular volume	6-24 hours 6 – 48 hours 2 – 5 days	*Increased CNS activity* tremor*, insomnia, nausea, vomiting, anxiety, tachycardia, hypertension, increased respirations Seizures, hyperreflexia *DELIRIUM TREMENS:* **altered sensorium:** tactile, visual or auditory hallucinations (ex. **formication – "something crawling" on them) especially at night,** altered mental status, seizures, coma, death. ***Often occurs when hospitalized for a nonrelated illness.***
STIMULANTS COCAINE AMPHETAMINES	• **Initial:** elevated/euphoric mood, restlessness, pressured speech • **Psychosis:** mild ⇔ anxiety. Paranoia, ***aggression, agitation,*** hallucinations (Ex. tactile, auditory) • *Treat cocaine intoxication with benzodiazepines,* neuroleptics & blood pressure reduction.	• **Neurologic:** ↑motor activity, headache, tremor, flushing, hyperthermia, cold sweats, nausea, vomiting, seizures • ***SYMPATHETIC STIMULATION:*** sweating, tachycardia, **hypertension, *pupillary dilation*,*** peripheral vasoconstriction, myocardial infarction. • Compulsive & stereotyped behavior (ex. picking at skin), rhabdomyolysis.	Varied onset	Craving with resultant dysphoria, agitation, anxiety, diaphoresis, **hypersomnia, increased appetite.** **Neurologic:** nightmares, ***suicide ideation*,*** headache, irritability, extreme fatigue, muscle cramps.
OPIOIDS & NARCOTICS	• **Euphoria & sedation:** drowsiness, impaired social functioning, impaired memory, slow or slurred speech. • *Naloxone (Narcan) used to treat opioid intoxication**	• ***Pupillary constriction**** *(narcotics are miotics).* • ***Respiratory depression,* bradycardia, hypotension,*** coma, nausea, vomiting, hypothermia. • Chronic: pruritus & constipation (opioid receptors in GI tract decreases motility).	6-24 hours (Methadone may take longer)	Neurologic: psychomotor agitation, anxiety, irritability, twitching, yawning dysphoria, insomnia, diaphoresis Vitals: hyperthermia, hypertension, tachycardia Flulike sx: ***rhinorrhea*,*** myalgias, chills, ***piloerections**** (Goosebumps). GI: nausea, vomiting, diarrhea Ocular: ***pupillary dilation*, tearing***
NICOTINE	• Nausea, vomiting, diarrhea, abdominal pain, headache	Tremor, tachycardia, salivation	Usually begin within 24h after last use	Psychomotor: anxiety, restlessness, bradycardia, increased appetite & craving
CANNABIS	• Euphoria, giddiness. • Psychosis in some cases.	Dry mouth (cotton-mouth), conjunctival erythema, tachycardia, hypotension	Usually on seen with heavy usage	Irritability insomnia, restlessness, diaphoresis, diarrhea, twitches.
PCP	• Impulsiveness, homicidality, psychosis, delirium, seizures, **nystagmus**			Depression, irritability, anxiety, sleep problems
LSD	• Visual hallucinations & synesthesias (seeing sound as color), delusions, pupillary dilation			

ALCOHOL WITHDRAWAL

CLINICAL MANIFESTATIONS

1. UNCOMPLICATED ALCOHOL WITHDRAWAL: 6 – 24 hours after last drink (time may vary).
   *Increased CNS activity:** tremors, anxiety, diaphoresis, palpitations, insomnia, GI (nausea, vomiting, diarrhea). Uncomplicated = no seizures, hallucinosis or delirium tremens.

2. WITHDRAWAL SEIZURES: 6 – 48 hours after last drink.
   Usually generalized tonic-clonic type. MC occurs as a single episode.

3. ALCOHOLIC HALLUCINOSIS: 12 – 48 hours after last drink.
   Visual auditory and/or tactile *hallucinations.*
   Patient has a *clear sensorium & normal vital signs.*

4. DELIRIUM TREMENS: *2 – 5 days after last drink.*
   Delirium (altered sensorium), hallucinations, agitation.
   Abnormal vital signs (ex. tachycardia, hypertension, fever). Patients often diaphoretic.

MANAGEMENT

Requires medical treatment & hospitalization. *Alcohol withdrawal can potentially be fatal.*

1. *IV Benzodiazepines:*
   Diazepam (Valium), *Lorazepam* (Ativan), *Chlordiazepoxide* (Librium), *Oxazepam*
   MOA: *potentiates GABA-mediated CNS inhibition.* ETOH mimics GABA at the receptor sites (GABA is the most abundant inhibitory neurotransmitter in the CNS) so ETOH withdrawal causes increased CNS activity. Benzodiazepines are titrated until they patient is slightly somnolent & then gradually tapered.
   Lorazepam or Oxazepam preferred in patients with advanced cirrhosis or alcoholic hepatitis (Chlordiazepoxide may cause over titration in these patients).

2. **IV fluids & supplementation:** *IV thiamine & magnesium (prior to glucose administration),* multivitamins (including B12/folate), IV fluids + dextrose. Intoxication may cause hypoglycemia. If glucose is given before thiamine, it may induce Korsakoff's syndrome in some patients (not really proven but the order may show up on exam questions).

3. Avoidance of medications that can lower seizure threshold if possible (ex. Bupropion, Haloperidol, anticonvulsants, Clonidine, beta-blockers)

ALCOHOL INTOXICATION

CLINICAL MANIFESTATIONS
1. Disinhibition, ***depression:*** slurred speech, impaired judgment & somnolence. Ataxia, impaired attention or memory. Labile mood: erratic behavior, aggression.

MANAGEMENT
1. **Acute intoxication:** *Observation* (allow for the drug to be metabolized).

2. Chronic patients or known alcohol-dependent patients: Observation. They should also receive thiamine & folate. ***IV thiamine & magnesium (prior to glucose administration),*** multivitamins (including B12/folate), IV fluids + dextrose. Intoxication may cause hypoglycemia. If glucose is given before thiamine, it may induce Korsakoff's syndrome in some patients (not really proven but the order may show up on exam questions).

3. **Psychosis or severe aggression:** Haloperidol. Patients should be sedated.

ALCOHOL DEPENDENCE

- Alcohol abuse becomes dependence when withdrawal symptoms develop or tolerance.

CAGE ALCOHOL SCREENING
≥2 considered a positive screen.

Cutdown	Have you felt the need to cut down on drinking?
Annoyed	Have people told you that they were annoyed at you when you drink?
Guilt	Have you ever felt guilty about your drinking?
Eye opener	Have you ever needed an eye opener to start your day or reduce jitteriness?

MANAGEMENT
1. Supportive: psychotherapy: ex individual, group (ex. Alcoholics Anonymous); Inpatient & residential rehabilitation programs.

2. ***Disulfiram (Antabuse)**** can be a deterrent to alcohol use.
    MOA: inhibits aldehyde dehydrogenase (enzyme needed to metabolize alcohol), leading to increased acetaldehyde when coupled with alcohol intake ⇨ uncomfortable symptoms including: hypotension, palpitations, flushing, hyperventilation, dizziness, nausea, vomiting and headache.
    CI: patients with cardiovascular disease, diabetes mellitus, hypothyroidism, epilepsy, kidney or liver disease.

3. ***Naltrexone:*** opioid antagonist that reduces alcohol craving & reduces alcohol-induced euphoria.

4. Gabapentin, Topiramate.

SUICIDE RISK FACTORS

- **Previous attempt or threat is the strongest single predictive factor** (since a majority of suicide attempts occur on the first try). If suspected, the patient should be directly asked if they have a plan.
- <u>Sex:</u> **females attempt suicide more than males, however males complete suicide more often** than women.
- <u>Age:</u> increases with age (but teenagers attempt it more often than older adults).
      Elderly white men have the highest suicide rate in the US.
- <u>Race:</u> whites > blacks.
- <u>Psychiatric disorders:</u> majority of people who attempt or commit suicide have underlying psychiatric disorders (especially depression, bipolar disorder, substance abuse, schizophrenia, anxiety disorders).
- <u>Substance abuse</u> associated with an increased risk.
- <u>Marital status:</u> alone > never married > widowed > separated or divorced > married without children > married with children (marriage is protective).
      <u>Others:</u> positive family history of suicide, history of impulsivity, or chronic illnesses. Among highly skilled workers, physicians are at an increased risk of suicide.

GRIEF REACTION

- Altered emotional state as a response to a major loss (ex. death of a loved one).
- Only persistent complex bereavement disorder is considered a mental disorder.

- **Normal grief: *resolves within 1 year*.** It peaks usually within the first couple months of the loss. May progress to major depressive disorder.

- <u>Abnormal grief:</u> severe symptoms, continued symptoms >1 year, positive suicide ideation.

- <u>Persistent complex bereavement disorder:</u> severe grief reactions that persists >1 year (or 6 months in children) after the death of the bereaved.

CLINICAL MANIFESTATIONS
1. **Normal grief:** sadness, irritability, intense yearning for a loved one, poor concentration, sleep disturbances, illusions/hallucinations (hearing or seeing the dead) but patient perceives the illusions/hallucinations as not being real.
   - Normal responses include denial, shock, confusion, sadness, numbness or guilt. May develop depressive symptoms.

2. **Abnormal grief:** suicide ideation, psychosis, psychomotor deficits, illusions/hallucinations (hearing or seeing the dead) but the patient perceives the illusions/hallucinations as being real.

MANAGEMENT
1. <u>Psychotherapy:</u> cognitive behavioral, supportive. Benzodiazepine may be used for insomnia.

SELECTED REFERENCES

Patel G, Fancher TL. In the clinic. Generalized anxiety disorder. Ann Intern Med. 2013;159(11):ITC6-1, ITC6-2, ITC6-3, ITC6-4, ITC6-5, ITC6-6, ITC6-7, ITC6-8, ITC6-9, ITC6-10, ITC6-11.
Nickel JC. Prostatitis. Can Urol Assoc J. 2011;5(5):306-15.

Price JS. Evolutionary aspects of anxiety disorders. Dialogues Clin Neurosci. 2003;5(3):223-36.

Lam RW, Levitan RD. Pathophysiology of seasonal affective disorder: a review. J Psychiatry Neurosci. 2000;25(5):469-80.

Mansell W, Pedley R. The ascent into mania: a review of psychological processes associated with the development of manic symptoms. Clin Psychol Rev. 2008;28(3):494-520.

Association AP. Diagnostic and Statistical Manual of Mental Disorders, Fifth Edition, DSM-V®. American Psychiatric Pub; 2013.

Strakowski SM, Adler CM, Almeida J, et al. The functional neuroanatomy of bipolar disorder: a consensus model. Bipolar Disord. 2012;14(4):313-25.

Sood AB, Razdan A, Weller EB, Weller RA. How to differentiate bipolar disorder from attention deficit hyperactivity disorder and other common psychiatric disorders: a guide for clinicians. Curr Psychiatry Rep. 2005;7(2):98-103.

Widiger TA. Personality disorder diagnosis. World Psychiatry. 2003;2(3):131-5.

Standage KF. The use of Schneider's typology for the diagnosis of personality disorders--an examination of reliability. Br J Psychiatry. 1979;135:238-42.

Tyrer P, Mitchard S, Methuen C, Ranger M. Treatment rejecting and treatment seeking personality disorders: Type R and Type S. J Pers Disord. 2003;17(3):263-8.

Villemarette-pittman NR, Stanford MS, Greve KW, Houston RJ, Mathias CW. Obsessive-compulsive personality disorder and behavioral disinhibition. J Psychol. 2004;138(1):5-22.

Halmi KA. Obsessive-compulsive personality disorder and eating disorders. Eat Disord. 2005;13(1):85-92.

Van os J, Kapur S. Schizophrenia. Lancet. 2009;374(9690):635-45.

Buckley PF, Miller BJ, Lehrer DS, Castle DJ. Psychiatric comorbidities and schizophrenia. Schizophr Bull. 2009;35(2):383-402.

Smith T, Weston C, Lieberman J. Schizophrenia (maintenance treatment). Am Fam Physician. 2010;82(4):338-9.

Hartling L, Abou-setta AM, Dursun S, Mousavi SS, Pasichnyk D, Newton AS. Antipsychotics in adults with schizophrenia: comparative effectiveness of first-generation versus second-generation medications: a systematic review and meta-analysis. Ann Intern Med. 2012;157(7):498-511.

Ananth J, Parameswaran S, Gunatilake S, Burgoyne K, Sidhom T. Neuroleptic malignant syndrome and atypical antipsychotic drugs. J Clin Psychiatry. 2004;65(4):464-70.

Rosen JC, Reiter J, Orosan P. Assessment of body image in eating disorders with the body dysmorphic disorder examination. Behav Res Ther. 1995;33(1):77-84.

Attia E, Walsh BT. Anorexia nervosa. Am J Psychiatry. 2007;164(12):1805-10.

Hay PJ, Claudino AM. Bulimia nervosa. Clin Evid (Online). 2010;2010

Caronna EB, Milunsky JM, Tager-flusberg H. Autism spectrum disorders: clinical and research frontiers. Arch Dis Child. 2008;93(6):518-23.

Rustad JK, Musselman DL, Nemeroff CB. The relationship of depression and diabetes: pathophysiological and treatment implications. Psychoneuroendocrinology. 2011;36(9):1276-86.

Francis K. Autism interventions: a critical update. Dev Med Child Neurol. 2005;47(7):493-9.

Walsh CA, Morrow EM, Rubenstein JL. Autism and brain development. Cell. 2008;135(3):396-400.

Fisher JA. Investigating the Barons: narrative and nomenclature in Munchausen syndrome. Perspect Biol Med. 2006;49(2):250-62.

Kroenke K. Efficacy of treatment for somatoform disorders: a review of randomized controlled trials. Psychosom Med. 2007;69(9):881-8.

Tsai MH, Huang YS. Attention-deficit/hyperactivity disorder and sleep disorders in children. Med Clin North Am. 2010;94(3):615-32.

Kumar R, Sachdev PS. Akathisia and second-generation antipsychotic drugs. Curr Opin Psychiatry. 2009;22(3):293-99.

Riederer P, Lachenmayer L, Laux G. Clinical applications of MAO-inhibitors. Curr Med Chem. 2004;11(15):2033-43.

Owens MJ, Morgan WN, Plott SJ, Nemeroff CB. Neurotransmitter receptor and transporter binding profile of antidepressants and their metabolites. J Pharmacol Exp Ther. 1997;283(3):1305-22.

Bymaster FP, Dreshfield-ahmad LJ, Threlkeld PG, et al. Comparative affinity of duloxetine and venlafaxine for serotonin and norepinephrine transporters in vitro and in vivo, human serotonin receptor subtypes, and other neuronal receptors. Neuropsychopharmacology. 2001;25(6):871-80.

CHAPTER 11 – DERMATOLOGIC DISORDERS

SKIN BASICS

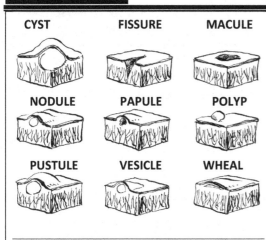

CYST   FISSURE   MACULE

NODULE   PAPULE   POLYP

PUSTULE   VESICLE   WHEAL

MACULE: flat nonpalpable lesion <10mm.
PATCH: flat nonpalpable lesion >10 mm.

PAPULE: solid, raised lesions <5mm in diameter.
NODULE: solid, raised lesions >5mm in diameter.

PLAQUE: raised, flat-topped lesion >10mm.

VESICLE: circumscribed, elevated fluid-filled lesion <5mm.
BULLA: circumscribed, elevated fluid-filled lesion >5mm.

PUSTULE: pus-filled vesicle or bulla.

WHEAL: transient, elevated lesion (local edema).

PETECHIAE: small punctate hemorrhages that don't blanch.

ALOPECIA AREATA

- *Nonscarring immune-mediated hair loss* targeting the anagen hair follicles. Scalp MC.

- Commonly **associated with other autoimmune disorders:** ex. thyroid, Addison's disease.

CLINICAL MANIFESTATIONS
1. **Smooth discrete circular patches of complete hair loss** that develops over a period of weeks.
   - **Exclamation point hairs*** short hairs broken off a few mm from the scalp at the margins
     of the patches with *tapering near the proximal hair shaft* (exclamation point)!
   - In some causes, it may be diffuse loss, hair regrowth may occur (fine white hair regrowth).
2. Nail abnormalities:
     pitting may be seen in ~30%, nail fissuring, trachyonychia (roughening of the nail plate) etc.
3. May spontaneously resolve or progress to alopecia totalis (complete scalp hair loss) or alopecia universalis (complete hair loss on the scalp & body – including the eyelashes).

MANAGEMENT
1. Local: intralesional corticosteroids. Extensive: topical corticosteroids.
2. May be observed in mild cases. Relapse is common.

ANDROGENETIC ALOPECIA

- Progressive loss of the terminal hairs on the scalp in a characteristic distribution (pattern).

- Dihydrotestosterone (DHT) is the key androgen leading to androgenetic alopecia.

CLINICAL MANIFESTATIONS
- Varying degrees of hair thinning & nonscarring hair loss MC affecting the temporal scalp, midfront scalp or vertex area of the scalp.

MANAGEMENT
1. **Minoxidil:** best used if recent onset alopecia involving a smaller area.

2. **Oral Finasteride: *5-α reductase inhibitor*** - androgen inhibitor (inhibits the conversion of testosterone to dihydrotestosterone). S/E: decreased libido, sexual or ejaculatory dysfunction.

ECZEMATOUS ERUPTIONS

ATOPIC DERMATITIS (ECZEMA)

- *Atopic disease association.* Atopic triad:* ❶*eczema* ❷*allergic rhinitis* ❸ *asthma.* Starts in childhood.

PATHOPHYSIOLOGY
1. *Altered immune reaction* in genetically susceptible people when exposed to certain triggers ⇨ T cell mediated immune activation & *↑IgE production.*

TRIGGERS: heat, perspiration, allergens & contact irritants (ex wool, nickel, food).

CLINICAL MANIFESTATIONS
pruritus hallmark
1. **Acute lesions:** erythematous, ill-defined blisters/papules/plaques; Later ⇨ dries, crusts over & scales (looks similar to psoriasis). *MC in flexor creases* (ex. antecubital & popliteal folds).
   - Dermatographism: localized development of hives when the skin is stroked.

2. *Nummular eczema: sharply defined discoid/COIN-SHAPED* lesions* especially on the dorsum of the hands, feet & extensor surfaces (knees, elbows).

MANAGEMENT
1. **Acute: *topical corticosteroids,* antihistamines for itching*** (diphenhydramine, hydroxyzine). Wet dressings (ex. Burrow's solution). Antibiotics if secondary infection develops.
   - Topical calcineurin inhibitors (ex. *Tacrolimus, Pimecrolimus*) are alternatives to steroids (no skin atrophy like steroids). S/E: irritation, possible lymphoma/skin cancer risk.

2. Chronic lesions: daily hydration & emollients. Oral antihistamines used for pruritus.

3. **Health maintenance:** avoid exacerbating factors or irritants (ex. soaps, detergents, frequent baths). Maintain skin hydration: skin emollients (ex. Eucerin, Aquaphor), tepid baths.

CONTACT DERMATITIS

- Irritants: chemicals, detergents, cleaners, acids, prolonged water exposure, metals etc.
- **Diaper rash:** prolonged exposure to urine &/or feces in infants.

CLINICAL MANIFESTATIONS
Burning, itching & erythema to the affected area, dry skin, eczematous eruption.

MANAGEMENT
1. Avoid irritants. Protective equipment, wet dressings (Burrow's solution). Topical corticosteroids.
2. Diaper rash: frequent diaper changes, topical petroleum or zinc oxide to the affected area.

DYSHIDROSIS (DYSHIDROTIC ECZEMA)   (POMPHOLYX)

Triggers: sweating, emotional stress, warm & humid weather, metals (ex. nickel).

CLINICAL:
Pruritic "tapioca-like" tense vesicles on the soles, palms & fingers (ex. *lateral digits*).

MANAGEMENT
Topical steroids (med-high) *ointments preferred,* cold compresses, Burrow's solution, tar soaks.

LICHEN SIMPLEX CHRONICUS (NEURODERMATITIS)

• *Skin thickening* in patients *with eczema* 2ry to *repetitive rubbing/scratching* -"itch-scratch" cycle.

CLINICAL MANIFESTATIONS
Scaly, well-demarcated, rough hyperkeratotic plaques *with exaggerated skin lines.*

MANAGEMENT
*avoid scratching the lesions, topical steroids** (high-strength), antihistamines, occlusive dressings.

PERIORAL DERMATITIS

• MC seen in young women. May have a history of topical corticosteroid use.
CLINICAL MANIFESTATIONS
Papulopustules on an erythematous base, which may become confluent into plaques with scales. May have satellite lesions. Classically spares the vermillion border.

MANAGEMENT
Topical: *Metronidazole or Erythromycin.* Oral: Tetracyclines. *Avoid topical corticosteroids.*

PAPULOSQUAMOUS DISEASES

LICHEN PLANUS

PATHOPHYSIOLOGY: idiopathic cell-mediated immune response. ↑*Incidence with Hepatitis C.**

CLINICAL MANIFESTATIONS
1. **5 P's: Purple, Polygonal, Planar, Pruritic Papules with fine scales** & irregular borders.
   - MC on flexor surfaces of extremities, *skin, mouth, scalp, genitals, nails* & mucous membranes.
   - May also develop *Koebner's phenomenon:* new lesions at sites of trauma (also seen in psoriasis).

   - *WICKHAM STRIAE:** fine white lines on the skin lesions or on the oral mucosa. Nail dystrophy.

MANAGEMENT
1. *Topical corticosteroid 1st line.** Symptomatic tx: antihistamines for pruritus, occlusive dressings.
2. 2nd line: PO steroids, UVB therapy, Retinoids. The rash usually resolves spontaneously in 8-12 months.

PITYRIASIS ROSEA

• Uncertain etiology (±associated with *viral infections–HHV7).* Primarily older *children/young adults.*
• ↑ in the spring/fall. Can mimic syphilis (so order RPR if the patient is sexually active).

CLINICAL MANIFESTATIONS
1. *HERALD PATCH** (solitary salmon-colored macule) on the trunk 2-6 cm in diameter ⇨ general exanthem 1-2 weeks later: smaller, very pruritic 1 cm round/oval *salmon-colored papules* with white circular *(collarette) scaling along cleavage lines** in a *Christmas Tree pattern.**
   - *Confined to trunk & proximal extremities* (face usually spared). Resolves in 6-12 weeks.

MANAGEMENT
1. *None needed.* Pruritus: PO antihistamines, topical corticosteroids, oatmeal baths.
2. ±UVB phototherapy if severe & started early on in the course.

PSORIASIS

- Chronic, multisystemic inflammatory immune disorder with genetic predisposition.

PATHOPHYSIOLOGY
Keratin hyperplasia *(proliferating cells in the **stratum basale + stratum spinosum** due to **T cell activation** & cytokine release* ⇨ greater epidermal thickness & increased epidermis turnover.*

CLINICAL MANIFESTATIONS
1. **PLAQUE:** *MC type. Raised, dark-red plaques/papules with* THICK SILVER/WHITE SCALES.*
   MC on the extensor surfaces of the elbows/knees, scalp, nape of the neck. Usually pruritic.
   Nail pitting (25%). *Yellow-brown discoloration under the nail (**oil spot**) pathognomonic.*
   - ***Auspitz sign:*** * punctate bleeding with removal of plaque/scale.   Auspitz sign is not specific to psoriasis (may be seen in actinic keratosis as well).
   - ***Koebner's phenomenon:*** new skin lesions at sites of trauma (also seen in eczema).

2. **Pustular:** deep, yellow non-infected pustules that evolve into red macules on palms/soles.

3. **GUTTATE:** *small, erythematous papules with fine scales, discrete lesions & confluent plaques.*

4. Inverse: erythematous (lacks scale). MC seen in body folds (ex. groin, gluteal fold, axilla).

5. Erythrodermic: generalized erythematous rash involving most of the skin (worst type).

6. **Psoriatic arthritis:** inflammatory arthritis associated with psoriasis.   Joint stiffness >30 minutes relieved with activity. "Sausage digits." Radiographs: "pencil in cup" deformity.*

MANAGEMENT
1. **Mild-Moderate: *topical steroids 1ˢᵗ line.*** * (high-strength) ± Vitamin D analogs (*Calcipotriene*), topical tar, topical Retinoids/Vitamin A analogs (ex. Tazarotene).

2. **Moderate-Severe:** *phototherapy: UVB,* PUVA (oral Psoralen followed by ultraviolet A).
   Systemic tx: ex. **Methotrexate**, Cyclosporine, Retinoids (Acitretin), biologic agents.

PITYRIASIS (TINEA) VERSICOLOR

- Overgrowth of the yeast ***Malassezia furfur*** (formerly Pityrosporum) - part of the normal skin flora.

CLINICAL MANIFESTATIONS
1. ***Hyper/hypopigmented***, well-demarcated round/oval macules with fine scaling. Often coalesce into patches on the trunk, face, extremities. The involved skin fails to tan with sun exposure.

DIAGNOSIS
1. **KOH prep** from skin scraping: ***hyphae & spores* "spaghetti & meatball"*** appearance.
2. **Wood's lamp:** ***yellow-green fluorescence*** (enhanced color variation seen with versicolor).

MANAGEMENT
1. **Topical antifungals: *Selenium sulfide,*** * *Sodium sulfacetamide, Zinc pyrithione, "azoles".*

2. Systemic therapy: Itraconazole or Fluconazole in adults if widespread or if failed topical tx.
   Must not shower for 8-12 hours afterwards because azoles are delivered to the skin via sweat.

SEBORRHEIC DERMATITIS

- Unclear etiology. Hypersensitivity to **Malassezia furfur** (formerly Pityrosporum ovale), a fungal skin commensal, may play a role. Adult men MC.
- Occurs in areas of **high sebaceous gland oversecretion** (ex scalp, face, eyebrows, body folds).
- Tends to worsen during winter months (UV light helpful) & during times of stress.

CLINICAL MANIFESTATIONS
1. **"Cradle Cap": infants.** Erythematous plaques with fine white scales.
2. **Adults:** erythematous plaques with fine white scales common on the scalp **(dandruff)**, eyelids, beard mustache, nasolabial folds, trunk (chest) & intertriginous regions of the groin.

MANAGEMENT
1. **Topical: Selenium sulfide, Sodium sulfacetamide, Ketoconazole** (shampoo or cream) or Ciclopirox, **steroids. Zinc pyrithione.** Calcineurin inhibitors (Pimecrolimus, Tacrolimus).
2. Systemic: oral antifungals (ex. Itraconazole, Fluconazole, Ketoconazole, Terbinafine).
3. Cradle cap: baby shampoo, Ketoconazole (cream or shampoo), topical corticosteroids.

HYPERSENSITIVITY REACTIONS

CUTANEOUS DRUG REACTIONS

- Medication-induced changes in the skin & mucous membranes. Most are hypersensitivity reactions.
- **Most cutaneous drug reactions are self-limited** if the offending drug is discontinued.
- **Triggers:** antigen from foods, insect bites, drugs, environmental, exercise-induced, infections.

PATHOPHYSIOLOGY:
1. **Type I: Ig-E mediated: ex. urticaria & angioedema**. Immediate.
2. **Type II: cytotoxic, Ab-mediated** (drugs in combo with cytotoxic antibodies cause cell lysis).
3. **Type III: immune antibody-antigen complex.** Ex. drug-mediated vasculitis & serum sickness.
4. **Type IV: delayed (cell mediated)** - morbiliform reaction ex: **Erythema Multiforme.**
5. Nonimmunologic: cutaneous drug reactions due to genetic incapability to detoxify certain medications (ex. anticonvulsants & sulfonamides).

CLINICAL MANIFESTATIONS
1. **Exanthematous/Morbiliform Rash: MC skin eruption.** Generalized distribution of **"bright-red" macules & papules that coalesce to form plaques.** Rash typically begins 2-14 days after medication initiation ex: antibiotics, NSAIDs, Allopurinol & thiazide diuretics.

2. **Urticarial:** 2nd MC type. Occurs usually within minutes to hours after drug administration.
   MC triggers: antibiotics, NSAIDs, opiates & radiocontrast media.

3. **Erythema Multiforme:** 3rd MC. Target lesions may not always be present in drug-induced EM.
   MC drugs: Sulfonamides, Penicillins, Phenobarbital, Dilantin.

4. **Fever, abdominal or joint pain may accompany the cutaneous drug reaction.***
5. Less common: acneiform, eczematous, exfoliative, photosensitivity & vasculitis.

MANAGEMENT
1. Discontinuation of the offending medication is the one of 1st steps in management.
2. **Exanthematous/Morbiliform:** oral antihistamines.
3. **Drug induced urticaria/angioedema: systemic corticosteroids, antihistamines.**
4. **Erythema Minor:** symptomatic therapy.
5. **Anaphylaxis: intramuscular epinephrine treatment of choice.***

URTICARIA (HIVES) & ANGIOEDEMA

- **Type I HSN (IgE)** or complement-mediated edematous reaction of the dermis &/or SQ tissues.
- **Triggers:** *foods, meds, infections*, insect bites, drugs, environmental, stress, heat, cold.

PATHOPHYSIOLOGY
Mast cells release ***histamine*** (causing vasodilation of venules ⇨ edema of dermis & SQ tissues).

CLINICAL MANIFESTATIONS
1. **Urticaria:** *blanchable, edematous pink papules, <u>wheals</u> or plaques* (oval, linear or irregular) that may coalesce. Hives often disappear within 24 hours & new crops often occur.
   - <u>Dermatographism:</u> local pressure to the skin may cause wheals in that area.
   - <u>Darier's sign:</u> localized urticaria appearing where the skin is rubbed (urticaria pigmentosa).

2. **Angioedema:** painless, deeper form of urticaria affecting the lips, tongue, eyelids, hands, feet & genitals. Anaphylaxis may occur.

MANAGEMENT:
Oral antihistamines tx of choice. Eliminate precipitant factors, corticosteroids. H_2 blockers.

ERYTHEMA MULTIFORME

- *Acute self-limited <u>type IV hypersensitivity reaction</u>.* MC in young adults 20-40y.
- Skin lesions usually evolve over 3-5 days & persist about 2 weeks.

ASSOCIATIONS: ***Herpes simplex virus MC,**** *Mycoplasma (especially children),* S. pneumo.
   Meds: *sulfa drugs, beta-lactams, Phenytoin, Phenobarbital etc. Malignancies, autoimmune.*

CLINICAL MANIFESTATIONS
*TARGET **(iris) lesions classic:*** ***dull "dusty-violet" red, purpuric macules/vesicles or bullae*** in the ***center*** surrounded by pale edematous rim & a peripheral red halo. Often febrile.
   1. **EM MINOR:** target lesions distributed acrally. ***No mucosal membrane lesions.****

   2. **EM MAJOR:** target lesions with ***involvement of ≥1 mucous membranes**** (oral, genital or ocular mucosa) <10% BSA acrally ⇨ centrally. ***No epidermal detachment.****

MANAGEMENT: *symptomatic:* discontinue offending drug, antihistamines, analgesics, skin care. ***Steroid***/lidocaine/Diphenhydramine mouthwash for oral lesions. Systemic steroids if severe.

STEVEN-JOHNSON SYNDROME (SJS) & TOXIC EPIDERMAL NECROLYSIS (TEN)

- *MC after drug eruptions*: especially ***sulfa & anticonvulsant meds,**** NSAIDs, Allopurinol, antibiotics; Infections less common: *ex. <u>Mycoplasma</u>,* HIV, HSV; *Malignancy,* idiopathic.

- **SJS** *= sloughing <10% body surface area;* **TEN** *= sloughing >30%.* May develop *skin necrosis.*

CLINICAL MANIFESTATIONS
1. fever & URI symptoms ⇨ *widespread blisters* begin on trunk/face, erythematous/pruritic macules ***≥1 mucous membrane*** involvement ***with epidermal detachment**** (⊕ *Nikolsky sign*).

MANAGEMENT: treat like severe burns: burn unit admission, pain control, prompt withdrawal of offending medications, fluid & electrolyte replacement, wound care (ex. gauze, petroleum).

ACNEIFORM LESIONS

ACNE VULGARIS

4 main pathophysiologic factors:
1. **Increased sebum production**: ↑*androgens* increase sebaceous gland activity.
   MC after puberty, ↑androgens (ex. Polycystic Ovarian Syndrome & Cushing's disease).
2. **Clogged sebaceous glands**: due to ↑proliferation of follicular keratinocytes.

3. ***Propionibacterium acne overgrowth:*** P. acne is part of the normal flora that overgrows in blocked pores ⇨ lipase production by P. acne which converts sebum into inflammatory fatty acids that damage healthy cells ⇨ inflammatory response.
4. **Inflammatory response.**

CLINICAL MANIFESTATIONS
Commonly seen in areas with ↑sebaceous glands (ex face, back, chest, upper arms).
1. ***Comedones:*** small, noniflammatory bumps from clogged pores.
   - ***Open comedones (blackheads)**** - incomplete blockage.
   - ***Closed comedones (whiteheads)**** - complete blockage.

2. **Inflammatory:** papules or pustules surrounded by inflammation.

3. **Nodular or cystic acne:** *often heals with scarring.*

DIAGNOSIS
1. **Mild:** comedones (± small amounts of papules &/or pustules).
2. **Moderate:** comedones, larger amounts of papules &/or pustules.
3. **Severe:** nodular (> 5 mm) or cystic acne.

MANAGEMENT
1. **MILD:** *topical retinoids, benzoyl peroxide, topical antibiotics, OCPs.*
   - **Topical retinoids:** *(ex Retin-A, Adapalene).*
     Ind: noninflammatory & inflammatory acne (antibacterial, decreases comedone formation & reduces inflammation). May be used alone or in combination with other meds.

   - **Benzoyl Peroxide: MOA:** decreases Propionibacterium concentration & reduces inflammation.
     S/E: erythema, dermatitis. Used alone or in combination with other meds.

   - **Topical antibiotics:** ex. Clindamycin. MC used with benzoyl peroxide to reduce resistance.
   - **OCPs:** decreases androgen production in pubertal women, reducing sebum production.

2. **MODERATE:** as above + ***oral antibiotics***, ±anti-androgen agents.
   - **Oral Antibiotics:** used in moderate to severe inflammatory acne. Tetracyclines such as ***Doxycycline or Minocycline.*** *Erythromycin, Clindamycin.*

   - **Spironolactone:** anti-androgen effects. Spironolactone is a K⁺-sparing diuretic.

3. **SEVERE (NODULAR OR CYSTIC ACNE):** *Isotretinoins**
   - **Isotretinoin:** MOA: affects all 4 of the pathophysiologic mechanisms of acne.
     S/E: *psych side effects, hepatitis & increased triglycerides/cholesterol, arthralgias, leukopenia, premature long bone closure, dry skin.* ***Highly teratogenic**** (must obtain at least 2 pregnancy tests prior to initiation of treatment & monthly while on treatment), must commit to 2 forms of contraception (used @ least 1 month prior to initiation & 1 month after it is discontinued).

ROSACEA

- Unclear etiology: persistent vasomotor instability with lesion formation. MC in males >30y.
- *Triggers: ETOH,* ↑temperature:* hot drinks, hot/cold weather, hot baths, spicy foods, meds.*

CLINICAL MANIFESTATIONS
1. *Acne-like rash + erythema, facial flushing, telangiectasia, skin coarsening, papulopustules with burning, stinging.* Red eyes. Symptoms due to increased capillary permeability.

2. *Absence of comedones (blackheads) in rosacea distinguishes it from acne.**

MANAGEMENT
1. **Topical: *Metronidazole 1st line,** *Azelaic acid, Ivermectin cream.* Sulfacetamide, anti-acne topical antibiotics.
2. Moderate-severe: oral antibiotics, Laser. Isotretinoin may be used in refractory cases.
3. **Lifestyle modifications:** *Sunscreen,* avoid toners, astringents menthols, camphor & triggers.

VERRUCOUS (WARTY) LESIONS

ACTINIC KERATOSIS

- MC seen in fair-skinned elderly with *prolonged sun exposure.*

- *Premalignant condition to squamous cell carcinoma (MC premalignant skin condition!)**

CLINICAL MANIFESTATIONS
Dry, rough, scaly "sandpaper" skin lesion or erythematous, hyperkeratotic (hyperpigmented) plaques* ±projection on the skin (horn).

DIAGNOSIS
Punch or shave biopsy:
Atypical epidermal keratinocytes & cells with large hyperchromatic pleomorphic nuclei from the basal layer upwards.

MANAGEMENT
Observation, surgical (***cryosurgery,**** dermabrasion); Medical (topical 5-fluorouracil, Imiquimod).

SEBORRHEIC KERATOSIS

- *MC benign skin tumor.* MC in fair-skinned elderly with prolonged sun exposure.

CLINICAL MANIFESTATIONS
Small papule/plaque velvety warty lesion with *"GREASY/STUCK ON APPEARANCE".**
Varied possible colors ex. flesh-colored, grey, brown & black.

MANAGEMENT
1. *No treatment needed (benign).*

2. Cosmetic management: ***cryotherapy,*** curettage or laser therapy.

HUMAN PAPILLOMAVIRUS INFECTIONS

- HPV infects keratinized skin, causing excessive proliferation & retention of the stratum corneum ⇨ papule formation.

- **Cutaneous HPV:** verruca (warts): common (vulgaris), plantar (plantaris), flat (plana).

- **Mucosal HPV:** *genital warts (condyloma acuminata), cervical dysplasia/cancer & anogenital carcinoma* (intraepithelial).

CLINICAL MANIFESTATIONS
1. **COMMON & PLANTAR WARTS (vulgaris & plantis):** firm, hyperkeratotic papules between 1-10 mm with red-brown punctations (***thrombosed capillaries** are pathognomonic*).
   - Borders ± be rounded or irregular. Common on the hands.

2. **FLAT WARTS (VERRUCA PLANA):** numerous, small, discrete, flesh-colored papules measuring 1-5 mm in diameter & 1-2mm in height. Typically seen on the face, hands, shins.

3. **GENITAL WARTS (CONDYLOMA ACUMINATA):** tiny, *painless* papules evolve into *soft, fleshy, cauliflower-like lesions** ranging from skin-colored to pink or red, occurring in clusters in the genital regions & oropharynx. Lesions persist for months & may spontaneously resolve, remain unchanged or grow if not treated.

DIAGNOSIS
*Mucosal HPV: **whitening of lesion with acetic acid application.*** Clinical, serologies.
   - Histology: koilocytic squamous cells with hyperplastic hyperkeratosis.

MANAGEMENT: *most warts resolve spontaneously within 2 years* if immunocompetent.
1. Verruca vulgaris & plantaris: topical over the counter salicylic acid & plasters. Cryotherapy (liquid nitrogen), electrocautery, CO_2, laser, intralesional bleomycin.

2. Condyloma acuminata: chemical, Salicylic acid, cryotherapy, laser & Podophyllin.

3. Gardasil vaccine: in women 11-26y protects vs. 70% of HPV strains (HPV 6, 11, 16, 18).
   - Gardasil 9: targets the same as Gardasil (6, 11, 16, 18) as well as HPV types 31, 33, 45, 52, & 58.

VITILIGO

- *Autoimmune destruction of melanocytes ⇨ skin depigmentation.*

CLINICAL MANIFESTATIONS
Irregular discrete macules & patches of total depigmentation.
   - commonly involves the dorsum of the hands, axilla, face, fingers, body folds & genitalia.

MANAGEMENT
1. Localized: Topical corticosteroids. Calcineurin inhibitors great for facial involvement.
2. Disseminated: systemic phototherapy (ex. narrow band UVB) may aid in repigmentation.
3. Laser therapy, grafts & cultured epidermal suspensions may be effective on limited areas.

NEOPLASMS

BASAL CELL CARCINOMA

- *MC type of skin cancer in US:** MC in fair-skinned with prolonged sun exposure, Xeroderma pigmentosum (genetic disorder with inability to repair damage caused by UV light exposure).

- *Slow growing:** locally invasive but *very low incidence of metastasis.*

CLINICAL MANIFESTATIONS
1. Flat firm area with *small, raised, TRANSLUCENT/PEARLY/WAXY PAPULE & CENTRAL ULCERATION** & *RAISED, ROLLED BORDERS. MC on face/nose/trunk.* Often friable *(bleeds easily).*

2. May have overlying *telangiectatic vessels.*

DIAGNOSIS
1. *Punch or shave biopsy:** basophilic palisading cells on histology.

MANAGEMENT
1. *Electrodesiccation/curettage* used MC in nonfacial tumors with low risk of recurrence.
2. ± *Mohs micrographic surgery for facial involvement*, difficult cases or recurrent cases.
3. Surgical excision used for tumors with either low or high risk of tumor recurrence.
4. Small superficial: Imiquimod & 5FU for superficial non-facial lesions. Cryosurgery.

MALIGNANT MELANOMA

- *UV radiation* associated with 80% of cases.
- *Aggressive* High METS potential. MC skin cancer-related death.*
- ↑in Caucasians & light hair/eye color, Xeroderma pigmentosum.

4 MAJOR SUBTYPES
1. **Superficial spreading:** MC type (70%). May arise de novo or from a pre-existing nevus.
2. Nodular: 2nd MC type. May be associated with rapid vertical growth phase.
3. Lentigo maligna
4. Acral lentiginous: MC type found in dark-skinned individuals.
5. Desmoplastic: most aggressive type.

CLINICAL MANIFESTATIONS
1. *"ABCDE"** **A**symmetry; **B**orders: irregular; **C**olor: variation (dark blue, black); *Diameter: usually ≥6mm, **E**volution* (suspect in a lesion with recent/rapid change in appearance)*.*

2. *Thickness most important prognostic factor for METS.**
   10 year survival rate: <1mm 95%, 1-2mm 80%; 2-4mm 55%, > 4mm 30%.

DIAGNOSIS
1. *full-thickness wide excisional biopsy + lymph node biopsy.** Shave biopsy discouraged.

MANAGEMENT
1. *Complete wide surgical excision* with lymph node biopsy or dissection.
2. ± Adjuvant therapy in some high risk: α-interferon, immune therapy or radiotherapy.

SQUAMOUS CELL CARCINOMA OF THE SKIN

- 2nd MC skin cancer. ***Often PRECEDED BY ACTINIC KERATOSIS,* *HPV infection,*** *sun & environmental exposure, Xeroderma pigmentosum, chronic wounds.* MC lips, hands, neck & head.
- Malignancy of keratinocytes of skin/mucous membranes: hyperkeratosis & ulceration.

- *Bowen's disease = squamous cell carcinoma in situ. **Slow growing** (rarely metastasizes).*

CLINICAL MANIFESTATIONS
Red, elevated thickened nodule with adherent *white scaly or crusted, bloody margins*.

DIAGNOSIS
Biopsy: atypical keratinocytes & malignant cells with large, pleomorphic, hyperchromatic nuclei in the epidermis, extending into the dermis. May form nodules with laminated centers ("epithelial/keratinous pearls").

MANAGEMENT
1. *Wide local surgical excision treatment of choice.*

2. Electrodessication & curettage, Mohs (recurrent/aggressive), radiation therapy.

KAPOSI SARCOMA

- Connective tissue cancer caused by *Human herpesvirus 8 (HHV-8).**
- *MC in immunosuppressed patients or HIV* (CD4 count <100/mm^3).

CLINICAL MANIFESTATIONS
1. *macular, papular, nodule(s), plaque-like brown/pink/red or violaceous lesions.*

MANAGEMENT
HAART therapy. Radiation therapy for local disease.

ERYTHEMA NODOSUM

- *Painful, erythematous inflammatory nodules seen on the anterior shins* (range in colors from pink, red to purple). Usually bilateral. May also occur on other parts of the body.

ETIOLOGIES:
1. **Estrogen exposure:** ex. OCPs, pregnancy.
2. Inflammatory disorders: *sarcoidosis,* inflammatory bowel disease, leukemia, Behçet disease.
3. Infections: streptococcal, TB, sarcoidosis, fungal (ex *Coccidioidomycosis*).

MANAGEMENT
The lesions are generally self-limited & usually resolve spontaneously within a few weeks (excellent prognosis).   Treat the underlying cause.

1. NSAIDs for pain.

2. Persistent: corticosteroids (if underlying cause is not infectious in nature).

INFECTIOUS SKIN LESIONS

IMPETIGO

- Highly contagious superficial vesiculopustular skin infection.

- Occurs typically at sites of superficial skin trauma (ex. insect bite), primarily on exposed surfaces of the **face** & extremities.
- Risk factors: warm, humid conditions, poor personal hygiene.

TYPES OF IMPETIGO
1. NONBULLOUS:
- Impetigo contagiosa: **vesicles, pustules** ⇨ characteristic **"honey-colored crust."*** *MC type.*
- Associated with regional lymphadenopathy. **Staph aureus MC.*** *GABHS (2nd MC).*

2. BULLOUS:
- Vesicles form large bullae (rapidly) ⇨ rupture ⇨ thin *"varnish-like crusts."* Fever, diarrhea.
- **Staph aureus MC.** Rare (usually seen in newborn/young children).

3. ECTHYMA: ulcerative pyoderma caused by **GABHS** (heals with scarring). Not common.

MANAGEMENT
1. **Mupirocin (Bactroban) topically drug of choice.*** tid x 10 days. Bacitracin.
   Wash the area gently with soap & water. Good skin hygiene.

2. **Extensive disease or systemic symptoms (ex. fever): *systemic antibiotics:***
   Cephalexin* (Keflex): 1st generation cephalosporin.
   Dicloxacillin (especially effective against S. aureus); Clindamycin.
   Erythromycin, Azithromycin (Zithromax) or Clarithromycin (Biaxin).

FOLLICULITIS, FURUNCLE, CARBUNCLE

FOLLICULITIS
- Superficial hair follicle infection with singular or clusters of small papules or pustules with surrounding erythema. Staph aureus MC.

- **MANAGEMENT: *topical Mupirocin, Clindamycin, Erythromycin.***
  Oral antibiotics: Cephalexin, Dicloxacillin for refractory/severe cases.

FURUNCLE (BOIL)
- Deeper infection of the hair follicle (in contrast to folliculitis which is superficial). Tender nodule
  - **fluctuant abscess with central plug** (may have surrounding cellulitis).

- **MANAGEMENT: *incision & drainage. Heat compresses,*** *oral antibiotics if associated with cellulitis.*
  May eradicate the source of Staphylococcus aureus by nasal application of Mupirocin.

CARBUNCLE
- Larger, more painful, **interlocking furuncles/*abscesses with multiple openings*** + cellulitis.

- **MANAGEMENT:** same as furuncle.

CELLULITIS

- Acute, spreading superficial infection of dermal, subcutaneous tissues.
- **MC caused by S. aureus & Group A beta hemolytic streptococcus (GABHS/S. pyogenes).**

- Usually occurs after a break in the skin: underlying skin problems (impetigo, viral lesions, tinea), trauma (bites, puncture wounds, pressure ulcers) and surgical wounds.

CLINICAL MANIFESTATIONS
1. **Local: *macular erythema*** (flat margins, **_not sharply demarcated),_** swelling, warmth, and tenderness.

2. **Systemic:** Not common - fever, chills, ±tender lymphadenopathy, ±lymphangitis (erythematous streaking), myalgias, vesicles, bullae, hemorrhage & necrosis may develop.

SPECIAL TYPES OF CELLULITIS
1. ERYSIPELAS: *group A strep (GABHS) MC cause.* **_Well demarcated margins_** of cellulitis, intensely erythematous (St. Anthony's fire).
   - *MC involves the face* or skin with impaired lymphatic drainage.
      Management: IV Penicillin. Vancomycin (if PCN allergic or MRSA is suspected).

2. LYMPHANGITIS: spread of the infection via the lymphatic vessels. Seen as **_streaking_** from the infected area following the lymph vessels. Complications include bacteremia.

MEDICAL MANAGEMENT
Antibiotics (usually 7-10 days):
- **Cephalexin; Dicloxacillin**
- Clindamycin or Erythromycin if PCN allergic.
- **MRSA:** IV Vancomycin or Linezolid. Oral options include: Trimethoprim-sulfamethoxazole (2nd best PO med for MRSA but doesn't cover strep well), Clindamycin. Doxycycline, Daptomycin. Linezolid is the best PO drug for MRSA (but usually reserved for severe cases).

- **_Cat bite (Pasteurella multocida)*_** ⇨ **_Amoxicillin/clavulanate;*_** Doxycycline if PCN allergic.

- Dog bite ⇨ *Amoxicillin/clavulanate.*
     2nd line: Clindamycin + either Ciprofloxacin or Trimethoprim-sulfamethoxazole.

- Human bite ⇨ **_Amoxicillin/clavulanate._**
     2nd line: Clindamycin + either Moxifloxacin or Trimethoprim-sulfamethoxazole.
- Puncture wound through a tennis shoe ⇨ Ciprofloxacin (covers Pseudomonas).

PARONYCHIA

- Infection of the nail margin. MC occurs after skin trauma (ex. biting nails, cuticle damage).
- **_Staph aureus MC_** (especially if rapid), GABHS. Candida if slow growing.
- **Felon:** closed-space infection of the fingertip pulp (a paronychia can progress to a felon).

CLINICAL MANIFESTATIONS: painful, red swollen area around the nail at the cuticle site.

MANAGEMENT
Warm soaks (reduces pain & swelling), **_antibiotics:_** ex. Cephalexin. **Incision & drainage.**

PARASTIC INFECTIONS OF THE SKIN & HAIR

SCABIES

- *Sarcoptes scabiei* are mites that are transmitted through prolonged, close skin-skin contact or fomites (clothing, bedding). They cannot survive off of the human body for >4 days.
- Female mites **burrow into the skin to lay eggs, feed & defecate** (scybala are the fecal particles that precipitate a hypersensitivity reaction in the skin).

CLINICAL MANIFESTATIONS
1. **Intensely pruritic lesions:*** papules, vesicles & _LINEAR BURROWS_* – commonly found in the **intertriginous zones** including **web spaces between fingers/toes, scalp.** Usually spares the neck & face. *Intense pruritus with minimal skin findings increased intensity at night.**

2. **Red itchy pruritic papules or nodules on the scrotum, glans or penile shaft, body folds pathognomonic for scabies.*** Infected patients ± remain without symptoms for up to 4-6 weeks.

DIAGNOSIS
1. Often a *clinical diagnosis.*
2. Skin scraping of the burrows with mineral oil to identify mites or eggs under microscopy.

MANAGEMENT:
1. **Permethrin topical** (Elimite, Nix) **drug of choice.*** Applied topically from the neck to the soles of the feet for 8-14 hours before showering. A repeat application after 1 week is recommended.
2. **Lindane:** cheaper. **DO NOT use after bath/shower (causes seizures*** due to increased absorption through open pores).
   CI: Teratogenic, not used in breastfeeding women, children <2y.

3. 6-10% sulfur in petroleum jelly for pregnant women/infants. *Oral Ivermectin if extensive.*
4. *All clothing, bedding etc. should be placed in a plastic bag @least 72h then washed & dried using heat.*

PEDICULOSIS (LICE)

- Head louse (*Pediculus humanus capitus*); Body louse (*Pediculus humanus corporis*);
  Pubic louse (*Phthirus pubis*).
- **Transmission:** person to person. Fomites (hats, headsets, clothing, bedding).

CLINICAL MANIFESTATIONS
1. **Intense itching*** (especially occipital area), **papular urticaria near the lice bites.**

2. **Nits:*** white oval-shaped egg capsules at the base of the hair shafts. Removed with a comb.

MANAGEMENT
1. **Permethrin topical drug of choice.*** Capitus: Permethrin shampoo left on x10 minutes.
   Pubis/Corporis: Permethrin lotion x at least 8-10 hours. Safe in children ≥2 years of age.

2. 2nd line: **Lindane. S/E: neurotoxic** *(headaches, seizures– do not use after showering).* Malathion. Oral Ivermectin can be used in cases that are refractory to topical therapies.

3. *Bedding/clothing are laundered in hot water with detergent & dried in hot drier for 20 minutes. Toys that cannot be washed should be placed in air-tight plastic bags x 14 days.**

MOLLUSCUM CONTAGIOSUM

- Benign viral infection (***poxviridae*** family). ***Highly contagious*** (skin to skin MC & fomites).

- MC in children, sexually active adults, patients with HIV.

CLINICAL MANIFESTATIONS
1. ***single or multiple <u>dome-shaped</u>, flesh-colored to pearly-white, waxy papules with <u>CENTRAL UMBILICATION.</u>*** Curd-like material may be expressed from the center if lesion is squeezed.

MANAGEMENT
1. ***No treatment needed in most cases*** (spontaneous resolution in 3-6 months usually).

2. *Curettage (rapid resolution),* Cryotherapy, Podophyllotoxin. electrodessication. ±Imiquimod.
3. Topical retinoids may be needed in severe cases.

DERMATOPHYTOSIS

- ***Fungal skin infections: Trichophyton,*** Microsporum, Epidermophyton.
  Infects keratinized tissues in the stratum corneum of the skin, hair & nails by ingesting keratin.

- <u>**Risk Factors:**</u> increased skin moisture (ex. occlusive gear), Immunodeficiency (HIV, DM), peripheral vascular disease.

CLINICAL MANIFESTATIONS
1. **TINEA CAPITUS:** varied presentation: annular, scaling lesions & broken hair shafts. Inflamed plaques with multiple pustules (kerion) with scarring & ***alopecia -*** *"ring worm"* common name.

   <u>**Management:**</u> ***PO Griseofulvin 1st line.*** PO Terbinafine, Itraconazole of Fluconazole 2nd line tx.

2. **TINEA BARBAE:** papules, pustules & hair follicles.

3. **TINEA PEDIS:** *"athlete's foot": pruritic scaly eruption rash between toes.*

   <u>**Management:**</u> ***Topical antifungal,*** PO Griseofulvin if ineffective.
   Clean shoes with antifungal spray, keep cool/dry.

4. **TINEA CRURIS:** *"Jock Itch":* diffusely red rash on the groin or on the scrotum.
   <u>**Management:**</u> ***topical antifungal.***   PO Griseofulvin if ineffective.

5. **TINEA CORPORIS:** erythematous plaques (circular rash with clear center & defined borders), scaling, cracking & vesicles. The ***<u>presence of scales in tinea corporis</u>*** distinguishes it from erythema migrans.
   <u>**Management:**</u> ***Topical antifungal,*** PO Griseofulvin if ineffective.

6. **ONYCHOMYCOSIS:** nail infection by various fungi (ex. tinea, candida). Occurs MC on great toe. Opaque, thickened, discolored & cracked nails with subungual hyperkeratinization.
   <u>**Management:**</u> Itraconazole & Terbinafine. Systemic antifungals: Griseofulvin, Itraconazole & Terbinafine & Griseofulvin associated with ***hepatotoxicity*** & drug interactions.
   Topical Ciclopirox.

<u>**DIAGNOSIS:**</u> ***KOH smear.*** <u>**Wood's lamp:**</u> ***green fluorescence if due to Microsporum.***

PEMPHIGUS VULGARIS

- **Autoimmune disorder** 2ʳʸ to **desmosome disruption*** (desmosomes link keratinocytes). Keratin serves as a barrier function of the **epidermis.** **Anti-desmosome/anti-epithelial Ab.** (Type II HSN).

- Desmosomes hold the skin together (epidermal cell junctions). MC young patients (30s-40s).

CLINICAL MANIFESTATIONS
1. *Oral mucosal membrane erosions & ulcerations 1ˢᵗ ⇨ **painful flaccid skin bullae (ruptures easily),*** leaving painful denuded skin erosions that bleed easily.

2. ⊕ NIKOLSKY SIGN* superficial **detachment of skin under pressure/trauma** (pulls off in sheets).

DIAGNOSIS
1. Skin biopsy (ex. punch): intraepithelial splitting with *acantholysis* (detached keratinocytes).
   Direct immunofluorescence: **IgG throughout the epidermis,** basal keratinocytes in a pattern that resembles a "row of tombstones".
2. ELISA: anti-desmoglein antibodies.

MANAGEMENT
Systemic: high-dose corticosteroids 1ˢᵗ line.* **Methotrexate,** Azathioprine. Cyclophosphamide.
Local wound care (treat like burns). Treat secondary infections with antibiotics.

BULLOUS PEMPHIGOID

- Chronic widespread autoimmune blistering skin disease **primarily of the elderly** (65-75y).
PATHOPHYSIOLOGY
- Type II HSN (IgG) autoimmune attack on the epithelial basement membrane causing **subepidermal blistering** (especially the groin, axilla, abdomen & flexural areas). ±Drug-induced.

CLINICAL MANIFESTATIONS
Urticarial plaques ⇨ **tense bullae (don't rupture easily)*** blister roof contains epidermis. *Pruritus.*
Lack of Nikolsky sign. *Subepidermal involvement distinguishes it from pemphigus vulgaris.*

MANAGEMENT: Systemic corticosteroids, antihistamines. Immunosuppressants (Azathioprine).
Topical corticosteroids may be used in mild disease or applied to early lesions to prevent blisters.

MELASMA (CHLOASMA)

- **Hypermelanosis (hyperpigmentation) of sun exposed areas** of the skin.
RISK FACTORS
- ↑ **estrogen exposure (OCPs, pregnancy),* sun exposure.** Women with darker complexions.

CLINICAL MANIFESTATIONS
Hypermelanotic (brown-pigment) symmetrical macules especially on the face & neck.

DIAGNOSIS
Wood's lamp: appearance is unchanged under black light in dermal melasma.
   - may be enhanced in epidermal melasma.

MANAGEMENT:
Sunscreen. Topical bleachers: ex. **Hydroquinone,** Azelaic acid. Topical retinoids. Chemical peels.

BROWN RECLUSE SPIDER BITES

- MC in Southwestern & Midwestern US.
- Brown recluse spiders (Loxosceles reclusa) may have a <u>violin pattern</u> on its anterior cephalothorax.

CLINICAL MANIFESTATIONS

1. **Local effects:** local burning & erythema at the bite site for 3-4 hours ⇨ blanched area (due to vasoconstriction) ⇨ erythematous margin the around ischemic center *"red halo"* ⇨ 24-72h after *hemorrhagic bullae that undergoes eschar formation* * ⇨ necrosis in ~10%.

MANAGEMENT

1. **Local wound care:** clean the affected area with soap & water, apply cold packs to the bite site (avoid freezing the tissue). If possible, keep the affected body part in elevated or neutral position. Most wounds heal spontaneously within days to weeks.

2. **Pain control:** ex. NSAIDs (or opioids if more severe). Tetanus prophylaxis if needed.

3. <u>Dermal necrosis:</u> debridement in some cases if it will lead to better wound healing. Dapsone has been used in the past. Antibiotics only if a secondary infection develops (treat like cellulitis).

BLACK WIDOW SPIDER BITES

- Usually have an event <8 hours of an event with contact with the spider (Latrodectus Hesperus) ex. outdoor activities, outdoor furniture use, gardening, sleeping outside, etc.

CLINICAL MANIFESTATIONS

1. <u>Latrodectism:</u> *local symptoms:* asymptomatic or pain at the bite site with the onset of generalized symptoms within 30 minutes to 2 hours ⇨ *systemic symptoms: muscle pain,* * *spasms & rigidity.* Muscle pain MC affects the extremities, back & abdomen. Usually self-limited with resolution within 1-3 days.

2. <u>Physical exam:</u> classic appearance is a blanched circular patch with a surrounding red perimeter and central punctum (target lesion).

MANAGEMENT

1. **Mild:** wound care & pain control: gently clean the area with mild soap & water. NSAIDs, opioids.
2. **Moderate to severe:** opioids ± muscle relaxants (ex. benzodiazepines, Methocarbamol).
   Antivenom reserved for patients not responsive to the above medications. Antivenom is not always readily available and if given, usually given after a consult with a toxicologist.

HIDRADENITIS SUPPURATIVA

- Chronic abscess of apocrine sweat glands or sebaceous cysts with tract formation.
  Red tender inflammatory nodules/abscesses.
- MC in obese women. MC areas: axilla, groin, under breasts or anogenital area.

MANAGEMENT

1. <u>Mild disease:</u> topical Clindamycin. Intralesional injections of Triamcinolone for small cysts.
2. **Deep, recurrent infections:** punch debridement if small, unroofing of larger ones with washout.
   Painful abscess: incision & drainage.
3. <u>Systemic Antibiotics:</u> Tetracycline, Cephalosporin, Clindamycin, Ciprofloxacin.
4. <u>Surgical excision of the apocrine glands:</u> may prevent recurrence if severe.
5. <u>Lifestyle:</u> dietary changes (avoid high glycemic foods), smoking cessation, local skin care

SEBACEOUS CYSTS

- Name commonly used to describe epidermoid or pilar cysts. Both secrete keratin (not sebum) and do not originate from the sebaceous glands.

CLINICAL MANIFESTATIONS
1. Mobile masses of fibrous tissue and keratinous (cottage cheese like) substance.

MANAGEMENT
No treatment needed. Cosmetic removal. Incision & drainage if it becomes infected.

BURN SIZE   Rule of Nines   Not used for 1st degree burns.

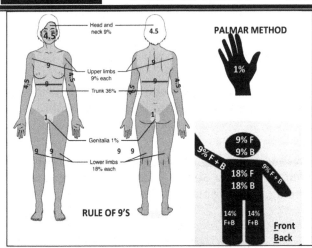

Palm size classically has been considered to represent 1% of TBSA (it accurately represents 0.4% with entire hand representing 0.8%)

Minor Burns: <10% TBSA burn* in adults*
<5%TBSA burn in young /old*
<2% full thickness burn
- Must be isolated injury
- Must <u>not</u> involve face, hands, perineum, feet
- Must <u>not</u> cross major joints. Must <u>not</u> be circumferential

MAJOR BURNS: >25% TBSA burn* in adults*
>20%TBSA burn in young/old*
>10% full thickness burn
- <u>Burns involving</u> the face, hands, perineum, feet
- Burns crossing major joints, circumferential burns

<u>Lund-Browder</u> chart is the most accurate method for estimating TBSA in both children & adults.

BURN MANAGEMENT

CLEANSING: wash the wound using only mild soap and water (skin disinfectants may actually inhibit healing). *Do **NOT** apply ice directly*. Cool compresses used to stop the thermal burning. **Chemical Burns***: irrigate profusely with running water for at least 20 minutes*.

DEBRIDEMENT: sloughed/necrotic skin may be debrided (may be done at the follow up visit). Escharotomy recommended for circumferential burns to prevent compartment syndrome.

BLISTERS: ruptured blisters should be removed. Management of clean intact blisters is controversial.

PAIN MANAGEMENT: Acetaminophen, NSAIDs alone or in combination with opioids.

ANTIBIOTICS: topical antibiotic should be applied to any nonsuperficial burn.
- *Silver sulfadiazine (SSD)* commonly used. Used on 2nd-3rd degree burns. *Silvadene CI if sulfa allergies, pregnancy, children <2 months, <u>NO</u> Silvadene on face (due to discoloration S/E).*
- Honey and modern membrane-like dressings have compared favorably to SSD.
- Aloe vera or topical antibiotic (ex. Bacitracin) used for superficial burns.

DRESSINGS: *superficial burns do not require dressings*. Partial and full-thickness burns are often covered with a sterile dressing to prevent infection - nonadherent gauze & elastic gauze (ex kerlix). *Fingers & toes should be individually wrapped* to prevent maceration and gauze should be placed in between them. Biologic & synthetic dressings may also be used.

INTRAVENOUS FLUID RESUSCITATION: PARKLAND FORMULA
- *Lactated Ringers* 4ml/kg/%TSA. IV x first 24 hours
$1/2$ in 1st 8 hours the other ½ over the remaining 16 hours.

	1ST DEGREE	2ND DEGREE		3RD DEGREE	4TH DEGREE
	SUPERFICIAL	SUPERFICIAL PARTIAL THICKNESS	DEEP PARTIAL THICKNESS	FULL THICKNESS	
DEPTH	• Epidermis (Intact epidermal barrier)	• Epidermis + Superficial portion of dermis (papillary)	• Epidermis into deep portion of dermis (reticular)	• Extends through entire skin	• Entire skin into underlying fat, muscle, bone.
APPEARANCE	• Erythematous (red) • Dry	• Erythematous, pink • Moist, weeping • ⊕ BLISTERING	• Red, yellow, pale white • Dry • ⊕ BLISTERING	• Waxy, white • Leathery, Dry	• Black, charred, eschar • Dry
SENSATION	• PAINFUL • Tender to touch	• Most PAINFUL of all burns • Very tender to touch	• Not usually painful ±pain with pressure. • May have decreased 2 point discrimination	• PAINLESS	• PAINLESS
CAPILLARY REFILL	• ⊕ refill intact: blanches with pressure	• ⊕ refill intact: blanches with pressure	• Absent capillary refill	• Absent	• Absent
PROGNOSIS	• Heals within 7 days • No scarring	• Heals within 14-21 days • No scarring (but ± leave pigment changes)	• 3 weeks – 2 months • Scarring common (may need skin graft or excision to prevent contractures)	• Months • Does not spontaneously heal well	• Does not heal well. • Usually needs debridement of tissues & tissue reconstruction.

453

SMOKE INHALATION INJURIES

• Must r/o upper airway obstruction & carbon monoxide toxicity with smoke inhalation injuries.

UPPER AIRWAY OBSTRUCTION:
- Smoke inhalation is usually limited to the upper airways (steam can travel to lower airways).
- **Signs of possible upper airway thermal injury:** *surface burns of the neck & face, hoarseness, singed nasal hair,* *soot in the mouth (or nose) or black sputum present.*
- Respiratory distress may not be apparent until hours later.

CARBON MONOXIDE TOXICITY
Carbon monoxide is an odorless, tasteless, colorless, nonirritating gas that has over 200 times the affinity for hemoglobin than oxygen.

CLINICAL MANIFESTATIONS: Neurologic: headache, nausea, malaise, altered mental status, seizures, brain hypoxia, coma; Cardiac: cardiac dysrhythmias, dyspnea, angina.

DIAGNOSIS: measure SaO_2, carboxyhemoglobin, methemoglobin.
- ↑*carboxyhemoglobin levels on ABG or VBG** (levels do not correspond with severity).
- Most pulse oximeters can't differentiate between HbO_2 and carboxyhemoglobin.

MANAGEMENT: *O_2 100% nonrebreather* 10-12L/min *until carboxyhemoglobin <10%.*
May need hyperbaric O_2 in severe cases (↑carboxyhemoglobin + acidosis, severe neuro sx).

CYANIDE POISONING
SYMPTOMS: rapidly developing coma, apnea (with severe lactic acidemia), cardiac derangements.
DIAGNOSIS: via history & physical examination. Cyanide levels.
MANAGEMENT: "cyanide kit" - Amyl nitrite for inhalation, IV sodium nitrite or thiosulfate.

HIGH VOLTAGE ELECTRIC INJURIES

• Determine current intensity (household usually ~110V), type of current (AC or DC), tissue resistance, duration & type of contact, area, "vertical" more dangerous than "horizontal", water immersion. DC current can often violently propel the victim from the current source (due to single, large muscle spasm) & posterior shoulder dislocations may occur.   AC currents can cause muscle contraction (causing patient to hold on tight to the source).

CLINICAL MANIFESTATIONS
1. **Cardiac arrest:** Low-voltage AC may produce ventricular fibrillation. High-voltage AC/DC may produce asystole. *ECG is recommended to look for cardiac changes.*
2. **Musculoskeletal:** *rhabdomyolysis* (urinalysis is performed to look for myoglobinuria).
3. Neurological.

MANAGEMENT
1. Thermal burn management as needed. Patients may need to be placed on telemetry.

2. Outpatient: asymptomatic patients with household burns may be discharged if normal ECG on presentation and normal physical examination.

3. Admission: if >600V ⇨ admit even if asymptomatic. Keep urine output at 100ml/hr & alkalinize the urine to protect the kidney.

PRESSURE ULCERS

Stage I	superficial, **nonblanchable redness** that does not dissipate after pressure is relieved.
Stage II	epidermal damage extending into the **dermis**. Resembles a **blister or abrasion**.
Stage III	full thickness of the skin and may extend into the **subcutaneous layer.**
Stage IV	Deepest. Extends beyond the fascia, extending into the **muscle, tendon or bone.**

MANAGEMENT
1. Wet to dry dressings, hydrogels.
2. I, II – local wound care, pain management. III and IV may need surgical debridement.

DERMATITIS HERPETIFORMIS

- Pruritic autoimmune skin disorder _STRONGLY ASSOCIATED WITH CELIAC DISEASE*_ ⇨ **IgA immune complex deposition in the dermal papillae.**

CLINICAL MANIFESTATIONS
1. Pruritic, papulovesicular rash on the extensor surfaces (including the forearms) & scalp.

MANAGEMENT: Gluten free diet. **Dapsone.**

KELOIDS

- Excess production of Type I & III collagen during wound healing. MC in African-Americans.

CLINICAL MANIFESTATIONS
- Grossly exaggerated scar that often grows pedunculated (especially on the earlobes, face & upper extremities).

MANAGEMENT
1. **Corticosteroid injections 1st line management** (ex. intralesional Triamcinolone).

2. 2nd line: intralesional 5-fluorouracil, silicone gel sheets, pressure therapy, cryotherapy.

PYOGENIC GRANULOMA

- AKA lobular capillary hemangioma. Misnomer - it is neither pyogenic nor a granuloma.
- MC in children & young adults especially after trauma. ↑**Incidence in pregnancy** (higher incidence of **gingival involvement).**

CLINICAL MANIFESTATIONS:
1. **Solitary glistening, friable red (raspberry-like) nodule or papule** **(may bleed or ulcerate).** Usually evolves over a period of weeks. MC on arms, hands, fingers, legs.

MANAGEMENT
1. Pedunculated: shave excision or curettage followed by cautery of the base.
2. Nonpedunculated (sessile): surgical excision.
3. Topical Imiquimod or Alitretinoin gel. Injectable sclerosing agents.

PYODERMA GANGRENOSUM

- Ulcerative skin lesion 2^{ry} to immune dysregulation (misnomer as it is not infectious nor gangrenous as the name implies). ± preceded by trauma.

- *Associated with inflammatory diseases: Inflammatory Bowel disease (Crohn, UC),* Rheumatoid arthritis,* spondyloarthropathies etc.

CLINICAL MANIFESTATIONS
1. Inflammatory, erythematous blue-red papules or pustules ⇨ *painful, necrotic ulcer with irregular purple/violet undermined borders and a purulent base.*

DIAGNOSIS
1. Clinical diagnosis in a majority of cases. <u>Biopsy</u>: neutrophilic infiltration (usually not needed).

MANAGEMENT
1. *Topical Corticosteroids (high potency)* or Tacrolimus (calcineurin inhibitor). Local wound care.
2. <u>2nd line</u>: systemic Corticosteroids or Cyclosporine if refractory to topical therapy.
3. <u>3rd line</u>: intravenous immunoglobulin (IVIG), Cyclophosphamide, Chlorambucil.

LIPOMA

- Subcutaneous benign tumor of adipose tissue. MC on the trunk & extremities.

CLINICAL MANIFESTATIONS
1. Soft, symmetric, painless easily mobile, palpable mass in the subcutaneous tissue.

MANAGEMENT
No treatment needed. May perform surgical removal for cosmetic reasons.

SELECTED REFERENCES

Jerant AF, Johnson JT, Sheridan CD, Caffrey TJ. Early detection and treatment of skin cancer. Am Fam Physician. 2000;62(2):357-68, 375-6, 381-2.
Fiddler IJ. Melanoma Metastasis. Cancer Control. 1995;2(5):398-404.

Friedman RJ, Rigel DS, Kopf AW. Early detection of malignant melanoma: the role of physician examination and self-examination of the skin. CA Cancer J Clin. 1985;35(3):130-51.

Wong CS, Strange RC, Lear JT. Basal cell carcinoma. BMJ. 2003;327(7418):794-8.

Bershad SV. In the clinic. Atopic dermatitis (eczema). Ann Intern Med. 2011;155(9):ITC51-15.

Caproni M, Bonciolini V, D'errico A, Antiga E, Fabbri P. Celiac disease and dermatologic manifestations: many skin clue to unfold gluten-sensitive enteropathy. Gastroenterol Res Pract. 2012;2012:952753.

Atkins D. Food allergy: diagnosis and management. Prim Care. 2008;35(1):119-40, vii.

Gambichler T. Management of atopic dermatitis using photo(chemo)therapy. Arch Dermatol Res. 2009;301(3):197-203.

Bewley A. Expert consensus: time for a change in the way we advise our patients to use topical corticosteroids. Br J Dermatol. 2008;158(5):917-20.

Thongprasom K, Carrozzo M, Furness S, Lodi G. Interventions for treating oral lichen planus. Cochrane Database Syst Rev. 2011;(7):CD001168.

Schlosser BJ. Lichen planus and lichenoid reactions of the oral mucosa. Dermatol Ther. 2010;23(3):251-67.

Arndt KA, Paul BS, Stern RS, Parrish JA. Treatment of pityriasis rosea with UV radiation. Arch Dermatol. 1983;119(5):381-2.

Langan SM, Smeeth L, Hubbard R, Fleming KM, Smith CJ, West J. Bullous pemphigoid and pemphigus vulgaris--incidence and mortality in the UK: population based cohort study. BMJ. 2008;337:a180.

Prajapati V, Barankin B. Dermacase. Actinic keratosis. Can Fam Physician. 2008;54(5):691, 699.

Menter A, Gottlieb A, Feldman SR, et al. Guidelines of care for the management of psoriasis and psoriatic arthritis: Section 1. Overview of psoriasis and guidelines of care for the treatment of psoriasis with biologics. J Am Acad Dermatol. 2008;58(5):826-50.

Axelrod S, Davis-lorton M. Urticaria and angioedema. Mt Sinai J Med. 2011;78(5):784-802.

Lamoreux MR, Sternbach MR, Hsu WT. Erythema multiforme. Am Fam Physician. 2006;74(11):1883-8.

Auquier-dunant A, Mockenhaupt M, Naldi L, et al. Correlations between clinical patterns and causes of erythema multiforme majus, Stevens-Johnson syndrome, and toxic epidermal necrolysis: results of an international prospective study. Arch Dermatol. 2002;138(8):1019-24.

Haberal M, Sakallioglu abali AE, Karakayali H. Fluid management in major burn injuries. Indian J Plast Surg. 2010;43(Suppl):S29-36.

Katz KA, Swetman GL. Imiquimod, molluscum, and the need for a better "best pharmaceuticals for children" act. Pediatrics. 2013;132(1):1-3.

Brooklyn T, Dunnill G, Probert C. Diagnosis and treatment of pyoderma gangrenosum. BMJ. 2006;333(7560):181-4.

Nthumba PM. Giant pyogenic granuloma of the thigh: a case report. J Med Case Rep. 2008;2:95.

Cancio LC. Airway management and smoke inhalation injury in the burn patient. Clin Plast Surg. 2009;36(4):555-67.

Tunzi M, Gray GR. Common skin conditions during pregnancy. Am Fam Physician. 2007;75(2):211-8.

Hay RJ. Scabies and pyodermas--diagnosis and treatment. Dermatol Ther. 2009;22(6):466-74.

Burgess IF. Human lice and their control. Annu Rev Entomol. 2004;49:457-81.

CHAPTER 12 – INFECTIOUS DISEASES

CELL WALL SYNTHESIS INHIBITORS

PENICILLINS

	INDICATIONS
NATURAL PENICILLINS Penicillin VK (oral) Penicillin G benzathine (IM) Penicillin G aqueous (IM,IV) Penicillin G potassium (IM, IV)	- *Gram-positive** (most potent gram ⊕ coverage of all PCNs). - Pen G good for *non β-lactamase* producing **gram-positive cocci**, (staph, strep, enterococci); Anthrax, **gram-positive anaerobes** (ex. *Clostridium sp*). **Meningococcus (although gram-negative).** **Ind:** *strep pharyngitis, oral/dental infections,* syphilis.**
PENICILLINASE-RESISTANT **"ANTI-STAPHYLOCOCCUS"** Nafcillin (IV) Dicloxacillin (PO) Oxacillin (IV) (Methicillin prototype). *Penicillinase = β-lactamase*	- Narrow spectrum of activity ⇨ *gram-positive** (designed primarily vs. β-lactamase producing staphylococcus).* Covers some streptococci. *NOT* active vs. MRSA, enterococcus or gram-negatives. - **Ind: staphylococcal skin/soft tissue infections.** - **Only PCNs effective vs. β-lactamase bacteria on their own.**
AMINO-PENICILLINS Amoxicillin (PO) Ampicillin (PO, IM, IV)	- *Gram positive & negative coverage.* Not active vs. β-lactamase. - **Ind:** UTIs in pregnancy, AOM, *active vs. enterococcus,* H. flu, E. coli, L. monocytogenes, strep spp (GBS), proteus, salmonella.
AMINO-PENICILLINS **"WITH β-LACTAMASE INHIBITOR"** Amoxicillin + Clavulanate (Augmentin) Ampicillin + Sulbactam (Unasyn)	- *Enhanced coverage including* ❶*β-lactamase producing* M. catarrhalis, H. influenza, E coli & B. fragilis ❷ *anaerobes.** - **Augmentin:** *AOM, sinusitis, ABECB, dental infections, bite wounds.* - **Unasyn:** *skin/soft tissue infections*, intrabdominal/peritonitis. Beta lactam inhibitor enhances staphylococcal coverage.
ANTI-PSEUDOMONAL **PENICILLINS** Piperacillin/Tazobactam (Zosyn) (IV) Ticarcillin/Clavulanate (Timentin) (IV) Carbenicillin (PO)	- *Broadest spectrum penicillins.* Reserved for severe infections or suspected Pseudomonal infections. Doesn't cover atypicals such as Legionella, Mycoplasma or Chlamydophila pneumoniae. - Carbenicillin (PO) – E coli, Proteus mirabilis, Pseudomonas. - Clavulanate, sulbactam & tazobactam are β-lactamase inhibitors.

CEPHALOSPORINS

1st GENERATION *Skin, soft tissue**	**Cephalexin** (Keflex) (PO), **Cefazolin** (Ancef) (IV), **Cefadroxil** (Duricef – PO) - *Gram-positive cocci (including β-lactamase)*, anaerobes, E. coli, H. flu. - **Ind:** *skin, soft tissue infections (staph, strep).* Surgical prophylaxis.
2nd GENERATION *Skin, Respiratory/ENT,* *UTI, Anaerobes*	**Cefaclor** (Ceclor), **Cefuroxime** (Ceftin PO or Zinacef IV, IM), **Cefoxitin** (IV), Cefotetan - *Broader gram-negative coverage:* H flu, Proteus, Neisseria, Moraxella. *Increasing level of gram-negative activity & loss of gram-positive as you go from 1st to 4th generation.* - **Ind:** AOM, Pneumonia, UTI. Abdominal infections (anaerobes), skin & soft tissue infections. Cefuroxime: acute epiglottitis, early Lyme disease.
3rd GENERATION *PNA, CNS, Gram negative* Broad Spectrum	*Ceftriaxone* (Rocephin) (IM/IV), *Ceftazidime,** Cefibuten, Cefotaxime, *Cefixime* - **Ind:** meningitis* (good CNS penetration), gonorrhea, CAP (hospitalized). - *Ceftazidime has coverage vs. Pseudomonas.*
4th GENERATION	*Cefepime* (Maxipime). Broad *coverage (including Pseudomonas).*
5TH GENERATION	Ceftaroline (Teflaro). *Broadest spectrum: positive (including MRSA) & negative.*

CARBAPENEMS	*Imipenem* (IV) *Meropenem* (IV)	*Broadest spectrum of all antibiotics!* Cilastatin added to Imipenem to reduce renal clearance of Imipenem. **S/E:** *associated with lowering of seizure threshold.**

MONOBACTAM	*Aztreonam* (IV)	• *Gram-negative aerobes only* including Pseudomonas. Beta lactam with *no cross reactivity with other beta lactams.* S/E: GI upset, vertigo.

459

VANCOMYCIN	• *Gram ⊕ only:** S. aureus, **MRSA,** S pneumoniae. Restricted use by CDC. • Inhibits phospholipids/***peptidoglycans***	IV: *MRSA, MRSE* infections. *PO: C. difficile colitis* (not absorbed).
BACITRACIN	• *Gram ⊕ mainly.** • Little effect vs. anaerobes, gram negative	*Nephrotoxic* so used primarily as a topical preparation for wounds.
POLYMYXIN	• *Gram negative coverage.* • Disrupt the cell membrane & outer membrane permeability of gram negatives.	• *IM/IV preparations are nephrotoxic & neurotoxic.* Others forms used MC. • Topical, ophthalmic & otic forms

PROTEIN SYNTHESIS INHIBITORS

MACROLIDES

Erythromycin	- Bacteria lacking cell walls: *Mycoplasma.* ***Atypicals: Legionella, Chlamydophila.*** - *Good vs. gram-negative & positive*: Strep pneumo & GABHS	- *Strep throat (if allergic to PCN).* - CAP. Used topically for acne. - *Safe in pregnancy.* - *S/E: poor GI tolerance.**
Azithromycin (Zithromax)	- Same as above plus H flu & Moraxella. - *Best atypical coverage (Mycoplasma, Chlamydia, Legionella).**	- CAP, ABECB - *1 time 1g dose for Chlamydia.* - *Anti-inflammatory in the lung.*
Clarithromycin (Biaxin)	- Same as above	- CAP, Legionella, H. pylori. - sinusitis, bronchitis, ABECB.
- Bind to 50S ribosomal unit. **GI side effects & many drug-drug interactions (especially with Erythromycin) - _inhibits cytochrome P450_** so _caution in patients taking Warfarin, Theophylline, Carbamazepine_ (may increase those drug levels). - **Caution if patient is on niacin or statins** (increased incidence of muscle toxicity). **PROLONGED QT INTERVAL.***		

TETRACYCLINES

Doxycycline	- *As above, chlamydia, Q fever, bubonic plague, cat scratch fever, RMSF, Lyme disease, PID.*
Tetracycline	- Acne.
Minocycline	- Acne.
MOA: binds to 30S ribosomal subunit *(bacteriostatic).* **Good vs. gram-positives & negatives, intracellular organisms.** **S/E:** GI disturbances, *photosensitivity, _dental staining_, _NOT_ used in children <8y old or in pregnancy, hepatotoxic.* *Cannot be given with dairy products*, *(Ca, Mg, Al, Fe).* Safe in patients with renal failure.	

CLINDAMYCIN (LINCOSAMIDE)

*Covers gram ⊕, most anaerobes above diaphragm** (little gram-negative). **May cause C. difficile colitis!**

AMINOGLYCOSIDES (AG)

➤ **_GRAM-NEGATIVE AEROBES ONLY_!** Not good for CNS penetration. **Bactericidal** (binds to 30S ribosomal unit).
➤ **_OTOTOXIC & NEPHROTOXIC_* (ATN).** Hearing loss is usually irreversible. Tinnitus, vertigo, ataxia.
➤ *Commonly used with penicillins for broad empiric coverage* (synergism allows for AG gram-positive activity).

Gentamicin	- *Gram-negative (including Pseudomonas).* Aminoglycosides don't reliably cover gram positives or anaerobes on their own. - Not commonly used for Neisseria infections.	- Used with Ampicillin in neonatal meningitis - Septic shock - Pyelonephritis & complicated UTI - Endocarditis (enterococcus) - Yersinia, Tularemia
Tobramycin	Slightly ↑activity vs. Pseudomonas	Topical (keratitis) Nosocomial pneumonia (given with 3rd gen. cephalosporin)
Neomycin	Same as above	- Bowel prep, part of Neosporin & Cortisporin. - Otitis externa (*don't use if TM is not visualized*).
Amikacin (Amikin)	Pseudomonas, Acinetobacter, Serratia	Restricted use by CDC (reserved for bad infections).
Streptomycin		*Tuberculosis, tularemia*, Yersinia pestis.

LINEZOLID	**Gram-positive only:** including MRSA, VRE, Enterococcus faecium and **faecalis.** Also covers atypicals: Mycoplasma, Chlamydophila, Legionella. VRE = Vancomycin-resistant Enterococcus.
	MOA: inhibits protein synthesis (50S ribosomal unit). Bacteriostatic vs. staph & enterococci (bactericidal vs. strep). S/E: GI: N/V/D, headache, thrombocytopenia (especially with treatment duration >2 weeks), MAO Inhibition.

CHLORAMPHENICOL	**Broad spectrum.** Usually indicated in severe anaerobic infections or unresponsive life-threatening infections. **Good CSF penetration.**
	MOA: inhibits protein synthesis (50S ribosomal unit). S/E: **bone marrow suppression:** reversible anemia, hemolytic anemia, aplastic anemia, **Gray baby syndrome.***

DNA OR RNA SYNTHESIS INHIBITORS

FLUOROQUINOLONES

Inhibits DNA gyrase (Bactericidal). **CI: pregnant females, <18y (interferes with articular cartilage).**		
Ciprofloxacin (Cipro)	- **Best gram-negative coverage of all FQ** (**enteric organisms,** H flu, Neisseria, Campylobacter). **Excellent v Pseudomonas.*** - **Not active vs. S. pneumo** (so *not used in CAP*).	- **UTI, pyelonephritis*** - **Gastroenteritis,*** PID - Malignant OE, sinusitis - Gonococcal arthritis
Norfloxacin (Norflox) Levofloxacin (Levaquin)	Better activity vs. gram positive. **Respiratory FQ – used for CAP (Pneumonia).**	- UTI, pyelonephritis, **CAP** - Gonococcal, Gastroenteritis
Moxifloxacin (Avelox)	**Best gram-positive, anaerobic & atypical coverage activity of all FQ**	- Respiratory: CAP, bronchitis, sinusitis - Intrabdominal infections - Ophthalmic, skin infections
Ofloxacin (Floxin)	Newer FQ: above plus enhanced coverage of Staphylococcal aureus, epidermis, saprophyticus. Streptococcus pneumoniae	- as above -CAP (community acquired pneumonia). -ABECB: acute bacterial exacerbations of chronic bronchitis
Gatifloxacin (Tequin)	Same as Ofloxacin	- ABECB, CAP
Lomefloxacin (Maxaquin)	Same as Ofloxacin	As above

METRONIDAZOLE (Flagyl)	**Effective only v. anaerobes/ protozoa.*** - **Anaerobes:** B. fragilis, C. Difficile. - **Protozoa:** Entamoeba histolytica, Giardia lamblia, Trichomonads.	- intraabdominal - vaginitis, vaginitis - pseudomembranous colitis - amoebic liver abscess
	MOA: inhibits DNA synthesis. Approved for 1st trimester. **Disulfiram-like reaction if used with ETOH, neurotoxicity.**	

DAPTOMYCIN	**Gram-positive only:** including MRSA, VRE, enterococcus faecium & faecalis. **Used in complicated skin infections.**
	MOA: binds & depolarizes bacterial membranes, causing inhibition of protein, DNA & RNA synthesis (cyclic lipopeptide). S/E: **muscle toxicity,** GI, arthralgias. Inactivated by surfactant so not used in pneumonia.

INHIBITORS OF ESSENTIAL METABOLITES

TRIMETHOPRIM/SULFAMETHOXAZOLE BACTRIM	**Effective vs. gram negative & Staph** **2nd best PO coverage vs. MRSA.*** (Linezolid is the 1st). - **Not active vs. group A strep.***	- UTI, AOM, ABECB (Acute Bacterial Exacerbation of Chronic Bronchitis). - **PCP - drug of choice.**
Inhibits folic acid synthesis therefore **avoid in pregnancy/infants.***		
S/E: GI upset, hepatitis, leukopenia, thrombocytopenia, Steven-Johnson syndrome, hemolysis if G6PD deficient.		

NITROFURANTOIN	Ind: **only used for cystitis** (not for pyelonephritis or other infections). Gram-positives, gram-negatives, enterococcus.
	MOA: **excreted in urine,** where its active metabolites attack multiple bacterial sites. **Safe in pregnancy** (except at term). S/E: **hypersensitivity pneumonitis, chronic pulmonary fibrosis.**

Quinupristin/Dalfopristin (Synercid)	MOA: Streptogramin class. Binds to 50S subunit to inhibit protein synthesis. Bacteriostatic (cidal to some bacteria). Name Synercid comes from the fact that the drug is a combination of 2 streptogramins (class A and B) that work "**syner**"gistically to become bacteri"**cid**"al.

- *Mainly GRAM-POSITIVE:* (*including MRSA & VRSA – Vancomycin-resistant Staphylococcal aureus*).
- Covers *Vancomycin-resistant Enterococcus faecium** only (*not Enterococcus faecalis*).
- Positive atypical coverage against Mycoplasma & Legionella.
- Has limited gram-negative activity.

S/E: *thrombophlebitis* (so only given via a central line).

SIDE EFFECTS, ADVERSE REACTIONS AND COMMENTS

PENICILLINS	*Hypersensitivity reaction.* Anaphylaxis in 0.05% (skin test does not predict it). Neurotoxicity. Hematologic side effects. *PCN & Cephalosporins associated* with *nephrotoxicity (Interstitial nephritis).**
AMPICILLIN	*Maculopapular rash in patients with infectious mononucleosis** >90%, diarrhea.
CEPHALOSPORINS	*10% cross reactivity in patients allergic to PCN. Disulfiram reaction (2nd/3rd),* diarrhea. Uncommon S/E: increased LFTs, neutropenia, thrombocytopenia.
AZTREONAM	Beta-lactam that has no cross reactivity with PCN or cephalosporins.
VANCOMYCIN	*"Red Man syndrome"** (Histamine release-occurs when infused too rapidly). Avoided with slow infusion over 1-2 hours. Ototoxic (reversible), nephrotoxic.
MACROLIDES	*GI upset* (less with newer ones). Cytochrome P450 inhibition, *PROLONGED QT INTERVAL.** **Caution if patient is on niacin or statins** (increased incidence of muscle toxicity).
FLUOROQUINOLONES	*Tendon rupture,* growth plate arrest, damage to articular cartilage *(not given if <18y or in pregnant women).** *May exacerbate Myasthenia Gravis.* Photosensitivity, *QT prolongation.** Ciprofloxacin inhibits the CP450 system.
CLINDAMYCIN	*May cause of C. difficile colitis.** Does not have good CSF penetration.
TETRACYCLINES	GI upset, *deposition in teeth* causing *teeth discoloration;* hepatotoxic. *(not given to children <8y or in pregnancy).** *Photosensitivity.* Not given simultaneously with dairy products, Ca, Al, Mg or iron.
SULFONAMIDES **Ex:** BACTRIM	Rash in 3-5%; *do not give after 2nd trimester:* may develop *kernicterus.* *Sulfa allergy, hemolysis if G6PD deficient.**
METRONIDAZOLE Flagyl	*Avoid ETOH during and 48h after; Disulfiram-like reaction, neurotoxicity,* metallic taste, possible carcinogenic potential, pancreatitis.
PHOTOSENSITIVITY	*Tetracyclines, Fluoroquinolones, Sulfonamides, Trimethoprim-sulfamethoxazole Pyrazinamide.*
AUGMENTIN	Augmentin is the penicillin with the highest occurrence of diarrhea.

ANTIFUNGAL MEDICATIONS

POLYENE ANTIFUNGALS   Nystatin (topical, oral); *Amphotericin B*

MOA: *binds to cell membrane sterols* (increasing the permeability/fragility of the cell membrane).

AMPHOTERICIN B:
1. **Indications:** *antifungal of choice* for most *invasive or life-threatening fungal infections.**
2. **SIDE EFFECTS:** *fever/chills during infusion,* electrolyte abnormalities *(↓K,↓Mg),* **nephrotoxicity** & hematologic toxicity (anemia), azotemia (↑BUN/creatinine), cardiac arrhythmias.
3. **Lipid-based Ampho B:** - advantages: high tissue concentrations, decreased infusion-related reactions, marked *decrease in nephrotoxicity* but VERY expensive.

NYSTATIN
1. **Indications:** used primarily topically (vaginal) & local treatment: *oral candidiasis (thrush).* Because of poor oral bioavailability. No significant drug interactions.

"AZOLES" ANTIFUNGALS

- Imidazoles: **Clotrimazole** (Lotrimin), **Ketoconazole** (Nizoral), **Econazole, Miconazole**
- Triazoles: **Fluconazole** (Diflucan), **Itraconazole, Voriconazole, Posaconazole**

MOA: *inhibits ergosterol synthesis* (ergosterols are essential for fungal cell membrane stability).

INDICATIONS: Candidiasis, Cryptococcus, Histoplasmosis, Coccidioidomycosis, Tinea (topical).
- **Fluconazole** – *drug of choice for noninvasive candida & Cryptococcal infections,* water soluble, *good for urine & CSF infections.** Fluconazole is eliminated by the kidney.
- **Voriconazole** EXTENDED spectrum (covers Aspergillus). *Voriconazole drug of choice for invasive aspergillis.** Does not cover Mucorales species well.
- **Itraconazole**: EXTENDED spectrum (covers Aspergillus). *Drug of choice for noninvasive Histoplasmosis, Blastomycosis, Coccidioidomycosis* (S/E: may cause CHF).
- **Ketoconazole & Itraconazole** - lipid soluble, **poor CSF penetration**, inhibits CP450.

SIDE EFFECTS
- **Fluconazole:** *hepatitis,* nausea, rash, alopecia, headache.
- **Ketoconazole:** *suppression of testosterone & cortisol* (used to treat refractory Cushing's). *↑LFTs*

ALLYLAMINES   Terbinafine (Lamisil); **Butenafine** (Mentax)

MOA: *inhibits ergosterol synthesis* (by inhibiting squalene epoxidase).
INDICATIONS: *dermatophyte infections:*
- Onychomycosis: Terbinafine PO
- Tinea (Corporis, Pedis, Cruris): Terbinafine or Butenafine topical

GRISEOFULVIN

MOA: *inhibits fungal cell mitosis preventing proliferation & function.*
INDICATIONS: *Tinea infection: capitus,* cruris, pedis, unguium.
   Give with fatty meals to increase absorption.
S/E: *Hepatitis, teratogenic:* (including males – males must avoid attempting to conceive for 6 months after treatment).

CASPOFUNGIN, ANIDULAFUNGIN, MICAFUNGIN

MOA: *Inhibits cell wall glucan synthesis.*   Echinocandins.
INDICATIONS: *includes azole- & AmB-resistant strains of Aspergillis & Candidiasis.*
S/E: fever, thrombophlebitis, headache, ↑LFTs, rash, flushing. *only IV* - very expensive.

FUNGAL DISEASES

CANDIDIASIS

- **Candida albicans** (yeast). Part of the normal GI & GU flora but **MC opportunistic pathogen.**

CLINICAL MANIFESTATIONS
1. ESOPHAGITIS: **MC manifestation.** Substernal odynophagia, gastroesophageal reflux, epigastric pain, nausea, vomiting, ±thrush. **Endoscopy: white linear plaques/erosions.***
   MANAGEMENT: Fluconazole PO 1st line treatment.*

2. ORAL THRUSH: **friable white plaques (± leave erythema or bleed if scraped).***
   MANAGEMENT: Nystatin tx of choice* swish & swallow. Clotrimazole troches.

3. VAGINAL CANDIDIASIS: **vulvar pruritus, burning, vaginal discharge (white, thick curd-like).***
   MANAGEMENT: Miconazole, Clotrimazole. Fluconazole weekly if persistent vaginitis.

4. INTERTRIGO: cutaneous infection MC in moist, macerated areas.
   Pruritic rash beefy red erythema* with **distinct, scalloped borders & satellite lesions.***
   MANAGEMENT: Clotrimazole topical, keep area dry.

5. FUNGEMIA, ENDOCARDITIS: seen in immunocompromised patients, ±indwelling catheters.
   MANAGEMENT: IV Amphotericin B. Caspofungin if severe. ±IV Fluconazole if mild.

DIAGNOSIS
Potassium Hydroxide (KOH) smear: budding yeast & pseudohyphae.* Clinical diagnosis.

CRYPTOCOCCOSIS

- **Cryptococcus neoformans** or C. gattii (_ENCAPSULATED,_* budding round yeast).
- **MC in immunocompromised** patients. **Transmission:** inhalation of _PIGEON/BIRD DROPPINGS._*

CLINICAL MANIFESTATIONS
1. MENINGOENCEPHALITIS: **MC cause of fungal meningitis.*** Headache, meningeal signs (neck stiffness, nausea, vomiting, photophobia). *Meningeal signs uncommon in patients with HIV.*

2. PNEUMONIA: cough, pleuritic chest pain, dyspnea. Skin lesions may be seen if disseminated.

DIAGNOSIS
1. **Lumbar puncture: Fungal CSF pattern:** ↑WBC (lymphocytes), ↓glucose, ↑protein. **India Ink stain** shows _encapsulated yeast_. Latex agglutination reveals **Cryptococcal antigen in CSF.***
2. May have ⊕ blood cultures in patients with HIV.

MANAGEMENT
1. **Amphotericin B plus Flucytosine*** x2 weeks **followed by oral Fluconazole** x 10 weeks.
2. Pneumonia if immunocompetent: *Fluconazole* or Itraconazole x 3- 6 months.

PROPHYLAXIS IN HIV:
Cryptococcus considered an AIDS defining illness. Routine prophylaxis is usually not indicated but in select persons, *Fluconazole* may be given *if CD4 ≤100* cells/μL.

HISTOPLASMOSIS

- **Histoplasma capsulatum** (dimorphic oval yeast). **AIDS-defining illness**. MC if CD4 ≤150 cells/μL.

- **Associated with soil containing BIRD/BAT DROPPINGS** in the **MISSISSIPPI & OHIO RIVER VALLEYS.*** Also seen with demolition, people who explore caves (spelunkers), excavators in those areas.

- Once inhaled, they are ingested by alveolar macrophages. *H. capsulatum grows within the phagosome* where they remain viable in macrophages & can disseminate via the macrophages.

CLINICAL MANIFESTATIONS
1. *Asymptomatic: most patients* (flu-like symptoms if they become symptomatic).

2. **Pneumonia** (atypical). Fever, nonproductive cough, myalgias.

3. **Dissemination:** *if immunocompromised*: hepatosplenomegaly, fever, oropharyngeal ulcers, bloody diarrhea, ±adrenal insufficiency if the adrenal gland is involved.

DIAGNOSIS
1. ↑ALP,↑LDH, pancytopenia. **CXR:** pulmonary infiltrates, hilar/mediastinal lymphadenopathy.

2. Cultures: ⊕ blood culture if disseminated/HIV; Sputum cultures or antigen by PCR. Urine Ag.

MANAGEMENT
1. **Mild-moderate disease: Itraconazole 1st line treatment.***

2. **Severe disease: Amphotericin B.** Also used if Itraconazole therapy is ineffective.

PNEUMOCYSTIS (PCP PNEUMONIA)

- **Pneumocystis jirovecii** (formerly carinii) is a yeast-like fungus (doesn't respond to antifungals).
- **Transmission:** inhalation. *MC opportunistic infection in HIV – especially if CD4 ≤200 cells/μL.*

CLINICAL MANIFESTATIONS
*Fever, dyspnea on exertion, nonproductive cough, O₂ desaturation with ambulation.**

DIAGNOSIS
1. **Chest radiographs: bilateral diffuse interstitial infiltrates.** May be normal.

2. ↑**LDH*** (>200U/L), fluid specimens.
3. Bronchoalveolar lavage specimen or induced sputum: **definitive diagnosis.**
   - *Direct fluorescent antibody staining to see both trophic & cyst forms.* MC technique used.
   - Trophic forms: Wright-Giemsa stain. Cysts: methenamine silver & toluidine blue stains.

MANAGEMENT
1. **Trimethoprim-sulfamethoxazole drug of choice*** x 21 days.
   ± **add Prednisone if hypoxic** (ex. PaO₂ <70 mmHg, A-a gradient ≥35mmHg).

2. Sulfa allergy ⇨ **Dapsone**-Trimethoprim, Pentamidine, Clindamcin-Primaquine, Atovaquone.

PCP PROPHYLAXIS IN HIV
CD4 ≤200 cells/μL ⇨ **Trimethoprim-sulfamethoxazole.***

ASPERGILLOSIS

- Aspergillus is a fungus commonly found in *garden and houseplant soil & compost.* Transmission is via inhalation. *MC affects lungs, sinuses & CNS.** Aspergillus produces *aflatoxin. Aflatoxin B1* is associated with an *increased risk of hepatocellular carcinoma.*
- Can cause disease in immunocompetent as well as immunosuppressed patients.

CLINICAL MANIFESTATIONS

1. ALLERGIC BRONCHOPULMONARY ASPERGILLOSIS: *MC in patients with asthma & cystic fibrosis.** Due to airway Type I hypersensitivity reaction to the fungus *(eosinophilia & ↑IgE).**
    Clinical: asthma sx, cough, thick brown sputum (mucus plugs), fever, pulmonary infiltrates.

2. ASPERGILLOMA: the fungus colonizes a preexisting pulmonary cavitary lesion. Can be an asymptomatic incidental finding on CXR or cough + *hemoptysis.** *"Fungal ball"* on CXR.

3. ACUTE INVASIVE ASPERGILLUS: fever, headache, toothache, epistaxis, *invasive chronic sinusitis.** Commonly involves the lungs ⇨ *hemoptysis, pleuritic chest pain, dyspnea.* ↑LDH. Often fatal.

4. CHRONIC INVASIVE (DISSEMINATED): immunocompromised/neutropenic patients. Pleuritic chest pain, cough, necrotizing skin lesions, wound infections, brain abscesses.

5. CHRONIC NECROTIZING PULMONARY: (rare). MC in immunocompromised (ex. stem cell transplants). Chronic pneumonia with nonproductive cough, dyspnea, pleuritic chest pain, fever, chills, weight loss. Cavitary lesions or fibrosis on CXR.

DIAGNOSIS

1. Galactomannan levels (found in the cell walls of Aspergillus - specific), β-D glucan assay, Culture.
2. ↑IgE & eosinophilia in allergic.

3. **Biopsy:** ex: *dusky, necrotic tissue* (ex. nose).
    - SEPTATE *hyphae with regular branching at wide angles** (45°). Distinguishes it from Mucor.

MANAGEMENT

1. **Allergic Bronchopulmonary Aspergillosis:**
    tapered corticosteroids, chest physiotherapy *± Itraconazole.*

2. **Severe/Invasive Aspergillus or Sinusitis:** *Voriconazole drug of choice,** high-dose Itraconazole, Amphotericin B, Caspofungin ⇨ surgical debridement if refractory.

3. **Aspergilloma:** *symptomatic: surgical resection.** *Asymptomatic: observation.*

MUCORMYCOSIS

- *MC Rhizopus,* Mucor & Rhizomucor. Other agents include Absidia & Cunninghamella.
- *MC seen in diabetic patients*, immunocompromised, patients with hyperglycemic acidosis.

CLINICAL: *rhino-orbital-cerebral infection*: ex. *sinusitis* that spreads to the orbits, palate & brain. *Black eschars** of the nasal mucosa, palate & cyanosis of the skin over the involved area.

DIAGNOSIS: biopsy: NON-SEPTATE broad hyphae with irregular right–angle branching (90°).

MANAGEMENT: *IV Amphotericin B 1st line treatment.** Posaconazole. May need surgical debridement.

BLASTOMYCOSIS

- *Blastomyces dermatitidis: pyogranulomatous fungal infection.* Fungus in nature, mold in tissues.
- Occurs MC in *immunocompetent men* **involved in outdoor activities (around _soil or decaying wood_) in close proximity to waterways** (ex. Mississippi & Ohio river basins or Great Lakes).

CLINICAL MANIFESTATIONS
1. PULMONARY: *MC site of involvement.* **Many are asymptomatic.** Chronic disease:
   Flu-like: cough with or without sputum production, dyspnea, headache, fever.
   Pneumonia: high fever, chest pain, productive cough.

2. CUTANEOUS: *papules* ⇨ **verrucous, crusted or ulcerated lesions*** which expand (may leave a central scar when healed). Skin MC site of extrapulmonary blastomycosis.

3. DISSEMINATED: **MC in lungs, skin, _bone_** (ribs or vertebral pain) & **_genitorurinary_ system** (*prostatitis or epididymitis*).

DIAGNOSIS
Sputum/pus/CSF or urine cultures: round broad-based budding yeast with thick, refractile double walls. CXR: consolidation. Nonspecific leukocytosis, anemia.

MANAGEMENT: *Itraconazole 1st line treatment of choice.*
_Amphotericin B if severe:_* (rapidly progressive, AIDS-related or CNS disease – ex meningitis).

COCCIDIOIDOMYCOSIS "Valley fever"

- *Coccidioides immitis* grows in **soil in arid/desert regions _Southwestern US, Mexico_**, South & Central America. Common opportunistic infection in HIV patients in endemic area.
- Transmission: inhalation of spores.

CLINICAL MANIFESTATIONS
1. PRIMARY PULMONARY DISEASE: 60-65% asymptomatic.
   Mild flu-like illness: fever, chills, nasopharyngitis, headache, cough, pleuritic chest pain.

2. VALLEY FEVER:* *fever, arthralgias (pain & swelling of the knees & ankles common),* *erythema nodosum* or *erythema multiforme.** Maculopapular rash, flu-like symptoms.

3. DISSEMINATED/EXTRAPULMONARY/PERSISTENT DISEASE: *CNS (ex. meningitis)* in 50%. Can affect any organ especially the lungs, skin, soft tissue, lymph nodes & joints.

DIAGNOSIS
Early: Enzyme-linked immunoassays for **IgM & IgG antibodies 1st test usually ordered** with immunodiffusion tests conducted only if the EIA is positive. **Cultures most definitive,** PCR, skin testing. Meningitis: CSF complement fixing antibodies, CSF shows lymphocytosis & ↓glucose.
Pulmonary: CXR: persistent cavitations, miliary pneumonia, abscesses & nodules.
Histology: *spherules* (thick-walled spherical structure containing endospores) seen in tissues.

MANAGEMENT
1. *Most cases asymptomatic/mild & are self limited* & require no treatment.
2. Localized lung disease is treated symptomatically in most cases.
3. *Fluconazole for CNS disease;* Amphotericin B (severe disease); Itraconazole, Ketoconazole.
Serial serologic complement fixation titers are used to monitor treatment.

GRAM NEGATIVE BACTERIAL DISEASES

CHLAMYDIA

Chlamydia trachomatis: most common overall bacterial cause of STDs in the US.*
CLINICAL MANIFESTATIONS
1. URETHRITIS: purulent or mucopurulent discharge, pruritus, dysuria, dyspareunia (pain with intercourse), hematuria. Up to 40% asymptomatic (especially men).

2. PELVIC INFLAMMATORY DISEASE (PID): abdominal pain, ⊕ *cervical motion tenderness.*

3. REACTIVE ARTHRITIS (REITER'S SYNDROME): *urethritis, uveitis, arthritis* (reactive arthritis is an *autoimmune* reaction). ⊕ *HLA-B27.**
4. LYMPHOGRANULOMA VENEREUM: genital/rectal lesion with softening, suppuration & lymphadenopathy.

DIAGNOSIS
1. *Nucleic acid amplification- test of choice for both gonorrhea & chlamydia** (vaginal swab or first-catch urine preferred).
2. Genetic probe methods, culture, antigen detection.

MANAGEMENT
1. *Azithromycin** (1 gram x1 dose) or *Doxycycline** 100mg bid for 10 days. Re-test in 3 weeks to ensure clearance of the organism. *Also treat for Gonorrhea (Ceftriaxone 250mg IM x 1 dose).*

GONORRHEA

• *Neisseria gonorrhoeae (gram-negative diplococci).* MC cause of urethritis in men <30y.* 2-8d IP.
CLINICAL MANIFESTATIONS
1. URETHRITIS & CERVICITIS: *anal, vaginal, penile, or pharyngeal discharge;* PID, epididymitis, prostatitis. Dx: culture shows gram negative diplococci in polymorphonuclear leukocytes

2. DISSEMINATION: *arthritis-dermatitis syndrome:* tendon pain (tenosynovitis), arthralgias (joint pain), rash (maculopapular, petechial). *Septic arthritis (especially of the knee).*

MANAGEMENT
1. *Ceftriaxone 250mg IM** *plus Doxycycline or Azithromycin* (for additional coverage for Gonorrhea as well as to cover possible Chlamydia). Cefixime alternative to Ceftriaxone. Azithromycin 2g can also be given as an alternative but associated with significant GI S/E.

CAT SCRATCH DISEASE

• *Bartonella henselae.** After a scratch or bite from a flea-infested cat (2-4 week incubation period).

CLINICAL MANIFESTATIONS: MC in children & young adults.
Brown/red papule/ulcer at the inoculation site. 1-7 weeks later ⇨ *fever,* headache, malaise ⇨ *lymphadenopathy* (erythema & warmth of the overlying skin) lasting 2-4 months.

MANAGEMENT
1. **Mild:** *symptomatic treatment* (usually self-limited): antipyretics, analgesics, warm compresses.

2. **Moderate:** *Azithromycin 1st line** *or Doxycycline.* Severe ⇨ Rifampin, Gentamicin, Ciprofloxacin.

3. Doxycycline preferred if optic neuritis or neurologic disease.

MENINGOCOCCAL MENINGITIS

- **Neisseria meningitidis (meningococcus)** - gram negative diplococci (kidney-bean shaped).

CLINICAL MANIFESTATIONS
1. Fever, headache, photophobia; *neck stiffness (rigidity)*, AMS, PURPURIC RASH* **(DIC).**
2. ⊕ *Kernig's sign:* inability to straighten the leg when the hip is flexed to 90°.
3. ⊕ *Brudzinski's sign:* neck flexion causes involuntary hip/knee flexion.

MANAGEMENT
Note: *most people are treated empirically for meningitis*
(ex. Ceftriaxone + Vancomycin in adults or Ampicillin + Cefotaxime in infants).

1. *Penicillin G tx of choice if susceptible.** Chloramphenicol, 3rd generation cephalosporin.

PROPHYLAXIS:
For patients exposed to those infected: *Ciprofloxacin* 500mg orally x 1 dose or *Rifampin.*

PREVENTION: vaccine may be given in patients >55y & high-risk patients (ex asplenia).

CHANCROID

- HAEMOPHILUS DUCREYI* (gram-negative fastidious coccobacillus). Incubation period 3-7days.
- 10% co-infection with HSV or syphilis in the US (rare in US).
- STD MC transmitted after a break in the skin.

CLINICAL MANIFESTATIONS
1. *PAINFUL* genital ulcers* (irregular borders, erythema) ⇨ *bubo formation (enlarged lymph nodes) that may rupture forming abscess pockets, painful inguinal lymphadenopathy,* ±vaginal discharge or fever.

DIAGNOSIS:
Clinical diagnosis usually (because it is difficult to culture). PCR or immunochromatography.

MANAGEMENT
1. *Azithromycin** 1g x 1 dose, *Ceftriaxone* 250mg IM x 1; Erythromycin 500mg tid x 7d, Ciprofloxacin.

HAEMOPHILUS INFLUENZAE

- *MC cause of epiglottitis.** *2nd MC cause of CAP.* *Often associated with sinusitis, otitis media.*

- **RISK FACTORS: underlying pulmonary disease:* COPD,* Bronchiectasis, Cystic Fibrosis,*** ETOH, Diabetes Mellitus, children <6y & the elderly.

MANAGEMENT
1. *Amoxicillin.* Amoxicillin/clavulanic acid (Augmentin) if positive for beta-lactamase. Fluoroquinolones, Trimethoprim-sulfamethoxazole (Bactrim).

2. *IV Ceftriaxone* for *epiglottitis, pneumonia or meningitis.*

TULAREMIA

- *Francisella tularensis* – gram negative coccobacillus MC seen in rodents & rabbits. IP 2-15d.
- *Transmission: tick/insect bite or handling animal tissues. Rabbits important reservoir.**

CLINICAL MANIFESTATIONS: most are asymptomatic.
1. **Ulceroglandular:** *MC type. Fever, headache nausea ⇨ single papule at the site of inoculation ⇨ ulceration of papule with central eschar & tender regional lymphadenopathy.** Ulcers of the hand or arm MC after animal exposure. Ulcers of the head/trunk/legs MC after tick exposure. Splenomegaly.
2. Glandular: tender regional lymphadenopathy with the absence of skin lesions.
3. Oculoglandular: if splashed in the eye with infected material ⇨ pain, photophobia, tearing.
4. Pharyngeal: due to ingestion of contaminated food/water ⇨ fever & sore throat.
5. Typhoidal: after ingestion of infected meat (ex *undercooked rabbit meat*) ⇨ fever & GI sx: nausea, vomiting, diarrhea.
6. Pneumonia, meningitis, pericarditis.

DIAGNOSIS: serologies, blood cultures.

MANAGEMENT: *Streptomycin drug of choice.** Gentamicin, Doxycycline.

| **DISEASES WITH ESCHARS:** Tularemia, Anthrax, Leishmaniasis, Coccidioidomycosis, Mucormycosis |

BRUCELLOSIS

- Gram-negative coccobacilli. MC lab-acquired infection (Category B biological weapon).
- *Goat, sheep, cattle hogs MC animal vector.* Rare in US. *Endemic in Mexico.**
Transmission: handling infected tissues or *ingestion of infected unpasteurized milk & cheese.**

CLINICAL MANIFESTATIONS: *nonspecific: absent or low-grade fever (MC sx)*, weakness, myalgias, arthralgias, headache, anorexia, weight loss, easy exhaustion. Hepatosplenomegaly.

DIAGNOSIS: culture, serologies, lymphocytosis.

MANAGEMENT: *Rifampin + Doxycycline.* Rifampin + Trimethoprim-sulfamethoxazole in children. Doxycycline plus (Streptomycin or Gentamicin) is an alternative treatment.

HOT TUB FOLLICULITIS

- *Pseudomonas aeruginosa.** Commonly seen in people who bathe in a *contaminated spa, swimming pool, or hot tub (especially if it is made of wood).**

CLINICAL MANIFESTATIONS
Small (2–10 mm) *pink to red bumps*, which may be filled with pus or covered with a scab appear 1-4 days after exposure to the source. Itchy, tender bumps located around hair follicles.

MANAGEMENT
1. *Usually spontaneously resolves within 7–14 days without treatment.**
2. *Ciprofloxacin orally if persistent.*

Suspect Pseudomonas in conjunctivitis in contact lens wearers or puncture wounds while wearing tennis shoes.*

Q FEVER

- **_Coxiella burnetii_**. Transmission is inhalation or ingestion. Gram negative.
- Exposure to **_sheep, goats, cattle & their products (ex. wool)._*

CLINICAL MANIFESTATIONS
1. **ACUTE:** **_pneumonia main manifestation of acute Q fever._*** _Influenza-like illness:_ severe headache, fever (with relative bradycardia), cough, abdominal pain, hepatitis, or encephalopathy.

2. **CHRONIC:** **_culture-negative endocarditis main manifestation of chronic Q fever._*** Vascular infection of the aorta, persistent low grade fever, rash (septic thromboembolism).

DIAGNOSIS
1. Acute: **_immunofluorescence IFA MC test used_** (Coxiella anti-phase II immunoglobulins). PCR
2. Chronic: Phase I IgG immunoglobulins.
3. Leukopenia, ↑LFTs. Weil-Felix testing was used prior to IFA.

MANAGEMENT
_Doxycycline tx of choice._* Fluoroquinolones, Macrolides, Trimethoprim-sulfamethoxazole. Rifampin may be used in chronic disease.

PLAGUE

- **_Yersinia pestis_**: gram-negative rod. Incubation period 2-10 days.

- **Transmission:** **_via infected rodents & their fleas;*_** **_person to person transmission via droplets._** Rare in US. (10-15 cases/year in US in states like Arizona, New Mexico, California, Colorado, Utah).

CLINICAL MANIFESTATIONS
Rapid onset of fever, chills, weakness, malaise, myalgias, tachycardia, severe headache & AMS. 3 forms:
1. **BUBONIC:** **_MC form (95%): acutely swollen, extremely, warm, red, painful nodes (buboes)_** 2-10cm in diameter in the **_groin, axilla & cervical regions._*** Lymphatic spread may lead to hematogenous spread.

2. **SEPTICEMIC:** subsequent, advanced disease characterized by **_DIC & gangrene_**. Plague without the presence of buboes. **_DIC: extensive purpura_** 'black death". **_Acral gangrene:_** distal extremities, nose or penis. _Patients often die from pneumonia or meningitis._

3. **PNEUMONIC:** tachypnea, productive cough, frothy **_blood-tinged sputum_** "red death", cyanosis.

DIAGNOSIS
Gram stain from tissue: ⇨ bipolar staining (**_SAFETY-PIN APPEARANCE of organisms)._*** Cultures.

MANAGEMENT:
1. **_Streptomycin or Gentamicin 1st line treatment._*** Doxycycline 2nd line.
    Place on strict respiratory isolation for at least 48 hours after initiating antibiotic therapy.

POST-EXPOSURE PROPHYLAXIS
Doxycycline or Tetracycline. Trimethoprim-sulfamethoxazole is an alternative.

GRAM POSITIVE BACTERIAL DISEASES

NECROTIZING FASCIITIS (FLESH EATING DISEASE)

- **MC GABHS (often polymicrobial).** Rapid progression of the infection through the fascia.

- **FOURNIER'S GANGRENE:** *necrotizing fasciitis of the **penis/scrotum** especially seen with **impaired immunity (ex. Diabetes Mellitus)** or after trauma to the area.*

CLINICAL MANIFESTATIONS
Erythema & ***extreme <u>pain out of proportion to physical exam</u>*** * ⇨ develop ***blue, <u>hemorrhagic bullae</u>* (blisters at site)** ⇨ ***gangrene*** ⇨ septic shock. Crepitus may be elicited.

MANAGEMENT
Surgical debridement + broad spectrum antibiotics:
ex. Ampicillin/sulbactam, Piperacillin/tazobactam, Imipenem.

DIPHTHERIA

- ***Corynebacterium diphtheriae*** (gram positive rod). Rare in US due to vaccination. IP 1-7d.

TRANSMISSION: inhalation of respiratory secretions. Exotoxin induces inflammatory response.

CLINICAL MANIFESTATIONS
1. ***Tonsillopharyngitis or laryngitis is the classic presentation.***
   - *<u>PSEUDOMEMBRANES:</u>* *<u>friable gray/white membrane on pharynx that bleeds if scraped.</u>* *
     Pseudomembranes are made up of WBCs, RBCs, fibrin & organisms.

   - ***<u>Bull neck:</u>*** * neck swelling due to enlarged cervical lymphadenopathy.

   - Fever & nasopharyngeal symptoms. Neuropathy.

2. *<u>MYOCARDITIS</u>, **arrhythmias or heart failure*** (exotoxin-induced inflammatory response).

DIAGNOSIS
Clinical diagnosis. PCR, culture to confirm. Isolate until 3 negative pharyngeal cultures.

MANAGEMENT
1. ***Diphtheria antitoxin (horse serum) most important + Erythromycin or Penicillin*** *x 2 weeks.*
   Clindamycin or Rifampin are alternatives. Penicillin + Aminoglycoside for endocarditis.
   - Antitoxin reduces sequelae & increase recovery time. Supplied by the CDC.
   - Antibiotics used to prevent the spread of diphtheria.

PROPHYLAXIS FOR CLOSE CONTACTS
Erythromycin x 7- 10 days or Penicillin benzathine G x 1 dose.

PREVENTION
DTaP schedule: 5 doses between 6 months & 7 years of age with booster at 11years:
Given at 2 mos, 4 mos, 6 mos & between 15-18 months, between 4-6y of age & booster 11-12y.

ERYSIPELOID

- Erysipelothrix rhusiopathiae (gram-positive bacillus).
- *Occupational disease follows skin abrasion, <u>puncture wound from raw fish, shellfish, raw meat/poultry</u>.*

CLINICAL MANIFESTATIONS

1. LOCALIZED CUTANEOUS: *limited to hands/fingers/webspaces:* severe pain/burning/tingling, **non-pitting edema, <u>purplish erythema</u> with sharp irregular margins extending peripherally but <u>clearing centrally</u>.**

2. DIFFUSE CUTANEOUS: may be associated with fever.
3. GENERALIZED: ±low grade fever. Endocarditis & bacteremia uncommon but serious sequelae.

DIAGNOSIS: Usually clinical. Culture from material obtained during biopsy.

MANAGEMENT: *Penicillin G or V*, Cephalosporins, Clindamycin.

TETANUS

- *Clostridium tetani* (gram-positive rod). Ubiquitous in soil germinates *especially in puncture* & crush wounds*. 5 day - 15 week incubation period (IP).

PATHOPHYSIOLOGY

- Neurotoxin (tetanospasmin) blocks neuron inhibition (via blocking acetylcholinesterase) ⇨ *severe muscle spasm* (Ach-mediated sustained contractions at the neuromuscular joint).

CLINICAL MANIFESTATIONS

1. GENERALIZED TETANUS: pain/tingling at the inoculation site ⇨ *early sx:* **local muscle spasms, neck/jaw stiffness,** TRISMUS* = *lockjaw – the MC presenting symptom,* dysphagia, hyperirritability (symptoms often occur within 7 days) ⇨ drooling, **risus sardonicus** (facial contractions), <u>opisthotonus</u> (arched back), muscle rigidity in descending fashion (hands & feet usually spared). These spasms **may affect the respiratory muscles. Spasm with minor stimulation, ↑deep tendon reflexes.** Autonomic dysfunction can lead to tachycardia, hyperpyrexia & hypertension (though bradycardia and hypotension may also be seen).

2. NEONATAL TETANUS: usually transferred from an unimmunized mother or unsanitary practices (such as using a soiled instrument in cutting of the umbilical cord).
3. LOCALIZED: uncommon variant - just the local muscles around the wound are affected.
4. CEPHALIC: cranial nerve involvement only.

MANAGEMENT

1. *Metronidazole** (or *Penicillin G*) **plus** IM **Tetanus immune globulin (**ex. **5,000 units).** Benzodiazepines to reduce spasms ex. **Diazepam**. Respiratory support if needed.

PROPHYLAXIS

1. *Previously vaccinated:* **Tdap*** *or* Td vaccine q10y (given if major cut occurs >5y since last booster).

2. Never vaccinated: Tetanus immune globulin 250u + initiation of tetanus toxoid vaccine, second dose between 4-8 weeks & third dose given between 6-12 months after the second.

GAS GANGRENE (MYONECROSIS)

- **Clostridium perfringens*** (other Clostridial species) causing a life-threatening infection.
- **Traumatic injury*** & IV drug injection use MC causes (*anaerobic conditions*).

CLINICAL MANIFESTATIONS
1. Sudden onset of pain & edema in an area of wound contamination, **systemic toxicity (shock).**
2. **Brown to blood-tinged watery exudates** with skin discoloration of the surrounding area.
3. **CREPITUS/GAS IN THE TISSUE PALPATED ON PHYSICAL EXAM.***

DIAGNOSIS:
1. Radiographs: **AIR IN THE SOFT TISSUES.*** CT/MRI gives more detail. Muscle involvement seen.
2. Culture or smear of exudates: gram-positive rods/bacilli (spore forming). Blood cultures.

MANAGEMENT:
1. **IV Penicillin** (ex. 2 million q 3 hours) + **IV Clindamycin, debridement.** May need amputation.
2. Tetracycline & Metronidazole other antibiotic alternatives.

BOTULISM

- **Clostridium botulinum** (gram-positive, spore-forming rods). Neurotoxin inhibits acetylcholine release at the neuromuscular junction ⇨ **weakness, flaccid paralysis, respiratory arrest.**

TRANSMISSION
1. ADULT: ingestion of preformed toxin in **canned/smoked/vacuum-packed foods.***
2. INFANT: **ingestion of honey*** or dust containing spores ⇨ active toxin production in the gut.
3. WOUND BOTULISM: Rare. MC after traumatic injury with soil contamination or in *IVDA.*

CLINICAL MANIFESTATIONS: symptoms occur 12-36 hours after ingestion (6-8h if <1 year old).
1. Sudden onset of **8 D's:** *Diplopia,* **Dilated, fixed pupils,*** *Dry mouth, Dysphagia, Dysarthria, Dysphonia,* **Descending Decreased muscle strength** ⇨ *flaccid* paralysis. GI symptoms (N/V). CN palsies.
2. **"Floppy baby syndrome:"** *newborn* ⇨ *lethargy, weakness, flaccid paralysis, weak cry, failure to thrive.*

MANAGEMENT
1. **ANTITOXINS IN ALL CASES:*** If >1y ⇨ equine-derived Botulism antitoxin heptavalent. If <1y ⇨ human-derived botulism immune globulin.
2. *Intubation if respiratory failure.*
3. *No antibiotics in foodborne type* (may worsen disease via toxin release from bacteria lysis).
4. Antibiotics ONLY used in wound botulism: *Penicillin G 1st line.* Metronidazole, Clindamycin.

LISTERIOSIS

- **Listeria monocytogenes** non-spore forming, *endotoxin-producing,* gram-positive bacilli.
- MC found in *contaminated food* ex. **cold deli meats** & **unpasteurized dairy products (ex. soft cheeses, milk).*** Highest in 3 populations: ❶children ❷elderly & ❸pregnant patients.

CLINICAL MANIFESTATIONS
1. **Listeriosis: bacteremia** (ex. in **infants <2 months & elderly).*** 3rd MC cause of meningitis.

2. **Pregnancy:** *3rd trimester* ⇨ febrile illness **associated with premature labor & stillbirth.***

MANAGEMENT
IV Ampicillin tx of choice.* **Gentamicin** is added in meningitis, endocarditis, immunocompromised.
   Trimethoprim-sulfamethoxazole is an alternative to Ampicillin if PCN allergic.

ANTHRAX

- *Bacillus anthracis* (gram-positive, spore-forming rod).
- *Naturally found in livestock:* ex. cattle, horses, goats, sheep & swine.

<u>Transmission:</u> inhalation, ingestion of spores or direct contact (ex. wool, handling animal hide or hair).

CLINICAL MANIFESTATIONS

1. <u>CUTANEOUS:</u> 5-14 days after exposure ⇨ erythematous papule at the inoculation site that ulcerates ⇨ *PAINLESS BLACK ESCHAR** with marked surrounding edema & vesicles. *MC type.*
2. <u>INHALATION ANTHRAX:</u> nonspecific flu-like symptoms rapidly progressing to dyspnea (pleural effusions), hypoxia & shock. Inhalation <5%.
   - **DIAGNOSIS:** *WIDENING OF THE MEDIASTINUM ON CXR** (due to hemorrhagic lymphadenitis).
3. <u>GI anthrax:</u> rare in US. Ingestion of meat with spores ⇨ GI bleeding, abdominal pain, N/V.

<u>MANAGEMENT:</u> *Ciprofloxacin for tx & exposure.** *Doxycycline.* Rifampin + Macrolide, Clindamycin.

SPIROCHETAL DISEASES

SYPHILIS

- Chronic infection caused by the spirochete **Treponema pallidum.** Known as *"the great imitator"* because the rash & disease can present in many different ways similar to other diseases.

TRANSMISSION

- **Direct contact:** of an infected lesion during *sexual activity* & contact with lesions (including mucous membranes). May also be transmitted to the fetus via the placenta.
- The organism enters tissues from direct contact, forming a chancre at the inoculation site and from there, goes to the regional lymph nodes before disseminating.

CLINICAL MANIFESTATIONS: incubation period is between 3 days to 3 months. 3 phases.

❶ **PRIMARY:**
   - *CHANCRE:** *painless ulcer at/near the inoculation site* with *raised indurated edges* (usually begins as a papule that ulcerates). Chancres heal spontaneously on average within 3-4 weeks (even without medical management).
   - Nontender regional lymphadenopathy near the chancre site lasting 3-4 weeks.

❷ **SECONDARY:**
   Secondary symptoms may occur a few weeks - 6 months after the initial symptoms.
   - *maculopapular rash** diffuse bilateral maculopapular lesions *(involvement of the palms/soles common).* Lesions may be pustular in some patients.

   - *CONDYLOMA LATA:** wart-like, moist lesions involving the mucous membranes & other moist areas. Especially near the chancre site. Highly contagious.
   - <u>Systemic sx:</u> fever, lymphadenopathy (may be tender), arthritis, meningitis, headache, hepatitis (elevated alkaline phosphatase).

❸ **TERTIARY (LATE):** may occur from 1 to >20 years after initial infection or after latent infection.
   - *GUMMA:* *noncancerous granulomas* on skin & body tissues (ex bones).
   - **Neurosyphilis:** headache, meningitis, dementia, vision/hearing loss, incontinence; **Tabes dorsalis** (demyelination of posterior columns ⇨ ataxia, areflexia burning pain, weakness).
   - *ARGYLL-ROBERTSON PUPIL:** small, irregular pupil that constricts normally to near accommodation but does not constrict/react to light.
   - **Cardiovascular: aortitis,** aortic regurgitation, aortic aneurysms.

- **Early syphilis:** clinical syndrome that occurs within the first year of infection: includes primary, secondary & early latent syphilis.

- **Latent syphilis:** *asymptomatic infection + normal physical exam but positive serologic testing.*
  Early latent: If <1 year (patients are usually highly infectious).
  Late latent: > 1 year. Associated with a lower transmission rate (except in fetal transmission).

CONGENITAL SYPHILIS
- *Hutchinson teeth* (notches on teeth), sensorineural hearing loss, CNS abnormalities.
- *Saddle-nose deformity.*
- ToRCH syndrome.

DIAGNOSIS
1. ***Darkfield microscopy:*** allows for direct visualization of the spirochete.
   Indications: *used in patients with a chancre or condyloma lata.*

2. **Screening tests:** *non treponemal testing via:*
   - *RPR* (Rapid Plasma Reagent). These tests look at titers (ex. positive test indicates a titer of 1:32 or greater). Changes in titers help to determine therapeutic response. However, these tests are nonspecific in initial testing and must be **confirmed** by more specific **treponemal testing (ex: FTA).** RPR is usually positive 4-6 weeks after infection.

   - *VDRL* (Venereal Disease Research Laboratory).

   - Screening tests are nonspecific. False positives can be seen with antiphospholipid syndrome, pregnancy, tuberculosis, rickettsial infections (ex. Rocky Mountain spotted fever).

3. **Confirmatory treponemal tests:** *FTA-ABS** (fluorescent treponemal antibody absorption) or Microhemagglutination test for *T. pallidum* antibodies.

MANAGEMENT
1. ***Penicillin G tx of choice* in all stages of syphilis.*** Penicillin preferred even in the penicillin allergic patient (so desensitization may be sometimes used for adequate management).
   - **Primary, secondary or early-latent:** Penicillin G benzathine IM 2.4 million units x 1 dose.

   - **Tertiary or late-latent:** Penicillin G benzathine 2.4 million units IM every week x 3 doses.

   - S/E of penicillin treatment: *Jarisch-Herxheimer reaction*: acute febrile response due to rapid lysis of many spirochetes with antibiotic administration. Associated with myalgias & headaches. Antipyretics during the 1st 24 hours reduces the incidence of the reaction.

2. PCN allergic: *Doxycycline* or Tetracycline, Macrolide, Ceftriaxone (none are as effective as PCN).

PATIENT FOLLOW UP
- All patients should be reexamined clinically and serologically at 6 months and 12 months after treatment.
- A 4-fold reduction in the titer of the nontreponemal antibody serologic tests within 6 months denotes adequate management. If not, it may indicate reinfection or treatment failure.
- All patients with syphilis should be tested for HIV.

LYME DISEASE

*Borrelia burgdorferi** (gram negative spirochete) that is spread by the vector *Ixodes (deer) tick.*

PATHOPHYSIOLOGY
- Most cases are transmitted by the *Ixodes scapularis tick* in the nymphal phase - MC sources are the *white-tailed deer* & white-footed mice. MC in the spring & summer (when the nymphs feed). MC in the Northeast, Midwest & Mid-Atlantic regions of the United States.

- The highest likelihood of transmission is if the tick is engorged and/or has been attached for at least 72 hours.

CLINICAL MANIFESTATIONS
1) EARLY LOCALIZED: *ERYTHEMA MIGRANS** (90%). *Expanding, warm, annular, erythematous rash* (classically seen with *central clearing or "bull's-eye"* appearance usually within a month of & around area of tick bite). The lesion usually expands slowly over days to weeks. May be accompanied with viral-like syndrome, headaches, fever, malaise or lymphadenopathy.

2) EARLY DISSEMINATED: (1-12 weeks) *rheumatologic*: arthritis (especially large joints); **neurologic**: headache, meningitis, weakness, CN palsies ex. *CN VII/Facial nerve palsy,** neuropathy; **cardiac: AV block,** pericarditis; Multiple erythema migrans lesions.

3) LATE DISEASE: persistent synovitis, persistent neurological symptoms, subacute encephalitis. Acrodermatitis chronica atrophicans: bluish discoloration of extremities seen in Europe.

DIAGNOSIS
1. **Clinical:** especially in early Lyme disease: presence of EM, history of tick bite, arthritis. This is because *patients with erythema migrans are often seronegative in the early stage.*

2. **Serologic testing:** *ELISA followed by Western Blot if ELISA is positive or equivocal.* IgM &/or IgG antibodies to *B. burgdorferi* are employed as an adjunct to patients with clinical symptoms suggestive of Lyme disease as it only tells if a patient has been infected with the spirochete (does not determine if the person has an active infection). Used in patients who traveled to an endemic area PLUS risk factor for exposure to ticks PLUS symptoms consistent with Lyme disease. *During the time that erythema migrans is present, serologic testing is often negative.*
    - False positive ELISA: other spirochetal diseases: syphilis, yaws; viral or bacterial illnesses & other Borrelial species.

MANAGEMENT
Early disease:
1. *Doxycycline** bid x 10-21 days *usually preferred** (early disseminated duration 14-28 days). Azithromycin or Erythromycin can be used if Doxycycline is contraindicated & PCN allergic.

2. *Amoxicillin (treatment of choice in children <8y, pregnancy)** x 14-21 days. Cefuroxime.

Late/severe disease:
1. *IV Ceftriaxone if 2nd/3rd AV heart block, syncope, dyspnea, chest pain, CNS disease* (OTHER than CN VII palsy). *ex. meningitis.*

PROPHYLAXIS
Doxycycline 200mg x1 dose *within 72h of Ixodes tick removal if the tick is present for ≥36h & >20% ticks infected in the area* where the tick bite occurred. If allergic, no prophylaxis given.

ROCKY MOUNTAIN SPOTTED FEVER

Potentially fatal but curable tick-borne disease caused by **_Rickettsia ricketsii* (spread by ticks)._**

PATHOPHYSIOLOGY
• *Rickettsia ricketsii:* gram negative, obligate intracellular bacterium with an affinity for vascular endothelial cells, leading to _vascular injury_, microhemorrhages & microinfarcts.

• **Vector: _Dermacentor andersoni/variabilis (wood/dog tick_ respectively) are the vectors.**
      MC in South-central & Southeastern United States (especially in the spring/summer).

CLINICAL MANIFESTATIONS
1. 2-14 days after tick bite. Fever/chills, myalgias, arthralgias, headache, N/V, lethargy, seizures
   ⇨ **_blanching, erythematous macular rash FIRST ON WRISTS/ANKLES* ⇨ palms/soles characteristic & spreading centrally over 2-3 days_** (10% don't develop a rash).
         ± faint macules ⇨ papules, **_petechiae._**

2. Patient may develop encephalitis, ARDS, cardiac or bleeding disorders.

DIAGNOSIS
1. **_Clinical diagnosis (don't wait for serologies)_** – fever, rash, history of tick bite.

2. **Serologies:** indirect immunofluorescent antibody test for IgM and IgG antibodies.
   • A fourfold rise in titers indicates acute disease.
   • A negative serology test in the first few days does not mean the patient is not infected so clinical suspicion must be take into consideration.

3. Skin biopsy. May develop thrombocytopenia or hyponatremia.

4. CSF: low glucose & pleocytosis (increased cell count).

MANAGEMENT
Ideally, treatment should begin ideally within 5 days of symptom onset to reduce mortality.
   1. **_Doxycycline (even in children)*_** x 5-14 days (dental staining not as likely with short course).

   2. **_Chloramphenicol 2nd line._** Chloramphenicol treatment of choice in pregnancy. Third trimester usage of Chloramphenicol associated with gray baby syndrome.

PARASITIC DISEASES

AMEBIASIS

Entamoeba histolytica (protozoan spread by fecal contamination of soil, water).

CLINICAL MANIFESTATIONS: _GI colitis, dysentery_ (bloody diarrhea), **_AMEBIC LIVER ABSCESS.*_**

DIAGNOSIS: stool O&P (ova & parasites), positive serologic tests in colitis (ELISA).

MANAGEMENT
1. **Colitis: _Metronidazole*_** *(Flagyl)* or Tinidazole followed by an intraluminal agent: ex. Paromomycin (anti-parasitic aminoglycoside) or Diloxanide furoate or Diiodohydroxyquin (Iodoquinol).
2. **Abscess:** Metronidazole or Tinidazole + intraluminal antiparasitic followed by Chloroquine.
      May need drainage if no response to medications after 3 days.

ACANTHAMOEBA KERATITIS

TRANSMISSION
Often minor ocular trauma: swimming with contact lens, infected contact lens solution.

CLINICAL MANIFESTATIONS
1. *keratitis (especially in contact lens wearers):** ocular pain, photophobia, tearing, blurred vision, conjunctival injection.
   Physical exam: **Corneal stromal ring infiltrate,** hypopyon.

2. Encephalitis & granulomatous disease seen in immunocompromised patients.

MANAGEMENT
Combination treatment: Biguanide-Chlorhexadine ±Propamidine or Hexamidine.

MALARIA

- *Red blood cell disease caused by Plasmodium* (falciparum, vivax, ovale, malariae) protozoa that are transmitted by the **female Anopheles mosquito.**
- *Falciparum most dangerous type.** *Sickle cell trait & thalassemia trait are protective vs. Malaria.*
  Plasmodium spp. infects red blood cells ⇨RBC lysis ⇨ cyclical fever.

CLINICAL MANIFESTATIONS
1. *Cyclical fever** (cold stage/chills ⇨ hot stage/fever ⇨ diaphoretic stage every other or 3rd day), **leukopenia, hemolytic anemia, thrombocytopenia** headache, myalgias, GI sx. Splenomegaly. Cyclical fever every 48h (P. vivax & P. ovale) & 72h (P. malariae). Irregular fever with P. falciparum.

2. *P. falciparum: cerebral malaria (coma* due to lysed RBCs occluding cerebral flow), blackwater fever = severe hemolysis + hemoglobinuria (dark urine) + renal failure.

DIAGNOSIS
*Giemsa stain peripheral smear (thin & thick):** parasites in RBCs. Thrombocytopenia, ↑LDH.

MANAGEMENT
1. **Chloroquine* 1st line in sensitive areas.** Quinidine.
2. **Multi drug-resistant area:** *Atovaquone (with Doxycycline or Clindamycin).*

BABESIOSIS

- *Babesia microti - Malaria-like protozoa that **attacks red blood cells.***
- *History of tick bite (Ixodes). Northeast US (Long Island, Massachusetts).**

CLINICAL MANIFESTATIONS
Fever & chills, **hemolytic anemia & jaundice,** arthralgia, myalgia.

DIAGNOSIS
Peripheral smear: parasites within the RBCs especially in *PATHOGNOMONIC TETRADS** (Maltese cross).

MANAGEMENT
Atovaquone plus Azithromycin OR Quinine plus Clindamycin.

TOXOPLASMOSIS

Toxoplasma gondii (protozoan) primarily transmitted by cats (including cat litter), raw pork, lamb.

CLINICAL MANIFESTATIONS

1. Primary infection: usually asymptomatic in immunocompetent patients.
   May develop a mono-like illness with cervical lymphadenopathy if symptomatic.

2. ENCEPHALITIS* & CHORIORETINITIS *in immunocompromised patients* (CD4 ≤100);* fever, lymphadenopathy (especially cervical), malaise, myalgias, headaches, arthritis.

3. CONGENITAL: part of the ToRCH syndrome: *To*xoplasmosis, *R*ubella, *C*ytomegalovirus, *H*erpes simplex 2: *blueberry muffin rash (TTP – Thrombotic Thrombocytopenia Purpura), hepatosplenomegaly, hearing loss, mental development delays.*

DIAGNOSIS

1.PCR. Head CT scan/MRI: ± show *RING-ENHANCING LESIONS* (may also be seen with CNS lymphoma).

MANAGEMENT

1. *Sulfadiazene (or Clindamycin) + Pyrimethamine (with folinic acid/leucovorin to prevent bone marrow suppression & reduce nephrotoxicity).* Spiramycin if pregnant.

PROPHYLAXIS

CD4 ≤100 cells/μL: *Trimethoprim-sulfamethoxazole.** Dapsone + Pyrimethamine & Leucovorin.

ENTEROBIASIS (PINWORM)

Enterobius vermicularis. **Transmission:** *feco-oral* (especially in *school-aged children*).

CLINICAL MANIFESTATIONS: *perianal itching esp. nocturnal* (eggs are laid at night).

DIAGNOSIS: *Scotch tape test* (early in AM) to look for eggs under a microscope

MANAGEMENT: *Albendazole,** Mebendazole. Pyrantel 2nd line. None are used in children ≤2y old.

CHAGAS DISEASE (AMERICAN TRYPANOSOMIASIS)

- Protozoa *Trypanosoma cruzi.* Symptoms MC in children. *Leading cause of CHF in Latin America.**
- Prevalent in Latin America northward to Texas. Vector is assassin bug (bites in the evening).

CLINICAL MANIFESTATIONS:

1. **Acute**: illness lasting 3 weeks to 3 months: fever, *UNILATERAL PERIORBITAL EDEMA,** lymphadenopathy, edema at the site of the bite, hepatosplenomegaly. Most asymptomatic.
   Romaña's sign: unilateral perioribital swelling. **Chagoma:** inflammatory nodule @ bite site.

2. **Latent phase**: destruction of nerve cell ganglia causes *cardiomyopathy, congestive heart failure (CHF),* arrhythmias, GI abnormalities (*megacolon & megaesophagus*).

DIAGNOSIS: peripheral blood smear or culture. Serology or muscle biopsy in the latent phase.
Echocardiogram: *cardiomegaly with apical atrophy/aneurysm.*

MANAGEMENT

Benznidazole or Nifurtimox for 90-120 days depending on age (obtained from CDC).

AFRICAN TRYPANOSOMIASIS (AFRICAN SLEEPING SICKNESS)

- Protozoa *T. brucei (rhodesiense & gambiense). Vector is TSETSE FLY.**
- Prevalent in sub-Sahara Africa & South/Central America.

CLINICAL MANIFESTATIONS: 2 stages:
1. **Early/Hemolymphatic stage:** *painless chancre at the bite site* 2-3 days after bite, increasing in size, resolving in 2-3 weeks. Intermittent ever, general malaise, headaches, joint pains & itching. *Generalized or regional lymphadenopathy (often extremely large).*
   Winterbottom sign – posterior cervical lymphadenopathy. Transient rash.

2. **Late/CNS stage:** persistent headache, *daytime sleepiness followed by nighttime insomnia* (tryptophol released by T. brucei induces sleep), behavioral changes, wasting syndrome, seizures in children.

DIAGNOSIS: peripheral blood smear or aspiration of an affected lymph node.
MANAGEMENT: infectious disease consult. Pentamidine (gambiense), Suramin (rhodesiense).

TRICHINOSIS (TRICHENELLOSIS)

- Trichenella species (especially *Trichenella spiralis)* - parasitic roundworm infection.
- *Transmitted by raw or undercooked meat (especially pork,* wild boar or bear).*

PATHOPHSYIOLOGY
Larvae cysts are ingested, go to the duodenum and jejunum to grow into adults & replicate. Adults are excreted in the stool & larva penetrate intestinal wall & *encapsulate in striated muscle tissue.* Severity of disease correlates with the number of ingested larvae.

CLINICAL MANIFESTATIONS
1. *Gastrointestinal phase:* abdominal pain, nausea, diarrhea, vomiting. *Week 1* ⇨ muscle phase progression...
2. *Muscle phase: myositis:** muscle pain, tenderness, swelling and weakness with high fever. Eye: *palpebral/circumorbital edema,** ± retinal hemorrhages; macular or urticarial rash, dyspnea, dysphagia, or conjunctivitis.
3. Cardiac: myocarditis (due to eosinophilia – they don't make cysts in cardiac tissues).
4. CNS: encephalitis or meningitis.
5. Pulmonary: pneumonia.

DIAGNOSIS
1. *Eosinophilia: hallmark,** ↑creatine kinase & ↑LDH* (due to muscle involvement).
2. Usually clinical & confirmed with serologies:
   - *consider in any patient with PERIORBITAL EDEMA, MYOSITIS & EOSINOPHILIA.**
3. Muscle biopsy: larvae seen in striated muscle (not commonly used). Definitive diagnosis.

MANAGEMENT
1. **Mild cases:** most cases are mild and self-limited & require only symptomatic treatment (analgesia and antipyretics).

2. **Severe cases:** *Albendazole** or Mebendazole (antiparasitic) plus Corticosteroids. Albendazole & Mebendazole are contraindicated in children ≤2y & in pregnancy.

ASCARIASIS

• *Ascaris lumbricoides (giant roundworm).* MC intestinal helminth worldwide. Contaminated soil.

CLINICAL MANIFESTATIONS
Small worm load: asymptomatic. Larger load: vague abdominal symptoms. High load: may migrate to pancreatic duct, bile duct, appendix, diverticula and cause symptoms at the site.

DIAGNOSIS: eggs in feces or large worm may be coughed, vomited, leave nose, anus or mouth. Stool O & P (ova & parasites), *Eosinophilia.*

MANAGEMENT: *Mebendazole, Albendazole; Pyrantel if pregnant (given after 1st trimester).**

LEISHMANIASIS

• Protozoa Leishmania species. *Spread by the bite of a FEMALE SANDFLY.**
• Prevalent in Mediterranean, Central & South America, Africa & Asia.

CLINICAL MANIFESTATIONS
1. **Cutaneous:** ❶ *small erythematous papules* with *ulceration or* ❷ *dry, indurated plaque* with *satellite pustules** that develops at the bite site weeks to months after infection. May crusts over in the center *leaving a raised, bordered scar.* ± become painful later but *not painful initially.* May be multiple if diffuse. *Regional lymphadenopathy.*
2. **Mucocutaneous:** *especially cartilaginous areas* of the nasal mucosa & the mouth.
3. **Visceral:** fulminant disease if organism migrates to vital organs. *Hepatosplenomegaly*

DIAGNOSIS: culture. Leishmania donovani has a higher incidence of causing visceral infection.
MANAGEMENT: Infectious disease consult. Sores usually heal spontaneously.

OTHER DISEASES

EHRLICHIOSIS

Gram negative intracellular bacteria that *infects & destroys white blood cells.* 2 types:
• ❶ **Human Granulocytic Anaplasma** phagocytophilum (HGA): transmitted by *Ixodes tick (same tick in Lyme disease).* Ixodes tick transmits **B**abesiosis **E**hrlichiosis & **L**yme disease (think of the cranial nerve 7 "BEL" palsy associated with Lyme disease). Seen especially in the summer.
• ❷ **Human Monocytic Ehrlichiosis** (HME): *Ehrlichia chaffeensis & canis* transmitted by *Lone star tick (Amblyommma americanum).*

CLINICAL MANIFESTATIONS
1. Symptoms usually begin 7-10 days after a tick bite with a prodrome of rigors, malaise & nausea ⇨ *high fever, toxicity, myalgia, headache. NO rash usually. ± splenomegaly.* Although rare, if rash does develops, it can be macular, maculopapular. Petechial rash reflects thrombocytopenia.

DIAGNOSIS:
1. Peripheral smear/**Buffy coat**: *morulae in WBCs** = Ehrlichia clusters in the cell vacuoles, forming large *mulberry-shaped aggregates* especially with HGA. Serologies (titers).
2. ↑LFTs, *thrombocytopenia. Leukopenia* (reflects the WBC destruction associated with infection).

MANAGEMENT
*Doxycycline 1st line treatment.** Rifampin. Chloramphenicol.

MYCOBACTERIUM AVIUM COMPLEX (MAC)

- Mycobacterium avium & intracellulare. Transmission: present in soil/water (not person to person).
- Sx occurs rarely in immunocompetent patients (↑ in bronchiectasis). Seen in HIV when **CD4 ≤50.***

CLINICAL MANIFESTATIONS:
1. **Pulmonary infection** in immunocompetent: cough with sputum, fever, weight loss, **Bronchiectasis.**
2. **Disseminated (in HIV patients):** FUO, sweating, weight loss, fatigue, diarrhea, dyspnea, RUQ pain.
3. **Lymphadenitis in children**: cervical submandibular/maxillary.

DIAGNOSIS: Acid fast bacillus staining & culture.

MANAGEMENT: **Clarithromycin + Ethambutol*** @ least 12 months (± Rifabutin or Rifampin).
HIV prophylaxis: if **CD4 ≤50 cells/microL** ⇨ Clarithromycin, Azithromycin. Rifabutin 2nd line.

MYCOBACTERIUM KANSAII

- Causes Tuberculosis-like disease. **Management:** Rifampin + Ethambutol.

MYCOBACTERIUM MARINUM   "Fish tank Granuloma"

- Atypical Mycobacterium found in fresh & salt water. Inoculation of a **skin abrasion or puncture in a patient with contact of an aquarium, salt water, or marine animals** (ex. fish & turtles).
- **Occupational hazard of aquarium handlers, marine workers, fisherman & seafood handlers*** aka "Fish tank Granuloma".

CLINICAL MANIFESTATIONS
1. Localized cutaneous disease: **erythematous bluish papule or nodule at the site of trauma*** that can ulcerate (history of exposure to non chlorinated water 2 – 3 weeks earlier). **Subsequent lesions may occur along the path of lymphatic drainage** over a period of months.

DIAGNOSIS: culture
MANAGEMENT: tetracyclines, fluoroquinolones, macrolides, sulfonamides. 4-6 week duration of tx.

LEPROSY (HANSEN's DISEASE)

- Mycobacterium leprae. **Primarily affects superficial tissues (especially skin & peripheral nerves)*** Endemic in subtropical areas. Requires long exposure (few months to 20-50 years IP).

CLINICAL MANIFESTATIONS
1. LEPROMATOUS: **nodular, plaque or papular skin lesions (lepromas)** with poorly defined border. Hypopigmented lesions can be seen especially in cooler areas of the body: face, ears, wrists, elbows, buttocks & knees. Loss of eyebrows & eyelashes. **Slowly evolving SYMMETRIC nerve involvement (SENSATION PRESERVED)*** paresthesias in the affected peripheral nerves. MC seen in immunocompromised patients.
2. TUBERCULOID: **limited dz:** sharply demarcated **hypopigmented macular lesions numb to the touch (LOSS OF SENSATION)*** with sudden onset of asymmetric nerve involvement. MC in immunocompetent patients (immune system reaction in the nerves causes the loss of sensation).
3. MONONEURITIS MULTIPLEX:* nerve damage: clawing (median & ulnar involvement), foot drop (common peroneal nerve). vibratory & proprioception preserved.

DIAGNOSIS: Acid fast bacillus smear performed on tissue obtained from a skin biopsy.

MANAGEMENT
1. Lepromatous: Dapsone, Rifampin, Clofazimine x 2-3 years.
2. Tuberculoid: Dapsone + Rifampin 6-12 months followed by Dapsone x 2 years.

VIRAL DISEASES

HUMAN HERPESVIRUS FAMILY
1. HSV-1 – oropharyngeal	3. Varicella Zoster	5. CMV	7. Pityriasis rosea
2. HSV-2 - genital	4. Epstein Barr	6. Roseola	8. Kaposi sarcoma

HERPES SIMPLEX VIRUS 1 & 2

CLINICAL MANIFESTATIONS
- *Prodromal symptoms 24h prior (burning, paresthesias, tingling)* ⇨ painful, grouped vesicles on an erythematous base.* HSV-1 (oral) HSV-2 (genital) both can interchange.

1. **ORAL LESIONS:**
   ACUTE HERPETIC GINGIVOSTOMATITIS: primary infection in children. Sudden onset of fever, anorexia ⇨ *gingivitis* (gum swelling, friable/bleeding gums);* vesicles in the mouth, tongue & lips ⇨ grey/yellow lesions. >90% of US population are infected with HSV-1.
   ACUTE HERPETIC PHARYNGOTONSILLITIS: primary infection in adults. Vesicles that rupture ⇨ ulcerative lesions with grayish exudates in posterior pharyngeal mucosa.
   HERPES LABIALIS: *2ry infection most often HSV-1. Cold sore, fever blister with stress/illness.*

2. GENITAL LESIONS: *most often HSV-2* (but can be HSV-1 as well). HSV-2 seen in 25% of population.
3. HERPES KERATITIS: usually unilateral. Slit lamp: *dendritic ulcers.*
   Management: *antiviral eye drops (ex. Trifluridine, Vidarabine, Ganciclovir). Oral Acyclovir.*
4. BELL PALSY: associated with HSV-1.
5. HSV ESOPHAGITIS: *small deep ulcers on EGD* seen primarily in the immunocompromised.
6. HERPETIC WHITLOW: HSV infection of the nail or finger.
7. ENCEPHALITIS: *HSV MC cause of encephalitis.*

DIAGNOSIS
1. *PCR most sensitive & specific test for HSV.* Clinical diagnosis.
2. **Tzanck smear:*** *multinucleated giant cells & intranuclear inclusion bodies.*

MANAGEMENT: *Acyclovir (IV for encephalitis),* Valacyclovir, Famciclovir.

CYTOMEGALOVIRUS   (HHV 5)

Present in most people (70% in US). *Clinical disease only in immunocompromised patients*

CLINICAL MANIFESTATIONS
1. **Primary disease:** *most asymptomatic. Mononucleosis-like illness* (if symptomatic).
2. CONGENITAL CMV: *sensorineural hearing loss common* & "blueberry muffin rash" (TTP) petechiae.* Hepatosplenomegaly, mental & motor dysfunction.
   Part of congenital ToRCH syndrome: Toxoplasmosis, other (Syphilis), Rubella, CMV, HSV.

CMV REACTIVATION: seen in the immunocompromised: HIV, steroid use, chemo, s/p transplant.
1. RETINITIS: hemorrhage with soft exudates: *scrambled eggs/ketchup appearance (pizza pie)** appearance on *funduscopy* if *CD4 ≤50;* Pneumonitis, Encephalitis; Colitis (CD4 ≤100).
2. ESOPHAGITIS: Odynophagia. *Large superficial ulcers on upper endoscopy.*
DIAGNOSIS: serologies (Antigen tests, IgM, IgG titers). PCR.
   Biopsy of tissues: *Owl's eye* appearance* (epithelial cells with enlarged nuclei surrounded by clear zone & cytoplasmic inclusions).

MANAGEMENT: *Ganciclovir* treatment of choice.* 2nd line: Foscarnet, Cidofovir. Valacyclovir.

VARICELLA ZOSTER VIRUS (HHV-3)

Transmission: respiratory droplets, direct contact. 10-20 day incubation period.

CLINICAL MANIFESTATIONS

1. **VARICELLA (CHICKEN POX):** *primary infection.* Fever, malaise. Clusters of **vesicles on an erythematous base "dew drops on a rose petal"** in *DIFFERENT STAGES** (macules, papules, vesicles, pustules & crusted lesions) at any given time beginning on the face, trunk ⇨ extremities. Usually pruritic. More severe presentation may occur in adults.

2. **HERPES ZOSTER (SHINGLES):** *VZV reactivation along one dermatome** of the dormant virus in the spinal root & cranial nerve ganglia. ± Disseminated in HIV.

3. **HERPES ZOSTER OPHTHALMICUS:** shingles involving 1st division of the ***trigeminal nerve (CN V).*** *Hutchinson's sign:* lesions on nose usually **heralding ocular involvement.***
    Dendritic lesions seen on slit lamp exam if keratoconjunctivitis is present.*

4. **HERPES ZOSTER OTICUS (RAMSAY-HUNT SYNDROME):** *facial nerve (CN VII) - otalgia, lesions on the ear, auditory canal & tympanic membrane, facial palsy, auditory sx:* tinnitus, vertigo, deafness, ataxia.

5. **POST HERPETIC NEURALGIA:** pain >3months, hyperesthesias or decreased sensation.

MANAGEMENT

1. **Chicken Pox:** symptomatic treatment
2. **Shingles:** *Acyclovir, Valacyclovir, Famciclovir (given within 72 hours to prevent PHN).*
3. **HZO:** *PO antivirals**; May add Trifluridine, Acyclovir or Vidarabine ophthalmic.
4. **Ramsay Hunt syndrome:** *oral Acyclovir plus Corticosteroids.*
5. **PHN:** *Gabapentin or Tricyclic antidepressants (TCAs).** Topical (Lidocaine gel, Capsaicin)

Complications of Chicken Pox: *Bacterial infection MC,* PNA, Encephalitis, Guillain Barré syndrome.

EPSTEIN-BARR VIRUS (INFECTIOUS MONONUCLEOSIS) – HHV-4

Transmission: *saliva* "kissing disease" esp. young adults 15-25y. 80% of adults are seropositive.

CLINICAL MANIFESTATIONS

❶ *fever* ❷ *sore throat* (±exudative), ❸ *POSTERIOR cervical lymphadenopathy* (but may be general), malaise, myalgias, general lymphadenopathy, *splenomegaly;* hepatomegaly.
    Petechial rash in ~5% *(especially if given Ampicillin).**

EBV infects B cells ⇨ associated with Hodgkin Lymphoma. May cause Burkitt's lymphoma & may cause CNS lymphoma in patients with AIDS.

DIAGNOSIS

1. *Heterophile (Monospot) Ab test* (positive within 4 weeks). Rapid Viral Capsid Antigen test.
2. Peripheral smear: >50% lymphocytes with >10% *atypical lymphocytes.** ↑LFTs.

MANAGEMENT

1. ***Supportive mainstay of tx:*** rest, analgesics, antipyretics. Symptoms may last for months.
2. Corticosteroids used ONLY if airway obstruction due to lymphadenopathy, hemolytic anemia or severe thrombocytopenia. Strep & EBV can coexist.
3. *Avoid trauma/contact sports at least 1 month if splenomegaly to prevent splenic rupture.**

RABIES

Life-threatening Rhabdovirus infection of the CNS (encephalitis of gray matter).

TRANSMISSION

Infected saliva from bites of rabid animals: **raccoons, bats, skunks, foxes, wolves,** (dogs cause >90% in developing countries). **NOT rodents** (only rodent that will survive long enough to transmit it is a woodchuck). If a person was **asleep in a room with a bat, they should be given prophylaxis _even if no visible bat bite_** is seen! Rhabdovirus goes through axons from the peripheral to the central nervous system. Incubation period usually 3-7 weeks (rarely ±be years).

CLINICAL MANIFESTATIONS

1. **Prodrome:** _pain, paresthesias, itching at the initial site of the bite pathognomonic_ ⇨ CNS phase.

2. **CNS phase:** encephalitis, aerophobia, **_hydrophobia*_** (painful laryngospasm after drinking liquids), numbness, paralysis. Patients may become sensitive to air currents (aerophobia) & changes in temperature. May develop rabid rage, hypersalivation (foaming at the mouth) with thick sputum ⇨ respiratory phase.

3. **Respiratory phase:** respiratory muscle paralysis (leading to death).

DIAGNOSIS

NEGRI BODIES* in brain of dead animals (especially in hippocampus). **Animal observation 7-10 days.***

MANAGEMENT: _once sx occurs, patients rarely survive._ Coma induction, Amantadine & Ribavirin.

POST EXPOSURE PROPHYLAXIS 1ST EPISODE

1. **_HDCV (Rabies Vaccine)_ days 0,3,7,14 + _Rabies Immune Globulin_** ½ wound, ½ IM (20u/kg). ideally started within 6 days of the exposure.
    If immunocompromised, include day 28 in the HDCV vaccine schedule.

Post exposure prophylaxis in subsequent exposures: Rabies vaccine day 0 & 3. No immunoglobulin

SMALLPOX (VARIOLA)

- Orthopox virus. Category A bioterrorism agent. IP 7-17d. Transmission: Inhalation. Virus migrates & multiplies in the lymph nodes, spleen & bone marrow.

CLINICAL MANIFESTATIONS

Flu like prodrome: abrupt onset of high fever & **severe head/back pain,*** chills, rigors, coryza and pharyngitis ⇨ **skin eruptions in the SAME STAGE SIMULTANEOUSLY:*** macules initially progressing to papules & umbilicated pustules with well defined borders ⇨ crusting over in about 2 weeks. **Palmar & plantar lesions common** (unlike varicella). Trunk to the extremities.

DIAGNOSIS: Lab confirmation of tissues from the lesions with an electron microscope.

MANAGEMENT

Supportive (antibiotics if secondary infection). Household & face to face contacts should be isolated & vaccinated within a few days after exposure.

Eczema, dermatitis & burns are contraindications to the smallpox vaccine.

WEST NILE FEVER

- *Flavivirus* transmitted by infected mosquitos (Arbovirus). *Birds are reservoir** (associated with the death of large number of birds). *Seen late summer & early fall.* The homeless are at increased susceptibility.

CLINICAL MANIFESTATIONS
Most patients are asymptomatic. Flu-like sx, pharyngitis, headache, fatigue, malaise, nausea, vomiting. May develop roseolar, maculopapular rash, stiff neck & mental status changes.

MANAGEMENT: intense supportive management.

SEVERE ACUTE RESPIRATORY SYNDROME (SARS)

- *Coronavirus.* Transmitted by respiratory droplets. Causes an ***atypical pneumonia.***

CLINICAL MANIFESTATIONS
Nonspp flu-like sx: persistent fever (>100.4), rigors, rhonchi, headache, malaise, pharyngitis ⇨ cough, dyspnea, rales, ***atypical pneumonia*** (±watery diarrhea late in the disease). Elderly may present with malaise & delirium. O_2 saturation usually <95%.

DIAGNOSIS
1. RT-PCR for SARS-CoV in urine, stool & nasal secretions. ***Stool is the 1st to be positive c/n 14d.****

2. **CT can:** ground glass opacities or focal consolidation (pneumonia).

MANAGEMENT: aggressive supportive management.

HANTAVIRUS (HEMORRHAGIC FEVER)

- *Rodents main vector (ex. **Deer mouse feces or rodent urine**).**

- *MC in **SW United States**.* Affects primarily young, healthy adults especially males.

CLINICAL MANIFESTATIONS: 3-week incubation period.
1. **Prodromal febrile phase:** The aerosolized virus enters the lung causing a prodromal febrile phase (fever, chills, *severe myalgias especially involving the back & legs*)* ⇨ nausea, vomiting, diarrhea, headache & weakness.

2. **Cardiopulmonary phase:** sudden respiratory distress & ***pulmonary edema**** (massive capillary leakage in the pulmonary vascular bed) may progress to ***cardiovascular collapse*** (shock & coagulopathy) & ***renal failure***. Lasts 2-7 days. In survivors, recovery is rapid.

MANAGEMENT: Supportive, ICU admission.

DENGUE FEVER

* *Flavivirus* transmitted by the **Aedes** mosquito.   Seen in the tropics mainly.   IP 7-10 days.

CLINICAL MANIFESTATIONS

1. **BIPHASIC FEVER PHASE:*** sudden onset of chills, ***initial high fever*** (3-7 days) ⇨ remission hours to 2 days ⇨ ***second fever phase*** (1-2 days), severe myalgias, *"break bone" joint pain, headache*, sore throat.

2. **BIPHASIC RASH:*** erythematous skin mottling, *flushed skin (sensitive & specific)* ⇨ defervescence with the onset of a ***maculopapular rash*** (spares palms & soles) ⇨ ***petechiae*** on the extensor surface of limbs.

3. **HEMORRHAGIC FEVER:** ecchymosis, gastrointestinal bleeding, epistaxis, pleural effusions, ascites & shock.   Hemorrhagic fever usually occurs in children in endemic areas. ***"tourniquet test":*** purpura from the pressure of the tourniquet placed on the arm. **Hepatitis.**

DIAGNOSIS

Leukopenia, elevated LFTs (*hepatitis is common*); IgM, IgG, ELISA.

MANAGEMENT

Volume support, pressors, **Acetaminophen** (instead of NSAIDs to reduce bleeding).

CREUTZFELDT-JAKOB DISEASE

Prion-mediated degenerative brain disease ⇨ rapidly progressive dementia (fatal within 1y).

PATHOPHYSIOLOGY

A prion is a misfolded protein that enters CNS cells, inducing abnormal folding of normal proteins ⇨ ***spongioform cortex*** *(holes in tissues).*   Idiopathic or transmitted from infected tissue (ex corneal transplant), contaminated beef with CNS tissue of infected animals ex "mad cow disease".

CLINICAL MANIFESTATIONS

Rapidly progressive dementia, marked gait abnormalities, myoclonus (especially if startled).

HOOKWORM

Ancylostoma duodenale or Necator americanus.   25% of the world is infected.   Occasional cases occur in United States (Southeast).

Skin exposure to larvae in soil contaminated by human feces.   The larvae penetrate the skin & migrate to the pulmonary capillaries. They are carried to the mouth via the mucociliary escalator & swallowed, where they enter the small bowel and suck blood (whole cycle about ~4 weeks).

CLINICAL MANIFESTATIONS

1. <u>Skin:</u> very pruritic erythematous dermatitis at the site of entry.
2. <u>Pulmonary:</u> asymptomatic. Low grade fever, blood-tinged sputum, wheezing, coughing
3. <u>Intestinal:</u> abdominal pain, ulcer-like symptoms, diarrhea, anorexia. Iron deficiency anemia.

DIAGNOSIS

1. <u>Stool:</u> eggs noted, positive guaiac, eosinophilia, hypochromic microcytic anemia.

MANAGEMENT

1. **Albendazole,** Mebendazole, Pyrantel. <u>Supportive:</u> iron supplementation, vitamins, proteins.

HUMAN IMMUNODEFICIENCY VIRUS (HIV)

- **HIV**: retrovirus (changes viral RNA into DNA via *reverse transcriptase*). HIV-1 (MC) & HIV-2.

- **Transmission**: *sexual intercourse, IV drug use* (shared needles etc.), mother to child transmission (during birth or breastfeeding), receipt of blood products before 1985, mucosal contact with infected blood or needle stick injuries.

CLINICAL MANIFESTATIONS
Patients may present at any stage and have varied presentations.
1. *Acute seroconversion*: *flu-like illness:* fever, malaise, generalized rash.   Generalized lymphadenopathy is common.

2. *AIDS:* defined as *CD4 count <200* cells/μL *or the development of an AIDS-defining illness* with or without HIV testing. Recurrent severe & potentially life-threatening opportunistic infections or malignancies. HIV wasting syndrome (chronic diarrhea & weight loss),   AIDS-associated neurologic changes (ex. encephalopathy or dementia).

DIAGNOSIS:
1. **Antibody Testing**
   - *ELISA: (screening test).* If reactive, the test is confirmed by Western Blot. Usually becomes reactive within 3 – 6 months of infection.
   - **Rapid testing:** blood or saliva test.

2. *Western Blot: confirmatory test.*

3. *HIV RNA viral load:* can be positive in the window period. Also used to monitor infectivity & treatment effectiveness in patients diagnosed with HIV.

OPPORTUNISTIC INFECTIONS:

CD4 Count cells/μL	DISEASE	1ST LINE PROPHYLAXIS	2ND LINE PROPHYLAXIS
700 – 1,500	Normal		
>500	Lymphadenopathy		
500-200	Tuberculosis	INH if latent TB	Rifampin
	Kaposi Sarcoma, Thrush, Lymphoma, Zoster		
≤ 200	**Pneumocystis (PCP)**	Trimethoprim/ sulfamethoxazole	Dapsone, Atovaquone, Pentamidine (aerosolized).
≤ 150	Histoplasmosis (select)	Itraconazole	Amphotericin B
≤ 100	**Toxoplasmosis**	TMP/SMX	Dapsone + Pyrimethamine + Folinic acid
	Cryptococcus (select)	Fluconazole	Amphotericin B
≤ 50	**MAC**	Azithromycin or Clarithromycin	Rifabutin (must obtain a CXR prior to use to r/o active Tuberculosis)
	CMV retinitis	Valganciclovir	Ganciclovir + Foscarnet

Others: Diarrhea (Cryptosporidium, Isospora, Microspora), Human Papilloma Virus.

Select = routine prophylaxis not recommended in general population. May be used in selected cases.

POST-EXPOSURE PROPHYLAXIS: in patients with high risk of infection (ex. occupational exposure) best started within 72 hours of incident (the earlier the better).

HAART REGIMENS FOR TREATMENT NAÏVE PATIENTS:

❶ NNRTI + 2 NRTIs OR	NNRTI = Non-nucleoside Reverse Transcriptase Inhibitor NRTI = Nucleos(t)ide Reverse Transcriptase Inhibitor
❷ PI + 2 NRTIs OR	Protease inhibitor (preferably boosted c ritonavir)
❸ INSTI + 2 NRTIs	INSTI = Integrase strand transfer inhibitor

NRTIs
Zidovudine (Retrovir)
Emtricitabine (Emtriva)
Abacavir (Ziagen)
Lamivudine (3TC/Epivir)
Didanosine (ddI)
Zalcitabine (ddC)
Stavudine (d4T)
Tenofivir (Viread)
	MOA: inhibits viral replication by interfering with HIV viral RNA-dependent DNA polymerase
	
	Truvada (Emtricitabine/Tenofovir)
	
	S/E: peripheral neuropathy, pancreatitis, hepatitis.
	    Zidovudine* ⇨ *bone marrow suppression, myopathy.
	    Emtricitabine may be associated with depigmentation of palms/soles.

NNRTIs *Efavirenz* (Sustiva) *Delavirdine* (Rescriptor) *Etravirine* (Intelence) *Nevirapine* (Viramune) *Rilpivirine* (Edurant)	**MOA:** inhibits viral replication by interfering c HIV viral RNA-dependent DNA polymerase. **S/E:** Rash. ***Efavirenz causes vivid dreams, depression & neurologic disturbances.****

PROTEASE
INHIBITORS
Atazanavir (Reyataz)
Darunavir (Prezista)
Lopinavir & Ritonavir
  (Kaletra)
Nelfinavir (Viracept)
Indinavir (Crixivan)
Ritonavir (Norvir)
Fosamprenavir (Lexiva)
Saquinavir (Invirase)
	MOA: inhibits HIV protease, leading to production of noninfectious, immature HIV particles.
	
	S/E: *GI:* N/V/diarrhea, ***Lipodystrophy,* Hyperlipidemia**.
	
	    Indinavir associated with renal stones.
	
	    Ritonavir associated with paresthesias.

INTI *Raltegravir* (Isentress) *Dolutegravir* (Tivicay)	**Integrase Inhibitors** **MOA:** prevents insertion of a DNA copy of the viral genome into the host DNA **S/E: *Hyperlipidemia***, GI sx: N/V, diarrhea, headache, hyperglycemia
FUSION INHIBITORS Enfuvirtide (Fuzeon)	**MOA:** disrupts the virus from fusing with healthy T cells **S/E: *Hyperlipidemia***, GI symptoms.
CCR5 ANTAGONISTS Maraviroc (Seizentry)	**MOA:** blocks viral entry into WBCs **S/E:** rash, cough

	PRODROME	RASH	MISCELLANEOUS
VARICELLA Chicken Pox	• Flu-like sx: fever, headache, malaise	• *Rash in DIFFERENT stages simultaneously* (macules, papules, vesicles, crusted lesions) • Face initially ➪ extremities.	• *Vesicles on erythematous base dew drops on a rose petal"** • Usually does not involve palms/soles
VARIOLA Smallpox	• Flu-like sx: fever, headache, malaise	• *Lesions appear in the SAME stage simultaneously* • Vesicles ➪ pustules ➪ scarring	• *Classically involves palms/soles*
RUBEOLA Measles	• URI prodrome: *3 C's:* - *Cough, Coryza, Conjunctivitis*	• *Maculopapular BRICK-RED* rash beginning @ hair line/face ➪ extremities. Lasts 7 days.*	• *Koplik spots on buccal mucosa** • *Otitis Media MC long term cx**, encephalitis, pneumonia in children
RUBELLA German Measles	• URI prodrome. • *Post cervical & postauricular lymphadenopathy*	• *Maculopapular pink-light red* spotted rash on face ➪ extremities. Lasts 3 days*	• *Photosensitivity & arthralgias (joint pains) especially in young women* • Not long term sequelae in children • *TERATOGENIC in 1st trimester:* (ToRCH)
ROSEOLA Sixth's disease	• 3 days of **high fevers** • *Child appears well during febrile phase.*	• *Pink maculopapular blanchable rash.* • *Only childhood viral exanthema that STARTS ON TRUNK/EXTREMITIES* then goes to face*	• Lasts 1-3 days. • Associated with HHV-6 & HHV-7
ERYTHEMA INFECTIOSUM 5th's disease	• Coryza, fever	• *Red flushed face "SLAPPED CHEEK APPEARANCE" with CIRCUMORAL PALLOR ➪ LACY RETICULAR RASH on the body*	• *Arthropathy in older adults* • *Aplastic crisis in Sickle Cell disease** • *Increased fetal loss in pregnancy* • *Parvovirus B-19*
COXSACKIE A VIRUS Hand Foot Mouth	• Fever, URI symptoms	• *Vesicular lesions on a reddened base with an erythematous halo in oral cavity ➪ vesicles on the hands/feet (includes palms & soles)*	• *Seen especially in summer* • Affects hands, feet, mouth & genitals
ENDEMIC TYPHUS	• Flu-like sx: fevers, chills, severe headache.	• Maculopapular rash trunk & axilla ➪ extremities (spares the face, palms & soles)	• *Flushed face, hearing loss (CN 8 involvement), conjunctivitis*
SCALDED SKIN SYNDROME	• Local S. aureus infection	• Fluid filled blisters with *positive Nikolsky sign: (sloughing of skin with gentle pressure)* • *Painful diffuse red rash begins centrally*	• *Seen in children <6y* • *Due to S. aureus exotoxin*
TOXIC SHOCK SYNDROME	• High fever, watery diarrhea • Sore throat, headache • *Staph aureus exotoxin*	• *Red rash (diffuse, maculopapular) with desquamation of palms & soles*	• *Seen in adults (ex tampon use, nasal packing left in too long) due to* • Management: IV Antibiotics
ROCKY MOUNTAIN SPOTTED FEVER	• Triad: fever, headache, rash	• *Red maculopapular rash first on wrists/ankles* ➪ central (eventually palms & soles). Petechiae*	• *Fever with relative bradycardia*
KAWASAKI	• Fever, conjunctivitis, cervical lymphadenopathy	• *Strawberry tongue, edema/desquamation of palms & soles.* Rash can present in different ways	• *Rare but dreaded complication is myocardial infarction & coronary artery involvement*
SCARLET FEVER		• *Strawberry tongue, sandpaper rash* facial flushing with circumoral pallor.* Desquamation can occur	• *Forchheimer spots: small red spots on the soft palate (resolves quickly)*

SELECTED REFERENCES

Deyell MW, Chiu B, Ross DB, Alvarez N. Q fever endocarditis: a case report and review of the literature. Can J Cardiol. 2006;22(9):781-5.

Centor RM, Witherspoon JM, Dalton HP, Brody CE, Link K. The diagnosis of strep throat in adults in the emergency room. Med Decis Making. 1981;1(3):239-46.

Mcisaac WJ, Kellner JD, Aufricht P, Vanjaka A, Low DE. Empirical validation of guidelines for the management of pharyngitis in children and adults. JAMA. 2004;291(13):1587-95.

Aliouat-denis CM, Chabé M, Demanche C, et al. Pneumocystis species, co-evolution and pathogenic power. Infect Genet Evol. 2008;8(5):708-26.

Morris A, Beard CB, Huang L. Update on the epidemiology and transmission of Pneumocystis carinii. Microbes Infect. 2002;4(1):95-103.

Smith NL, Denning DW. Underlying conditions in chronic pulmonary aspergillosis including simple aspergilloma. Eur Respir J. 2011;37(4):865-72.

Kitchen MS, Reiber CD, Eastin GB. An urban epidemic of North American blastomycosis. Am Rev Respir Dis. 1977;115(6):1063-6.

Hector RF, Laniado-laborin R. Coccidioidomycosis--a fungal disease of the Americas. PLoS Med. 2005;2(1):e2.

Kotrappa KS, Bansal RS, Amin NM. Necrotizing fasciitis. Am Fam Physician. 1996;53(5):1691-7.

Brooke CJ, Riley TV. Erysipelothrix rhusiopathiae: bacteriology, epidemiology and clinical manifestations of an occupational pathogen. J Med Microbiol. 1999;48(9):789-99.

Sobel J. Botulism. Clin Infect Dis. 2005;41(8):1167-73.

Tularemia--United States, 1990-2000. MMWR Morb Mortal Wkly Rep. 2002;51(9):181-4.

Feder HM, Johnson BJ, O'connell S, et al. A critical appraisal of "chronic Lyme disease". N Engl J Med. 2007;357(14):1422-30.

Swanson SJ, Neitzel D, Reed KD, Belongia EA. Coinfections acquired from ixodes ticks. Clin Microbiol Rev. 2006;19(4):708-27.

Johnston SP, Sriram R, Qvarnstrom Y, et al. Resistance of Acanthamoeba cysts to disinfection in multiple contact lens solutions. J Clin Microbiol. 2009;47(7):2040-5.

Chuenkova MV, Pereiraperrin M. Trypanosoma cruzi targets Akt in host cells as an intracellular antiapoptotic strategy. Sci Signal. 2009;2(97):ra74.

Kennedy PG. Clinical features, diagnosis, and treatment of human African trypanosomiasis (sleeping sickness). Lancet Neurol. 2013;12(2):186-94.

Sundar S, Chakravarty J. Leishmaniasis: an update of current pharmacotherapy. Expert Opin Pharmacother. 2013;14(1):53-63

"Warm + Cream" in Kawasaki Disease. Available at: http://sketchymedicine.com/2012/07/kawasaki-disease/. Accessed February 24, 2014.

Slama TG, Amin A, Brunton SA, et al. A clinician's guide to the appropriate and accurate use of antibiotics: the Council for Appropriate and Rational Antibiotic Therapy (CARAT) criteria. Am J Med. 2005;118 Suppl 7A:1S-6S.

Kourkoumpetis T, Manolakaki D, Velmahos G, et al. Candida infection and colonization among non-trauma emergency surgery patients. Virulence. 2010;1(5):359-66.

Ecevit IZ, Clancy CJ, Schmalfuss IM, Nguyen MH. The poor prognosis of central nervous system cryptococcosis among nonimmunosuppressed patients: a call for better disease recognition and evaluation of adjuncts to antifungal therapy. Clin Infect Dis. 2006;42(10):1443-7.

Kauffman CA. Histoplasmosis: a clinical and laboratory update. Clin Microbiol Rev. 2007;20(1):115-32.

Pääkkönen M, Kallio MJ, Kallio PE, Peltola H. Sensitivity of erythrocyte sedimentation rate and C-reactive protein in childhood bone and joint infections. Clin Orthop Relat Res. 2010;468(3):861-6.

Lozano R, Naghavi M, Foreman K, et al. Global and regional mortality from 235 causes of death for 20 age groups in 1990 and 2010: a systematic analysis for the Global Burden of Disease Study 2010. Lancet. 2012;380(9859):2095-128.

Riedo FX, Plikaytis BD, Broome CV. Epidemiology and prevention of meningococcal disease. Pediatr Infect Dis J. 1995;14(8):643-57.

Workowski KA - MMWR Recomm Rep (2006) Sexually transmitted diseases treatment guidelines 2006.pdf

Stamm LV. Global challenge of antibiotic-resistant Treponema pallidum. Antimicrob Agents Chemother. 2010;54(2):583-9.

Arnott A, Barry AE, Reeder JC. Understanding the population genetics of Plasmodium vivax is essential for malaria control and elimination. Malar J. 2012;11:14.

Rassi A, Rassi A, Marcondes de rezende J. American trypanosomiasis (Chagas disease). Infect Dis Clin North Am. 2012;26(2):275-91.

Bialecki C, Feder HM, Grant-kels JM. The six classic childhood exanthems: a review and update. J Am Acad Dermatol. 1989;21(5 Pt 1):891-903.

Edgeworth JA, Farmer M, Sicilia A, et al. Detection of prion infection in variant Creutzfeldt-Jakob disease: a blood-based assay. Lancet. 2011;377(9764):487-93.

Cook GC. Enterobius vermicularis infection. Gut. 1994;35(9):1159-62.

Tolle MA, Schwarzwald HL. Postexposure prophylaxis against human immunodeficiency virus. Am Fam Physician. 2010;82(2):161-6.

Das K, Arnold E. HIV-1 reverse transcriptase and antiviral drug resistance. Part 1. Curr Opin Virol. 2013;3(2):111-8.

Dalldorf G, Gifford R. Clinical and epidemiologic observations of Coxsackie-virus infection. N Engl J Med. 1951;244(23):868-73

CHAPTER 13 – HEMATOLOGIC DISORDERS

BASICS OF HEMATOLOGY

RED BLOOD CELLS NEED IRON FOR HEMOGLOBIN PRODUCTION

- **RED BLOOD CELLS:** have the role of delivering oxygen for use by all tissues of the body via hemoglobin.

  Heme component: iron (Fe) is part of heme and functions to bind & release oxygen as needed.

  Globin component: consists of 4 subunits. Ex. In adult hemoglobin (HgbA), there are 2 alpha chains & 2 beta chains that make up the globin unit of HgbA.

IRON (Fe) REGULATION

- Total body Fe is regulated primarily by regulation of Fe absorption. Not enough iron will lead to anemia & decreased oxygen carrying ability of RBCs.
- Humans rely so much on Fe that there is not an efficient system of Fe excretion from the body (so states of iron overload can be toxic (ex. hemochromatosis or multiple transfusions). Too much free iron is toxic to cells as it causes free radical production, leading to cell damage & death.
- Chelation therapy is used in patients who receive frequent transfusions to remove excess Fe.

TRANSFERRIN & TOTAL IRON BINDING CAPACITY (TIBC): Transferrin binds to free Fe to reduce the oxidative damage associated with free Fe. ***Transferrin transports Fe throughout the body*** to be used. ***TIBC is an indirect way to measure transferrin levels.*** Disease states associated with:
- ↑**Transferrin** & ↑**TIBC:** *Fe deficiency* - more transferrin leads to ↓*transferrin saturation %.*
- ↓**Transferrin** & ↓**TIBC:** Anemia of chronic disease. Transferrin is an acute phase reactant aimed at decreasing Fe availability to microbes. May also be decreased in iron-overload states.

FERRITIN: Most Fe that is not used for hemoglobin synthesis is stored in the ferritin protein molecule, so ***Ferritin = Fe stores*** *"Ferrit IN storage".* Fe is also stored as hemosiderin in the macrophages.
- ↓**Ferritin:** *Fe deficiency anemia. In patients with reduced Fe, they use up their stores first, leading to ↓Fe stores (↓Ferritin).*
- ↑**Ferritin:** *anemia of chronic disease.* Thought to be part of the body's defense mechanism against invasion of organisms such as bacteria (which also rely on iron, obtaining it from the human host). States of infection or inflammation cause the first responders of the innate immune system (macrophages & neutrophils) to release cytokines (such as interleukins & tumor necrosis factor) that stimulate hepatic release of ***acute phase reactants.*** Acute phase reactants inhibit the growth of pathogenic organisms via:

  ↑**Ferritin:** ↑ferritin & ↑hepatic hepcidin production sequesters iron, reducing serum Fe levels & making it unavailable for use by bacteria.

  ↑**Haptoglobin:** binds free hemoglobin, reducing iron availability for microbes.

  ↑**C-reactive protein (CRP):** nonspecific marker of inflammation or infection. CRP causes microbial destruction by increasing opsonization (the process of marking a cell for destruction via macrophage ingestion).

  ↑**Hepcidin:** prevents iron release from macrophages, reducing Fe availability for microbes. Plays a major role in the progression of anemia of chronic disease.

  These responses are meant as an acute response but in chronic diseases, they persist, ultimately leading to anemia due to reduced serum Fe & decreased Fe availability for Hgb production.

SERUM FE: measures the amount of Fe bound to transferrin.
- ↓**Serum Fe:** seen commonly with both *Fe deficiency anemia* (due to decreased total body Fe) as well as *anemia of chronic disease* (due to induced lowering of serum iron by the acute phase reactant process described above). ***The best way to distinguish between Fe deficiency & anemia of chronic disease is by the TIBC & Ferritin levels.***

Fe deficiency anemia:	↓*serum Fe* (iron)	↓*ferritin*	↑*TIBC*
Anemia of Chronic Disease:	↓*serum Fe* (iron)	↑*ferritin*	↓*TIBC*
↑**Serum Fe:** *Fe overload states (ex hemochromatosis, thalassemias)*			

UNDERSTANDING HEMOLYTIC ANEMIAS

- **Hemolytic anemia**: anemia caused by ↑RBC destruction when the rate of destruction exceeds the bone marrow's ability to replace the destroyed cells. There are two types: intrinsic & extrinsic.
  - **Intrinsic (inherited disorders)**:
    - ex. Sickle cell anemia, Thalassemia, G6PD deficiency, Hereditary spherocytosis.
  - **Extrinsic (acquired disorders):** autoimmune hemolytic anemia, DIC, TTP, HUS, Paroxysmal nocturnal hemoglobinuria, Hypersplenism.

HEMOLYTIC ANEMIAS (BOTH INTRINSIC & EXTRINSIC) HAVE THE FOLLOWING FINDINGS IN COMMON:

Reticulocytosis: occurs if the bone marrow responds to the increased RBC destruction by trying to match it with increased RBC production. The bone marrow will release more ***immature RBCs (reticulocytes)*** in attempt to replenish the depleted RBC population, leading to a *reticulocytosis.*

↑LDH: LDH is an enzyme found in abundance in RBCs. ↑RBC destruction leads to ↑serum LDH.

↑Indirect Bilirubin: if ↑RBC destruction overwhelms the liver's UGT enzyme conjugating ability, there will be an ↑indirect bilirubin. Elevated levels may lead to ***jaundice.***
- ↑Direct (conjugated) bilirubin may also occur and can lead to ***dark urine*** production.

↓Haptoglobin: ↑RBC destruction leads to ↑free Hgb. Haptoglobin binds to free Hgb to reduce its oxidative toxicity. Over time, haptoglobin stores are used up, leading to low haptoglobin levels.

⊕ Schistocytes on peripheral smear: schistocytes are fragmented RBCs resulting from ↑RBC destruction in the spleen, liver or small blood vessels (ex small vessel thrombosis - DIC, TTP, HUS). These fragmented cells lead to further hemolysis of the damaged cells.

LOOK FOR THE FOLLOWING TO HELP DISTINGUISH BETWEEN THE HEMOLYTIC ANEMIAS:

SICKLE CELL ANEMIA: *sickled cells on peripheral smear, Hgb S* on hemoglobin electrophoresis.

THALASSEMIA: *microcytic anemia with normal/↑ serum Fe or no response to Fe tx.* Thalassemias are also associated with severe anemia & abnormal peripheral smear for a given hematocrit level.
- **Alpha Thalassemia:** *hemoglobin electrophoresis with **normal Hgb ratios** of HgbA, A_2 & F.* Alpha thalassemia is a diagnosis of exclusion (since the peripheral smear is normal).
- **Beta Thalassemia:** *hemoglobin electrophoresis:* ↓***HgbA,*** ↑HgbA$_2$, ↑***HgbF.****

G6PD DEFICIENCY: *EPISODIC hemolytic anemia associated with sulfa drugs, fava beans, infections.*

HEREDITARY SPHEROCYTOSIS: *microspherocytes, Coombs NEGATIVE,* ⊕ *osmotic fragility test.*

AUTOIMMUNE HEMOLYTIC ANEMIA: *microspherocytes, Coombs POSITIVE.*

TTP & HUS: *normal coags* (unable to distinguish between TTP & HUS via labs).
- **TTP: Pentad:** *Thrombocytopenia, hemolytic anemia, kidney damage, neurologic symptoms, fever.**

- **HUS: Triad:** thrombocytopenia, hemolytic anemia, & kidney damage. HUS MC seen in children (especially with diarrhea prodrome). HUS has a higher association with kidney involvement than TTP & does not classically have fever or neurologic symptoms.

DISSEMINATED INTRAVASCULAR COAGULATION (DIC): abnormal coags (prolonged PT & PTT).

PAROXYSMAL NOCTURNAL HEMOGLOBINURIA: dark urine (worse in the morning).

ROULEAUX FORMATION

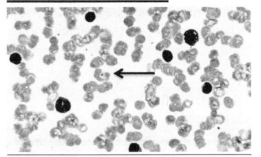

- RBCs stick together like a ***"stack of coins"*** due to ↑plasma proteins (such as immunoglobulins or fibrinogen).
- The increased density of the RBCs stuck together cause them to settle in the tube faster = ↑***ESR*** (Erythrocyte Sedimentation Rate).
- <u>Diseases:</u> high protein (***Multiple Myeloma***). disorders with ↑fibrinogen:
   Infections (acute/chronic).

AUTO AGGLUTINATION

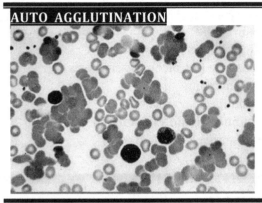

- ***Clumping of RBCs*** due to IgM auto-antibodies coating the surface of RBCs, leading to ↑RBC destruction by macrophages.
- *Cold IgM Ab agglutinins are reactive at colder temperatures* (ex 28-31°C).

DISEASES
- ***Cold agglutinin autoimmune hemolytic anemia***
   (ex. Mycoplasma pneumoniae, Epstein-Barr virus)*
- Cryoglobulinemia
- Ag-Ab reaction if blood not typed & cross-matched.

HOWELL-JOLLY BODIES

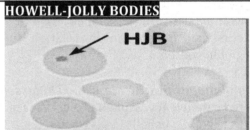

- Small dense basophilic RBC inclusions (usually removed by the spleen).

DISEASES
- ***Decreased splenic function:*** autosplenectomy (ex. sickle cell disease), post splenectomy
- Severe hemolytic anemia, megaloblastic anemia

HEMOLYTIC CELLS

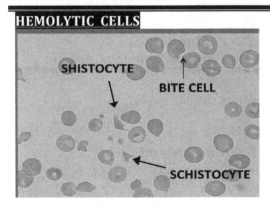

- <u>BITE CELLS</u> (degmacyte) = bite-like deformity due to phagocyte removal of denatured Hgb.
   - Thalassemia, G6PD deficiency

- <u>SCHISTOCYTES:</u> Fragmented RBCs.
   - Hemolytic anemias, Microangiopathic diseases

- <u>KERATOCYTES</u> "Helmet-shaped" RBCs.
   - Mechanical RBC damage in small vessels (microangiopathic diseases - ex. TTP, HUS, DIC, prosthetic valves)

BASOPHILIC STIPPLING

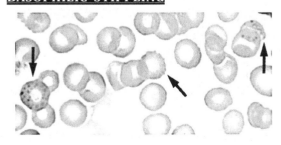

- Coarse blue granules in RBCs (residual RNA in RBCs – looks similar to reticulocytes but ***basophilic stippling is evenly distributed throughout the RBC.***

MC Acquired:
- ***Sideroblastic anemia,*** heavy metal poisoning (ex ***lead,*** arsenic), TTP
- Hemoglobinopathies: ***ex. Thalassemias***
- Myelodysplasia, chronic alcohol use

ECHINOCYTES "Burr cells"

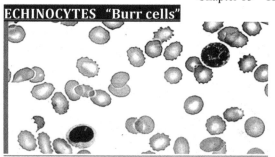

- RBCs with numerous, small, evenly spaced projections due to abnormal cell membrane.

DISEASES
- *Uremia*
- Pyruvate kinase deficiency
- Hypophosphatemia

ACANTHOCYTES "Spur cells"

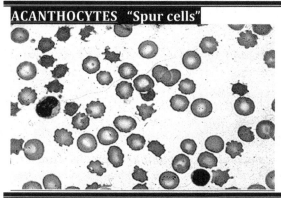

- Few large spiny, irregular projections on the RBC membrane.

DISEASES
- Liver disease (ex. alcoholic cirrhosis)
- Post splenectomy
- Thalassemia
- Autoimmune Hemolytic Anemia
- Renal disease

TARGET CELLS (Codocytes) & SPHEROCYTES

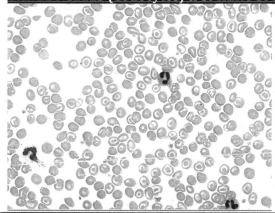

TARGET CELL: hypochromic RBC with round area of central pigment "target-shaped." Seen if there is excess cell membrane in relation to the hemoglobin content.

DISEASES
- *Hemoglobinopathies: sickle cell, Thalassemia,* severe Fe deficiency, asplenia, liver disease.

SPHEROCYTES: usually associated with hyperchromia (often with microcytosis).

DISEASES
- *Hereditary Spherocytosis*
- *Warm Autoimmune Hemolytic Anemia*

HYPERSEGMENTED NEUTROPHILS

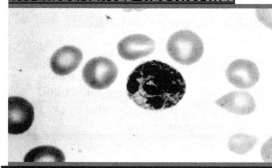

- Neutrophils with >5 lobes

DISEASES
- *B_{12} & Folate deficiencies*
  (especially if macrocytosis is present)*

AUER RODS

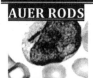

Acute Myelogenous Leukemia:
Seen in promyelocytic variant
Myeloperoxidase positive

REED-STERNBERG CELL

Hodgkin Lymphoma

APPROACH TO ANEMIA

- 3 etiologic causes of anemia: ❶↑*blood loss*, ❷↑ *RBC destruction* & ❸↓*RBC production*.
- Anemia may be mixed: ex. excessive menstruation (microcytic) + B_{12} deficiency (macrocytic).

CLINICAL MANIFESTATIONS OF ANEMIA
1. **Cardiovascular:** palpitations, tachycardia, high output heart failure, orthostatic hypotension, dizziness & syncope. **Pulmonary:** shortness of breath, tachypnea, chest pain.
2. **Skin:** pallor (↓color of the palmar creases, pale conjunctiva), purpura, petechiae, jaundice, retinal hemorrhage. **General:** fatigue, weakness.
3. **Neurologic:** headache, neuropathies, AMS, vertigo.
4. *Abdomen:* hepatosplenomegaly, ascites, ⊕hemoccult blood.

ANEMIA WORKUP
1. CBC with RBC indices: hemoglobin, hematocrit, MCV, MCH, RDW, RBC count.
2. Peripheral blood smear. Bone marrow biopsy gold standard (not usually needed).

RETICULOCYTE COUNT
*1st step in the workup of anemia** determined by CBC. It reflects the body's response to anemia.
   ↑**reticulocytes: *brisk bone marrow response to hemolysis or blood loss.****
   ↓ **reticulocytes: *deficient RBC production*** (ex. reduced marrow response).

MORPHOLOGIC APPROACH

Normal MCV is 80-100 fL.

Anemia with a low reticulocyte count can be separated (via Mean Corpuscular Volume [MCV]) into Normocytic (80 – 100), Microcytic (<80), or Macrocytic (>100).

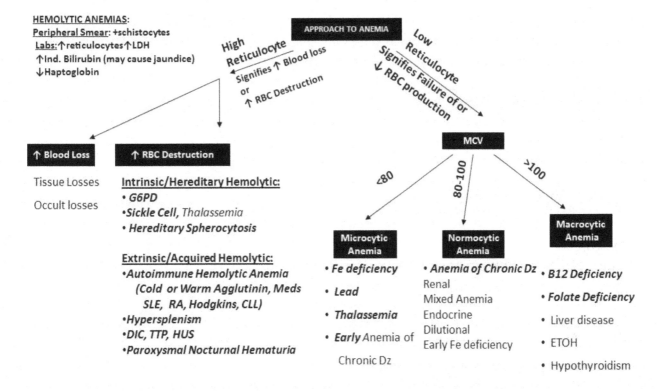

MACROCYTIC ANEMIAS

B12 (COBALAMIN) DEFICIENCY:

- *Animal food is the primary natural source of B12 (milk, cheese, eggs, meat).* Stomach acids release B12 from food & binds it to intrinsic factor for later absorption in the **terminal ileum**.
- Vitamin *B12* deficiency causes **abnormal synthesis of DNA**, nucleic acid & abnormal metabolism of erythroid precursors. B12 is needed to convert homocysteine ⇨ methionine for **DNA synthesis**. B12 body stores last for years but folate stores only last for ~4 months.

ETIOLOGIES

1. *Pernicious anemia:* **autoimmune destruction/loss of gastric parietal cells*** that secrete intrinsic factor ⇨ B12 deficiency. Accompanied by achlorhydria & atrophic gastritis.
2. **Strict vegans** (lack of animal sources in the diet if B12 is not supplemented).
3. *Malabsorption: ETOHism,* diseases affecting the ileum (*ex. **Celiac disease, Crohn**).*
4. ↓intrinsic factor production: *acid-reducing drugs (PPIs & H2RA reduces absorption), gastric bypass surgery. atrophic gastritis.* Zidovudine, Hydroxyurea.

CLINICAL MANIFESTATIONS

1. *neurologic symptoms:* **paresthesias, gait abnormalities, memory loss, dementia** (due to degeneration of the posterolateral of spinal cord). **GI:** anorexia, diarrhea, glossitis. Anemia.

DIAGNOSIS

1. **Peripheral smear:** *↑MCV >115 almost exclusively seen in B12 or Folate deficiency* (especially if *HYPERSEGMENTED NEUTROPHILS** are present). ⊕ Macroovalocytosis.
2. ↑**serum homocysteine,** ↑**methylmalonic acid.*** ↓B12 levels <170 pg/mL (normal >240).
3. **Pernicious Anemia:** ⊕intrinsic factor Ab, parietal cell Ab, ↑gastrin levels. ⊕ *Schilling test.*

MANAGEMENT

B12 replacement: **start with IM B12 - watch for signs of hypokalemia* with treatment.**
- Replacement leads to reticulocytosis with new cells taking up large amounts of potassium.
- Treatment results in increased reticulocyte count within 7 days. Oral B12 for mild disease.

FOLATE (VITAMIN B9) DEFICIENCY

Folate absorption occurs in the jejunum. Folate required for DNA synthesis. Stores last ~4 months.

ETIOLOGIES

Malabsorption, pregnancy, hemolysis (↑cell turnover), meds: Methotrexate, Bactrim, Phenytoin.

CLINICAL MANIFESTATIONS

Similar to B12 but *NOT ASSOCIATED WITH NEUROLOGIC ABNORMALITIES.** Glossitis.

DIAGNOSIS:

↑*MCV >115, HYPERSEGMENTED NEUTROPHILS,* ↓folate, normal B12, ↑serum homocysteine only.

MANAGEMENT

Folic acid 1mg PO daily. *Folate deficiency in pregnancy associated with neural tube defects.*
Replacing folate if it is B12 deficiency will correct the anemia but neurologic sx will worsen.*

OTHER CAUSES OF MACROCYTIC ANEMIA

ETOH abuse, liver disease & hypothyroidism; Myelodysplastic syndrome, acute leukemia.

MICROCYTIC ANEMIAS

ETIOLOGIES: 3MC clinically are _**iron deficiency, alpha/beta thalassemia, early anemia of chronic disease (ACD).**_ _**Lead poisoning is also in the differential.**_ ❶↓**iron availability:** severe iron deficiency, anemia of chronic disease, copper disease ❷↓**heme production:** lead poisoning, sideroblastic anemia ❸↓**globin production:** thalassemia & hemoglobinopathies (ex sickle cell, Hgb SC). _They all usually present with **hypochromic, microcytic anemia.**_

IRON DEFICIENCY ANEMIA

- Causes approximately half of the causes of anemia worldwide. _**MC due to bleeding.**_

ETIOLOGIES
1. _**Chronic blood loss:**_* excessive menstruation, _**occult (colon cancer, parasitic hookworms).**_
2. Dietary deficiency/↑requirements: pregnancy, rapid growth, infants that are breastfed.

CLINICAL MANIFESTATIONS
1. Anemia symptoms, _**pagophagia (ice craving), pica**_ (appetite for non food substances ex. clay & chalk), _**angular cheilitis, koilonychia**_ (nail spooning).

2. _**Plummer-Vinson syndrome: dysphagia + esophageal webs + atrophic glossitis**_ + Fe deficiency.*

DIAGNOSIS
↓_ferritin,_* ↑_TIBC,_ ↓_serum iron (Fe)._
↑_**RDW,**_* ↓RBC count/Hgb/Hct, ±↓MCV
↓_**Transferrin saturation**_ <15% ↓Reticulocytes

	SERUM FE	TIBC	FERRITIN
FE DEFICIENCY	↓(<30μg/dL)	↑*	↓* (<20μg/dL)
ANEMIA OF CHRONIC DZ	↓(<50μg/dL)	↓	↑ or normal

MANAGEMENT
1. **Iron replacement:** ex. Ferrous sulfate 325mg orally daily. Best absorbed on an empty stomach. _**Vitamin C increases Fe absorption.**_ Replacement is associated with GI S/E: nausea, vomiting, constipation & cramps so start with low dose & gradually increase it. Supplementation leads to an increase in the reticulocyte count within 7 days.

LEAD POISONING ANEMIA (PLUMBISM)

- Lead poisoning causes cell death, shortens the lifespan of RBCs & inhibits multiple enzymes needed for heme synthesis ⇨ _**acquired sideroblastic anemia.**_ _**MC in children.**_

CLINICAL MANIFESTATIONS
1. _**abdominal pain with constipation,**_ _**neurologic symptoms:**_* _(ex ataxia, fatigue, learning disabilities,_ coma, shock), anemia symptoms, metabolic acidosis. ± Asymptomatic.

DIAGNOSIS
1. ↑_**serum lead & ↑serum Fe,**_* ↓TIBC, ±↑Ferritin (looks similar to anemia of chronic disease except lead poisoning is associated with ↑serum Fe, ACD is associated with ↓serum Fe).

2. Peripheral smear: _**microcytic, hypochromic anemia with**_ BASOPHILIC STIPPLING* (dots of denatured RNA seen in RBCs) & _RINGED SIDEROBLASTS_* in bone marrow (iron accumulation in mitochondria due to failure of incorporation of iron into Hgb). May be normocytic.

3. X ray: _"lead lines"_* linear hyperdensities @ metaphyseal plates. _**Lead lines in gums**_ (adults).

MANAGEMENT
Remove source of lead. Chelation therapy may be needed if severe (ex. Succimer, CaNa2EDTA).

THALASSEMIA OVERVIEW

THALASSEMIA: *decreased production of globin chains.* Distribution of Thalassemia follows Plasmodium falciparum – thought to be *genetic benefit vs. malaria*). Most adults are heterozygotes.

- *Normally after 6 months of age, adult Hgb is the predominant Hgb produced:*

HgbA (Adult):	2 alphas, 2 betas *(ααββ)*	*95%*
HgbA$_2$:	2 alphas, 2 deltas (αα/δδ)	1.5-3%
HgbF (Fetal):	2 alphas, 2 gammas (ααγγ)	trace amounts

- *Think Thalassemia if microcytic anemia with normal/↑ serum Fe or no response to Fe tx.****

ALPHA THALASSEMIA

- *Decreased α-globin chain production.* 4 genes determine it.

- *MC in SE Asian* 68%, Africans 30%, Mediterranean (5-10%).

Disease	Abnormal Alleles	CLINICAL MANIFESTATIONS
Silent Carrier State	1/4	Clinically normal (usually asymptomatic).
Alpha Thalassemia minor (trait)	2/4	Mild microcytic anemia.
Alpha Thalassemia Intermedia (Hemoglobin H disease)	3/4	*Presents similar to β-Thalassemia major* ⇨ chronic anemia, pallor, hepatosplenomegaly, frontal & maxilla bony overgrowth, pathologic fractures, pigmented gallstones, iron overload.
Hydrops Fetalis	4/4	*Associated with stillbirth* or death shortly after birth *Hgb Barts:* gamma tetramers (γγγγ)*

DIAGNOSIS

1. **CBC:** hypochromic, microcytic anemia (↓MCV ex. 60-75– more pronounced than Fe deficiency). Normal or ↑RBC count; Normal or ↑serum iron & iron stores. Hgb may be as low as 3-6.

   - Peripheral smear: *target cells,** teardrop cells, basophilic stippling.
   - *Heinz bodies in Hemoglobin H disease** - insoluble β-chain tetramers (ββββ)/HgbH* ⇨ inclusions inside the RBCs.

2. **Hgb electrophoresis:** normal hemoglobin ratios in adults. Ratios stay the same because all 3 Hgb types contain 2 alpha chains so decreased alpha production affects all 3 proportionately.

MANAGEMENT

- **Mild thalassemia (α-trait):** no treatment needed.

- **Moderate disease:** folate (if reticulocyte count is high), avoid oxidative stress (ex. sulfa drugs) & avoid iron supplementation (patients are naturally iron overloaded).

- **Severe disease:**
   1. Blood transfusions: weekly (to correct anemia). Vitamin C, folate supplementation.

   2. Iron chelating agents: IV Deferoxamine, PO Deferasirox. **MOA:** prevents iron overload & removes excess iron in patients on chronic transfusion therapy.

   3. Splenectomy in some cases (stops RBC destruction).
   4. Allogeneic bone marrow transplantation is the definitive management of major.

BETA THALASSEMIA

- Decreased production of β-globin chains ⇨ excess α-chains.
- **_MC in Mediterranean_*** (ex. Greek, Italian), **_Africans_**, Indians, Asians.

Disease	Abnormal Alleles
β-Thalassemia trait (minor)	½
β-Thalassemia Major (Cooley's Anemia)	²/₂
β-Thalassemia Intermedia	Mild homozygous form

CLINICAL MANIFESTATIONS

1. **β-Thalassemia trait (minor):** usually asymptomatic. May have a mild to moderate anemia. Only one gene is defective (leading to ~50% decrease in β-chain synthesis).

2. β-Thalassemia Intermedia: milder symptoms compared to major.
   - associated with anemia, hepatosplenomegaly & bony disease.

3. **β-Thalassemia Major (Cooley's Anemia):** Patients usually asymptomatic at birth (due to the presence of fetal hgbF) but **_become symptomatic at 6 months_*** (when HgbF declines). Deficient β-chains ⇨ excess α-chains not able to form tetramers ⇨ ineffective erythropoiesis, erythroid hyperplasia & *extramedullary hematopoiesis **(frontal bossing** & maxillary overgrowth).* **Hepatosplenomegaly, severe hemolytic anemia** (jaundice, dyspnea, pallor), osteopenia (pathologic fractures), iron overload & pigmented gallstones.

DIAGNOSIS

1. **CBC:** hypochromic, microcytic anemia (↓MCV), normal or ↑RBC count, normal or ↑serum iron. Hgb usually about 6g/dL.
   - Peripheral smear: **_target cells,_*** teardrop cells, basophilic stippling, nucleated RBCs.

2. **Hemoglobin electrophoresis:**

	Hgb F	HgbA₂	HgbA
β-Thal trait (minor):	↑	↑	↓ *(due to ↓beta chain production).*
β-Thal Major (Cooley's):	↑ *up to 90%**	↑	*Little to no HgbA*

The ↑HgbA₂ & ↑HgbF are due to ↓β chains, causing excess α-chain coupling with δ & γ.

3. **Skull X-rays:** bossing with *"hair on end appearance"* (due to extramedullary hematopoiesis).

MANAGEMENT:

1. **β-Thalassemia trait (minor):** No medical care usually. Offer genetic counseling.

2. **β-Thalassemia major/severe anemia:**
   - Periodic blood transfusions. Vitamin C, folate supplementation. Avoid excess Fe intake.
   - Iron chelating agents: IV Deferoxamine, PO Deferasirox. **MOA:** prevents iron overload & removes excess iron in patients on chronic transfusion therapy.
   - Splenectomy if refractory. Allogeneic Bone marrow transplantation definitive treatment.

	MCV	RDW	FERRITIN	SERUM FE	HGB ELECTROPHORESIS
FE DEFICIENCY	Low	*High**	*Low**	*Low**	*Normal.* ± ↓HgbA₂, ↓RBC count
α- THALASSEMIA	Low	Normal	Normal	*Normal/↑*	*Adults: normal ratios* of HgbA, A₂, F. ↑*RBC count with normal or ↑Fe & Fe stores* Newborns: nml (α-trait); ±*HgH (Heinz) or Hgb Barts*
β – THALASSEMIA	Low	Normal (↑ in 50%)	Normal	*Normal/↑*	↑*HgbA₂,** ↑*HgbF,** ↑*RBC count*

NORMOCYTIC ANEMIAS

ETIOLOGIES: *anemia of chronic disease (MC),* renal, mixed disorders (ex iron + B_{12} deficiency); endocrine, early iron deficiency, asplenia, dilutional, sickle cell, G6PD.

ANEMIA OF CHRONIC DISEASE

ETIOLOGIES
- *chronic inflammatory conditions:* infection, inflammation, autoimmune disorders, malignancy.

PATHOPHYSIOLOGY
↓*serum Fe* is a consequence of ❶↑hepcidin produced by the liver in infectious/inflammatory states (which inhibits macrophage Fe release), *increased ferritin (as an acute phase reactant)* which *sequesters iron into storage* & cytokine inhibition of erythropoietin.

DIAGNOSIS
- *normal or ↑ ferritin* +↓TIBC*, ↓serum Fe. Mild normochromic normocytic anemia.* (early phase ± present with microcytic, hypochromic anemia). Hgb usually not <9-10mg/dL.

MANAGEMENT: treat underlying disease. Erythropoietin-α if due to renal disease.

GLUCOSE-6-PHOSPHATE DEHYDROGENASE (G6PD) DEFICIENCY

- X-linked recessive trait *affects primarily males,* 10-15% of *African-American males,** Mediterranean, African, Middle Eastern, SE Asian populations.

PATHOPHYSIOLOGY
- G6PD is a protective RBC enzyme against oxidative stress. In G6PDD, oxidative stress oxidizes Hgb into methemoglobin (which does not carry oxygen well) ⇨ ↑RBC membrane damage/fragility & denatured Hgb. *The denatured Hgb precipitates as Heinz bodies* & are targeted for destruction by splenic macrophages ⇨ *episodic hemolytic anemia.*

CLINICAL MANIFESTATIONS
1. Most patients are asymptomatic until times of oxidative stress. Sx begins 2-4 days after exposure.

2. *EPISODIC,* nonimmune *acute hemolytic anemia:** back or abdominal pain, symptoms of anemia, jaundice (↑indirect & direct bilirubin, dark urine), *splenomegaly.* Splenic RBC sequestration ⇨ hemolytic crisis. *RBCs rupture under oxidative stresses such as:*
   - *Infections (MC cause)* ex. pneumonia etc.
   - *Fava beans (broad beans):* contain oxidants which cause RBC damage.
   - Medications: *sulfa drugs* (ex Trimethoprim-sulfamethoxazole),* antimalarials, Methylene blue, INH, Fluoroquinolones, Nitrofurantoin, Aspirin, Dapsone, moth balls.
3. *Neonatal jaundice.* Acute renal failure in severe cases.

DIAGNOSIS
1. **Peripheral smear:** *during crisis shows normocytic hemolytic anemia: schistocytes ("bite" or fragmented cells – cells that look like they had a bite taken out of them).*
   ±HEINZ BODIES.* Smear usually normal when not in the acute stage.
2. **Labs:** ↑reticulocytes, ↑Ind bilirubin; ↓haptoglobin. *G6PD Enzyme assay:* ex. fluorescent spot test.

MANAGEMENT
1. Usually self-limited. Avoid offending food & drugs. Maintain adequate hydration.
2. **Severe Anemia:** Iron/Folic acid supplementation. ±blood transfusions if severe.

SICKLE CELL DISEASE

- **SICKLE CELL DISEASE:** autosomal recessive genetic disorder of HgbSS.
  Occurs when valine substitutes for glutamic acid on the β-chain.   0.15% of African-Americans.
- **SICKLE CELL TRAIT:** *Heterozygous HgbS (AS):* 8% of African-Americans. Sickle cell trait *confers some resistance to Plasmodium falciparum (malaria).* Usually asymptomatic unless exposed to severe hypoxia/dehydration. ***May have episodic hematuria & inability to concentrate urine.****
  Up to 50% of their Hgb is HgbS.

PATHOPHYSIOLOGY: ↓*solubility of HgbS under hypoxic conditions* ⇨ ❶*RBC sickling* causing *micro thrombosis** (± organ damage). ❷*hemolytic anemia* - sickled cells are destroyed by the spleen.

CLINICAL MANIFESTATIONS

1. **Early signs:** *begin @ 6 months* (when HgbSS replaces fetal hemoglobin). *DACTYLITIS MC 1st presentation @ 6-9 months** = swelling of the digits. Delayed growth & development.

2. **INFECTIONS:** *Osteomyelitis (esp Salmonella*). Functional asplenia* early in life (↑'es risk of infection with encapsulated organisms like S. pneumo H. flu, N. meningitidis, Klebsiella, Salmonella); *Aplastic crisis associated with Parvovirus B19 infections.** Folate deficiency.
3. Hemolytic anemia: jaundice, gallstones (pigmented, black).

4. **SIGNS OF MICROTHROMBOSIS (INFARCTIONS):**
   - **SKELETAL:** *"H"-shaped vertebrae** (vertebrae with central endplate depressions giving them an "H" shape), avascular (ischemic) necrosis of bones (ex. femoral or humeral head).

   - **SPLENIC SEQUESTRATION CRISIS:** vasoocclusion in spleen & RBC pooling in spleen ⇨*acute splenomegaly & rapidly* ↓*'ing Hgb* (± fatal) ⇨ **Splenic infarction: *functional asplenia.***
   - **Skin Ulcers:** especially on the tibia.

   - **PAINFUL OCCLUSIVE CRISES:** triggered by cold weather, hypoxia, infection, dehydration, ETOH, pregnancy. Associated with abrupt onset of pain *(acute chest syndrome, back, abdominal, bone pain).* Renal or hepatic dysfunction. *Priapism common** (low flow ischemic type).
   - Decreased O_2 affinity of HgbS ⇨ pulmonary HTN, congestive heart failure, symptoms of fatigue, shortness of breath. May cause renal medullary infarctions ⇨ inability to concentrate urine.

DIAGNOSIS

1. CBC with peripheral smear: ↓Hemoglobin (5-9 g/dL), ↓Hematocrit (17-29%). ↑Reticulocytes. target cells, *sickled erythrocytes.* ± *HOWELL-JOLLY BODIES** (indicates functional asplenia).

2. **Hemoglobin electrophoresis:**   **Sickle cell disease:** HgbS,   no HgbA, ↑HgbF
                                      Sickle Cell trait: HgbS, ↓HgbA

MANAGEMENT:

1. **PAIN CONTROL:** *IV hydration & oxygen 1st step in management of pain crisis** (reverses/prevents sickling). *Narcotics for adequate pain control. Avoid Meperidine* (high doses can cause seizures).
2. **HYDROXYUREA:** *reduces the frequency of pain crises.**
   MOA: ↑RBC water & ↓RBC sickling deformity & ↑'es HgbF (HgbF is resistant to sickling).
3. **FOLIC ACID** – Folic acid is needed for RBC production & DNA synthesis.
4. ***Children should be immunized for S. pneumococcus Haemophilus influenzae type B, & N. meningococcus (SHiN)* & should receive prophylactic penicillin from 4 months up until the age 6y.
5. ±RBC transfusion therapy ±indicated in the management of severe sickle cell crisis (ex. acute chest syndrome, splenic sequestration, preoperative transfusion) but is not used in mild crisis.
6. Allogeneic stem cell transplant: the only possibly curative management for sickle cell disease but associated with significant side effects.

HEREDITARY SPHEROCYTOSIS (HS)

- Autosomal dominant <u>intrinsic hemolytic anemia</u> (RBC defect). MC in N. Europeans.

PATHOPHYSIOLOGY

- ***RBC membrane/cytoskeleton defect*** (spectrin) ⇨ ***↑cell fragility & sphere-shaped RBCs*** ⇨ ↑RBC hemolysis in spleen by splenic macrophages. Aplastic crisis if infected with Parvovirus B19.

CLINICAL MANIFESTATIONS

- Hemolysis: anemia, jaundice, ***splenomegaly,*** pigmented black gallstones (calcium bilirubinate).

DIAGNOSIS:

1. **Blood smear**: ***HypERchromic microcytosis - 80% spherocytes*** (round RBCs ***lacking central pallor***)* ↑RDW.
2. ⊕***OSMOTIC FRAGILITY TEST**** (easy cell lysis), ***Coombs negative.**** ↑MCHC (mean corpuscular hemoglobin concentration)

MANAGEMENT:

1. <u>Folic acid</u> (not curative but helpful). Folate helps maintain RBC production & DNA synthesis.
2. **Splenectomy: *treatment of choice in severe disease**** (stops splenic RBC destruction).

AUTOIMMUNE HEMOLYTIC ANEMIA (AIHA)

- ***Antibodies vs. own RBC's surface*** ⇨↑RBC destruction by macrophages, spleen & complement. ***Idiopathic MC cause overall***. Meds ±warm or cold (ex ***PCN, methyldopa – hapten formation***).

WARM AGGLUTININS: ***IgG Ab**** causes <u>splenic macrophage RBC destruction</u> via phagocytosis (@ core body temp. 98.6°F). **Etiologies: *Autoimmune* (*SLE most common*,** RA), malignancy (***CLL***). The RBCs may be partially ingested by macrophages ⇨ spherocytes that are often destroyed.

COLD AGGLUTININS: ***IgM Ab**** vs. RBC induces intravascular <u>complement-mediated RBC lysis </u>especially at ***colder temperatures*** (<39°F). May follow infection (ex ***Mycoplasma, EBV***, HIV), malignancy.
- **CLINICAL:** anemia, ***acrocyanosis,*** fatigue, weakness, dyspnea, hemoglobinuria, ±Raynauds.

DIAGNOSIS: ⊕***Direct Coombs test,**** Cold agglutinin study, Peripheral smear: ***microspherocytes,*** polychromasia, RBC <u>agglutination</u>. ⊕ ***Coombs distinguishes AIHA from hereditary spherocytosis.****

MANAGEMENT

1. WARM: ***corticosteroids 1st line**** ⇨ <u>Splenectomy</u> or Rituximab ⇨ immunosuppressants. IVIG.
2. COLD: ***avoid cold exposure.*** Rituximab if treatment is needed. Plasmapheresis if refractory.

PAROXYSMAL NOCTURNAL HEMOGLOBINURIA

- ***Rare, <u>acquired</u> stem cell mutation*** ⇨RBCs deficient in GPI anchor surface protein that protects RBC from complement ⇨ ***↑complement-mediated RBC destruction (hemolysis) + thrombosis.****

CLINICAL MANIFESTATIONS

1. HEMOLYTIC ANEMIA: due to complement-induced RBC lysis. ***Dark cola-colored urine during the night or early in AM with partial clearing during the day.****
2. VENOUS THROMBOSIS of large vessels: free Hgb circulates & bind irreversibly with nitric oxide. Decreased NO leads to a hypercoagulable state. Thrombosis occurs in uncommon veins for ***thrombosis: ex: hepatic, mesenteric***, cerebral & subdermal veins.
3. PANCYTOPENIA: protein deficiency seen in RBCs, WBCs & platelets derived from stem cells ⇨ bone marrow failure. Often occur after bone marrow injury. *Hypercoagulability despite pancytopenia.*

DIAGNOSIS

1. ***Flow cytometry best screening test.**** Hemosiderinuria, sucrose test (cells lyse in hypotonic solution).
2. Osmotic fragility test, ↑RDW, Coombs negative. PNH may progress to myelodysplasia & AML.

MANAGEMENT *Eculizumab* (anti-complement C5 Ab). Prednisone ↓'es hemolysis. Marrow transplant.

BASICS OF HEMATOLOGY

HEMOSTASIS

The process to stop bleeding (prevents exsanguination during injuries). 2 phases:

PRIMARY HEMOSTASIS: *PLATELETS* form a plug at the site of vascular injury: **platelet adhesion, activation & aggregation**. Platelets adhere to site of the injury becoming activated, sending out ADP & Thromboxane A_2, which attracts other platelets to aggregate, ***forming a platelet plug.***
- **Disease examples:** thrombocytopenia (ITP, TTP, HUS, DIC, von Willebrand deficiency).
- ***Disorders that affect platelets will affect primary hemostasis,*** bleeding time (ex immediate bleeding after surgery) but ***PT & PTT usually unaffected*** (clotting factors are unaffected).
- These diseases classically cause ***petechiae & mucocutaneous bleeding*** (oral, GI, menorrhagia).

SECONDARY HEMOSTASIS: *CLOTTING FACTORS* (proteins) respond in a cascade to form ***fibrin strands which strengthens the platelet plug*** (that was formed during primary hemostasis).
- **Disease examples:** Hemophilia, DIC & von Willebrand disease.
- Disorders that affect the extrinsic pathway (prolongs PT) and intrinsic pathway (prolongs PTT).
- These diseases classically cause ***deep delayed bleeding (ex. hemarthrosis = bleeding into the joints & muscles)*** & ***delayed bleeding after surgery.***

PRIMARY HEMOSTASIS
PLATELET adhesion, activation, aggregation.

SECONDARY HEMOSTASIS
CLOTTING FACTORS leading to fibrin formation.

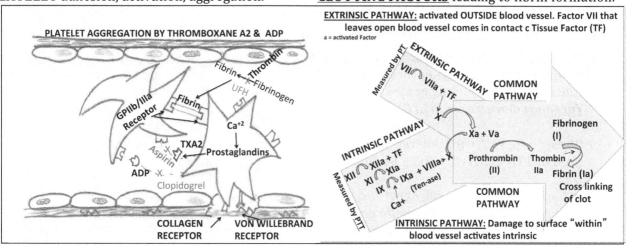

PTT (Partial Thromboplastin Time): measures efficacy of the ***INTRINSIC*** & common coagulation pathway. Normal PTT times require the presence of Factors I, II, V, ***VIII, IX****, X, *XI* and *XII*.

Factors 1, 2, 5, **8, 9**, *11 & 12.*

> **Prolonged PTT:** *Heparin,* DIC, vWD, Hemophilia A & B* & *antiphospholipid antibodies* (which paradoxically ↑'es thrombogenicity).
> ***Heparin overdose antidote: Protamine sulfate.****

PT (Prothrombin Time):

Measures the ***EXTRINSIC (tissue factor) pathway*** & common pathway.
Normal PT times primarily require the presence of Factors I, II, V, ***VII*** & *X* (1, 2, 5, *7 & 10*).

> **Prolonged PT:** *Warfarin therapy, Vitamin K deficiency, DIC.*
> ***Warfarin overdose antidote: Vitamin K.****

THROMBOTIC THROMBOCYTOPENIC PURPURA (TTP)

<u>Pentad:</u> ❶*Thrombocytopenia* (*petechiae,* bruising, purpura, *mucocutaneous bleeding* involving the skin, oral, epistaxis, GI, GU-menorrhagia) ❷*microangiopathic hemolytic anemia* (anemia, jaundice, fragmented RBCs/schistocytes on peripheral smear) ❸*kidney failure/uremia* (*not as common*) ❹*neurologic symptoms** (headache, CVA, AMS) ❺ *fever* (rare).

ETIOLOGIES
- **Primary TTP**: *idiopathic (autoimmune). Antibodies vs. ADAMTS13** ⇨ ↓ADAMTS13*
- **2ry TTP**: 2ry to malignancy, marrow transplantation, **SLE,** estrogen, pregnancy, *HIV₁* (↑incidence).

PATHOPHYSIOLOGY: ↓ADAMTS13 (a vWF cleaving protease) ⇨ large vWF multimers adhere to platelets & causes endothelial platelet adhesion ⇨ *small vessel thrombosis** ⇨ RBCs become sheared (damaged) as they circulate in the partially occluded small vessels ⇨ *hemolytic anemia*.

DIAGNOSIS
1. **Labs:** *thrombocytopenia, normal coags** (PT/PTT). Same labs as HUS. Since the problem is ↓platelets & not clotting factors, normal coags in TTP & HUS differentiate them from DIC.*
2. **Hemolytic anemia:** peripheral smear: ↑reticulocytes, schistocytes (bite/fragmented cells); ↑LDH, ↑Indirect bilirubin; ↓haptoglobin. Coombs negative. **Splenomegaly.**

MANAGEMENT
1. *PLASMAPHERESIS treatment of choice!** MOA: removes the antibodies vs. ADAMTS13 & adds missing ADAMTS13 to serum. Monitor LDH/platelets until normal x 2 days.

2. **Immunosuppression:** *Corticosteroids,* Cyclophosphamide etc. No platelet transfusions (may cause thrombi formation). ± Splenectomy if refractory to plasmapheresis & Corticosteroids.

HEMOLYTIC UREMIC SYNDROME

- **Triad:**❶*Thrombocytopenia* (bruising, purpura bleeding) ❷*microangiopathic hemolytic anemia* (anemia, jaundice, fragmented RBC's/schistocytes on peripheral smear) ❸*kidney failure (uremia) more common in HUS than TTP.*

- HUS associated MC with children, higher incidence of renal failure, *lacks the fever & neurologic sx seen in TTP** however, HUS ± be difficult to distinguish from TTP because labs are similar.

- *Predominantly seen in CHILDREN* (usually preceded by ENTEROHEMORRHAGIC E. coli O157:H7** (5-10 days), *Shigella or Salmonella gastroenteritis.** When it occurs in adults, it is seen with HIV, SLE, antiphospholipid syndrome. *Suspect HUS if renal failure in children with diarrhea prodrome.*

PATHOPHYSIOLOGY
1. *Platelet activation by exotoxins** (ex. Shigella toxin & Shiga-like toxin in E. coli O157:H7). The toxins enters the blood where it damages the vascular endothelium & activates platelets (microthrombi formation) ⇨ eventual platelet depletion ⇨ thrombocytopenia. The toxins preferentially damage the kidney (causing uremia & hypertension). The small vessel thrombosis causes RBC damage as they circulate through these vessels ⇨ hemolytic anemia.

DIAGNOSIS
- same labs/peripheral smear as TTP (hemolytic anemia, normal coags). ↑*BUN/creatinine.**

MANAGEMENT
1. *Observation in most children** (usually self limited): IV fluids to maintain renal perfusion.
2. *Plasmapheresis* (±FFP) if severe, neurologic complications or nonrenal complications.
- *Antibiotics may worsen the condition** (due to increased verotoxin release as a result of cell lysis).

DISSEMINATED INTRAVASCULAR COAGULATION (DIC)

- *Pathological activation of coagulation system* ⇨ ❶ *widespread microthrombi* which consumes coagulation proteins (V, VIII, fibrinogen) & platelets ⇨ ❷ *severe thrombocytopenia: diffuse bleeding* from skin, respiratory tract, GI tract.

ETIOLOGIES
1. *Infections: ex. gram negative sepsis MC,** endotoxins.
2. *Malignancies:* acute myelogenous leukemia, lung or GI cancers, prostate cancer etc.
3. *Obstetric*: preeclampsia, abruptio placentae, septic abortion, amniotic embolus.
4. Massive tissue injury (ex. burns); RMSF, liver disease, viral, aortic aneurysm, ARDS.

CLINICAL MANIFESTATIONS
patients usually acutely ill with:
1. *widespread hemorrhage: venipuncture sites,** mouth, nose, extensive bruising.

2. *thrombosis:* renal, hepatic, respiratory dysfunction, *gangrene* (clots block circulation).

DIAGNOSIS
1. ↑thrombin formation: ↓*fibrinogen, ↑PTT/PT/INR.** *Severe thrombocytopenia.*
   Peripheral smear: fragmented RBCs (schistocytes).
2. ↑*fibrinolysis:* ↑*D-dimer.**

MANAGEMENT
1. *Treat the underlying cause* is the most important step in the management of DIC.
2. Bleeding: *FFP if severe bleeding* (replaces coagulation factors). Cryoprecipitate (replaces fibrinogen). ±Platelet transfusion (in certain cases if platelet count <20,000/μL).
3. Thrombosis: ±Heparin in selected cases of _severe_ thrombosis.

IDIOPATHIC (AUTOIMMUNE) THROMBOCYTOPENIC PURPURA (ITP)

- Acquired, abnormal *isolated thrombocytopenia** (low platelet count) of idiopathic cause.
- 1ry ITP: idiopathic.   2ry: immune-mediated & associated with underlying d/o (*SLE, HIV, HCV* etc).

Acute ITP: *MC in children after a viral infection** (often self limited).
Chronic ITP: *MC in adults* (often recurrent). Women <40y MC. Males >70y.

PATHOPHYSIOLOGY
*Autoimmune antibody reaction vs. platelets** with splenic platelet destruction* often *following acute infection (ex viral)** ⇨ antibody vs. GPIIb/IIIa receptor found on platelets.

CLINICAL MANIFESTATIONS
1. Often asymptomatic.
2. ↑*mucocutaneous bleeding:* purpura, bruises, petechiae, bullae, epistaxis, menorrhagia, bleeding of the tooth & gums *(NO splenomegaly).**

DIAGNOSIS
isolated thrombocytopenia with *normal coag tests.** Normal coags because it is a platelet disorder not a coagulation disorder. Smear may show megakaryocytes or large-sized platelets.

MANAGEMENT
1. CHILDREN: *observation** (~80% resolve without treatment within 6 months) ⇨ *±IVIG.*
2. ADULTS: *Corticosteroids** (blunts the immune response)⇨**IVIG**⇨ *splenectomy if refractory.**
   Platelet transfusion only if <20,000/μL to prevent spontaneous intracranial hemorrhage.*

	ITP	TTP	HUS	DIC
Pathophysiology	• Autoimmune-Antibody reaction vs. platelets* with splenic platelet destruction ⇨ consumptive thrombocytopenia	• Auto-Ab vs. ADAMTS13* (vWF-cleaving protease) ⇨ unusual large vWF multimers ⇨ micro thrombosis of small vessels ⇨ thrombocytopenia (consumptive) & hemolytic anemia.	• Exotoxins (Shiga-like & Shiga toxins) damages vascular endothelium*, activating platelets ⇨ microthrombosis of small vessels ⇨ consumptive thrombocytopenia and hemolytic anemia. • ADAMTS13 normal	• Pathologic clotting cascade activation ⇨ widespread thrombi ⇨ consumption of platelets ⇨ diffuse bleeding
Incidence	• Predominantly young children 2-4y. Often 1-3 weeks following acute viral infection.* Often self-limited in children. • Adult: young women <40y idiopathic. Often recurrent	• Young adults 20-50y • MC women	• Predominantly seen in children with diarrhea prodrome*. Enterohem. E coli O157:H7 (80%). Shigella, Salmonella, • Adults: seen with HIV, SLE, Anti phospholipid syndrome.	• MC in young or elderly • MC gram negative sepsis* • OB emergencies • Malignancy • Massive tissue trauma.
Clinical Manifestations	• Often asymptomatic. • ↑mucocutaneous bleeding: petechiae, bruising, purpura, bullae, bleeding of tooth & gums, menorrhagia. • NO SPLENOMEGALY*	PENTAD* 1. Thrombocytopenia: bruising, purpura, bleeding. 2. Microangiopathic hemolytic anemia: anemia, jaundice. 3. Kidney failure/uremia: (not as common as in HUS. 4. Neuro sx:* headache, CVA, AMS 5. Fever	TRIAD 1. Thrombocytopenia: bruising, purpura, bleeding 2. Microangiopathic hemolytic anemia: anemia, jaundice 3. Kidney failure/uremia: predominant feature.* Suspect HUS if renal failure in children with diarrhea prodrome*.	• Diffuse hemorrhage: venipuncture sites, mouth, nose; extensive bruising. • Thrombosis: renal failure, gangrene (as clots block circulation). • Patients usually acutely ill
Diagnosis	• ISOLATED THROMBOCYTOPENIA* • Normal coag tests (PT, PTT)	• Thrombocytopenia Hemolytic anemia: • Peripheral smear: ↑reticulocytes, schistocytes ("bite or fragmented cells) • LFTs: ↑Ind bili; ↓haptoglobin • Normal coag tests (PT, PTT)	• Labs & peripheral smear in TTP & HUS look the same. • ↑BUN/Creatinine* (Renal failure) • Normal coags (PT, PTT) distinguish TTP & HUS from DIC*	Hemolytic anemia: • Peripheral smear: ↑reticulocytes, schistocytes ("bite or fragmented cells) • LFTs: ↑Ind bili; ↓haptoglobin • ABNORMAL COAG TESTS*: ↓fibrinogen, ↑D-dimer, ↑PT, PTT. severe thrombocytopenia.
Management	• CHILDREN: observation ~80% resolve without tx within 6 months. ±Intravenous immunoglobulin. • ADULTS: CORTICOSTEROIDS* (blunts the immune response) ⇨ IVIG ⇨ SPLENECTOMY IN REFRACTORY CASES.*	• PLASMAPHERESIS mainstay* (↓es mortality). Removes Ab & adds ADAMTS13 • Immunosuppression: steroids, Cyclophosphamides etc.	• Observation in most children (usually self-limited). • Plasmapheresis ±FFP if severe, • NO antibiotics* - may worsen the disease (↑toxin release).	• Reversal of the underlying cause mainstay of tx* ±Platelet transfusion (if <20,000) ±Fresh frozen plasma ±Heparin in select cases.

HEMOPHILIA A (Factor VIII 8 Deficiency)

- The MC type of hemophilia (80%). X-linked recessive trait _occurs almost only in males_* (rarely homozygous females). Can also be caused by spontaneous mutation. 1st episode usually <18y.

- _Lack of Factor VIII affects the INTRINSIC PATHWAY_ of the clotting cascade ⇨ _failure to form hematomas._

CLINICAL MANIFESTATIONS
1. _HEMARTHROSIS_* (80%): ±bleed in weight-bearing joints (ex _ankles,_ knees, elbows) ⇨ _ARTHROPATHY._

2. _Excessive hemorrhage in response to trauma & surgery/incisional bleeding_* (ex. tooth extraction). Epistaxis, bruising. _GI_/urinary tract hemorrhage (blood in stool/urine).

3. _Hemophilias less commonly presents with purpura/petechiae_* (platelet function is normal). _Spontaneous hemorrhage less common_ (only seen with severe form).

DIAGNOSIS
1. _Low Factor VIII, prolonged PTT._* Normal PT/bleeding time/fibrinogen levels, _normal platelet levels._ _Mixing study (with normal plasma) will correct/normalize PTT._

MANAGEMENT
1. _Factor VIII infusion_* to levels 25-100% as needed.

2. _Desmopressin (DDAVP):_* transiently ↑'es _Factor VIII & vWF_ release so may be used prior to procedures to prevent bleeding.

HEMOPHILIA B (Christmas Disease) (Factor IX/9 Deficiency)

- X-linked recessive trait: _almost exclusively in males_ (homozygous females - rare).

CLINICAL MANIFESTATIONS
Clinically indistinguishable from Hemophilia A (same symptoms). _Deep tissue bleeding._*

DIAGNOSIS
- ↓serum Factor IX, _prolonged PTT. PTT corrects with mixing study._

MANAGEMENT
- Factor IX infusion. _Desmopressin NOT useful_ (Desmopressin only used in Hemophilia A & vWD)

MIXING STUDY
Distinguishes factor deficiencies (vWD, hemophilias) from ⊕ factor inhibitors (ex lupus anticoagulant, Ab vs Factor VIII). 50% normal factors should normalize the PT/PTT.

- If affected blood is mixed with normal plasma & PT/PTT corrects ⇨ factor deficiency.

- _If PTT doesn't correct with mixing study_ ⇨ ⊕ _presence of factor inhibitors (ex. ⊕ lupus anticoagulant, antiphospholipid syndrome)._

VON WILLEBRAND DISEASE

- **_Ineffective platelet adhesion_*** due to autosomal dominant disorder associated with **_deficient/defective von Willebrand Factor_** (platelet aggregation is normal – only platelet adhesion is affected). MC in women.

- **_MC hereditary bleeding disorder_*** (1% of population). May also be acquired.
- vWF is necessary for *initial platelet adhesion & prevents Factor VIII degradation.* vWF is produced by endothelial cells & megakaryocytes.

CLINICAL MANIFESTATIONS
1. **_Mucocutaneous bleeding:* easy bruising, epistaxis, gums, GI, menorrhagia_**. Varying degrees of bleeding. **_Bleeding after minor lacerations.*_**
   Incisional bleeding less common in vWF disease than in hemophilia.

2. **_Petechiae:* common in vWF_** but in rare in Hemophilias (normal platelets in hemophilia).

DIAGNOSIS
1. **↓*vWF levels, ±prolonged PTT_** (±↓factor VIII). **_Bleeding time & PTT prolongation worse with aspirin.*_** Factor 8 & 9 are part of intrinsic pathway ⇨ ↑PTT. *PTT corrects with mixing study.*

   - stress, surgery, pregnancy and oral contraceptives may increase vWF levels.

2. **↓*Ristocetin activity test gold standard:*** no platelet aggregation with Ristocetin (Ristocetin is an antibiotic that causes platelet agglutination in vitro).
   Hypoactivity is associated with vWF deficiency.

MANAGEMENT
Avoid aspirin. Important to assess bleeding times immediately before procedures.

1. **_Type I - quantitative deficiency (MC type_** 75%):

MILD DISEASE	*No treatment needed*
MODERATE	*DDAVP (Desmopressin)* **MOA:** synthetic ADH (↑vWF, Factor VIII levels)
SEVERE	vWF-containing products ex. Factor VIII concentrates (also contains vwF), recombinant vWF.

2. Type II (qualitative deficiency) ⇨ ***DDAVP*** (***vWF + Factor VIII prior to procedures***).

3. *Type III (severe, absent vwF - rare disorder)* ⇨ ***vWF + Factor VIII (8).*** *DDAVP not helpful in III.*

DISORDERS	PT	PTT	BLEEDING TIME	PLATELET count
THROMBOCYTOPENIA	Unaffected	Unaffected	**Prolonged**	Decreased
HEMOPHILIA	Unaffected	*Prolonged*	Unaffected (normal platelets)	Unaffected
VON WILLEBRAND DISEASE	Unaffected	*Prolonged*	*Prolonged (especially with aspirin challenge).*	Unaffected
VITAMIN K DEFICIENCY (EX. WARFARIN)	*Prolonged*	Normal or minor prolongation.	Unaffected	Unaffected
DIC	*Prolonged*	*Prolonged*	*Prolonged*	*Decreased*

HODGKIN DISEASE   (HODGKIN'S LYMPHOMA)

- Lymphocyte neoplasm. *Bimodal:* peaks @20* then again *>50y.*
- *Associated with Epstein-Barr virus.** MC in males (Nodular sclerosing MC in females).*
- Upper body lymph nodes ex. neck, axilla, shoulder, abdomen.
  - *Contiguous, orderly spread via lymph nodes.*

Types: Nodular sclerosing, Mixed cellularity, lymphocyte-rich, lymphocyte-depleted.

CLINICAL MANIFESTATIONS
1. *PAINLESS LYMPHADENOPATHY* – firm, nontender, freely mobile (especially supraclavicular, cervical & mediastinal). *ALCOHOL MAY INDUCE LYMPH NODE PAIN.** Hepatosplenomegaly.

2. **Systemic "B" symptoms (advanced disease):** ↑cytokines ⇨ *Pel-Ebstein fever* (cyclical fever that increase & decrease over a period of 1-2 weeks, *night sweats*), *weight loss*, anemia, pruritus.

DIAGNOSIS
1. **Excisional biopsy:** *REED-STERNBERG CELL pathognomonic!*** (large cells with bilobed or multilobar nucleus - *"owl-eye appearance"* with inclusions in the nucleoli). CD15+, CD30+.
   - *only seen with Hodgkin Lymphoma.* Associated with clonal B-cell proliferation.

2. *Mediastinal lymphadenopathy.* PET/CT scan for staging.

MANAGEMENT
1. Local disease (stage I, II, IIIA): radiation therapy.
2. Stage IIIB, IV: combination chemotherapy. May also be used in earlier stages.
   (ex. ABVD – Adriamycin (Doxorubicin), Bleomycin, Vinblastine, Dacarbazine).
Hodgkin Lymphoma is highly curable (compared to NHL).

NON HODGKIN LYMPHOMA

- Lymphocyte neoplasm: Diffuse B cell, T cell, follicular, etc. MC >50y. *PERIPHERAL lymph nodes MC.**

- **Risk Factors:** ↑*age, immunosuppression* (*HIV,* viral infections), connective tissue disease, family history, history of radiation therapy (XRT).

CLINICAL MANIFESTATIONS
1. Variable. *Local: painless lymphadenopathy,** splenomegaly.
   - *Extranodal sites common: GI, skin & CNS MC,* testicular enlargement, mediastinal masses.

   - **Burkitt Lymphoma:** often presents with abdominal pain (sporadic type), jaw involvement (African type). Histology in Burkitt shows "starry sky" appearance.
   - Systemic "B" symptoms (fever, night sweats, weight loss, anemia, pruritus) rarer in NHL (± seen in advanced disease). PET/CT scan used for staging.

MANAGEMENT
Unpredictable course.
1. Follicular: indolent form (but not curable generally). *Rituximab: antibody vs. CD20 on B cells.*

2. Diffuse Large B cell: MC type & most aggressive type (but curable with chemotherapy often).
   Ex. R-CHOP Rituximab (antibody vs. CD20), Cyclophosphamide, Hydroxydaunorubicin, Oncovorin/Vincristine, Prednisone.

WALDENSTRÖM MACROGLOBULINEMIA

- Lymphoplasmacytic B-cell lymphoma that ***produces excess IgM*** paraprotein (considered an indolent type of Non Hodgkin's lymphoma). Incurable but treatable.

PATHOPHYSIOLOGY
- ***Clonal B-cell IgM production*** (postgerminal center IgM memory B cell that has failed to switch isotype class) ⇨ ↑abnormal monoclonal IgM.

CLINICAL MANIFESTATIONS
- Often asymptomatic (aka smoldering). Associated with "OVA" **O**rganomegaly, **V**iscosity, **A**nemia.
- ***Organomegaly:*** **lymphadenopathy,** splenomegaly, hepatomegaly (30-40%).
- ***Hyperviscosity syndrome:*** large IgM molecules increase serum viscosity, slowing the passage of blood through the capillaries ⇨ *blurred vision, headache, vertigo, nystagmus, dizziness, tinnitus, diplopia, ataxia.* Complications include retinal hemorrhages & CVA.
- ***Anemia:*** weakness, fatigue, weight loss, pallor. Anemia is due to bone marrow failure.
- ***Chronic, oozing blood from nose, gums:*** IgM interacts with platelets & inhibits fibrin formation.
- Peripheral neuropathy (10%) especially due to IgM acting as an autoantibody vs. myelin-associated glycoproteins in nerves & other nerve components.
- ***Cryoglobulinemia:*** IgM precipitates out of the serum in cold temperatures, resulting in Raynaud's phenomenon, urticaria, acral cyanosis, and/or tissue necrosis.

DIAGNOSIS
1. **SERUM PROTEIN ELECTROPHORESIS:** *IgM monoclonal spike* (macroglobulinemia).
   Differs from Multiple myeloma, which is classically an IgG or IgA spike.

2. **BONE MARROW BIOPSY:** **≥*10% lymphoplasmacytic infiltrate*** (must exclude CLL). Dutcher bodies.
3. Anemia, thrombocytopenia, neutropenia. Elevated beta-2 microglobulin level.

MANAGEMENT
1. Highly responsive to chemotherapy but rarely curative: Rituximab, Chlorambucil, Cyclophosphamide, Vincristine. CHOP therapy may be used.
2. Rituximab (monoclonal Ab vs CD20) may be used alone if mild symptoms are present.
3. ***Plasmapheresis*** used to ***treat severe hyperviscosity syndrome with complications.***

MONOCLONAL GAMMOPATHY OF UNDERTERMINED SIGNIFICANCE (MGUS)

- ↑***immunoglobulins*** (monoclonal proteins) ***WITHOUT CLINICAL MANIFESTATIONS/ORGAN DAMAGE.***
- 1% of adults. 3% of adults >70y. 1% yearly risk of developing multiple myeloma or lymphoma.
- ***MC IgG*** (69%), *IgM* (17%), *IgA* (11%), IgD. Kappa light chains (62%), lambda light chains (38%).
- May be associated with other diseases, infection, autoimmune disorders (ex SLE, ITP).

CLINICAL MANIFESTATIONS
- ***Asymptomatic by definition**** (often found while being worked up for another reason).

DIAGNOSIS:
1. **SERUM PROTEIN ELECTROPHORESIS:** *monoclonal spike (ex. IgG)* - elevated but usually <3g/dL.
   Monoclonal spike is usually stable over time (usually does not progress).
2. URINE PROTEIN ELECTROPHORESIS: none or stable amounts of Bence-Jones proteins.
3. **BONE MARROW BIOPSY:** *<10%* plasmacytoid or plasma cells (definitive diagnosis).
4. ABSENCE of hypercalcemia, anemia, renal failure, lytic bone lesions (seen in multiple myeloma).

MANAGEMENT
1. **Conservative or observation:** low malignant potential risk.

MULTIPLE MYELOMA (PLASMACYTOMA)

- Cancer associated with proliferation of a **_single clone of plasma cells*_** ⇨ ↑**_monoclonal Ab (especially IgG, IgA)._**

- Monoclonal Ab accumulate in bone marrow, interrupting marrow's normal cell production.
- ↑**RISK:** **_elderly >65y, African-Americans, men,*_** ?exposure to herpes virus, benzene.

CLINICAL MANIFESTATIONS
Bones "BREAK" in Multiple Myeloma – helpful mnemonic.
Bone pain: *especially spine** & ribs* due to **osteolytic, destructive lesions** & *osteopenic fractures, spinal cord compression* (plasma cells can form a tumor), radiculopathy.
Recurrent infections: (Strep pneumo, gram negative) from **leukopenia.** Hyperviscosity.
Elevated Calcium (hypercalcemia): only heme malignancy associated with bone destruction.
Anemia: fatigue, pallor, weakness, weight loss, hepatosplenomegaly, soft tissue masses.
Kidney Failure* - antibody light-chain protein deposition in the kidney. Neurologic involvement.

DIAGNOSIS
1. Serum Protein Electrophoresis: **_monoclonal (M) protein spike._*** IgG 60%, IgA (20%).

2. Urine Protein Electrophoresis: **_Bence-Jones proteins:_*** kappa or lambda light chains.

3. CBC: **_Rouleaux formation:_*** RBCs stick together due to ↑plasma protein ⇨ ↑**ESR.**

4. Skull Radiographs: **_"punched-out" lytic lesions._*** *Bone scans NOT helpful!*
5. Bone Marrow biopsy: **_Plasmacytosis_** >10%

MANAGEMENT
1. **Autologous stem cell transplant definitive treatment.** ±Preceded by chemotherapy ex. Thalidomide or alkylating agents ex. Melphalan). Bisphosphonates for bony destruction.

ACUTE LYMPHOCYTIC LEUKEMIA (ALL)

- Malignancy of lymphoid stem cells in bone marrow ⇨ lymph nodes, spleen, liver, other organs.
- **_MC childhood malignancy*_** **(peak age 3-7y).** B cell, T cell, null type (non B/T cell).
- **Down syndrome** *in children >5y old* ⇨ ↑*ALL (<5y* ⇨ *Megakaryoblastic acute myelogenous leukemia).*

CLINICAL MANIFESTATIONS
1. Pancytopenia symptoms: ex. **fever MC symptom**, fatigue, lethargy. Bone pain.
2. **_CNS symptoms:_*** headache, stiff neck, visual changes, vomiting. CNS & testes MC site for METS.

PHYSICAL EXAMINATION
Pallor, fatigue, petechiae, bruising, **hepatosplenomegaly, lymphadenopathy,** ± *mediastinal mass.*

DIAGNOSIS
Bone marrow: **hypercellular with >20% blasts;** WBC: 5-100,000/μL, anemia, thrombocytopenia.

MANAGEMENT
1. Oral chemotherapy (ex. Hydroxyurea). **Highly responsive to combination chemotherapy** (remission >90%). Imatinib used if Philadelphia chromosome ⊕.
2. Stem cell transplant if relapse. **Intrathecal Methotrexate for CNS disease.**

CHRONIC LYMPHOCYTIC LEUKEMIA (CLL) (B Cell)

B cell clonal malignancy. MC >50y, males, Caucasians. **CLL MC leukemia in adults overall.***

CLINICAL MANIFESTATIONS
1. Most are asymptomatic (often incidental finding of leukocytosis on routine blood testing).
2. *Fatigue MC,* dyspnea on exertion, ↑infections. *Lymphadenopathy,* hepatosplenomegaly.

DIAGNOSIS
1. Peripheral smear: incompetent, **well-differentiated, lymphocytes with scattered "SMUDGE CELLS".***
   (fragile B cells that often smudge during slide preparation). Lymphocytosis >20,000/µL.
2. Pancytopenia: thrombocytopenia, anemia. Flow cytometry: CD5, CD19, CD20 & CD23 ⊕ B cells.

MANAGEMENT
1. Observation if indolent.
2. Chemotherapy if symptomatic or progressive (ex. **Fludarabine*** ± Rituximab, Chlorambucil).
3. Allogeneic stem cell transplant is curative. Poorer prognosis: ZAP-70 ⊕, del(17p), del(11q).

ACUTE MYELOGENOUS LEUKEMIA (AML)

- **MC ACUTE form of leukemia in adults** (80% of cases). Majority of patients **>50y.**

CLINICAL MANIFESTATIONS
1. **Pancytopenia:** *anemia, thrombocytopenia, neutropenia.* **Splenomegaly, gingival hyperplasia** (monocytic), bone pain. Megakaryoblastic MC in children <5y with Down Syndrome.
2. **±Leukostasis (WBC >100,000/µL):** *CNS deficits: headaches, confusion, TIA, CVA)* Pulm: *respiratory distress, dyspnea.* Leukostasis management: leukapheresis or chemotherapy.

DIAGNOSIS
1. **Bone marrow:** *AUER RODS** (rods of cytoplasmic granules in promyelocytic) & **>20% blasts.***

MANAGEMENT
1. **Combination chemotherapy.** Induction tx - aim to reduce cell population ex. Cytarabine + anthracycline (Daunorubicin) ⇨ Consolidation (short-term intensive tx to sustain remission).
2. ±Allogeneic bone marrow transplant after remission. All-trans-retinoic acid if promyelocytic.

TUMOR LYSIS SYNDROME: complication 48-72h after induction tx - large # of cells being destroyed ⇨ *hyperuricemia, ↑K, ↓Ca, ↑Phosphate, acute renal Failure.* **MANAGEMENT:** *Allopurinol, IV fluids.***

CHRONIC MYELOGENOUS LEUKEMIA (CML)

- Well differentiated WBCs – granulocyte proliferation). Patients usually >50y.

CLINICAL MANIFESTATIONS
1. Most asymptomatic until they develop **blastic crisis** (acute leukemia), **SPLENOMEGALY.***

DIAGNOSIS
1. Cytogenetics or FISH: ⊕**PHILADELPHIA CHROMOSOME*** = translocation between chromosome 9 & 22, causing a fusion gene bcr-abl. Think "Philadelphia Cre**M** cheese".
2. **Strikingly ↑WBC counts** (ex. 100,000), ↑LDH, **↓LAP (leukocyte alkaline phosphatase)** score.
   Chronic: <5% blasts, Accelerated: >5% to 30% blasts; Acute blast crisis: >30% blasts.

MANAGEMENT
- Chemotherapy: ex. Hydroxyurea.
   Imatinib BCR-ABL tyrosine kinase inhibitor (**Philadelphia** ⊕). Others: Dasatinib, Ponatinib.
- Allogeneic stem cell transplant in severe disease or if failed chemotherapy.

	HODGKINS DISEASE (HD) LYMPHOMA	NON HODGKINS LYMPHOMA (NHL)
AGE	• Bimodal* peaks in 20s then in 50s	• >50y, Increased risk with immunosuppression: ex HIV, viral infection
CELL TYPE	• REED STERNBERG CELLS pathognomonic* B cell proliferation with bilobed or multilobar nucleus "owl eye."	• B CELL: Diffuse large B cell MC (more aggressive). Follicular (indolent but less curable); Mantle Cell, Burkitt's, Marginal zone MALT lymphoma is an extranodal type of marginal zone lymphoma), small cell lymphoma (SCL) & CLL thought to be same disease with different presentations (SCL primarily in the lymph nodes, CLL in the bone marrow/peripheral blood). • T cell: (T cell, T lymphoblastic), Natural Killer Cells.
LYMPH NODE INVOLVEMENT	• UPPER LYMPH NODE INVOLVEMENT*: neck, axilla, shoulder, chest (mediastinum). ± painful lymph nodes c ETOH ingestion* Usually painless lymph nodes. • CONTIGUOUS spread to LOCAL LYMPH NODES. Usually Localized, single group of nodes (extranodal rare).	• PERIPHERAL MULTIPLE NODE INVOLVEMENT*: axillary, abdominal, pelvic, inguinal, femoral. Waldeyer's ring (tonsils, base of tongue, nasopharynx) • NONCONTIGUOUS EXTRANODAL SPREAD*: GI MC, Skin 2nd MC (especially T cell), testes, bone marrow, GU, liver, spleen, thyroid, kidney, spine, CNS (headache, lethargy, spinal cord compression, focal neurologic symptoms).
ASSOCIATED SYMPTOMS	• B sx: fever, weight loss, anorexia, night sweats. Associated with a poorer prognosis. • PEL EBSTEIN FEVER: intermittent cyclical fevers x1-2 weeks*	• B symptoms not as common on presentation (but may be seen with advanced disease or aggressive disease). • Leukemic phase can be seen at times with NHL.
EBV ASSOCIATION (EPSTEIN-BARR VIRUS)	• ↑associated with Epstein-Barr Virus* (40%)	• Rare in most types of NHL. • EBV common in Burkitt's lymphoma – ❶ Endemic (Africa): associated with jaw involvement. ❷ Immunodeficient: ex. post transplant lymphoma & AIDS-associated lymphoma. ❸Sporadic (not associated with EBV).
MANAGEMENT	• Excellent 5y cure rate (60%)	• Variable.

	AML	CML	ALL	CLL
EPIDEMIOLOGY	• MC acute form of leukemia. >50y	• Older males	• MC children* (peaks 3-7y)	• MC Leukemia in adults
DIAGNOSIS	>20% blasts (immature WBCs). • PROMYELOCYTIC - ⊕AUER RODS* - Sudan Black & Myeloperoxidase ⊕ • ACUTE MONOCYTIC: - Gingival infiltration/hyperplasia • MEGAKARYOCYTIC: ↑Down syndrome	• PHILADELPHIA CHROMOSOME* • Striking ↑WBC: >100,00 • Chronic <5% blasts • Accelerated 5-30% blasts • Acute >30% blasts	• >30% blasts. PAS ⊕ • Precursor B-cell ALL (~85%) associated with CNS sx. • Precursor T cell MC associated with adolescents with mediastinal mass & CNS sx	• SMUDGE (SMEAR) CELLS* • Well differentiated lymphocytes • ZAP-70 ⊕ ⇔ 8y survival. ZAP-70 negative ⇔ >25y.
MANAGEMENT	• Chemotherapy. • Stem cell Transplant. • Tumor Lysis syndrome c chemotx: ↑K, ↓Ca, ↑Phos, Hyperuricemia & renal failure. Tx: Allopurinol, IV fluids.	• PO Chemotherapy (ex. Hydroxyurea, Imatinib). • Imatinib BCR-ABL tyrosine kinase inhibitor (Philadelphia ⊕).	• PO Chemotx in Philadelphia ⊕ • Induction: kills detectable disease for complete remission. • Consolidation: short term intensive therapy to sustain remission. • Maintenance: low dose to eradicate any remaining undetectable cells.	• Indolent: observation. • Symptomatic or progressive: Chemotherapy. • Allogeneic stem cell transplant is curative

	Bleeding Syndrome	Petechiae	Ecchymosis	Bleed after minor cuts	Bleeding after surgery
THROMBOCYTOPENIA (Quantitative/Qualitative)	Mucocutaneous bleeding* (oral, nasal, GI, GU), petechiae	Common*	Small superficial	Yes	Immediate
FACTOR DEFICIENCY: Hemophilias	Deep bleeding* (joint, muscles)	Uncommon	Large hematomas	Not usually	Delayed*

POLYCYTHEMIA VERA (PRIMARY ERYTHROCYTOSIS)

- Acquired myeloproliferative disorder with **_overproduction of all 3 MYELOID cell lines._*** (***primarily*** ↑**RBCs***,** but also associated with ↑WBCs & ↑platelets). *Lymphocyte line normal.**
- ***Peaks 50-60y.*** *MC in men* (60%). Caused by **JAK2 mutation.**
- ***Primary erythrocytosis = ↑hematocrit in the absence of hypoxia.*** Mature myeloid cells.

CLINICAL MANIFESTATIONS

- Symptoms due to ↑**_RBC mass: hyperviscosity or thrombosis:_**
1. Headache, dizziness, tinnitus, blurred vision, **pruritus (especially after hot bath),*** fatigue, epistaxis, thrombosis. Erythromelalgia: episodic burning/throbbing of hands & feet with edema.

2. **Physical exam:** **_splenomegaly, facial plethora (flushed face),_** engorged retinal veins.

3. **Spent phase:** *splenomegaly, marrow fibrosis with marked pancytopenia.* 15% of patients present in the spent phase.

DIAGNOSIS

1. **Major criteria:** ❶ ↑**_RBC mass:*_** ↑*hematocrit,* ↑*Hgb* ❷ Bone marrow biopsy: hypercellularity (*erythroid, granulocytic & megakaryocytic proliferation*), ❸JAK2 mutation presence.
2. **Minor criteria:** ↓ **_serum erythropoietin levels._*** All 3 major or 1st 2 major + minor = PV.
3. ***Normal O₂ sat,*** ↑WBC, ↑platelets, ↑B₁₂, ↑LAP (Leukocyte alkaline phosphatase is an enzyme produced by WBCs). ±Fe deficiency despite polycythemia. ±progress to CML or myelofibrosis.

MANAGEMENT

1. ***Phlebotomy management of choice!*** Done until hematocrit <45% (to reduce the high risk of venous thrombosis ex Budd Chiari syndrome). Low-dose Aspirin (prevents thrombosis).
2. Myelosuppression: **_Hydroxyurea_** (inhibits cells with a high division rate), Interferon-α.
3. Allopurinol (if patients are hyperuricemic). Ruxolitinib is a JAK inhibitor.

SECONDARY ERYTHROCYTOSIS

- Major cause of ↑RBC mass. MC in obese, history of cigarette smoking.
- ***Secondary erythrocytosis = ↑hematocrit as a response to another process.***

ETIOLOGIES *3 major causes:*

1. Reactive (physiologic): due to **_hypoxia*_** ex. **_pulmonary disease (COPD),*_** high altitude, tobacco smokers, cyanotic heart disease. ***Reactive MC type.***
2. Pathologic: no underlying tissue hypoxia. Ex. renal disease (ex renal cell CA), fibroids, hepatoma.
3. Relative polycythemia: normal RBC mass in the setting of ↓plasma volume, dehydration.

CLINICAL MANIFESTATIONS

1. Symptoms related to the underlying precipitating cause (ex COPD, renal disease, cyanosis etc).
2. Physical Exam: cyanosis, clubbing, hypertension, hepatosplenomegaly, ±heart murmur.

DIAGNOSIS:

1. ↑**RBCs/_hematocrit with normal WBC & platelets,_*** normal erythropoietin levels (RBC mass normal in reactive polycythemia due to ↓ plasma volume).
   Normal WBC/platelets distinguishes 2ʳʸ from 1ʳʸ (Polycythemia Vera).

MANAGEMENT

1. Treat underlying disorder. Smoking cessation.

HEREDITARY HEMOCHROMATOSIS

- *Excess iron deposition* in parenchymal cells of the *heart, liver, pancreas & endocrine organs.*
- Autosomal recessive *disorder of ↑iron storage & ↑Fe absorption* especially in *men* (5x MC).
- Among Caucasians 1/200 with *C282Y HFE genotype** ⇨ ↑intestinal Fe absorption & decreased hepcidin production (Hepcidin normally inhibits Fe absorption, preventing Fe excess).

**PATHOPHYSIOLOGY: *increased intestinal Fe absorption* ⇨ ↑*serum Fe* & ↑Fe deposition in the liver, heart, pancreas, adrenal glands, testes, kidney & other tissues. Symptoms due to organ dysfunction:

CLINICAL MANIFESTATIONS
- *May be asymptomatic in early stages. Symptoms usually begin after 40y.* Nonspp sx: fatigue.
1. **Liver** dysfunction: abdominal pain, *cirrhosis,* fatigue, weakness, hepatomegaly, arthraglias.
2. **Heart failure: *cardiomyopathy, arrhythmias,*** heart failure & heart block.
3. **Hypogonadism**: testicular atrophy & impotence. Joints: synovitis, polyarthritis.
4. **Pancreatic Insufficiency:** deposition of Fe in pancreas ⇨ beta cell damage ⇨ diabetes.
   Physical Examination: *metallic or bronze skin = "BRONZE DIABETES."**

DIAGNOSIS:
1. ↑*serum iron** (>200 µg/dL), ↑*serum transferrin saturation* (>70%), normal /↓TIBC. ↑ *Ferritin.**
   *Fe storage overload = ↑Ferritin + ↑Fe = seen with either hemochromatosis or lead poisoning.**

2. ±↑LFTs, Genetic testing for HFE gene. ↑risk of hepatocellular carcinoma.
3. **Liver biopsy: *gold standard:** ↑liver parenchymal *hemosiderin* (↑Fe storage).

MANAGEMENT
1. *Phlebotomy:** weekly phlebotomy until depletion of iron (↓ferritin, ↓transferrin saturation or mild anemia) ⇨ Maintenance phlebotomy ~3-4 times a year for life.
2. *Chelating agents:* ONLY if unable to do phlebotomy (ex anemia). Usually not needed.
3. Treat complications, test blood relatives, genetic counseling. No iron pills, ETOH or vitamin C.

COAGULOPATHY OF ADVANCED LIVER DISEASE

- *Advanced liver disease associated with ↓production of coagulation factors.* Liver produces all coagulation factors (except Factor VIII & vwF produced by megakaryocytes & endothelial cells). Malabsorption of Vitamin K with liver disease. Portal HTN ⇨ splenomegaly ⇨ thrombocytopenia.

ETIOLOGIES: cirrhosis, end stage liver disease, ETOH, hemochromatosis, hepatitis, ischemia.

CLINICAL MANIFESTATIONS:
1. Bleeding is the classic finding (especially GI). Signs of liver disease.

DIAGNOSIS:
1. ↑*PT,** Often *low albumin.** *As disease advances ↑ in both PT & ↑PTT.** No response to Vitamin K. PT/PTT corrects with mixing study. ↓fibrinogen, ± thrombocytopenia.
2. Peripheral smear: ±target cells.

MANAGEMENT:
1. *Fresh Frozen Plasma:** if active bleeding or if undergoing an invasive procedure* (replaces deficient coagulation factors). Vitamin K does not correct the coagulopathy.

2. Cryoprecipitate: if ↓fibrinogen present. Cryoprecipitate contains fibrinogen, Factor VIII & vWF.

3. Correct the underlying disorder if possible. Avoid alcohol.

FACTOR V LEIDEN MUTATION

- *MC inherited cause of hypercoagulability.** 5% of US population. Due to a mutation of Factor V.

PATHOPHYSIOLOGY
- Mutated Factor V is resistant to breakdown by activated Protein C *(aProtein C resistance)* ⇨ *hypercoagulability* ⇨ *↑DVTs & PE especially in young patients.* Hepatic vein thrombosis.
  - Not associated with an increased incidence of myocardial infarctions or CVA.

DIAGNOSIS
Activated protein C resistance assay. If positive, confirm with DNA testing. Normal PT/PTT.

MANAGEMENT
1. High risk ⇨ indefinite anticoagulation.
   May need thrombophylaxis during pregnancy to prevent miscarriages.

2. Moderate risk (ex 1 thrombotic event with a prothrombotic stimulus or asymptomatic) ⇨ prophylaxis during high-risk procedures.

PROTEIN C DEFICIENCY

- Autosomal dominant inherited hypercoagulable disorder.

PATHOPHYSIOLOGY
Protein C is a vitamin K-dependent anticoagulant protein (produced by the liver) that stimulates fibrinolysis & clot lysis (inactivates Factor V & VIII). Protein C's anticoagulant effect is potentiated by Protein S. Protein C deficiency causes ↑risk of recurrent DVT & pulmonary embolism.

CLINICAL MANIFESTATIONS
1. *Recurrent DVTs or pulmonary emboli.* May have a family history. 70% of clots are spontaneous & 30% are have predisposing risk factors (ex. pregnancy, OCPs, surgery, trauma).

MANAGEMENT
1. Heparin ⇨ oral anticoagulation for life. May develop *warfarin-induced skin necrosis.**

ANTITHROMBIN III DEFICIENCY

Hypercoagulable disorder:
- Inherited: autosomal dominant or
- Acquired: ex. liver disease, nephrotic syndrome, DIC, chemotherapy.

PATHOPHYSIOLOGY
- Antithrombin III inactivates surplus thrombin. Antithrombin III activity is potentiated by Heparin. *Antithrombin III deficiency results in venous thrombosis.*

CLINICAL MANIFESTATIONS
1. *Recurrent DVTs or pulmonary emboli*. 1st episode often occurs between 20-30y

MANAGEMENT
1. Asymptomatic patients require anticoagulation only before surgical procedures.

2. Patients with a thrombotic event may receive *high-dose IV heparin* then oral anticoagulation indefinitely.

SELECTED REFERENCES

Evans DL, Edelsohn GA, Golden RN. Organic psychosis without anemia or spinal cord symptoms in patients with vitamin B12 deficiency. Am J Psychiatry. 1983;140(2):218-21.

Wambua S, Mwangi TW, Kortok M, et al. The effect of alpha+-thalassaemia on the incidence of malaria and other diseases in children living on the coast of Kenya. PLoS Med. 2006;3(5):e158.

Rossi E. Low level environmental lead exposure--a continuing challenge. Clin Biochem Rev. 2008;29(2):63-70.

Camaschella C. Recent advances in the understanding of inherited sideroblastic anaemia. Br J Haematol. 2008;143(1):27-38.

Pearson HA. Sickle cell anemia and severe infections due to encapsulated bacteria. J Infect Dis. 1977;136 Suppl:S25-30.

Jadavji T, Prober CG. Dactylitis in a child with sickle cell trait. Can Med Assoc J. 1985;132(7):814-5.

Slavov SN, Kashima S, Pinto AC, Covas DT. Human parvovirus B19: general considerations and impact on patients with sickle-cell disease and thalassemia and on blood transfusions. FEMS Immunol Med Microbiol. 2011;62(3):247-62.

Frank JE. Diagnosis and management of G6PD deficiency. Am Fam Physician. 2005;72(7):1277-82.

Parker CJ. Historical aspects of paroxysmal nocturnal haemoglobinuria: 'defining the disease'. Br J Haematol. 2002;117(1):3-22.

Moake JL. Thrombotic microangiopathies. N Engl J Med. 2002;347(8):589-600.

Sadler JE. A revised classification of von Willebrand disease. For the Subcommittee on von Willebrand Factor of the Scientific and Standardization Committee of the International Society on Thrombosis and Haemostasis. Thromb Haemost. 1994;71(4):520-5.

Colvin GA, Elfenbein GJ. The latest treatment advances for acute myelogenous leukemia. Med Health R I. 2003;86(8):243-6.

Franchini M. Hereditary iron overload: update on pathophysiology, diagnosis, and treatment. Am J Hematol. 2006;81(3):202-9.

Egeberg O. INHERITED ANTITHROMBIN DEFICIENCY CAUSING THROMBOPHILIA. Thromb Diath Haemorrh. 1965;13:516-30.

Michiels JJ. Erythromelalgia and vascular complications in polycythemia vera. Semin Thromb Hemost. 1997;23(5):441-54.

Peveling-oberhag J, Arcaini L, Hansmann ML, Zeuzem S. Hepatitis C-associated B-cell non-Hodgkin lymphomas. Epidemiology, molecular signature and clinical management. J Hepatol. 2013;59(1):169-77.

PHOTO CREDITS

CHAPTER 14 – PHARMACOLOGY

MEDICATIONS IN OTHER CHAPTERS

PERIPHERAL NERVOUS SYSTEM:

1. **SOMATIC:** controls voluntary skeletal muscles.

2. **AUTONOMIC:** controls involuntary functions (includes sympathetic & parasympathetic).
   - A. **Sympathetic nervous system (SNS):** adrenergic - *norepinephrine & epinephrine*.

   - B. **Parasympathetic nervous system (PNS):** cholinergic - *Acetylcholine* (Ach).
     - i. **Nicotinic receptor activation:**
       located at the synapse of the neuromuscular junction (excitatory function).

     - ii. **Muscarinic receptor activation:** also located at the synapse of the neuromuscular junction. Found in the periphery as well. Affects *cardiac muscle (↓SA/AV node & heart rate), ↑smooth muscle contraction of the bladder & bronchial tissue (bronchoconstriction) ↑secretory gland activity (↑saliva & GI secretions).*
       "SLUDD-C": ↑**S**alivation, **L**acrimation, **U**rination, **D**efecation, **D**igestion, pupil **C**onstriction

AUTONOMIC AGENTS

Agents affecting the autonomic nervous system

MUSCARINIC AGENTS

DIRECT AGONISTS (CHOLINERGICS):

- **Pilocarpine, Cevimeline, Methacholine, Carbachol, Bethanecol** (Urecholine)

MOA: stimulate the parasympathetic nervous system (via muscarinic acetylcholine receptors).

Indications (Ind): *acute angle glaucoma:* Pilocarpine & Carbachol causes constriction of pupil & decreases ocular pressure; *post-op ileus:* Bethanecol stimulates GI tract; *post-partum urinary retention:* Bethanecol; *dry mouth, Sjögren syndrome:* Pilocarpine, Cevimeline. Methacoline is used in provocation testing for the diagnosis of asthma (it causes bronchoconstriction).

Side Effects (S/E): *bradycardia, diarrhea, nausea, vomiting, incontinence, blurred vision.*

Contraindications (CI)/Caution: *cardiovascular disease, asthma* (bronchoconstriction).

INDIRECT AGONISTS:

- **Edrophonium, Neostigmine, Pyridostigmine, Rivastigmine**
- *Organophosphates (Sarin gas, Insecticides)*

MOA: *acetylcholinesterase inhibitor* (acetylcholinesterase is an enzyme that breaks down acetylcholine in the synapse. Inhibition leads to ↑*Ach* (both nicotinic & muscarinic receptors).

Ind: *Myasthenia Gravis:* Neostigmine, Pyridostigmine; *Alzheimer disease:* Donepezil, Tacrine; *Glaucoma:* Echothiopate, Demecarium; antidote for *atropine poisoning:* Pyridostigmine.

S/E: *dyspnea, muscle fasciculations, prolonged contractions, bradycardia, diarrhea, nausea, vomiting.*

Organophosphate Toxicity: *acetylcholinesterase inhibitors* ⇨ ↑*Ach* (continuous stimulation of nerve) *muscarinic & nicotinic S/E.* Sarin gas toxicity or insecticides may have any combination.

- **Muscarinic S/E: "SLUDD-C":** ↑salivation, lacrimation, urination, diarrhea, emesis, miosis (visual changes), cardiovascular (bradycardia, hypotension), respiratory: bronchospasm, rhinorrhea.
- **Nicotinic S/E:** muscle fasciculations, cramping, weakness, diaphragmatic failure. Autonomic: hypertension, tachycardia, mydriasis, pallor, diaphoresis.

Management of toxicity: *Atropine* (anticholinergic) **+ Pralidoxime** (reactivates cholinesterase).

MUSCARINIC ANTAGONISTS (ANTICHOLINERGICS):

- **Ipratropium** (Atrovent); **Tiotropium** (Spiriva), **Atropine, Scopolamine, Benztropine, Trihexyphenidyl, Oxybutynin** (Ditropan), **Tolterodine** (Detrol); **Propantheline**
- Ophthalmic (topical): **Cyclopentolate & Homatropine** (mydriatics)
- GI: Hyoscyamine/Atropine/Scopolamine (Donnatal), **Dicyclomine** (Bentyl).

Indications: _COPD:_ Ipratropium - bronchodilation; _Bradycardia:_ Atropine increases heart rate; _Motion sickness:_ Scopolamine; _Parkinson disease:_ Benztropine & Trihexyphenidyl especially for tremor;* _urge incontinence:_ Oxybutynin, Tolterodine – relaxes bladder neck smooth muscle & relaxes detrusor muscle spasm; _Diarrhea/GI spasm:_ Donnatal – slows GI motility.

ANTICHOLINERGIC S/E: _dry mouth, blurred vision (dilated pupils), urinary retention, constipation, dry skin, flushing, tachycardia, fever (hyperthermia), HTN, delirium._

CI/Caution: _acute narrow angle glaucoma, BPH with urinary retention_ (worsens both).

NICOTINIC ANTAGONISTS (NEUROMUSCULAR BLOCKING AGENTS)

- **Pancuronium, Rocuronium** (Nondepolarizing);   **Succinylcholine** (Depolarizing)

MOA: centrally acting anticholinergic ⇨ skeletal muscle paralysis.
   Depolarizing: produces persistent depolarization, making skeletal muscle resistant to acetylcholine activation.
   Nondepolarizing: blocks nicotinic receptor neurotransmission in skeletal muscle ⇨ ↓acetylcholine ⇨ skeletal muscle paralysis.

Indications: muscle relaxation during surgery, intubation.
S/E: _hypotension, respiratory arrest._

ADRENERGIC AGENTS

- Adrenergic agents affect the adrenergic receptors (α_1 α_2, β_1, β_2).

1. CATECHOLAMINES:

   Norepinephrine (Levophed) primarily affects the α_1 receptors to **elevate blood pressure** in the setting of acute hypotension, cardiac arrest (to raise blood pressure & heart rate).

   Epinephrine: affects α_1 α_2, β_1, β_2. **Ind:** cardiac arrest (↑'es heart rate), PEA (pulseless electrical activity), anaphylaxis (drug of choice – reduces laryngeal edema & inhibits anaphylaxis mediators), asthma, croup (racemic), part of local anesthetic (added to lidocaine to prolong its effect & reduces bleeding via $\alpha\text{-}_1$ vasoconstriction).

   Dopamine:
   Low doses: produce renal vasodilation via D_1 receptors (mild diuretic).

   High doses: β_1 activation (↑HR/contractility) & ↑α_1-mediated vasoconstriction. Used in the emergent management of severe congestive heart failure & shock (causes vasoconstriction, leading to an increased blood pressure).

2. α-1 RECEPTOR AGONISTS:
- **Phenylephrine** (Neo-synephrine), **Midodrine, Epinephrine**
- **Oxymetazoline** (Afrin), **Pseudoephedrine** (Sudafed)
- **Methylphenidate** (Ritalin for ADHD – Norepinephrine modulates attention in CNS).

MOA: α-1 mediated vasoconstriction ⇨ increases blood pressure, decreases bleeding. Causes mydriasis (pupil dilation) during eye examination, reduces nasal congestion.

Indications: <u>orthostatic hypotension</u>: Midodrine; <u>Weight loss</u> suppressants. Phenylephrine: direct injection for priapism, ophthalmic for mydriasis during eye exam, glaucoma; Brimonidine: glaucoma. Pseudoephedrine: decongestant, <u>stress incontinence</u> - α$_1$ activation increases urethral tone.

S/E: *syncope, tachycardia, HTN* (cautious use in patients with a history of hypertension).

3. α-1 RECEPTOR ANTAGONISTS (α-1 BLOCKERS)
- **Prazosin** (Minipress); **Terazosin** (Hytrin), **Doxazosin** (Cardura); **Tamsulosin** (Flomax)

MOA: α-1 blockade ⇨ vasodilation. Relaxes the prostate & bladder neck.

Ind: hypertension, benign prostatic hypertrophy (BPH). Tamsulosin is the most uroselective.

S/E: *vasodilation ⇨ 1st dose hypotension (syncope),* postural (orthostatic) hypotension, dizziness, reflex tachycardia, nasal congestion; Sexual dysfunction.

4. α-2 AGONISTS
- **Clonidine** (Catapres); **Methyldopa** (Aldomet)

MOA: stimulates central α-2 receptors ⇨ ↓sympathetic nervous system activity.

Indications: HTN. Methyldopa safe for use in pregnancy or with renal insufficiency.

S/E: *dry mouth, sedation, fatigue,* postural hypotension.

<u>Methyldopa</u> may cause autoimmune hemolytic anemia (positive Coombs), lactation (↑prolactin).

<u>Clonidine</u> headache. Can cause rebound *hypertensive crisis with abrupt withdrawal* that mimics pheochromocytoma (should be gradually withdrawn over 7-10 days)* if it is to be discontinued.

5. NONSELECTIVE α-RECEPTOR ANTAGONISTS (α-1 & α-2 BLOCKERS)
- **Phentolamine; Phenoxybenzamine**

MOA: blocks both α-1 & α-2 receptors ⇨ antihypertensive (vasodilation).

Ind: Phentolamine (pheochromocytoma preoperatively, Epi-pen injection reversal – reverses constriction by epinephrine), Phenoxybenzamine (pheochromocytoma).

S/E: orthostatic hypotension, reflex tachycardia, flushing, nasal congestion, diarrhea, nausea, vomiting, priapism, peptic ulcers, myocardial infarction, stroke, arrhythmias, fluid retention.

6. β-1 RECEPTOR AGONISTS
- **Dopamine, Dobutamine**

MOA: stimulates the heart & kidney. *Positive inotrope*, ↑'es renin release & ↑'es renal blood flow.

Ind: severe congestive heart failure (CHF), stress testing (positive inotrope). **S/E:** tachycardia.

7. β-2 RECEPTOR AGONISTS

- **Albuterol** (Proventil); **Terbutaline** (Brethine); **Salmeterol** (Serevent); **Metaproterenol** (Alupent)

MOA: *stimulates β-2 receptor ⇨ bronchodilation & uterine relaxation.*

Ind: asthma & COPD: bronchodilation; <u>delay premature labor:</u> Terbutaline. Priapism: Terbutaline – contraction of cavernous artery smooth muscle increases venous outflow.

S/E: *β-1 cross reactivity ⇨ tachycardia, muscle tremor, nervousness, palpitations.*

8. β-RECEPTOR ANTAGONISTS (BETA BLOCKERS)

TYPES
1. CARDIOSELECTIVE (β-1 only): **Metoprolol** (most cardioselective), **Atenolol, Esmolol, Bisoprolol**

2. NONSELECTIVE (β-1 & β-2): **Propranolol, Nadolol, Sotalol, Timolol.**

3. NONSELECTIVE + ALPHA α-1, β-1 & β-2: **Labetalol, Carvedilol**

4. ⊕INTRINSIC SYMPATHETIC ACTIVITY: Pindolol, Penbutolol. Acebutolol (cardioselective).

MOA: β-receptor blockade ⇨ decreases cardiac output, heart rate & contractility (except those with intrinsic sympathetic activity); decreases renin secretion, decreases post myocardial infarction-induced ventricular remodeling.

Ind: hypertension, tachyarrhythmias (Atenolol & Metoprolol are Class II antiarrhythmics), heart failure, angina, acute myocardial infarction, migraine prophylaxis, thyrotoxicosis-associated palpitations, acute angle glaucoma (Timolol), benign essential tremor, prophylaxis for esophageal variceal bleeding (Labetalol, Nadolol), aortic dissection.

S/E: fatigue, depression, impotence. Glucagon can be used as part of the management of toxicity.

CI & Caution:
Caution in patients with diabetes mellitus (masks the signs of hypoglycemia); caution in asthma/COPD (especially nonselective agents because they may cause bronchospasms).

2nd/3rd degree heart block (due to AV node blockade), cocaine-induced myocardial infarction (causes unopposed α-1 – mediated vasoconstriction), may worsen peripheral vascular disease & Raynaud's phenomenon, hypotension, decompensated heart failure (CHF).

Note: although beta-blockers have been shown to reduce mortality in patients with compensated heart failure, if the patient decompensates (congestive heart failure) then beta-blockers should either be discontinued or reduced until CHF is effectively managed.

Note: Atenolol & Metoprolol are Class II antiarrhythmics.
    Sotalol is a Class III antiarrhythmic.

Note: if beta-blockers must be used in patients with bronchospastic disorders (asthma/COPD), cardioselectives are the safest type of beta-blockers in these patients (less β2 cross-reactivity).

ANGIOTENSIN-CONVERTING ENZYME INHIBITORS

- Capto**pril** (Capoten), Enala**pril** (Vasotec), Rami**pril** (Altace), Benaze**pril** (Lotensin), Quina**pril**, Lisino**pril**, Trandola**pril.**

MOA: inhibits angiotensin-converting enzyme (ACE) ⇨ decreased synthesis/production of angiotensin II & aldosterone ⇨ ↓preload/afterload/blood pressure. Potentiates other vasodilators (ex. bradykinin, prostaglandins, nitric oxide).

Indications: hypertension, **_heart failure, post myocardial infarction_** (to prevent ventricular remodeling), **_diabetic nephropathy_** (initiate once microalbuminuria is present), **_proteinuria_** (causes efferent arteriole dilation, which reduces protein filtration at the glomerulus), hyperaldosteronism (blocks aldosterone production).

S/E: 1st dose hypotension; **_cough & angioedema (due to ↑ bradykinin),_** azotemia/renal insufficiency (especially if creatinine > 3.0 mg/dL or creatinine clearance <30) **_hyperkalemia_** (can be ameliorated with diuretics), neutropenia.

CI: pregnancy (teratogenic), bilateral renal artery stenosis (may induce renal failure).

DIGOXIN/DIGITALIS

MOA: cardiac glycoside
1. ⊕ **_inotropic:_** – Na^+/K^+ ATPase pump inhibition (decreases intracellular potassium & increases intracellular sodium). The increased intracellular sodium prevents calcium expulsion via the sodium-calcium antiporter ⇨ increased intracellular calcium-mediated contraction.
2. **Increased vagal tone:** ⇨ **_negative chronotrope_** (decreases heart rate), **_negative dromotrope_** (slows conduction velocity) due to cholinergic effects.

Ind: heart failure with left ventricular systolic dysfunction (positive inotrope that ↓hospitalization but has no mortality benefit). Atrial fibrillation in some patients (ex. hypotensive or in CHF).

S/E: narrow therapeutic index. Symptoms include:
1. CNS: seizures, dizziness.
2. GI: anorexia, nausea, vomiting, diarrhea (cholinergic effects).
3. Visual: double/blurred vision, objects appear green/yellow, halos around lights.
4. Gynecomastia
5. Digitalis effect: T wave inversion or flattening, shortened QT interval, scooped, downsloping sagging ST segment, junctional rhythms.

Digitalis Toxicity:
1. **ECG:** May show digitalis effect (described above), premature ventricular contractions (most common) or a wide range of tachy or bradyarrhythmias.

2. **Electrolyte abnormalities:**
   - Acute toxicity: may cause hyperkalemia (inhibition of the Na^+/K^+ ATP-ase pump increases extracellular potassium).
   - Chronic toxicity: hypokalemia hypomagnesemia, hypercalcemia, Verapamil, Amiodarone, Quinidine, Ticagrelor, renal failure & hypothyroidism may worsen toxicity.
   - Serum digoxin levels: levels don't always correlate with toxicity.

3. **Management:** antidote digoxin-specific antibody (Fab) fragments (Digibind).

Note: acute toxicity directly causes hyperkalemia but hypokalemia increases the risk of Dig toxicity.

CALCIUM CHANNEL BLOCKERS

- **Dihydropyridines:** Nife**dipine** (Procardia XL), Amlo**dipine** (Norvasc), Nicar**dipine,** Felo**dipine**

- **Non-dihydropyridines: Verapamil, Diltiazem** (Cardizem CD)

MOA:

1. **Dihydropyridines:** are potent vasodilators (little to no effect on cardiac contractility or conduction).

2. **Non-dihydropyridines:** affect cardiac contractility & conduction (negative chronotrope & inotrope), potent vasodilators, reduces vascular permeability. *Class IV antiarrhythmics.*

Indications: hypertension, angina, achalasia, vasospastic disorders (ex. prinzmetal angina, Raynaud's phenomenon, cocaine-induced myocardial infarction), atrial flutter, atrial fibrillation, migraine prophylaxis. Verapamil is 1st line for the prophylaxis of cluster headaches.

S/E: vasodilation: headache, dizziness, lightheadedness, flushing, peripheral edema, weakness, bradycardia. Antimuscarinic S/E with ***Verapamil (constipation,*** dizziness, flushing).

CI/Cautions: cautious use in patients already on beta-blockers. CHF with ventricular systolic dysfunction (especially nondihydropyridines), 2nd/3rd heart block (due to AV node blockade).

SODIUM NITROPRUSSIDE

MOA: arterial & venous dilation via the activation of cyclic guanosine monophosphate (cGMP).

Indications: hypertensive emergencies (short acting).

S/E: *cyanide toxicity* from its metabolite if used in high doses or with prolonged use, nausea, tachycardia, sweating.

NITROGLYCERIN/NITRATES

PO, sublingual, IV, topical. Nitroglycerin, Isosorbide dinitrate, Isosorbide mononitrate, Nitroprusside

MOA: nitric oxide activates guanylyl cyclase ⇨ ↑cyclic guanosine monophosphate (cGMP) & subsequent decreases in cytosolic free calcium. This leads to ↓***preload by venodilation & ↓afterload*** via arterial dilation (***vein dilation >>arterial***). ↑myocardial blood supply: ↑O_2 & ↑collateral blood flow to ischemic myocardium, reduces coronary vasospasm & ↑'es coronary artery dilation.

Indications: angina, acute coronary syndrome, pulmonary edema, heart failure, hypertensive emergencies, vasospastic disorders, topical for anal fissures, esophageal disorders (prophylaxis in esophageal varices, achalasia, diffuse esophageal spasms, nutcracker esophagus).

S/E: headache (dilation of cerebral arteries), flushing, tolerance, hypotension, peripheral edema, tachyphylaxis after 24 hours (allow nitrate-free period for 8 hours to prevent it), reflex tachycardia. Deteriorates with moisture, light, air.

CI: *SBP <90* mm Hg, ***right ventricular infarction, use of Sildenafil & other PDE-5 inhibitors.****

ANTI-ARRHYTHMIC AGENTS

CLASS I **NA+ CHANNEL BLOCKERS**	Decreases sodium conduction (especially depolarized cells). Affects phase 4 depolarization (by blocking Na+ channel opening, it reduces sinoatrial node automaticity & causes membrane stabilization).
Class IA: *Procainamide* *Quinidine* Disopyramide	**MOA:** decreases conduction velocity, *prolongs repolarization* & *refractory period.* *PROLONGS ACTION POTENTIAL* & increases excitation threshold. **Ind:** *atrial AND ventricular arrhythmias* (ex. *SVT, reentrant tachycardias, VT* esp if resistant to other meds). *Procainamide is 1st line tx for Wolff-Parkinson-White.* * **S/E:** Torsades de pointes, hypotension, tachycardia, tinnitus. Caution if kidney disease. Quinidine may enhance Digoxin toxicity. *Procainamide & Quinidine associated with drug-induced lupus syndrome.*
Class IB: *Lidocaine* Tocainide	**MOA: decreases conduction velocity & underlinesshortens repolarization,** *shortens action potential (affects ischemic as well as depolarized ventricular tissue – most useful in abnormal tissue as seen post myocardial infarction arrhythmias)* **Ind:** *Stable VT* (alternative). **CI:** *narrow complex supraventricular tachycardia (SVT).* **S/E of lidocaine:** *neurotoxicity* (especially if underlying CHF or renal disease).
Class IC: *Flecainide* Propafenone Encainide	**MOA:** significantly decreases conduction velocity (↑QRS prolongation). Affects ventricular tissue in healthy cells. No affect on action potential duration. **Ind:** ventricular tachycardia (used as last line management).
CLASS II **BETA- BLOCKERS**	Antagonizes beta-adrenergic receptors to different degrees by decreasing the slope of phase 4 (decreased calcium currents – ↓*SA & AV node conduction*)
Cardio selective (β₁): *Atenolol, Metoprolol,* *Esmolol* Nonselective (β₁, β₂): Propranolol, Timolol	**Ind:** *rate control of atrial flutter, atrial fibrillation,* PSVT, ventricular tachycardias. Post MI prophylaxis, ± PVCs. **S/E:** bradycardia, AV blocks, hypotension, CNS (fatigue, depression, sexual dysfunction) may mask the symptoms of hypoglycemia* (use with caution in diabetics). **CI:** sinus bradycardia, 2nd/3rd heart block, shock, CHF. **Caution:** DM, peripheral vascular disease. *Nonselectives may cause bronchospasm in patients with asthma & COPD.* Tx overdose with glucagon.
CLASS III **K+ CHANNEL BLOCKERS** *Amiodarone* Ibutilide Dofetilide Sotalol Bretylium	**MOA:** blocks K+ efflux during phase 3 ⇨ *action potential prolongation* * & prolongation of the effective refractory period, QT interval prolongation. • *Amiodarone (Class III but possess characteristics of class I through IV)* **Ind:** *atrial AND ventricular arrhythmias;* refractory SVT. **S/E of Amiodarone:** *pulmonary fibrosis,* * *thyroid disorders* * (contains iodine so can cause hyperthyroidism/hypothyroidism), corneal deposits (>6 month use), *hepatotoxicity,* blue-green skin discoloration. Monitor TFTs, PFTs & LFTs in patients on long-term Amiodarone.
CLASS IV **Ca+2 CHANNEL BLOCKERS**	*Slows SA node & AV node conduction* (decreases L-type Ca+2 channels ⇨ decreased conduction speed, ↑PR interval, prolonged effective refractory period.
Verapamil *Diltiazem*	**Ind:** *atrial arrhythmias:* * atrial flutter, atrial fibrillation, PSVT. **S/E:** *peripheral edema,* antimuscarinic S/E with *verapamil (constipation* dizziness, flushing), bradycardia, AV blocks.
Class V (Other)	Digoxin (cardiac glycoside). **Ind: A fib, heart failure.** **MOA:** inhibit ATP-ase ⇨ positive inotrope, negative chronotrope/dromotrope.

Nets play in **B** **K** for the **C**hampionship (Useful mnemonic to help remember the classes).

Also Note: Class I and III used primarily for rhythm control. Class II & IV primarily for rate control.

OTHER AGENTS USED TO TREAT BRADY & TACHYARRHYTHMIAS

1. ADENOSINE

MOA: *temporarily decreases SA node automaticity & blocks AV node conduction pathways* (by opening K+ channels). *Short ½ life ~10 seconds** (must administer *rapid bolus* to be effective).

Indications: *drug of choice for SVT** (especially caused by AV node reentry) & *narrow, REGULAR, complex tachycardia.* May be used to slow down rhythm to differentiate SVT from atrial flutter.

S/E: *transient flushing, chest pressure/pain. May cause bronchospasm in asthma/COPD.**

CI/Cautions: not used in atrial flutter, A. fib, or tachycardia not caused by AV-nodal reentry.

2. AMIODARONE

MOA: *Class III antiarrhythmic* but *has properties of Class I through IV.* Class III: *inhibits K+ efflux* ⇨ *↑QT duration;* Increases QRS duration via inhibition of the Na+ channel (Class I properties); produces vasodilation & slows AV-node conduction via α-$_1$ & β- blockade (Class II properties). *Prolongs the action potential.**

Indications: *Atrial AND ventricular arrhythmias;* refractory SVT.

S/E: *hypotension MC, bradycardia, vasodilation, heart block or polymorphic VT.
   Long term use: *thyroid disorders** (contains iodine), *pulmonary fibrosis*, corneal deposits (>90% of patients with >6 month use), ↑LFTs, blue-green discoloration of the skin.

Caution: Procainamide & Amiodarone are not used together generally.

3. MAGNESIUM SULFATE

MOA: terminates torsades de pointes by decreasing the influx of calcium & suppressing early after depolarizations seen with long QT syndrome.
Ind: *torsades de pointes.*

COMMON DRUGS THAT AFFECT THE CYTOCHROME P450 SYSTEM

Cytochrome P450 is a set of liver enzymes responsible for metabolizing drugs.

CYTOCHROME P450 INDUCERS
- Carbamazepine, Rifampin, Alcohol (chronic), Phenytoin, Phenobarbital, Sulfonylureas, St. John's Wort, Griseofulvin.
- *P450 inducers may decrease the effectiveness of other drugs:*
     ex. decreased serum levels of Theophylline, Phenytoin, Warfarin.

CYTOCHROME P450 INHIBITORS
- Sodium valproate, Isoniazid, Cimetidine, Ketoconazole, Amiodarone, Fluconazole, Quinidine, Ciprofloxacin, Alcohol (acute), Sulfonamides, Omeprazole, Grapefruit juice, Metronidazole, Ritonavir, Macrolides.
- *P450 inhibitors may increase the effectiveness of other drugs:*
     ex. increased serum levels of Theophylline, Phenytoin, Warfarin.

UNFRACTIONATED HEPARIN (UFH)

MOA: *potentiates antithrombin III* (inhibits conversion of fibrinogen to fibrin) by *indirectly inactivating factor Xa & IIa (thrombin).* Also releases tissue factor pathway inhibitor. Prevents new clot formation (however, *Heparin does not dissolve already existing clots*).

IND: thrombosis, pulmonary embolism (PE), deep venous thrombosis (DVT), PE/DVT prophylaxis, coagulopathies, acute coronary syndromes, peripheral arterial embolism, certain cases of disseminated intravascular coagulation.

Does not cross placenta so it is safe in pregnancy. Usually given as an IV bolus & continuous drip.

MONITORING: Must be monitored because dosing is unpredictable (heparin can bind to endothelial cells & other plasma proteins & platelet factor 4).
- *Half-life ranges from 30-60 minutes* depending on binding to other molecules. Once drip is discontinued, patient is back to their pretreatment baseline ~1 hour.
- a*PTT* (partial thromboplastin time). Titrate to PTT 1.5-2 times the normal value.
- Antifactor Xa levels may be monitored in heparin-resistant patients.

S/E:
1. hemorrhage, hyperkalemia, osteoporosis, transaminase elevations.

2. *Heparin Induced Thrombocytopenia*/HIT (because Heparin is highly negatively charged, may bind to positively-charged platelet factor 4, becoming a hapten). Antibodies bind/activate platelets ⇨ hypercoagulable state with simultaneous thrombocytopenia. Occurs MC 5-10 days after therapy initiation. Suspect if platelet <100,000/μL or ↓>50% from pretreatment.

CI/CAUTIONS: severe thrombocytopenia, prior HIT, hemophilia, severe HTN, recent surgery on the eyes, spine or brain. UFH is safer than LMWH in patients with kidney disease.

ANTIDOTE: *protamine sulfate* (positively charged particle binds to negatively charged heparin). If severe bleeding, may need to administer fresh frozen plasma.

LOW MOLECULAR WEIGHT HEPARIN (LMWH)

- **Enoxaparin** (Lovenox), **Dalteparin** (Fragmin)

MOA: *potentiates antithrombin III* (inhibits conversion of fibrinogen to fibrin), causing *inactivation of factor Xa* (more anti-Xa activity than UFH) but less inhibition of factor IIa (thrombin) because many of the molecules are too short to bridge thrombin & antithrombin. 2:1 to 4:1 Xa-IIa ratios. Given subcutaneously.

IND: thrombosis, PE, coagulopathies, DVT, clot prevention, ACS. More predictable, less side effects & longer half-life, lack of monitoring compared to UFH so may be better in most cases.

MONITORING: *no need to monitor PTT. Longer half-life (12 hours).* Factor Xa levels can be monitored if needed (ex. patients with renal insufficiency, obesity).

S/E: hemorrhage, anemia, thrombocytopenia (all less than UFH), osteoporosis, HIT 5x less likely.

CI/CAUTIONS: *renal failure* (renally cleared), elderly patients. Not as easily reversible as UFH.

WARFARIN (COUMADIN)

MOA: *vitamin K antagonist* ⇨ ***inhibits vitamin K-dependent clotting factors II*** (prothrombin), ***VII, IX & X (2, 7, 9, 10).*** It reduces the functional levels of factor X & prothrombin (which have half lives of 24 hours & 72 hours respectively).

MONITORING: affects common & extrinsic pathways so ***monitored via prothrombin time (PT)*** & *International Normalized Ratio (INR).* INR usually between 2.0 – 3.0 (mechanical heart valves 2.5 – 3.5). Often measured every 3-4 weeks once therapeutic (more often measurements when initiating therapy).

SIDE EFFECTS

1. **bleeding** *(especially when INR is above therapeutic range).* If INR <10, dose is withheld until back in therapeutic range. If INR >10, ***Vitamin K*** (plus FFP) should be administered.

2. ***Warfarin induced skin necrosis*** (Warfarin also inhibits vitamin K dependent anticoagulant proteins C and S, which have shorter half-lives than the Vitamin K dependent clotting factors, so for the first 2-5 days after the initiation of warfarin therapy, patients are actually procoagulant – ***must be bridged with heparin*** for at least 5 days even if INR is within therapeutic range & after 48 hours of INR being therapeutic.

3. ***Teratogenicity:*** crosses the placenta.

4. Cautious use in alcoholic or patients with fall risk.

INTERACTIONS: food containing Vitamin K (cruciferous vegetables such as spinach & kale) may reduce its effectiveness. Inhibitors of the CP450 system may increase Warfarin levels. Inducers of the CP450 system may decrease Warfarin levels.

DIRECT THOMBIN INHIBITORS

- **Dabigatran** (Pradaxa) oral; Parenteral: **Argatroban, Bivalirudin,** Lepirudin, Desirudin

MOA: binds & inhibits thrombin directly.

IND: DVT, PE, atrial fibrillation, prevention of thromboembolism (including CVA). Lepirudin & ***Argatroban tx of choice for heparin-induced thrombocytopenia (HIT).*** Bivalirudin is an alternative to Heparin in patients undergoing PCI, thromboprophylaxis after elective hip arthroplasty, some patients with HIT.

S/E: bleeding, dyspepsia, abdominal pain, ↑LFTs.
Idarucizumab is the reversible agent for Dabigatran.

CI/CAUTIONS: acute bleeding (no specific reversing agents for most), renal dosing.

MONITORING: Lepirudin monitored by aPTT (not the ideal test however).

FACTOR Xa INHIBITORS

- **Fondaparinux** (SQ), **Rivaroxaban** (oral), **Apixaban** (oral)

MOA: synthetic *selective Factor Xa inhibitor* (selectively binds only to antithrombin III). It is too short to bridge thrombin so it does not significantly inhibit factor IIa formation.
Fondaparinux does not bind to plasma proteins nor platelet factor 4 so its half-life is 17 hours (usually given as a once daily subcutaneous injection).

IND: DVT/PE/CVA prophylaxis (ex. in patients with atrial fibrillation). DVT/PE treatment (similar efficacy to UFH & LMWH); May be used in acute coronary syndromes (however there is an increased risk of catheter thrombosis). Can be used to treat HIT (it does not bind to platelet factor 4).

S/E: bleeding.

Caution: creatinine clearance <30ml/min.

ADP INHIBITORS

- **Clopidogrel** (Plavix), Prasugrel, Ticlopidine

MOA: *inhibits ADP-mediated platelet aggregation & activation.* Irreversibly blocks $P2Y_{12}$ (the key ADP receptor on platelets). Increases the bleeding time.

Indications: *antiplatelet use in patients with an aspirin allergy.* Acute coronary syndromes (unstable angina, non ST elevation MI, ST elevation MI) - given if conservative strategy or if PCI is planned. Patients are often on Clopidogrel for at least 1 year after stent placement. Peripheral arterial disease. Prasugrel is 10x stronger than Clopidogrel.

CI: Prasugrel CI if history of TIA or stroke. Caution if CABG or surgery is planned within 7days, hepatic/renal impairment, bleeding.

S/E: bleeding (especially with Prasugrel) both stopped 5-7 days before major surgery, hematologic S/E (rare): TTP, neutropenia, thrombocytopenia. Proton pump inhibitors may decrease the effectiveness of Clopidogrel.

TICAGRELOR

MOA: Oral $P2Y_{12}$ receptor antagonist (reversible inhibition of ADP). More predictable inhibition compared to Clopidogrel. More effective than Clopidogrel in the reduction of cardiovascular death.

IND: prevention of thrombotic attacks (ex. CVA, MI), STEMI.

Caution: hepatic impairment. Increased plasma levels of Ticagrelor when used with inhibitors of the liver enzyme CYP450: 3A4 (Ketoconazole, grapefruit juice), CABG surgery.
Ticagrelor may increase plasma Digoxin levels.

S/E: bleeding, *dyspnea*, asymptomatic ventricular pauses of 3 seconds in the first week of treatment.

CI: history of intracranial bleed or pathological bleeding.

GLYCOPROTEIN IIB/IIIA INHIBITORS

- **Eptifibatide** (Integrilin), **Tirofiban** (Aggrastat), **Abciximab** (Reopro)

MOA: inhibits the final pathway for platelet aggregation (GP IIb/IIIa receptor on platelets).
- Abciximab: antibody that targets the activated GP IIb/IIIa receptor.
- Eptifibatide: reversibly binds to the GP IIb/IIIa receptor.
- Tirofiban: reversibly binds to GP IIb/IIIa receptor.

Indications: patients undergoing PTCA (especially if not pretreated with an ADP receptor antagonist). Tirofiban good for high-risk UA. Can be used with Aspirin & Heparin.

S/E: internal bleeding thrombocytopenia (immune-mediated) more likely with Abciximab.

CI: internal bleeding within 30 days; Major trauma/surgery.

ANTI- EMETIC AGENTS

Nausea & vomiting is caused by sensory conflict **mediated by the neurotransmitters *GABA, acetylcholine, histamine, dopamine & serotonin.***
Therefore, antiemetics work primarily by blocking these transmitters.

SEROTONIN ANTAGONISTS **Ondansetron** (Zofran) **Granisetron** **Dolasetron**	**MOA:** *blocks serotonin receptors* (5-HT3) both peripherally & centrally in the chemoreceptor trigger zone of the medulla (suppressing the vomiting center). **S/E:** neurologic: headache, fatigue. GI sx: nausea, constipation. Cardiac: prolonged QT interval & cardiac arrhythmias.

DOPAMINE BLOCKERS
Prochlorperazine
(Compazine)
 	
Promethazine
(Phenergan)
 	
Metoclopramide
(Reglan)
	MOA: *blocks CNS dopamine receptors ($D_1 D_2$)* in the brain's vomiting center.
	Ind: nausea/vomiting, motion sickness.
	S/E: *QT prolongation, sedation,* constipation.
	Extrapyramidal Sx (EPS): *rigidity, bradykinesia, tremor, akathisia (restlessness).*
	  3 EPS syndromes include:
	   1. **Dystonic Reactions (Dyskinesia):** reversible EPS *hours-days after initiation* ⇨ intermittent, spasmodic, sustained involuntary contractions *(trismus, protrusions of tongue, forced jaw opening, difficulty speaking, facial grimacing, torticollis).**
	     Mgmt: *Diphenhydramine IV* or add *anticholinergic agent* (ex Benztropine).
	
	   2. **Tardive Dyskinesia:** repetitive involuntary movements mostly involving extremities & face – lip smacking, teeth grinding, rolling of tongue.* Seen with long-term use.*
	
	   3. **Parkinsonism:** (due to ↓dopamine in nigrostriatal pathways) – rigidity, tremor.
	
	Neuroleptic Malignant Syndrome (NMS): life threatening disorder due to D_2 inhibition in basal ganglia: *mental status changes, extreme muscle rigidity, tremor, fever,* autonomic instability (tachycardia,* blood pressure changes, tachypnea, profuse diaphoresis, incontinence, dyspnea). Ice to axilla/groin, ventilatory support. *Dopamine Agonists: Bromocriptine,* Amantadine, Levodopa/Carbidopa.

ANTIHISTAMINES/ ANTICHOLINERGICS **Diphenhydramine** (Benadryl) **Meclizine** (Antivert) **Scopolamine** - anticholinergic	**MOA:** acts on the brain's control center for nausea, vomiting & dizziness. **Ind:** nausea/vomiting, vertigo, motion sickness. **S/E:** *dry mouth, blurred vision (dilated pupils), urinary retention, constipation, dry skin, flushing, tachycardia, fever, delirium.* **CI/Caution:** *acute narrow angle glaucoma, BPH with urinary retention.*

ANTIHISTAMINES (H$_1$ RECEPTOR BLOCKERS)

Histamine is produced by mast cells (basophils & eosinophils). H$_1$ receptors are found in:
- **the brain: maintains a sense of wakefulness, plays a role in nausea & vomiting.** The chemoreceptor trigger zone in the medulla sends signals to the vomiting center of the brain to cause vomiting (based on neurotransmitters like histamine, serotonin & acetylcholine).
- **Respiratory airways: causes bronchoconstriction** *(wheezing).*
- **Blood vessels & endothelial cells: causes leaky capillaries** – ex. hives & hypotension.

1st GENERATION ANTIHISTAMINES:
Diphenhydramine, Hydroxyzine, Chlorpheniramine, Promethazine, Cyproheptadine, Meclizine, Dimenhydrinate (Dramamine)

Ophthalmic: **Pheniramine** (Visine-A, Naphcon-A) & **Olopatadine** (Patanol). Reduces ocular pruritus & congestion by inhibiting histamine release from mast cells.

INDICATIONS: *allergic reaction reduction* by inhibiting mast cell-mediated histamine release ⇨ relieves pruritus, rhinorrhea, watery eyes & sneezing. Used in ***urticaria*** for similar reasons. 1st generation also used to treat nausea, vomiting, motion sickness & as a sleep aid.

SIDE EFFECTS
- ***Sedation, fatigue & dizziness.**** Histamine is a CNS transmitter that maintains wakefulness so antihistamines that are centrally acting can cause sedation. 1st generation antihistamines can easily cross the blood brain barrier. Codeine & Promethazine are used as a recreational drug for some - known as "sizzurp, purple drank, lean".

- ***Anticholinergic (antimuscarinic) side effects:**** *dry mouth, blurred vision (dilated pupils), urinary retention, constipation, dry skin, flushing, tachycardia, fever (hyperthermia), HTN, delirium.* Remember acetylcholine muscarinic effects = SLUDD-C (Salivation, Lacrimation, Urination, Digestion, Defecation, pupillary Constriction) so anticholinergics have the opposite effect.

CONTRAINDICATIONS/CAUTIONS
- Porphyria, liver or kidney disease.
    Other relative contraindications are a direct cause of its anticholinergic effects on the body:
- ***Glaucoma:*** causes dilation of the pupil (due to its anticholinergic effects), closing off a preexisting narrow angle in susceptible patients.
- ***benign prostatic hypertrophy:*** due to urinary retention. Cautious use with antidepressants.

2nd GENERATION ANTIHISTAMINES:
- **Desloratadine, Loratadine** (Claritin), **Cetirizine** (Zyrtec), **Fexofenadine** (Allegra).

INDICATIONS: *reduces allergic reactions* by inhibiting mast cell-mediated histamine release ⇨ relieves pruritus, rhinorrhea, watery eyes & sneezing.

S/E: doesn't cross the blood brain barrier so much less likely to cause sedation & anticholinergic side effects.

MIGRAINE ABORTIVE MEDICATIONS

• Includes aspirin or combination aspirin/caffeine/butalbital (Fiorinal), Ergotamines, Triptans.

ERGOTAMINES

Dihydroergotamine (nasal spray, IM or IV), **Dihydroergotamine/caffeine** (Cafergot)
   MOA: *nonselective serotonin (5-HT) agonists* ⇨ vasoconstriction of cranial vessels.

   S/E: *chest tightness from constriction.* Nausea, vomiting, abdominal cramps, vertigo, paresthesias, *coronary vasospasm.*

   CI: *coronary artery or peripheral vascular disease, uncontrolled HTN* (because it causes vasoconstriction); Hepatic or renal disease. Pregnancy. Increased ergot toxicity if used with macrolides.

TRIPTANS

 Sumatriptan (PO, injectable, nasal), **Zolmitriptan** (PO, nasal), Rizatriptan, Frovatriptan.
   MOA: *serotonin 5-HT-$_{1B/1D}$ agonists* ⇨ vasoconstriction of cranial vessels.

   S/E: *chest tightness from constriction.* Nausea, vomiting, vertigo, paresthesias, flushing. *Coronary vasospasms.* Serotonin syndrome if used with SSRIs.

   CI: *coronary artery or peripheral vascular disease, uncontrolled HTN (due to vasoconstriction);* MAOI use, use of ergotamine within the previous 24 hours.

OTOTOXIC DRUGS

1. **Antibiotics:** *Aminoglycosides (permanent),* Vancomycin, Macrolides.
2. *Loop diuretics:* Furosemide, *Ethacrynic acid (more ototoxic* than Furosemide).
3. **Chemotherapeutic agents:** *Platinum agents* (permanent), *Cytarabine.*
4. Temporary causes: *NSAIDs, Aspirin, Quinine.*

CHEMOTHERAPEUTIC AGENTS FOR CANCER

Most cells undergo oxidative DNA damage so they continuously repair their DNA. Malignant cells usually undergo rapid replication (and often have reduced DNA repair mechanisms). Most chemotherapeutic agents work on the premise that these cells rapidly replicate & have impaired repair of their DNA. Other normally rapidly dividing cells of the body are most susceptible to changes induced by chemotherapeutic agents:

• **Hematopoetic stem cells:** *most chemotherapeutic agents cause bone marrow suppression (myelosuppression).*

• **Reproductive:** infertility

• **Renal:** nephrotoxicity

• **Endothelial cells:** mucositis

CHEMOTHERAPEUTIC AGENTS FOR CANCER

ALKYLATING AGENTS

Cyclophosphamide (Cytoxan)	**MOA:** inhibits DNA replication (by alkylating DNA). **Ind:** leukemias, lymphomas, multiple myeloma, ovarian & breast cancers, retinoblastoma, neuroblastoma, sarcoma. **S/E: _hemorrhagic cystitis & bladder cancer,* emesis, myelosuppression, GI mucosal damage (diarrhea),_** SIADH. Hemorrhagic cystitis prevented by increasing water intake.

PLATINUM AGENTS   (Alkylating Like Agents)

	MOA: inhibits DNA similar to alkylating agents (binds & crosslinks DNA).
Cisplatin (Platinol) **Carboplatin** (Paraplatin)	**Ind:** Cisplatin: advanced metastatic testicular, ovarian & bladder cancers. Carboplatin: advanced ovarian cancer. **S/E: _neurotoxicity_** (ototoxicity, neuropathy), **_renal failure*_** (prevent with IV saline & Amifostine), **_hypomagnesemia, highly emetogenic._**

ANTIMETABOLITES

MOA: pyrimide analogs that inhibit tumor growth via enzyme inhibition of DNA replication.

Methotrexate (Cytoxan)	**MOA: _folic antagonist.*_** **Ind:** non-Hodgkin lymphoma, trophoblastic tumors (ex choriocarcinoma, hydatidiform mole), lung, breast, head & neck cancers, osteosarcoma. CNS lymphoma (intrathecal). **S/E: _hepatotoxicity,_** GI: _stomatitis,_ diarrhea. **_Leukopenia (especially with high-dose Methotrexate – prevented by giving leucovorin),_** myelosuppression, **_renal toxicity_** (reduced with IV hydration & alkalinization of the urine with sodium bicarbonate or acetazolamide), nausea, vomiting, pulmonary toxicity (interstitial pneumonitis), neurotoxicity. **CI:** _pregnancy,_ severe renal or liver disease. **Caution:** patient should have good function of the bone marrow, liver & kidneys prior to the initiation of Methotrexate.
Fluorouracil (5-FU)	**MOA:** inhibits RNA synthesis in cancer cells by uracil antagonism (uracil is essential for RNA synthesis). Low emetogenic potential. **Ind:** topical (superficial basal cell cancer, actinic keratosis); Metastatic colon & breast cancers. **S/E:** teratogenic, dermatitis, photosensitivity, cardiotoxicity, ocular toxicity.
Cytarabine	**MOA:** inhibits DNA & RNA synthesis. **Ind:** great vs. hematologic cancers (AML, ALL, blastic phase of CML), NHL. Poor activity vs. solid tumors. **S/E: _CNS neurotoxicity_** (cerebellar syndrome), myelosuppression, stomatitis, emetogenic, sloughing off of the skin on the palms & soles, **_ocular toxicity, ototoxicity._**
Gemcitabine	**MOA:** inhibits DNA synthesis. **Ind:** advanced breast, ovarian, pancreatic & non small cell lung cancers. **S/E:** emetogenic, hepatitis, myelosuppression.

MITOSIS INHIBITORS

MOA: destabilizes microtubules, preventing mitosis & cell division.	
Vincristine (Oncovin)	**Ind:** leukemia. **S/E: _neurotoxicity_** (neuropathy, CN palsies, demyelination).
Vinblastine (Velban)	**Ind:** lymphoma, testicular cancer. **S/E: _neurotoxicity._**
Paclitaxel (Taxol)	**Ind:** advanced ovarian, breast & non small-cell lung cancers.
Docetaxel	**Ind:** advanced & metastatic breast, prostate, stomach, squamous cell, head, neck & non small lung cancers.

R-CHOP <u>R</u>ituximab (antibody vs. CD20), <u>C</u>yclophosphamide, <u>H</u>ydroxydaunorubicin, <u>O</u>ncovorin/Vincristine, <u>P</u>rednisone. Used in non-Hodgkin lymphoma.

ABVD <u>A</u>driamycin (Doxorubicin), <u>B</u>leomycin, <u>V</u>inblastine, <u>D</u>acarbazine. Used in Hodgkin lymphoma

MOPP <u>M</u>ustargen, <u>O</u>nocovorin, <u>P</u>rocarbazine, <u>P</u>rednisone. Older regimen for Hodgkin lymphoma

CHEMOTHERAPEUTIC AGENTS FOR CANCER

ANTHRACYCLINES (INTERCALATING AGENTS)

MOA: inhibits nucleic acid & protein synthesis by intercalating & binding with DNA.	
Doxorubicin (Adriamycin)	**Ind:** AML, ALL, solid tumors. **S/E:** *cardiotoxicity (dilated cardiomyopathy)** bone marrow suppression, alopecia, GI S/E. Obtain an echocardiogram or MUGA scan prior to initiation (to document ejection fraction). Dexrazoxane is a cardioprotective agent against the toxic effects of anthracyclines - used in select patients.
Daunorubicin (Cerubidine)	**Ind:** AML

OTHER CHEMOTHERAPEUTIC AGENTS

Bleomycin	**MOA:** unknown **Ind:** *malignant pleural effusions (also used for pleurodesis),* NHL, HL, squamous cell & testicular cancers. **S/E:** *pulmonary fibrosis.**
Hydroxyurea	**MOA:** inhibits DNA synthesis. **Ind:** solid tumors, squamous cell, head, neck cancers, refractory CML, essential thrombocytopenia, polycythemia vera.

GENERAL CHEMOTOXICITIES

Gastrointestinal
- **Nausea/Vomiting:** Doxorubicin, Cytarabine, Cyclophosphamide, Methotrexate, Cisplatin.
- **Mucositis:** 5FU, Methotrexate.

Cardiovascular
- *Anthracyclines (ex. Doxorubicin) cause dilated cardiomyopathy.**

Pulmonary: Bleomycin (fibrosis), Methotrexate.

Neurologic: Vincristine, Methotrexate, Cytarabine, Cisplatin.

Renal: high-dose Methotrexate, Cisplatin (renal failure), Cyclophosphamide (bladder cancer & hemorrhagic cystitis)

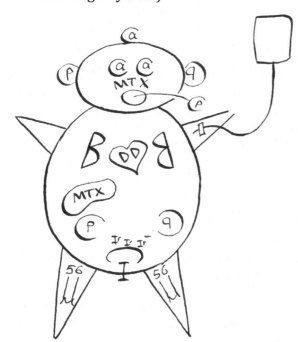

Ca = Cytarabine
- CNS toxicity, Ototoxicity

Cp = Cisplatin
- ototoxicity, highly emetogenic, renal failure

B = Bleomycin (pulmonary fibrosis)

MTX = Methotrexate
- Stomatitis, hepatotoxic,

D – Daunorubicin, Doxorubicin
- Dilated cardiomyopathy

C I = Cyclophosphamide, Ifosfamide
- Hemorrhagic cystitis

Irinotecan = acute & delayed diarrhea

Bone marrow toxicity:

5 = 5-FU; 6 = 6-Mercaptopurine, M = methotrexate

V of the arms & legs = Vincristine for peripheral neuropathy.

ANALGESICS

ACETAMINOPHEN Oral, rectal, IV	**MOA:** analgesia via inhibition of prostaglandin synthesis in the CNS. Blocks pain impulse generation peripherally. Antipyretic via inhibition of the hypothalamic heat-regulating center. No anti-inflammatory activity. **Metabolism:** maximum daily dose 4g/day (3g/day in chronic use). Metabolized in the liver, excreted in the urine. Cautious use in patients with hepatic impairment. **Ind:** analgesia, antipyretic (preferred analgesic in pregnancy/breastfeeding). **S/E:** hepatotoxicity or nephrotoxicity in high doses, rash. ***N-acetylcysteine is the antidote for toxicity***

NSAIDs
NONSELECTIVE
  Ibuprofen (Motrin)
  Indomethacin
    (Indocin)
  Naproxen (Naprosyn)
  Ketorolac (Toradol)
  Diclofenac (Voltaren)
  Etodolac (Lodine)
  Nabumetone
  Piroxicam (Feldene)
	MOA: *inhibits prostaglandin synthesis by blocking cyclooxygenase (COX-$_1$ & $_2$).*
	
	Ind: pain, antipyretic, anti-inflammatory.
	
	Monitoring: CBC, fecal occult blood test, LFTs
	
	S/E: *GI ulcers or bleeding* (especially Indomethacin & Piroxicam),
	    Renal toxicity.
	
	CI/Caution: active GI bleed, renal insufficiency, anticoagulant use, aspirin allergy, liver dysfunction, asthma.

ASPIRIN	**MOA:** *irreversibly* inhibits COX1 & COX2 (reduces prostaglandin & thromboxanes).
	Ind: analgesic, antipyretic. antiplatelet (low dose <300mg/day).
	  Anti-inflammatory (high-dose 2.1 to 7.3 g/day in divided doses) off-label use.
	S/E: *Reye syndrome* in children with viral infections (encephalopathy & fulminant hepatitis). Renal: *acute renal failure, interstitial nephritis,* bleeding (platelet dysfunction), *gastric mucosal injury* (gastritis, gastric ulcers, upper GI bleeding). Asthma exacerbation (arachidonic acid is converted to leukotriene production).
	CI: pregnancy. Discontinue drug 1 week prior to surgery, hemophilia. May cause hemolytic anemia if G6PD deficient.
	Toxicity: *initial signs*: vertigo, tinnitus, hearing loss, nausea, vomiting, diarrhea & *respiratory alkalosis & hyperepnea* (stimulates respiratory center). High anion gap metabolic acidosis, hypokalemia, hyperthermia, noncardiac pulmonary edema, altered mental status & liver injury.
	    Management: ABC (resuscitation). <u>Decontamination:</u> *activated charcoal* absorbs Aspirin and is usually given if alert or intubated (not given if AMS or not intubated). Gastric lavage not usually used (but may be employed if ingestion is < 1 hour). *Alkalinization of serum & urine* (with *sodium bicarbonate* – hypokalemia must be corrected or prevented for maximum effect). *IV fluids.* Supplemental glucose. *Hemodialysis* if severe, AMS, nonresponsive to other therapies, cerebral or pulmonary edema.
	Drug Interactions: enhances the effect of Lithium, Warfarin, Heparin & Digoxin.

COX-2 INHIBITORS
  Celecoxib
    (Celebrex)
	MOA: *reversibly* inhibits COX-2 only (prostaglandin inhibition). Since it does not inhibit COX-1, it is associated with less GI toxicity & does not inhibit platelets.
	Ind: used when an NSAID is needed but the patient has low platelets, GI ulcers, is on anticoagulation or corticosteroid therapy.
	  Chronic pain for rheumatoid arthritis, osteoarthritis.
	CI: sulfa or sulfonamide allergy. Avoid in renal insufficiency, severe heart disease, dehydration or liver failure. *May increase cardiovascular risk of thrombosis, MI & stroke.* **S/E:** thrombosis (endothelial cell dysfunction).

TRAMADOL (Ultram)	**MOA:** Binds to mu-opiate receptors (weak). Also inhibits norepinephrine & serotonin uptake. **S/E:** nausea, vomiting, constipation, dizziness, may lower seizure threshold. Serotonin syndrome when used with MAOI, TCAs or SSRIs.

OPIOIDS
  Fentanyl
    (Duragesic patch)
  Hydromorphone
    (Dilaudid)
  Methadone
  Morphine
  Meperidine (Demerol)
  Oxycodone
  Hydrocodone
  Codeine
  Loperamide
	MOA: *mu-opioid receptor agonist in the CNS.*
	Ind: analgesia, cough suppression (Codeine), diarrhea (Loperamide). Methadone used for opiate addiction management.
	S/E: sedation, dizziness, *constipation,* nausea, vomiting, allergic reactions, addiction. Meperidine is associated with seizures & serotonin syndrome (when used with MAOIs/SSRIs. Hallucinations with hydromorphone.
	CI/Cautions: potential for abuse, alcohol abuse. *Decreased GI motility*: paralytic ileus. GI obstruction, *constipation* (stimulation of opioid receptors in the GI tract slows down GI motility).
	Cautious use of Methadone with antidepressants.
	Toxicity: Overdose: *miosis (narcotics are miotics),* respiratory depression, coma,* hypotension, bradycardia.
	Antidote: Naloxone (Narcan)
	Withdrawal S/E: lacrimation, rhinorrhea, salivation, muscle spasms, diaphoresis, mydriasis & piloerections.

OPIOID-LIKE AGENT *Tapentadol* (Nucynta)	**MOA:** *centrally acting opioid analgesic.* **S/E:** nausea, vomiting, sweating, itching, drowsiness & constipation.

POISONS	TREATMENT	NOTES
Tricyclic antidepressants	*Sodium bicarbonate* may be used for cardiotoxicity.	Cardiotoxicity = prolonged QT interval.
Amphetamines	Ammonium chloride	
Opioids	*Naloxone, Naltrexone*	May be needed if severe (ex. respiratory depression).
Benzodiazepines	*Flumazenil*	Only used in severe cases.
Beta blockers	*Glucagon*	Usually given as an IM injection.
Theophylline	*Beta blockers*	Overdose symptoms usually due to ↑sympathetic activity.
Digitalis	*Digibind*	May need IV Magnesium.
Methemoglobin	Methylene blue, Vitamin C	
tPA, streptokinase	Aminocaproic acid	
Warfarin	*Vitamin K & fresh frozen plasma* Cryoprecipitate if continued bleeding	Especially if INR >10
Heparin	*Protamine sulfate*	
Ethylene glycol (Antifreeze)	*IV ethanol infusion* Fomepizole	

TOXINS	CLINICAL EXAM	WORKUP	ANTIDOTES/MGMT
ACETAMINOPHEN	Toxicity overwhelms the enzyme capability of the liver ⇨ ↓glutathione ⇨ **hepatic necrosis** • Anorexia, N/V, diaphoresis ⇨ RUQ pain, jaundice, coagulation abnormalities.	• APAP levels Follow nomogram • LFTs • PT/PTT/INR • UA, ECG	• **_N-acetylcysteine antidote_*** (glutathione substitute). • ***Activated charcoal*** especially within 1 hour of ingestion.

SALICYLATES
- **Aspirin**
- **Pepto Bismol**
- Ben Gay
- Oil of Wintergreen
	• ***Respiratory alkalosis**** due to respiratory stimulation ⇨ ***high anion gap metabolic acidosis*** occurs later. Fever.
	• **CNS:** seizures, coma, encephalopathy.
	• Renal failure, pulmonary edema.
		• Salicylates levels
		• Metabolic acidosis
		• ***Hypokalemia*** (from ↑urinary K+ loss)
			• Resuscitation (ABCs)
			• GI decontamination:
			  Activated charcoal, gastric lavage
			• Alkalinization:
			  sodium bicarbonate
			• Glucose helps with CNS sx
			• IV fluids
			• Hemodialysis (if severe).

BASES - **Oven cleaner** - **Drain cleaner** - **Bleach**	• Esophageal or gastric perforation, epiglottitis. • Respiratory distress. • Irritated mucous membranes.	• EGD to assess for damage.	• Supportive care • Emesis prevention • ±small amount of H_2O or milk as a diluent. • *Gastric lavage or acids contraindicated!* (will worsen symptoms).
HYDROCARBONS - Gasoline - Benzene - Petroleum - Kerosene, Motor oil	• ***Aspiration pneumonitis*** • Tachycardia, fever • CNS depression • Mucosal irritation • Vomiting, bloody diarrhea	• CXR: ± pneumonia, pneumothorax of pleural effusion). • UA • ECG	• Supportive treatment • ±antibiotics if pneumonia • *Avoid emetics or lavage*
ANTICHOLINERGICS - **Antihistamines** - Atropine - **Tricyclic antidepressants (TCA's)** Anticholinergics have antimuscarinic effects	**Sympathetic Stimulation:** • ***Hyperthermia (no sweating)*** • ***Tachycardia**, HTN* • ***Hot, flushed, dry skin & mucous membranes.**** • ***Mydriasis,**** visual changes • Urinary retention, ileus **CNS** • confusion, delirium, coma, seizure, respiratory depression	• ECG with TCA: **_wide QRS,_*** **_prolonged QT,_*** heart block, asystole, brady & tachyarrhythmias, ventricular arrhythmia (due to **_Na channel blocker effects of TCA's_**)	• Activated charcoal • Whole bowel irrigation • ***Physiostigmine*** (acetylcholinesterase inhibitor) • **TCA toxicity:** supportive. ***Sodium bicarbonate antidote.**** Diazepam for seizures.

CHOLINERGICS
- Organophosphates
 	
- **Insecticides & Pesticides**
  Chlorthion, Diazinon, Malathion
 	
- Sarin gas
	Muscarinic S/E: "SLUDD-C":
	↑**s**alivation, **l**acrimation, **u**rination, ↑GI: **d**iarrhea, emesis, miosis.
	CV: *bradycardia*, hypotension, Respiratory: bronchospasm and rhinorrhea.
	Nicotinic S/E: mydriasis, tachycardia, weakness, HTN, fasciculations. ***Children usually present with nicotinic S/E***
	"Garlic" breath (also seen c arsenic)
		• RBC cholinesterase levels
		
		• Blood glucose levels
			• ***Atropine + Pralidoxime***
			  - Atropine (anticholinergic)
			  - Pralidoxime reactivates the cholinesterase enzyme
			
			• Remove contaminated clothes

IRON	**GI:** nausea, vomiting, abdominal pain, shock, coagulopathy, red urine.	• RBC indices. LFTs • Metabolic acidosis • UA: assess for renal damage	• Emesis with gastric lavage • Whole bowel irrigation • ***Deferoxamine*** • Hemodialysis

SELECTED REFERENCES

Tai CH, Wu RM. Catechol-O-methyltransferase and Parkinson's disease. Acta Med Okayama. 2002;56(1):1-6.

Di nisio M, Middeldorp S, Büller HR. Direct thrombin inhibitors. N Engl J Med. 2005;353(10):1028-40.

Harrow M, Jobe TH. Does long-term treatment of schizophrenia with antipsychotic medications facilitate recovery?. Schizophr Bull. 2013;39(5):962-5.

Mirakhur RK. Preanaesthetic medication: a survey of current usage. J R Soc Med. 1991;84(8):481-3.

Varon J, Marik PE. The diagnosis and management of hypertensive crises. Chest. 2000;118(1):214-27.

Abou-khalil BW. Comparative monotherapy trials and the clinical treatment of epilepsy. Epilepsy Curr. 2007;7(5):127-9.

Makin G, Hickman JA. Apoptosis and cancer chemotherapy. Cell Tissue Res. 2000;301(1):143-52.

Parker WB. Enzymology of purine and pyrimidine antimetabolites used in the treatment of cancer. Chem Rev. 2009;109(7):2880-93.

Weitz JI. New anticoagulants for treatment of venous thromboembolism. Circulation. 2004;110(9 Suppl 1):I19-26.

Barnhart K, Coutifaris C, Esposito M. The pharmacology of methotrexate. Expert Opin Pharmacother. 2001;2(3):409-17.

Monroe EW, Daly AF, Shalhoub RF. Appraisal of the validity of histamine-induced wheal and flare to predict the clinical efficacy of antihistamines. J Allergy Clin Immunol. 1997;99(2):S798-806.

Milne JR, Hellestrand KJ, Bexton RS, Burnett PJ, Debbas NM, Camm AJ. Class 1 antiarrhythmic drugs--characteristic electrocardiographic differences when assessed by atrial and ventricular pacing. Eur Heart J. 1984;5(2):99-107.

Vaughan williams EM. Classifying antiarrhythmic actions: by facts or speculation. J Clin Pharmacol. 1992;32(11):964-77.

CHAPTER 15 – PEDIATRIC BLUEPRINT TOPICS

EXAMINATION OF THE NEWBORN

EXAMINATION OF THE HEAD

1. <u>Fontanelles:</u> anterior: 1 to 4 cm in size in both directions. Usually closes around 10-26 months of age. Posterior: 1cm in size on average (closes around 1 – 3 months). A third fontanelle may be seen with Trisomy 21 (Down syndrome).

2. <u>Caput succedaneum:</u> birth trauma related fluid accumulation under the scalp. Crosses the midline.

EXAMINATION OF THE GENITALIA & ANUS

1. <u>Anal patency:</u> assessed via rectal thermometer or observed stool. Delayed stool >48 hours after birth (meconium ileus) may indicate *Hirschsprung disease*, Cystic Fibrosis or imperforate anus.
2. <u>Hypospadia:</u> abnormal urethral placement (proximal & ventral). <u>Epispadia:</u> dorsal displacement.
3. Vaginal leukorrhea (or bloody discharge) as well as edema of the labia may be seen as a result of response to maternal estrogens. Usually self-limited.

NEUROLOGIC REFLEXES

1. **Suckling & Rooting:** instinctive suckling of anything that touches the roof of their mouth. Rooting = newborn will turn its head towards anything that strokes its cheek or mouth.
2. **Moro (startle):** shoulder abduction with spreading & extension of the fingers followed by the opposite (adduction & flexion). Peaks in the 1st month of life (disappears 2-4 months of age).
3. **Palmar grasp:** fingers will close when an object is placed in the infant's hand & their palm is stroked. Seen at birth & usually disappears around 5-6 months of age.
4. **Babinski:** upgoing plantar reflex – dorsiflexion of the foot (angles towards the shin) & big toe extension (curls upward) is normal and may be normally seen up to 2 years of age.

DEVELOPMENTAL HIP DISLOCATIONS OR DYSPLASIA

ORTOLANI MANEUVER:
Reduces the hip

BARLOW MANEUVER:
Dislocates the hip

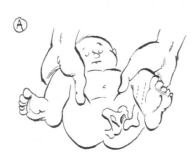
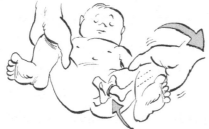

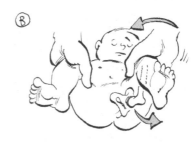
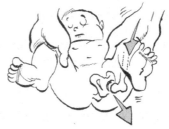

Examiner grasps the medial aspect of the knee & abducts the hips while applying anterior force to the femur, resulting in **reduction of the hip joint** (may feel a clunk).

Examiner adducts the fully flexed hip while applying posterior force to the femur, **resulting in dislocation of the hip.**

NORMAL FETAL CIRCULATION

FETAL CARDIAC PHYSIOLOGY

- **FETAL CIRCULATION USES RIGHT TO LEFT SHUNTS.** The *fetus receives its nutrients & oxygen from the placenta* (not the fetal lungs). The oxygenated & nutrient-rich blood goes from the placenta to the right atrium. There are 2 right to left shunts that bypass the nonfunctioning fetal lungs:

  1. **FORAMEN OVALE:** *which shunts* about 2/3 of the blood *from the right atrium directly into the left atrium.* The remaining 1/3 passes into the right ventricle. Most of the remaining 1/3 goes through the right ventricle and gets pumped into the pulmonary artery.

  2. **DUCTUS ARTERIOSUS:** *shunts blood from the pulmonary artery directly into the aorta* (systemic circulation), bypassing the fetal lungs.

Note: *as a baby takes its first breath, left side pressure becomes > right side pressure, promoting closure of these openings.*

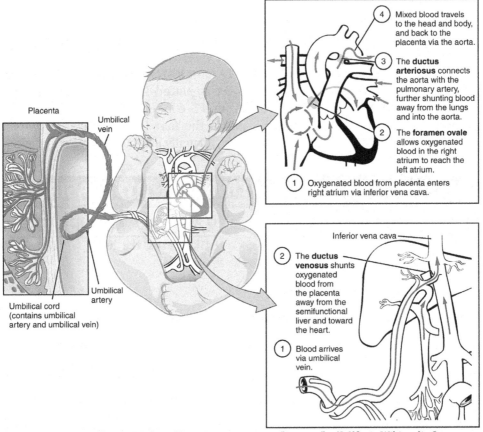

By OpenStax College [CC BY 3.0 (http://creativecommons.org/licenses/by/3.0)], via Wikimedia Commons

CLINICAL CORRELATION

Prostaglandins keep the ductus arteriosus patent (prostaglandins are vasodilators).

1. To *close a patent ductus arteriosus*, a *prostaglandin inhibitor* is given (ex. *IV indomethacin** or Ibuprofen). MC used in preterm infants or within the 1st 10-14 days of life.

2. To *keep the ductus arteriosus open, administer prostaglandins.* In severe cyanotic diseases (ex severe coarctation of the aorta, tetralogy of Fallot or transposition of the great vessels), a patent ductus arteriosus allows for mixing of the blood to improve cyanosis. *Prostaglandin E1 analogs* (ex. Alprostadil) maintains the ductus arteriosus open, reducing the cyanosis and improves circulation until surgical correction can be performed.

PEDIATRIC FUNCTIONAL MURMURS

Innocent (functional, physiologic) murmurs: non-pathologic, "functioning" murmurs caused by blood moving through the chambers. Innocent murmurs tend to be soft, not associated with symptoms, position-dependent, often occurs during systole & seen in up to 40% of children at some point in their lives.

Systolic murmurs may be innocent or pathologic. *Diastolic murmurs are almost always pathological.*

1. **STILL'S MURMUR:** MC innocent murmur. Usually heard from 2 years of age - preadolescence. ***Early to mid-systolic*** **musical, vibratory,* noisy, twanging, high-pitched** murmur, loudest in the inferior aspect of the **left lower sternal border & apex**. May radiate to the carotids. Thought to be due to vibration of the valve leaflets. Other murmurs may mimic it [ex. small VSD or subaortic stenosis (HCM)].
   - Diminishes with sitting, standing or Valsalva.
   - Accentuated with fever, supine position.

2. **VENOUS HUM:** 2nd MC innocent murmur. Due to the sound of the blood flowing from the head & neck (via the jugular veins) returning to the heart. Grade I or II, harsh, systolic ejection murmur (may be continuous). Localizes to the upper right or left sternal border (infraclavicular). May be diastolic (only non-pathologic diastolic murmur).
   - accentuated with: patient upright or seated with the head extended.
   - diminished with: Valsalva, gentle pressure on the jugular veins, supine position or when the head is turned fully to the contralateral shoulder.

3. **PULMONARY EJECTION MURMUR:** due to blood flowing across the pulmonary valve into the pulmonary artery. Commonly heard in in older children & adolescents. Best heard in *mid-systole* in the **second left intercostal space** (or superior aspect of the left lower sternal border). Harsh in quality.

CONGENITAL CYANOTIC HEART DISEASES

<u>5 Ts:</u>
1. **T**RUNCUS ARTERIOSUS *1 vessel* instead of 2 normal vessels (aorta & pulmonary artery)

2. **T**RANSPOSITION OF GREAT ARTERIES *2 vessels switched* (aorta & pulmonary artery).

3. **T**RICUSPID ATRESIA (*3= tri*) absence of the **tri**cuspid valve leads to a hypoplastic right ventricle. An ASD & VSD must be present for blood to flow out of the right atrium.

4. **T**ETRALOGY OF **F**ALLOT (*4- tetra*): 4 problems: ❶ right ventricular outflow obstruction ex. pulmonary stenosis ❷ right ventricular hypertrophy ❸ overriding aorta & ❹ ventricular septal defect (large, unrestrictive).

5. **T**OTAL **A**NOMALOUS **P**ULMONARY **V**ENOUS **R**ETURN (*5 vessels involved*): all 4 pulmonary veins connect to 1 vessel (superior vena cava) instead of the left atrium.

Hypoplastic left heart syndrome is often associated with mitral valve &/or aortic valve atresia.

VENTRICULAR SEPTAL DEFECT (VSD)

- **Hole in the ventricular septum** causing opening between the right & left ventricles.
- May occur alone or with other congenital heart diseases (ex. tetralogy of Fallot, transposition of the great arteries). **MC type of congenital heart disease.**

TYPES OF VSDs
1. **Perimembranous:** *MC type* (80%). Hole in LV outflow tract near the tricuspid valve.
2. **Muscular:** 5-20%. usually multiple holes in a **"swiss cheese"** pattern.
3. Inlet (posterior): 10%. Located posterior to the septal leaflet of the tricuspid valve.
4. Supacristal (outlet): 5%. Beneath the pulmonic valve. ± aortic valve insufficiency.

PATHOPHYSIOLOGY
- **Left to Right Shunt:** blood flows from the left ventricle (higher pressure) ⇨ right ventricle (lower pressure).

CLINICAL MANIFESTATIONS
1. Small (restrictive) VSD: asymptomatic or mild. MC found incidentally due to murmur. Small VSDs may close with time spontaneously (80% of muscular, 40% perimembranous). **Restrictive = normal pressure between ventricles maintained*** if defect is < 0.5 cm^2

2. Moderate VSD: *excessive sweating or fatigue especially during feeds* (due to ↑SNS activity from ↓CO), fatigue with feeding, lack of adequate growth, frequent respiratory infections.

3. **Large VSD:** more severe symptoms than moderate. *Non=restrictive = no pressure difference.*

4. **Eisenmenger's syndrome:** *in nonrestrictive.* In non-restrictive, the blood takes the path of least resistance (flows to the right side). Over time, when the pulmonary pressure becomes > systemic pressure ⇨ *RIGHT TO LEFT SHUNT.* Asymptomatic at rest but ± **cyanosis**, exertional dyspnea, chest pain & syncope.

PHYSICAL EXAMINATION
1. **Loud high-pitched harsh, holosystolic murmur** at the **lower left sternal border.**
   Classic isolated VSD is not usually associated with cyanosis.
2. Moderate: ± thrill, diastolic rumble at the mitral area (increased flow across the mitral valve).
3. Large VSD: signs of CHF (tachycardia, tachypnea, rales, cardiomegaly).

DIAGNOSIS
1. CXR: varies. May be normal or show left atrial enlargement, RV hypertrophy.
2. **Echocardiogram:** determines size & location of VSD. **Echo preferred over catheterization.**

3. **ECG: LVH with mild to moderate VSD,** normal with small VSD, **±combined RVH/LVH** (large equiphasic waves >50% in precordial leads – Katz-Wachtel phenomenon). LAE/RAE.
4. MRI: only used of echo nondiagnostic. MRI gives the same diagnostic info as catheterization.
5. Cardiac Catheterization: done if other tests are nondiagnostic or pulmonary HTN.

MANAGEMENT
Restrictive VSD (left > right-sided pressure) associated with good prognosis.
1. Most small VSDs will close spontaneously within 10 years.

2. Surgery: patch closure if symptomatic infants or uncontrolled CHF, growth delay, recurrent respiratory infections. Larger shunts repaired by age of 2y to prevent pulmonary HTN

TRANSPOSITION OF THE GREAT ARTERIES (TOGA)

- *MC cyanotic heart disease <u>presenting in the neonatal period</u> (dextro).*   8% of all CHD.
- Associated with other cardiac abnormalities: VSD 50%, ASD, PDA, PFO.

<u>DEXTRO (D)-TRANSPOSITION TGA</u>*: aorta arises from the right ventricle & pulmonary artery arises from the left ventricle ⇨ severe cyanosis.*

<u>LEVO (L) -TRANSPOSITION</u> *is usually acyanotic.* The right atrium (RA) sends blood to the morphologic left ventricle (LV), which is on the right side physically. This morphologic LV sends blood to pulmonary system. The left atrium (LA) sends blood to morphologic right ventricle (RV) located on the left side; The morphologic right ventricle sends blood to the systemic circulation.

PATHOPHYSIOLOGY
2 parallel circulations: 1st deoxygenated systemic venous blood drains from the RA to the RV and back to systemic circulation via the aorta. Oxygenated blood from pulmonary vein into LA and into LV and is recirculated to the pulmonary circulation. ***This dual parallel circulation is <u>incompatible with life unless mixing of circulation is present</u>*** via an atrial and/or ventricular septal defect, patent foramen ovale, bronchopulmonary collateral circulation or patent ductus arteriosus. ***The less mixing of the circulation, the more profound the hypoxia.***

CLINICAL MANIFESTATIONS
1. ***If the infant has an intact ventricular septum ⇨ cyanosis & tachypnea in the newborn*** (especially when the PDA closes).   The cyanosis is unchanged with the use of supplemental oxygen. Acidosis, tachypnea >60 breaths per minute.

2. The presence of a large VSD is associated with less severe cyanosis (but may present with CHF symptoms due to LVH volume overload).

DIAGNOSIS
1. **CXR:** classic triad: ❶ ***"egg on a string"**** or ***"egg on its side" appearance***   (due to great arteries forming a narrowed pedicle when transposed).   ❷ mildly increased pulmonary vascular congestion (despite hypoxemia) and ❸ mild cardiomegaly.

2. **Echocardiogram:** *primary means of diagnosis.* Evaluates structure & function of the heart, assesses for other congenital heart abnormalities.

3. **Catheterization (Angiogram):** seldom required to make the diagnosis but used in preparation for therapeutic treatment (balloon atrial septostomy).

MANAGEMENT
1. ***Surgical repair:*** arterial switch operation is the surgical treatment of choice.

2. **Temporary intercirculatory mixing prior to surgery:**
    - ***Prostaglandin E₁ analog*** (Alprostadil) maintains the patency of the ductus arteriosus, promoting intercirculatory mixing until surgical repair is performed.
    - ***Balloon atrial septostomy***: promotes intercirculatory mixing.   Once the infant is stabilized, corrective surgery is optimally performed in the first weeks of life.

Without treatment, 90% die by 1 year. 5 year survival rate after surgery >80%.

	ATRIAL SEPTAL DEFECT	PATENT DUCTUS ARTERIOSUS	COARCTATION OF AORTA	TETRALOGY OF FALLOT
DEFINITION	Hole in atrial septum (opening between right & left atrium).	Communication between descending thoracic aorta & pulmonary artery	Congenital narrowing of descending thoracic aorta. Male:female 2:1	MC cyanotic congenital heart disease
SHUNT	Left to Right (Noncyanotic)	Left to Right (Noncyanotic)	Noncyanotic usually	Right to Left (Cyanotic)*
ETIOLOGIES PATHOPHYSIOLOGY	• Ostium secundum MC* (80%) • Ostium primum – associated with mitral regurgitation • Sinus venosus, coronary sinus • ASD 2nd MC cause of CHD (VSD MC)	Prematurity, perinatal distress & hypoxia delays closure, Rubella infection in the 1st trimester. Continued Prostaglandin E₂ production promotes patency	↑LV afterload with SNS activity & RAAS activation ⇨ HTN, LVH, CHF. 70% ALSO HAVE BICUSPID AORTIC VALVE*	❶ RV outflow obstruction – pulmonary artery stenosis ❷ RV Hypertrophy ❸ VSD (large unrestrictive) ❹ overriding aorta – between ventricles
CLINICAL MANIFESTATIONS	• Most patients asymptomatic or minimal in childhood until >30y. • Infants/young children: recurrent respiratory infections, failure to thrive, exertional dyspnea. • Adolescents/Adults: exertional dyspnea, easy fatigability, palpitations, atrial arrhythmias, syncope, heart failure. • Stroke (paroxysmal embolus)	• Most asymptomatic • Poor feeding, weight loss, frequent lower respiratory tract infections, pulmonary congestion • Eisenmenger's syndrome: pulmonary HTN ⇨ left to right shunt switches & becomes right to left shunt (cyanotic)	• Secondary HTN* • bilateral claudication, dyspnea on exertion, syncope. • Infants: failure to thrive, poor feeding, shock. Types • Infantile: preductal • Adult: postductal	• Blue Baby syndrome (cyanosis) • Older: exertional dyspnea, cyanosis worsens with age. • "Tet-spells"*: paroxysms of cyanosis – older children relieve spells by squatting*. • Eisenmenger's syndrome: seen with PDA, VSD, TOF (±ASD)
PHYSICAL EXAM FINDINGS	• Systolic ejection crescendo-decrescendo flow murmur @ pulmonic area* (left upper sternal border). Sounds like PS (functional flow murmur). • WIDELY SPLIT FIXED S₂;* DOES NOT VARY WITH RESPIRATIONS.* • Loud S₁, hyperdynamic RV*	• CONTINUOUS MACHINERY MURMUR* loudest @ pulmonic area. • Wide pulse pressure: BOUNDING PERIPHERAL PULSES* LOUD S2 • Eisenmenger: normal hands (upper extremities) with cyanotic lower extremities (clubbed, blue toes)	• Systolic murmur that radiates to the back/scapula/chest* • ↑BP upper > lower extremities*. • Delayed/weak femoral pulses* ↓flow distal to obstruction in the lower extremities.	• Harsh holosystolic murmur @ left upper sternal border (sounds like PS). • Right ventricular heave. • Digital clubbing

DIAGNOSIS	• CXR:
	  -cardiomegaly
	• ECG:
	  -Incomplete RBB (rsR' in V₁ RAD)
	  -Crochetage sign: notching of the peak of the R wave in inferior leads.
	• Echocardiogram: gold standard
		• CXR:
		  Normal or cardiomegaly
		
		• ECG:
		  LVH, left atrial enlargement
		
		• Echocardiogram: gold standard
			• CXR:
			  - Rib notching*: ↑collateral circulation via intercostal arteries.
			  - "3 sign".* Narrowed aorta looks like the notch of the number 3
			• ECG: LVH
			
			• Angiogram: gold standard.* CT scan
				• CXR:
				  - Boot-shaped heart*
				  - Prominent right ventricle
				• ECG:
				  Right ventricular hypertrophy* Right atrial enlargement (RAE)
				• Echocardiogram: gold standard

MANAGEMENT	• Spontaneous closure likely in 1st year so may observe if small. • Surgical correction if symptomatic (usually between 2-4y)	• IV indomethacin 1st line tx* (closes the PDA) • Surgical correction if indomethacin fails. Best if done before 1-3y of age.	• Surgical Correction • Balloon angioplasty ± stent • Prostaglandin E₁ (PGE₁) preoperatively (reduces symptoms, improves lower extremity blood flow)	Surgical repair performed in the first 4 – 12 months of life. PGE1 infusion: prevents ductal closure if patient in cyanotic patients prior to surgery.

ATRIAL SEPTAL DEFECT

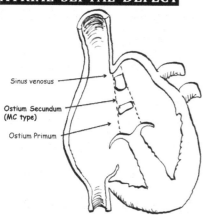

Sinus venosus

Ostium Secundum
(MC type)

Ostium Primum

HALLMARKS

- Usually asymptomatic until >30y

- *Systolic ejection murmur* best heard at the pulmonic area.
- May develop stroke due to paradoxic emboli.
- *Widely fixed, split S2 (doesn't vary with respirations).**

PATENT DUCTUS ARTERIOSUS

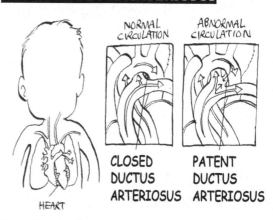

HALLMARKS

- *Continuous machinery murmur* loudest at pulmonic area

- Wide pulse pressure - *bounding pulses*

- *IV Indomethacin 1st line to close a PDA in infants* (prostaglandin inhibition).

TETRALOGY OF FALLOT

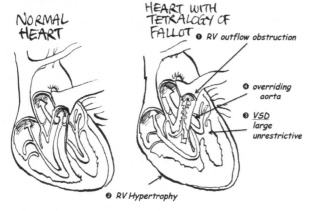

HALLMARKS

- MC cyanotic heart disease overall.

- Cyanosis in infants, **Tet spells** in older children (*periodic episodes of cyanosis relived with squatting* or putting an infant's knees to its chest).

- CXR: *boot-shaped heart*

- Management: surgical correction. Prostaglandin E1 prior to surgery to maintain patency of the ductus arteriosus.

COARCTATION OF THE AORTA

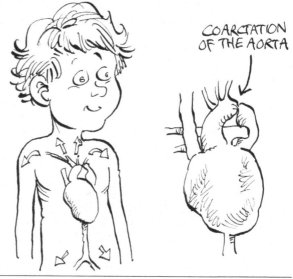

HALLMARKS

- 70% have a *bicuspid aortic valve.*
- Suspect in a child with 2ry *hypertension*, bilateral lower extremity claudication.
- Systolic murmur that radiates to the back, scapula or chest.
- *Systolic blood pressure in upper extremities > lower extremities.*
- Delayed or weak femoral pulses.
- CXR: *rib notching* (due to dilation of the intercostal arteries),
  "3" sign (shape of the coarctation).

PATENT FORAMEN OVALE

- Covered but not sealed open communication between the right and left atria; however, a PFO is not considered an ASD because no septal tissue is missing (it is due to failed septal fusion).

CLINICAL MANIFESTATIONS
1. **Most asymptomatic** but may develop **TIA** or **cryptogenic stroke** (stroke in the absence of a large vessel or cardioembolic source), systemic emboli, acute MI, migraine headaches. Neurologic decompression sickness may be seen in scuba divers with a PFO.
2. Physical examination: no abnormal cardiac findings associated with an isolated PFO.

PULMONARY ATRESIA

- Pulmonary atresia with intact intraventricular septum (PA/IVS) is characterized by **complete obstruction to right ventricular outflow** with varying degrees of right ventricular & tricuspid valve hypoplasia – **blood is unable to flow from the right ventricle into the pulmonary artery & the lungs.**

Valvular (membranous): atretic pulmonary valve, small valve annulus with fused valve leaflets leading to a thin, intact membrane that causes right ventricular outflow tract obstruction.

Muscular: obliteration of the muscular infundibulum. It is associated with severe right ventricular hypoplasia and increased coronary artery abnormalities.

CLINICAL MANIFESTATIONS
1. Cyanosis due to right-to-left shunting at the atrial level. Improved survival if there is a patent ductus arteriosus.
2. Single heart sound (due to a single semilunar valve – the aortic valve).
3. Systolic murmur of tricuspid regurgitation

MANAGEMENT
1. Maintain the patency of the ductus arteriosus (ex. prostaglandin E1 analog Alprostadil) to stabilize initially. Balloon atrial septostomy to improve the right to left atrial shunting.
2. Surgical repair: definitive. If untreated, approximately 50% of these children die within 2 weeks of birth & 85% by six months.

TRICUSPID ATRESIA

- 2% of all congenital heart disease. Absence of the tricuspid valve leads to a hypoplastic right ventricle. A PDA or VSD is necessary for pulmonary blood flow and survival.

CLINICAL MANIFESTATIONS
1. Cyanosis due to right-to-left shunting. Improved survival if there is a patent ductus arteriosus.
2. Single heart sound (S_2).

DIAGNOSIS
1. ECG: left ventricular hypertrophy.
2. CXR: normal or enlarged cardiac silhouette with _decreased_ pulmonary flow.

MANAGEMENT
1. Maintain the patency of the ductus arteriosus (ex. prostaglandin E1 analog Alprostadil) to stabilize initially. Presence of VSD improves oxygenation of blood.
2. Surgical repair: definitive. Subclavian artery to pulmonary shunt followed by a 2-staged surgical correction to direct systemic venous return directly to the pulmonary arteries.

HYPOPLASTIC LEFT HEART SYNDROME

- Failure of the development of the mitral valve, aortic valve or the aortic arch ⇨ small ventricle unable to supply the normal systemic circulation requirements. 1% of all congenital heart disease.

CLINICAL MANIFESTATIONS
Symptoms begin when the ductus arteriosus constricts, leading to cyanosis and heart failure.

DIAGNOSIS
ECG: right ventricular hypertrophy. CXR: cardiomegaly.

MANAGEMENT
Prostaglandin E1 to open the ductus arteriosus followed by surgical repair.

INFANT RESPIRATORY DISTRESS SYNDROME

IRDS (hyaline membrane disease): *disease of* PREMATURE INFANTS 2ry to ***insufficiency of surfactant*** production & lung structural immaturity ⇨ atelectasis & perfusion without ventilation. MC single cause of death in 1st month of life.

Surfactant production begins 24 – 28 weeks. By 35 weeks, enough surfactant is produced.

RISK FACTORS
Caucasian, males (2x MC), C-section delivery (infant stress during delivery causes cortisol production in infant), *perinatal infections, multiple births* (especially if ***premature)***, *maternal diabetes* (high insulin delays surfactant production).

CLINICAL MANIFESTATIONS
1. Usually *presents shortly postpartum with **respiratory distress***: tachypnea, tachycardia, chest wall retractions, expiratory grunting, nasal flaring & cyanosis.
2. Infant may develop respiratory failure & apnea.
- Clinical course is usually 2-3 days (with or without treatment).

DIAGNOSIS
1. CXR: bilateral diffuse **_reticular ground-glass opacities + air bronchograms,_*** poor expansion. Domed diaphragms.

2. ABG: hypoxia (usually responsive to supplemental oxygen). Normal or slightly ↑PCO_2.

3. Postmortem histopathology: waxy appearing layers lining the collapsed alveoli. May show airway distention.

MANAGEMENT
Exogenous surfactant given to open alveoli (via endotracheal tube).   Continuous Positive Airway Pressure (CPAP).

PREVENTION
Corticosteroids given to mature lungs if premature delivery expected (between 24 – 36 weeks).

- 90% survival rate with treatment and normal return of lung function within 1 month.

MECONIUM ASPIRATION

- Perinatal asphyxia of meconium-contaminated amniotic fluid ⇨ respiratory distress, hypoxia & acidosis.
- **_Increased incidence in postterm infants_*** & small for gestational age infants.

CLINICAL MANIFESTATIONS
1. Signs of respiratory distress (usually immediately after birth): cyanosis, severe tachypnea, use of accessory muscles, intercostal retractions, nasal flaring.

DIAGNOSIS
1. Evidence of meconium-stained amniotic fluid. May be present in the trachea, vernix or on the umbilical cord.
2. Respiratory distress at or shortly after birth.
3. CXR: streaky linear densities, diffuse patchy infiltrates with lung hyperinflation (flattened diaphragms, increased AP diameter). May show pneumothorax.

MANAGEMENT
1. **_Prevention is the most effective therapy_: _prevention of postmature delivery_** (> 41 weeks gestation) via labor induction & prevention of fetal hypoxia (via fetal heart monitoring).

2. Supportive management: maintain adequate oxygenation & ventilation (may need mechanical ventilation), empirical antibiotic therapy, correction of metabolic abnormalities.

Persistent pulmonary hypertension of the newborn is a potential complication of meconium aspiration or if the child becomes agitated during the management.

SUDDEN INFANT DEATH SYNDROME

- Defined as sudden death of an infant <1 year of age that is unexplained:
  - after investigation
  - performance of a complete autopsy
  - review of the medical history
  - examination of the death scene.

The leading cause of death between 1 month and 1 year in the United States.

RISK FACTORS
- **_Infants sleeping in the prone position (strongest modifiable risk factor),_** sleeping on a soft surface and/or with bedding accessories. overheating, low birth weight, prematurity, inadequate prenatal care, maternal smoking or drug use during pregnancy, bed sharing with the parent(s) & infant.

REDUCED RISK
- Supine position for sleeping
- Using a firm mattress
- Room-sharing (without bed-sharing)
- Pacifier use.

JAUNDICE IN THE NEWBORN

1. PHYSIOLOGIC:
- Usually due to increased indirect (unconjugated) bilirubin (the immature liver of a newborn is unable to efficiently conjugate bilirubin due to decreased UGT enzyme activity).
- Indirect bilirubin rises in days 3-5 days & falls in about half of the neonates during the 1st week of

2. PATHOLOGIC:
- May be suggestive if jaundice occurs in the first 24 hours of life (usually indicates hemolysis or hereditary spherocytosis), persistent jaundice 10-14 days, increased direct (conjugated) bilirubin > 2mg/dL, total bilirubin >12 mg/dL. Increased indirect may be physiologic or pathologic. Increased direct is always pathologic.
- Bilirubin >20 mg/dL can lead to kernicterus and neurotoxicity (from irreversible deposition of bilirubin in the basal ganglia, pons & cerebellum).
- **Increase indirect (unconjugated):** Most common causes are physiologic (after 24 hours & peaks 3-5 days), prematurity & breast-feeding jaundice (2nd-3rd day of life). Others include: Crigler-Najjar, Gilberts, Cretinism & hemolytic anemia (hemolytic presents within the 1st 24h of life).
- **Increased direct (conjugated):** Dubin-Johnson syndrome, Rotor syndrome, infections.

CLINICAL MANIFESTATIONS
1. Jaundice: yellowing of the skin, mucous membranes & sclera especially when bilirubin levels >5.0 mg/dL in neonates. Jaundice usually progresses from head to toe with increasing bilirubin levels.

2. **Kernicterus:** *cerebral dysfunction & encephalopathy* as a result of bilirubin deposition in the brain tissues (seizures, lethargy, irritability, hearing loss and mental development disorders). *Infants are at risk for kernicterus when bilirubin is >20* - 25 mg/dL.

MANAGEMENT
1. **Phototherapy** used in all types. Used in physiologic jaundice or jaundice associated with beastfeeding, when bilirubin is >15 mg/dL or if the levels fail to decrease.
2. **Exchange transfusion** used in severe cases, ABO incompatibility, RH isoimmunization & hemolysis.

PYLORIC STENOSIS

PATHOPHYSIOLOGY
Hypertrophy & hyperplasia of the muscular layers of the pylorus (causing a *functional outlet obstruction).* MC cause of intestinal obstruction in infancy. ↑incidence with Erythromycin use.
- *95% present in 1st 3-12 weeks of life* (rare >6 months).
- MC in Caucasians. Males 4:1. If seen in adults, it is associated with chronic ulcer disease.

CLINICAL MANIFESTATIONS
1. *NON-bilious vomiting/regurgitation* ⇨ *projectile** (70%) after feeding. Child remains hungry.
2. Signs of dehydration & malnutrition, *hypochloremic metabolic alkalosis* (from vomiting), jaundice.

3. *"OLIVE-SHAPED"* nontender, mobile, hard pylorus** 1-2cm in diameter (palpated especially after the infant has vomited), hyperperistalsis.

DIAGNOSIS
1. **Ultrasound:** *1st line test:** elongation/thickening of pylorus. *More sensitive & no radiation risk.*
2. **Upper GI contrast:** *STRING SIGN** (dye through narrowed channel) & delayed gastric emptying.

MANAGEMENT
1. **Initial management:** *rehydration (IV fluids),** potassium repletion if hypokalemic from vomiting.
2. **Pyloromyotomy** is the *definitive management.*

INTUSSUSCEPTION

- *intestinal segment invaginates/"telescopes" into adjoining intestinal lumen⇨ bowel obstruction.*
  - Commonly seen in children. ²/₃ of patients are between 6 months - 18 months of age.   MC in males.
  - MC occurs at the ileocolic junction. Often occurs after viral infection.
- Lead points: Meckel diverticulum, enlarged mesenteric lymph node, hyperplasia of Peyer's patches, benign/malignant tumor, submucosal hematomas (Henoch-Schonlein purpura), foreign body.

CLINICAL MANIFESTATIONS
1. **Classic triad: ❶vomiting ❷ abdominal pain & ❸ passage of blood per rectum** "CURRANT JELLY STOOL"* (stool mixed with blood & mucus).
2. Abdominal pain is usually colicky in nature, may present with lethargy.

PHYSICAL EXAM
1. *Dance's sign = SAUSAGE-SHAPED MASS* in the right upper quadrant or hypochondrium & emptiness in the right lower quadrant* (due to telescoping of the bowel).

DIAGNOSIS
*BARIUM CONTRAST ENEMA (OFTEN DIAGNOSTIC & THERAPEUTIC),** Radiographs: lack of gas in the bowels.

MANAGEMENT
Barium or air insufflation. Hydration (IV fluids).   Surgical resection if refractory to insufflation.

HIRSCHSPRUNG DISEASE

- *Congenital absence of ganglion cells ⇨ functional obstruction. MC in distal colon & rectum* (75%).
- May occur in other parts of the GI tract. Increased incidence in males & children with Down syndrome.

PATHYOPHYSIOLOGY
1. **Absence of enteric ganglion cells:** failure of complete neural crest migration during fetal development ⇨ absence of enteric ganglion cells (Auerbach & Meissner plexuses).
2. **Functional obstruction:** *due to failure of relaxation of the aganglionic segment.*   MC affects the distal colon (often with a transitional zone in the rectosigmoid colon).
3. Enterocolitis: vomiting, diarrhea signs of toxic **megacolon.**

CLINICAL MANIFESTATIONS
1. *Neonatal intestinal obstruction: meconium ileus (failure of meconium passage >48 hours)* in a full term infant (most full term infants usually pass meconium within 24 hours, may be delayed in preterm infants normally). *Bilious vomiting, abdominal distention.* Failure to thrive.
2. Enterocolitis: vomiting, diarrhea signs of toxic megacolon (looks similar to sepsis).
3. Chronic constipation.

DIAGNOSIS:
1. **Anorectal manometry:** lack of relaxation of the internal sphincter with balloon rectal distention. *Often used as initial screening test.* ↑pressure of the anal sphincter.
2. Contrast enema: transition zone (caliber change) at the area between normal & affected bowel.
3. Abdominal radiographs: signs of obstruction: decreased or absence of air in the rectum & dilated bowel loops. Not specific.
4. **Rectal biopsy:** *definitive diagnosis.* Shows the absence of ganglion cells. *Rectal suction biopsy* is less invasive (done without anesthesia). Full thickness biopsy done if suction is nondiagnostic.

MANAGEMENT
1. Surgical resection of the affected bowel.

ESOPHAGEAL ATRESIA

- Complete absence or closure of the esophagus.
- *MC associated with tracheoesophageal fistula.* Polyhydramnios commonly seen during pregnancy.

CLINICAL MANIFESTATIONS
1. Presents *immediately after birth with excessive oral secretions* that leads to choking, drooling, inability to feed, respiratory distress and coughing (especially when attempting to feed). May present later in life (depending on the degree of the atresia).
2. Gastric distention may occur. Aspiration pneumonia (reflux of gastric contents).

DIAGNOSIS
1. Inability to pass a nasogastric tube further than 10-15cm (coiling in the esophagus).
2. <u>Fluoroscopy:</u> small amount of water-soluble contrast may reveal it (but must be removed promptly to avoid aspiration). Barium should not be used (caustic if it leaks).

MANAGEMENT
1. Surgical ligation of the fistula with primary anastomosis of the esophageal segments may be done in stages if the distance between the two segments is large.

DUODENAL ATRESIA

- Complete absence or closure of a portion of the duodenum ⇨ gastric outlet obstruction.
- Polyhydramnios (increased amniotic fluid) is commonly seen during pregnancy. Increased incidence in Down syndrome. May be associated with other congenital deformities.

CLINICAL MANIFESTATIONS
Intestinal obstruction shortly after birth: abdominal distention, *bilious vomiting*.

DIAGNOSIS
1. <u>Abdominal radiographs:</u> distended duodenum & distended separated by the pyloric valve, causing a *"double-bubble" sign.**

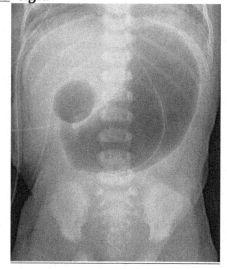

MANAGEMENT
1. Decompression of the GI tract. Electrolyte and IV fluid replacement.
2. Duodenoduodenostomy (surgical repair or anastomosis).

DIAPER RASH (DERMATITIS)

POSSIBLE ETIOLOGIES
1. **Wearing diapers:** contact dermatitis, miliaria, candida.
2. Rash in the diaper area as well as other areas: atopic dermatitis, seborrheic dermatitis.
3. Affects diaper area irrespective of diaper use: scabies, bullous impetigo.

RISK FACTORS
1. Friction and moisture from urine & feces.

MANAGEMENT
1. Frequent diaper changes every 2 hours or when soiled. Open air exposure. Topical Zinc oxide or petroleum jelly. 1% Hydrocortisone (use for <2 weeks). May need topical antibiotics.

ROSEOLA INFANTUM (SIXTH'S DISEASE)   Human Herpes virus 6 or 7

TRANSMISSION: respiratory droplets. Occurs MC <5y of age. ~10 day incubation period (IP).

CLINICAL MANIFESTATIONS
1. *Prodrome of HIGH FEVER 3-5 days* ⇨ fever resolves before the onset of a ***rose, pink*** maculopapular, blanchable rash on the ***trunk/back*** ⇨ ***face.*** Rash lasts hours (up to 1-2 days).
    - *ONLY CHILDHOOD VIRAL EXANTHEM THAT STARTS ON TRUNK* & spreads to face.
2. ***Child appears "well" & alert during the febrile phase.**** May be irritable during febrile phase.

MANAGEMENT: supportive, anti-inflammatories, antipyretics (to prevent febrile seizures).

COXSACKIE VIRUS

- ***Coxsackie virus*** part of the enterovirus family. ***MC in children <5y.*** Spread feco-oral and oral-orally. ***MC late summer/early fall.*** Two types - Coxsackie A & B.

BOTH A & B:
1. ***Aseptic meningitis,*** rashes, common cold symptoms or no symptoms.

PRIMARILY COXSACKIE A:
1. HAND FOOT & MOUTH DISEASE: mild fever, URI sx, decreased appetite starting 3-5d after exposure ⇨ oral enanthem: ***vesicular lesions with erythematous halos*** in the oral cavity (especially buccal mucosa & tongue) ⇨ exanthem 1-2 days afterwards - vesicular, macular or maculopapular lesions on the distal extremities (often includes the palms & soles).
2. HERPANGINA: sudden onset of high fevers, ***stomatitis:*** small vesicles on the soft palate, uvula & tonsillar pillars that ulcerate before healing, sore throat. 3-5 days. MC in children 3-10y.

MANAGEMENT: supportive (antipyretics, topical lidocaine).

PRIMARILY COXSACKIE B:
1. PERICARDITIS & MYOCARDITIS: *Coxsackie MC viral cause of pericarditis & myocarditis.*
2. PLEURODYNIA: fever, severe pleuritic chest pain & paroxysmal spasms of the chest/abdominal muscles including the diaphragm (may have swelling over the diaphragm), headache.

---

*RASHES THAT AFFECTS THE PALMS & SOLES: Coxsackie (Hand Foot & Mouth), RMSF (especially if wrist/ankles involved), Syphilis (secondary), Janeway lesions, Kawasaki, Measles, Toxic Shock Syndrome, Reactive Arthritis (Keratoderma Blenorrhagica), Meningococcemia.

MUMPS

*Paramyxovirus.** <u>Transmission</u>: respiratory droplets. ~12-14d IP. ↑incidence in the spring. Patients are usually infectious 48 hours prior to and 9 days after the onset of parotid swelling.

CLINICAL MANIFESTATIONS
1. Low grade fever, myalgias, headache ⇨ ***parotid gland pain & swelling.****

DIAGNOSIS: serologies. ↑amylase. Often clinical diagnosis.

MANAGEMENT: Supportive, anti-inflammatories. Symptoms usually lasts 7-10 days

COMPLICATIONS OF MUMPS: *MC seen in older patients:*
1. ***Orchitis in males**** (usually unilateral), oophoritis, encephalitis, aseptic meningitis.
2. ***Mumps MC cause of acute pancreatitis in children.*** Deafness, arthritis, infertility.

PREVENTION: **MMR Vaccine:** given at 12-15 months with a second dose at age 4-6y.

RUBEOLA (MEASLES)

<u>Transmission</u>: respiratory droplets, person to person, airborne. *Paramyxovirus.* ~10-12day IP.

CLINICAL MANIFESTATIONS
1. **URI prodrome:** *high fever, <u>3 Cs</u>: <u>C</u>ough, <u>C</u>oryza, <u>C</u>onjunctivitis ⇨ Kᴏᴘʟɪᴋ sᴘᴏᴛs* (small red spots in buccal mucosa with pale blue/white center)* precedes rash by 24-48h, lasts 2-3 days ⇨ *morbiliform (maculopapular) <u>brick-red</u>* rash on face beginning @ hairline* ⇨ extremities (palms & soles involvement usually seen last if it occurs) that darkens & coalesces.
2. ***Rash usually lasts 7 days*** fading from top to bottom. Fever often concurrent with the rash.

MANAGEMENT: Supportive, anti-inflammatories (no specific treatment).
Vitamin A reduces mortality in all children with measles (decreased morbidity & mortality).

COMPLICATIONS: *diarrhea, otitis media,* pneumonia, conjunctivitis & encephalitis.

RUBELLA (GERMAN MEASLES)

Rubella virus (Togavirus family). <u>Transmission</u>: respiratory droplets. ***"3 day rash."**** 2-3 week IP.

CLINICAL MANIFESTATIONS
1. *<u>Low-grade</u> fever, cough, anorexia, **lymphadenopathy (posterior cervical, posterior auricular)** ⇨ **pink, light-red spotted maculopapular rash** on face ⇨ extremities (lasts **3 days**).* Compared to rubeola, rubella spreads more rapidly & does not darken or coalesce.

   - <u>Forchheimer spots</u>: small red macules or petechiae on soft palate. (also seen in Scarlet fever).

2. ***Transient photosensitivity & joint pains may be seen (especially in young women).****

DIAGNOSIS: Clinical. Rubella-specific IgM antibody via enzyme immunoassay (MC used).

MANAGEMENT: anti-inflammatories, supportive.
   Generally no complications in children with Rubella (compared to Rubeola).

Teratogenic esp 1ˢᵗ trimester:* *congenital syndrome**- <u>sensorineural deafness</u>, cataracts, TTP ("blueberry muffin rash"), mental retardation,* heart defects (part of the TO<u>R</u>CH syndrome).

ERYTHEMA INFECTIOSUM (FIFTH DISEASE)

Parvovirus B19.* MC <10y. Transmission: respiratory droplets. 4-14 day incubation period (IP).

CLINICAL MANIFESTATIONS
1. Coryza, fever ⇨ ***"slapped cheek"**** rash on face with circumoral pallor 2-4 days ⇨ ***lacy reticular rash*** on extremities (especially upper). Spares the palms & soles. Resolves in 2-3 weeks.

2. ***Arthropathy/arthralgias: older children & adults.****
3. *Associated with ↑**fetal loss in pregnancy** (fetal hydrops, CHF, spontaneous abortion).*

DIAGNOSIS: serologies.

MANAGEMENT: supportive, anti-inflammatories.

PVB19 may cause aplastic crisis in patients with sickle cell disease* or G6PD deficiency.

Infectious diseases associated with arthropathy: *Erythema Infectiosum in older adults, Rubella (especially in young women), Coccidiomycosis (Valley fever also associated c erythema nodosum).*

ERYTHEMA TOXICUM

Thought to be due to immune system activation. Seen in up to 70% of neonates.

CLINICAL MANIFESTATIONS
Small erythematous macules or papules ⇨ pustules on erythematous bases 3-5 days after birth. Does not involve the palms or soles. Individual lesions may spontaneously disappear.

MANAGEMENT: self-limited. Usually resolves spontaneously in 1-2 weeks.

MILIARIA

- ***Blockage of eccrine sweat glands*** (especially in hot & humid conditions). This leads to sweat into the epidermis & dermis. Increased counts of skin flora (S. epidermis, S. aureus).

TYPES
1. **Miliaria crystallina:** tiny, friable clear vesicles (due to sweat in the superficial stratum corneum). ***MC in neonates*** (especially in 1 week old neonates).

2. **Miliaria rubra:** severely pruritic papules (may develop pustules). Deeper in the epidermis.

3. **Miliaria profunda:** flesh-colored papules (due to sweating in the papillary dermis).

MILIA

- ***1-2mm pearly white-yellow papules*** (due to keratin retention within the dermis of immature skin) ***especially seen on the cheeks, forehead, chin & nose***.

MANAGEMENT: none. Usually disappears by the 1st month of life (may be seen up to 3 months).

CAFÉ AU LAIT MACULES

- Uniformly hyperpigmented macules or patches with sharp demarcation. Either present at birth (or developing early in childhood). Varying colors from light brown to chocolate brown.

- Due to increased number of melanocytes & melanin in the epidermis.

- **Children with ≥6 Café au lait macules** (especially when accompanied with axillary or inguinal freckling) *should be evaluated for* **possible Neurofibromatosis type I.**

PORT-WINE STAINS (CAPILLARY MALFORMATION, NEVUS FLAMMEUS)

- Vascular malformations of the skin (due to superficial dilated dermal capillaries).

CLINICAL MANIFESTATIONS
Pink-red sharply demarcated, blanchable macules or papules in infancy. **Over time, they grow & darken to a purple (port-wine) color and may develop a thickened surface.**
- They occur most commonly on the head and neck. Usually unilateral or segmental.
- MC seen on the face but may occur anywhere. May be associated with other abnormalities (ex. glaucoma, spinal abnormalities).

MANAGEMENT
Pulse dye laser treatment (best if used in infancy for best outcomes).

STURGE-WEBER SYNDROME: *congenital disorder associated with* **classic triad: ❶facial port wine stain** (especially along trigeminal distribution area & around the eyelids) **❷leptomeningeal angiomatosis** & **❸ocular involvement** (ex. glaucoma). May develop hemiparesis contralateral to the facial lesion, seizures or intracranial calcification & learning disabilities.

MONGOLIAN SPOTS

- Congenital dermal melanocytosis due to mid-dermal melanocytes (melanin producing cells) that fail to migrate to the epidermis from the neural crest.
- May be seen in >80% of Asians & East Indian infants. Increased in African-Americans.

CLINICAL MANIFESTATIONS
Blue or slate gray pigmented macular lesions most commonly seen in presacral/sacral-gluteal area (may be seen on the shoulders, legs, back and posterior thighs as well) with indefinite borders. May be solitary or multiple.

Spots usually fade over the first few years of life (before 10 years of age).

NEVUS SIMPLEX (STORK BITE)

Areas of surface capillary dilation. MC seen on the nape of the neck, eyelids & forehead.
MANAGEMENT
1. Observation: most will resolve spontaneously by age 2 & don't usually darken over time.
2. Laser therapy will reduce the appearance of the lesions.

STAPHYLOCOCCAL SCALDED SKIN SYNDROME (RITTER DISEASE)

- **MC seen in infants** or children <5 years of age.

PATHOPHYSIOLOGY
- **Disseminated exfoliative exotoxins produced by Staphylococcus aureus** (esp. strains 71 & 55). These toxins may cause proteolysis & destruction of the intraepidermal desmosomes of the skin.

CLINICAL MANIFESTATIONS
1. Malaise, fever, irritability, extreme skin tenderness ⇨ **cutaneous, blanching erythema** - bright skin erythema often starting centrally & around the mouth before spreading diffusely. Erythema is worse in the flexor areas and around orifices – especially the mouth. After 1-2 days ⇨ develop sterile, flaccid **blisters** especially in areas of mechanical stress (hands, feet, flexural areas & buttocks ⇨ _POSITIVE NIKOLSKY SIGN:_* **separation of the dermis & rupture of the fragile blisters when gentle pressure is applied to the skin.** **Desquamative phase** – skin that easily ruptures, leaving moist, denuded skin before healing.

2. Inflamed conjunctiva may be seen (may become purulent) but _mucous membranes are not involved._

DIAGNOSIS
1. Clinical diagnosis. Intact bullae are sterile.
2. Cultures from urine, blood & nasopharynx. Skin biopsy: lower stratum granulosum layer splitting.

COMPLICATIONS
- Secondary infections: sepsis, pneumonia, cellulitis; Excessive fluid loss; Electrolyte imbalances

MANAGEMENT
1. Antibiotics: _**Penicillinase-resistant penicillin 1st line:**_* **Nafcillin or Oxacillin** ± Clindamycin Vancomycin if MRSA is suspected of if failed penicillin treatment.
2. Supportive skin care: maintain clean & moist skin, emollients to improve barrier function.
3. Fluid & electrolyte replacement.

SCARLET FEVER (SCARLATINA)

- Diffuse skin eruption that occurs in the setting of **GABHS (Streptococcus pyogenes) infection.**
- Due to Type IV (delayed) hypersensitivity reaction to a pyrogenic (erythrogenic toxin A, B or C).

CLINICAL MANIFESTATIONS
1. Fever, chills, **pharyngitis** ("Strep throat").

2. **Rash:** diffuse erythema that blanches with pressure plus many small (1 – 2 mm) papular elevations that feels like _**"SANDPAPER"**_ when palpated "sunburn with goosebumps". MC starts in the groin & axillae then rapidly spreads to the trunk and then the extremities. The _**rash often desquamates**_ over time (usually spares the palms & soles).
   - Often associated with a **flushed face with** CIRCUMORAL PALLOR & STRAWBERRY TONGUE.*
   - **Pastia's lines** = linear petechial lesions seen at pressure points, axillary, antecubital, abdominal or inguinal areas.

MANAGEMENT
Same as strep pharyngitis. May return to school 24 hours after antibiotic initiation.
1. **Penicillin G or VK 1st line.** Amoxicillin, Amoxicillin/clavulanic acid (Augmentin).
2. **Macrolides if PCN allergic.** Other alternatives include Clindamycin, Cephalosporins.

TURNER'S SYNDROME

- *Group of X chromosome abnormalities.* **Females with an absent/nonfunctional X sex chromosome.**
- 1 in every 2500 female newborns.

- **HALLMARKS:** hypogonadism ⇨ *primary amenorrhea or early ovarian failure,* * *delayed secondary sex characteristics* (absence of breasts), infertility, *short stature* (with normal growth hormone levels), *webbed neck, edema, low hairline, low set ears, widely spaced nipples.* Renal & cardiovascular abnormalities.

PATHOPHYSIOLOGY
- **Mosaicism:** (67-90%). Some cells have a combination of *X monosomy* (*45,XO* – missing X chromosome), some cells that are normal (46,XX), cells with partial monosomies (X/abnormal X), or cells that have a Y chromosome (46,XY).
- 45, X0 = absence/nonfunction of 1 of the X chromosome ⇨ gonadal dysgenesis.

CLINICAL MANIFESTATIONS
- **Hypogonadism:** absent/nonfunctional sex chromosome (45XO) ⇨ gonadal dysgenesis ⇨ rudimentary, fibrosed ovaries ⇨ *primary amenorrhea** in 80% (menopause before menarche) or *early ovarian failure* with secondary amenorrhea (20%), *delayed secondary sex characteristics* (absence of breasts), infertility in a majority of patients.

- **Physical Examination:** short stature, webbed neck, prominent ears, low posterior hairline, broad chest with hypoplastic widely-spaced nipples, (congenital lymphedema seen in neonates), short 4th metacarpals, high-arched palate, nail dysplasia. May have hearing loss.
- **Cardiovascular:** coarctation of the aorta (30%), mitral valve prolapse, bicuspid aortic valves, aortic dissection, hypertension.
- **Renal:** congenital abnormalities (ex horseshoe kidney), hydronephrosis.
- Endocrine: osteoporosis, hypothyroidism, Diabetes Mellitus, dyslipidemias.
- GI: telangiectasias (may present with GI bleeding), IBD, colon cancer, liver disease.

DIAGNOSIS:
1. *Karyotyping – definite diagnosis.* 45, XO, mosaicism, or X chromosome abnormalities.
2. High serum FSH & LH levels.

MANAGEMENT
1. Growth hormone replacement (may increase final height).
2. Estrogen/Progesterone replacement to cause pubertal development.

KLINEFELTER'S SYNDROME

- *Males with an extra X chromosome = 47, XXY* karyotype 80% (extra sex chromosome due to failure of separation of sex chromosome or translocation) ⇨ *males with HYPOGONADISM & SMALL TESTES.* *
- 1:800 births. MC chromosomal abnormality with hypogonadism.

CLINICAL MANIFESTATIONS
- Normal appearance before puberty onset ⇨ *tall stature* (thin & long-limbed with Eunochoid features). In adulthood, they become obese. ±scoliosis, ataxia, mild development delays, expressive language disorders. Increased risk of testicular cancer.
- *Hypogonadism: small testicles* & infertility (azoospermia), gynecomastia, scarce pubic hair.

DIAGNOSIS
- 47, XXY karyotype, low serum testosterone. Testosterone may help with secondary sex characteristics.

FRAGILE X SYNDROME

- X-linked genetic disorder that is the MC gene related cause of autism. The loss of function of the fragile X mental retardation 1 gene ⇨ lack of the production of the Fragile X mental retardation protein.

CLINICAL MANIFESTATIONS
- Younger males: mitral valve prolapse, hyperextensible joints, hypotonia, soft skin, flexible flat feet, macrocephaly.
- Older males: long and narrow face, prominent forehead & chin, large ears, *macroorchidism** (enlarged testicles).
- Behavioral: wide range of manifestations expressive language deficits > receptive.

DOWN SYNDROME (TRISOMY 21)

- Three copies of chromosome 21 (Trisomy 21) or 3 copies of a region of the long arm of chromosome 21.

CLINICAL MANIFESTATIONS
- Head & neck: low-set small ears, flat facial profile/flat nasal bridge, open mouth, protruding tongue, upslanting palpebral fissures, folded or dysplastic ears, brachycephalic, epicanthic folds, excessive skin at the nape of the neck, short neck. **Brushfield spots:** white/gray/brown spots on the iris.
- Extremities: transverse, single *palmar (Simian) crease,** hyperflexibility of the joints, short broad hands, increased space between the 1st & 2nd toes (sandal gap).
- Neonates: Poor Moro reflex, dysplasia of the pelvis, hypotonia, anomalous ears. May develop a transient neonatal leukemia.
- Intellectual impairment: wide range of presentation.
- *Congenital heart disease: atrioventricular septal defects*, ventricular septal defect, atrial septal defect, tetralogy of Fallot, patent ductus arteriosus.
- GI: duodenal atresia or stenosis, Hirschsprung disease.

EHLERS DANLOS SYNDROME (EDS)

- *Genetic disorder of collagen synthesis* leading to *skin hyperextensibility, fragile connective tissue, joint hypermobility.*
- 6 major types (ex classic, hypermobility, vascular, kyphoscoliosis, arthrochalasia, dermatosparaxis).

PATHOPHYSIOLOGY
1. *Abnormal production of collagen* (especially type IV) affecting tendons, ligaments, skin, blood vessels, eyes & other organs. *Aneurysm rupture is a common cause of death.*

CLINICAL MANIFESTATIONS
1. *SKIN HYPEREXTENSIBILITY** (ability to stretch skin >4cm in areas such as neck & forearm). Hyperextensibility increases with age.

2. **Fragile connective tissue:** *mitral valve prolapse.* Classic skin findings: *smooth velvety/doughy fragile skin** (*skin bruises easily** or may split with trauma, widened atrophic scars, delayed wound healing). Upper eyelid may evert easily (**Metenier's sign**).

3. *Joint hypermobility:* joint dislocations & subluxations, pes planus, pectus excavatum. May develop myopia.

MARFAN SYNDROME

- Systemic connective tissue disease (autosomal dominant) ⇨ *cardiovascular, ocular & musculoskeletal findings* in addition to multi-systemic involvement. Autosomal-dominant.

PATHOPHYSIOLOGY

- Mutation of the fibrillin-1 gene ⇨ TGFb (transforming growth factor beta) mutation & misfolding of the protein fibrillin-1, leading to **weakened connective tissues**.

CLINICAL MANIFESTATIONS

1. **Cardiovascular:** *mitral valve prolapse* (85%), **aortic root dilation** ⇨ *aortic regurgitation, aortic dissection & aortic aneurysms. Associated with progressive aortic dilation.**
2. **Musculoskeletal:** *TALL STATURE**, arachnodactyly (*long, lanky fingers, arms & legs*), scoliosis, anterior chest deformities: *PECTUS CARINATUM** (protrusion of chest and ribs/pigeon chest) or excavatum (breastbone appears sunken in chest). Spontaneous pneumothorax. *Joint laxity*
3. **Ocular:** *ECTOPIA LENTIS** (malposition or dislocation of the lens of the eyes) ⇨ reduced vision extreme nearsightedness (**myopia**).

Common in MS & EDS: aortic dilation, scoliosis, joint hypermobility/laxity, autosomal dominance.
Marfan only: tall stature, lens dislocation, pectus carinatum, overgrowth of the long bones, lack of the classic skin findings seen in EDS.

FETAL ALCOHOL SYNDROME

- Due to maternal alcohol use during pregnancy.

CLINICAL MANIFESTATIONS

- Children are often born small and remain relatively small throughout their lifetime. Associated with developmental delays & congenital abnormalities of internal organs.
- **Small physical findings:** microcephaly, thin upper lip, long & smooth philtrum, small palpebral fissures & small distal phalanges.

NEURAL TUBE DEFECTS

- *Associated with maternal folate deficiency* - decreased maternal folate intake, medications that inhibit folate (ex. Methotrexate, Valproic acid, Phenytoin, Sulfasalazine).

CLINICAL MANIFESTATIONS: sensory deficits, paralysis, hydrocephalus, hypotonia.

ANENCEPHALY: failure of closure of the portion of the neural tube that becomes the cerebrum.
SPINA BIFIDA:
- Incomplete closure of the embryonic neural tube ⇨ non-fusion of some of the vertebrae overlying the spinal cord ⇨ may lead to protrusion of the spinal cord through the opening. MC seen at the lumbar & sacral areas of the spine. 3 types:
- **Spina bifida with myelomeningocele:** *MC type. Meninges & spinal cord herniates through* the gap in the vertebrae. Often leads to disability in most cases.
- Spina bifida occulta: mildest form. No herniation of the spinal cord (the defects are too small for the spinal cord to herniate through). Overlying skin ± normal, have some hair growing over it, dimpling of the skin or birthmark over the affected area.
- Spina bifida with meningocele: only meninges herniate through the gap in the vertebrae.

DETECTION

↑*maternal serum α–fetoprotein* ⇨ amniocentesis: ↑*α–fetoprotein* & ↑*acetylcholinesterase*.

PRADER-WILLI SYNDROME

- Characterized by *prenatal hypotonia, postnatal growth delay, development disabilities, hypogonadotrophic hypogonadism & obesity after infancy.*

PATHOPHYSIOLOGY

- 75% occurs due to *small deletion/inexpression of genes on the paternal chromosome 15* (15q 11-13) from loss of *paternal copy* of a region of chromosome 15 is seen in up to 75%. The maternal copy of the gene is silenced through imprinting. Majority of cases occur sporadically.

- 25% occurs due to maternal uniparental disomy (a person receives 2 copies of a chromosome or part of a chromosome from one parent & no copies from the other parent).

CLINICAL MANIFESTATIONS

1. **Prenatal:** breech positioning, polyhadramnios (excess amniotic fluid) & reduced fetal movement.

2. **Neonates:** *severe hypotonia*: *floppy baby*, weak cry, newborns have *feeding difficulties:* trouble swallowing & suckling, making nasogastric feeding a necessity. Genital hypoplasia, *cryptorchidism*, depigmentation of the skin & eyes, excessive sleeping, strabismus. Usually small for gestational age and often have almond-shaped eyes.

3. **Early childhood:** during the first year of life, muscle tone improves and children develop a voracious appetite/*hyperphagia* (may have aggressive behavior especially related to eating) that leads to *obesity* if food intake is not controlled. Major milestone & intellectual delays. They often have short stature and reduced levels of growth hormone production. They often develop behavioral & learning difficulties. Skin picking is increased in these patients. Patients may have lighter skin & hair (relative to other family members).

4. **Late childhood/adolescence:** premature development of pubic & axillary hair with delay of the other secondary sex characteristics. Increased incidence of epilepsy & scoliosis.

5. **Adulthood:** sterility is almost universal in women.

PHYSICAL EXAMINATION

- Almond-shaped eyes, high/narrow forehead, thin upper lip with small, down-turned mouth; prominent nasal bridges. Small feet & hands (with tapering of the fingers). Soft skin that easily bruises (may have extreme flexibility). Excess fat (especially *truncal obesity*).

DIAGNOSIS

- DNA testing (DNA-based methylation studies).

MANAGEMENT

Growth hormone replacement, obesity control by monitoring food intake

BECKWITH-WIEDEMANN SYNDROME

- Abnormal gene expression affecting the chromosome 11p15.5 region.
- Large for gestational age, organomegaly, macroglossia, hypoglycemia in infancy, earlobe creases & pits, asymmetric limbs. *Increased risk of the hepatoblastoma & Wilm's tumor.*

NEUROBLASTOMA

- Cancer of the peripheral sympathetic nervous system. 3rd MC pediatric cancer (90% diagnosed by age 5y. ***MC in adrenal medulla & paraspinal region.***

CLINICAL MANIFESTATIONS: depends on tumor site. MC in abdomen (firm, irregular, nodular abdomen or flank mass), ***ataxia, opsoclonus myoclonus syndrome*** (hypsarrhythmia/rapid "dancing eyes" & myoclonus/"dancing feet" – jerky movements), hypertension (especially diastolic), diarrhea.
DIAGNOSIS: CT scan: tumor often with calcification & hemorrhaging. ↑vanillylmandelic acid.
MANAGEMENT: surgery, chemotherapy or radiation depending on stage of disease & site of the tumor.

NEUROFIBROMATOSIS TYPE 1 (von Recklinghausen's disease)

- Autosomal dominant ***neurocutaneous disorder*** due to a mutated NF1 gene (chromosome 17q11.2 region) encoding for the protein neurofibromin (a tumor suppressor). ***MC type*** (90%).

PATHOPHYSIOLOGY:
- Loss of neurofibromin ⇨ increased risk of developing benign and malignant tumors. Mutations are highly variable between patients with NF1 and can appear at any age.

CLINICAL MANIFESTATIONS
- requires at least 2 of the following:
  - ***≥6 café-au-lait spots***: flat, uniformly hypopigmented macules that appear during the first year of birth and increase in number during early childhood.
  - ***Freckling:*** *especially* ***axillary or inguinal*** *freckling.* May also be seen in intertriginous areas, & the neckline. Not usually present at birth but often appears by age 3 to 5 years.
  - ***Lisch nodules of the iris****:* hamartomas of the iris seen on slit lamp examination.* Often elevated and tan-colored.
  - *≥2 neurofibromas or ≥1 plexiform neurofibroma.* Neurofibromas are focal, benign peripheral nerve sheath tumors (often a combination of Schwann cells, fibroblasts, perineural cells and mast cells) described as small, rubbery lesions with a slight purplish discoloration of the overlying skin. Neurofibromas typically involve the skin but may be seen along peripheral nerves, blood vessels and viscera. Plexiform neurofibromas are located longitudinally along a nerve and involve multiple fascicles (may produce an overgrowth of an extremity).
  - ***Optic pathway gliomas***: may involve the optic nerve, optic chiasm, and/or postchiasmal optic tracts. Most commonly occurs in younger children (ex. <6 years of age). May develop an afferent pupillary defect. If the tumor is large and involves the hypothalamus, it may be associated with delayed or premature onset of puberty.
  - Others: osseous lesions: scoliosis is common (especially thoracic spine), sphenoid dysplasia, long bone abnormalities. 1st degree relative with NF1 or short stature.

NEUROIMAGING
- **MRI:** *unidentified bright objects* = hyperintense T2-weighted signals (may be due to demyelination or focal areas of increased water content). Seen most commonly in the basal ganglia, brainstem, cerebellum and subcortical white matter. There are no associated neurologic deficits. Increased brain volume often seen.

MANAGEMENT
- Optic pathway glioma: regular annual ophthalmologic screening. If any symptoms occur, an MRI of the brain & orbits should be performed.
- Neurofibromas: not removed unless there are associated complications.

NEUROFIBROMATOSIS TYPE 2

- Autosomal dominant associated with multiple CNS tumors *[bilateral CN VIII tumors* (also known as schwannomas, vestibular neuromas or acoustic neuromas), spinal tumors & intracranial tumors.

PATHOPHYSIOLOGY
- Mutation of the NF2 tumor suppressor gene (which normally produces the protein schwannomin aka merlin).

CLINICAL MANIFESTATIONS
1. **Neurologic lesions:**
   - *BILATERAL VESTIBULAR SCHWANNOMAS** (95%). Most develop by 30 years of age - hearing loss (usually gradual & progressive), tinnitus, and balance disturbances. Over a period of time, they can expand, causing hydrocephalus & brainstem compression.
   - Meningiomas: often multiple (especially in childhood), spinal & intramedullary tumors, neuropathy.
2. **Optic lesions:** cataracts (may cause visual impairment early in childhood), retinal hamartomas.
3. **Skin lesions:**
   - Cutaneous tumors, skin plaques (slightly raised and may be hyperpigmented), subcutaneous tumors that presents as nodules. Café-au-lait spots are seen with less frequency in NF2.

MANAGEMENT
1. **Vestibular schwannomas:**
   - Surgery may be needed for complicated or symptomatic tumors.
   - Bevacizumab: may cause shrinkage of the tumor and improvement in hearing.
     MOA: monoclonal antibody against vascular endothelial growth factor (VEGF).

TAY-SACHS DISEASE

- Rare, autosomal recessive genetic disorder most common in Ashkenazi Jewish families of Eastern European descent, Cajuns in Southern Louisiana & French Canadians.

PATHOPHYSIOLOGY
- Mutation of the HEXA gene on chromosome 15 ⇨ deficiency in β-hexosaminidase A ⇨ accumulation of gangliosides in the brain ⇨ premature neuron death & progressive degeneration of neurons.

CLINICAL MANIFESTATIONS
- **Infantile onset:** increased startle reaction, loss of motor skills. At 4-5 months of age ⇨ decreased eye contact, hyperacusis (exaggerated startle reaction to noise), paralysis, blindness, progressive developmental retardation & dementia. 2nd year: seizures and neurodegeneration. Death usually occurs between 3-4 years.
- **Juvenile onset:** symptoms occur between the ages of 2-10y ⇨ cognitive and motor skill deterioration, dysphagia, ataxia, spasticity. Death often occurs between the ages of 5-15y.
- **Adult onset:** usually develops symptoms during the 30s and 40s. Usually presents with unsteady, spastic gait and progressive neurological deterioration (leading to speech, swallowing difficulties), psychosis.

PHYSICAL EXAMINATION
- Retinal examination: *cherry-red spots with macular pallor.* Macrocephaly.

DIAGNOSIS: enzymatic assay.

MANAGEMENT
- No effective treatment.

TYPES OF VACCINES

1. LIVE, ATTENUATED VACCINES:

Contains a live, weakened version of the organism. Because it is the safest, closest thing to actually having the infection, it induces a good immune response of both *humoral (antibody) immunity* & *cell-mediated immunity*. No booster usually need. Cons: they are unstable & must be refrigerated. Because they may become virulent, **live attenuated vaccines are not given to immunocompromised or pregnant patients.***

- **_MMR._** *The only live, attenuated vaccine that can be given to HIV patients (if CD4 >200/µL).*
- **_Chicken pox (Varicella Zoster), Rotavirus._**
- Smallpox, yellow fever, oral typhoid, Franciscella tularensis, oral polio.

2. KILLED (INACTIVATED) VACCINES:

Killed organisms. These stimulate a weaker immune response compared to live attenuated vaccines so they only induce a humoral (antibody) immunity - may need booster shots.

- **_Influenza, Rabies, Polio Sal<u>K</u> (K= killed_** - this is the primary form used in US), Vibrio cholerae, **_Hepatitis A Vaccine._**

3. SUBUNIT CONJUGATE VACCINES:

Presents only the essential antigens needed to induce an immune system response (instead of giving the whole organism). Often contain multiple antigens that are linked or "conjugated" to toxoids or antigens that the immature immune system will recognize to identify bacterium that use their polysaccharide outer coating as a defense. **Made of capsular polysaccharides** so often used for many **_encapsulated organisms "SHiN"._**

- **_S._** *pneumococcal* (infant version is conjugated so induces a helper T cell response).
- **_H_** *influenza* (capsular polysaccharide), **_N._** *meningitidis*, PCV13 (pneumococcal vaccine).

4. SUBUNIT RECOMBINANT VACCINES:

A type of subunit vaccine in which recombinant DNA technology is used to manufacture the antigen molecules. Genes that encode for the important antigens are placed into Baker's yeast. The yeast reproduces the antigens that are processed & purified.

- **_Hepatitis B vaccine_** (HBsAg), **_HPV vaccine_** (6,11,16 & 18).

5. TOXOID VACCINES:

Chemically modified inactivated toxins from toxin-producing organisms to allow the body to recognize the harmless toxin. Later it has the ability to attack the natural toxin if exposed to it.

- **_Tetanus, Diphtheria, Pertussis_**

VACCINE CONTRAINDICATIONS

- **Baker's yeast:** *Hepatitis B*** should be avoided (Think <u>B</u> for <u>B</u>aker's yeast & Hepatitis <u>B</u>).
- **Eggs:** influenza vaccine should be avoided.
- **Gelatin:** avoid varicella, influenza vaccines.
- **Thimerosal:** preservative used in vaccines so should be avoided in multi-dose vaccines.
- **Neomycin & Streptomycin allergy:** _MMR_ (Measles Mumps Rubella) & **_inactivated Polio vaccine_** should be avoided (Neomycin & Streptomycin are preservatives in these vaccines).

PREGNANCY

Only vaccines safely given in pregnancy: diphtheria, tetanus, inactivated influenza, HBV.

Avoid live vaccines:

- *Live vaccines:* MMR, Varicella, Polio.
- *Live attenuated vaccines: intranasal influenza vaccine.*

Figure 1. Recommended immunization schedule for persons aged 0 through 18 years – United States, 2016.
(FOR THOSE WHO FALL BEHIND OR START LATE, SEE THE CATCH-UP SCHEDULE [FIGURE 2]).
These recommendations must be read with the footnotes that follow. For those who fall behind or start late, provide catch-up vaccination at the earliest opportunity as indicated by the green bars in Figure 1.
To determine minimum intervals between doses, see the catch-up schedule (Figure 2). School entry and adolescent vaccine age groups are shaded.

Vaccine	Birth	1 mo	2 mos	4 mos	6 mos	9 mos	12 mos	15 mos	18 mos	19–23 mos	2-3 yrs	4-6 yrs	7-10 yrs	11–12 yrs	13–15 yrs	16–18 yrs
Hepatitis B¹ (HepB)	1ˢᵗ dose	←— 2ⁿᵈ dose —→			←———————— 3ʳᵈ dose ————————————→											
Rotavirus² (RV) RV1 (2-dose series); RV5 (3-dose series)			1ˢᵗ dose	2ⁿᵈ dose	See footnote 2											
Diphtheria, tetanus, & acellular pertussis³ (DTaP: <7 yrs)			1ˢᵗ dose	2ⁿᵈ dose	3ʳᵈ dose		←———— 4ᵗʰ dose ————→					5ᵗʰ dose				
Haemophilus influenzae type b⁴ (Hib)			1ˢᵗ dose	2ⁿᵈ dose	See footnote 4		3ʳᵈ or 4ᵗʰ dose, See footnote 4									
Pneumococcal conjugate⁵ (PCV13)			1ˢᵗ dose	2ⁿᵈ dose	3ʳᵈ dose		←———— 4ᵗʰ dose ————→									
Inactivated poliovirus⁶ (IPV: <18 yrs)			1ˢᵗ dose	2ⁿᵈ dose	←——————————— 3ʳᵈ dose ———————————→							4ᵗʰ dose				
Influenza⁷ (IIV; LAIV)					←———————— Annual vaccination (IIV only) 1 or 2 doses ————————→						←— Annual vaccination (LAIV or IIV) 1 or 2 doses —→		←——— Annual vaccination (LAIV or IIV) 1 dose only ———→			
Measles, mumps, rubella⁸ (MMR)						See footnote 8	←—— 1ˢᵗ dose ——→					2ⁿᵈ dose				
Varicella⁹ (VAR)							←—— 1ˢᵗ dose ——→					2ⁿᵈ dose				
Hepatitis A¹⁰ (HepA)						←————— 2-dose series, See footnote 10 ————→										
Meningococcal¹¹ (Hib-MenCY ≥ 6 weeks; MenACWY-D ≥9 mos; MenACWY-CRM ≥ 2 mos)			←——————————————— See footnote 11 ———————————————→											1ˢᵗ dose		Booster
Tetanus, diphtheria, & acellular pertussis¹² (Tdap: ≥7 yrs)														(Tdap)		
Human papillomavirus¹³ (2vHPV: females only; 4vHPV, 9vHPV: males and females)														(3-dose series)		
Meningococcal B¹¹														←——— See footnote 11 ———→		
Pneumococcal polysaccharide⁵ (PPSV23)												←——————— See footnote 5 ———————→				

	Range of recommended ages for all children		Range of recommended ages for catch-up immunization		Range of recommended ages for certain high-risk groups		Range of recommended ages for non-high-risk groups that may receive vaccine, subject to individual clinical decision making		No recommendation

This schedule includes recommendations in effect as of January 1, 2016. Any dose not administered at the recommended age should be administered at a subsequent visit, when indicated and feasible. The use of a combination vaccine generally is preferred over separate injections of its equivalent component vaccines. Vaccination providers should consult the relevant Advisory Committee on Immunization Practices (ACIP) statement for detailed recommendations, available online at http://www.cdc.gov/vaccines/hcp/acip-recs/index.html. Clinically significant adverse events that follow vaccination should be reported to the Vaccine Adverse Event Reporting System (VAERS) online (http://www.vaers.hhs.gov) or by telephone (800-822-7967). Suspected cases of vaccine-preventable diseases should be reported to the state or local health department. Additional information, including precautions and contraindications for vaccination, is available from CDC online

TANNER STAGE	2	3	4	5
Males	Age 11 - 12	Age 13	Age 14 – 15	Age 16-17
Pubic hair	Straight pubic hair at the base of penis	Coarse dark and curly pubic hair	Hair is almost completely full	Pubic hair achieves adult appearance
Females	Age 11	Age 12	Age 13	Age 14-15
Pubic Hair	Minimal straight pubic hair (long, downy)	Increased pubic hair (dark & coarse) lateral extension	Adult-like extends across pubis	Adult appearance (extends to medial thighs)
Breast	Breast buds palpable, areola enlarge	Elevation of areola contour, areola enlargement	Secondary mound of areola & papilla	Adult breast contour

TANNER STAGES

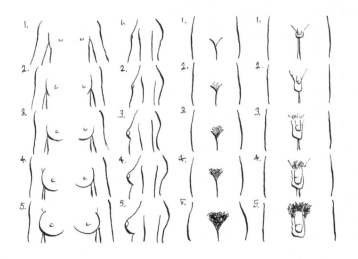

INDEX

Check out the interactive website www.pancepreppearls.com for extra chapters, radiology case studies, practice questions, blogs, videos and more to come!

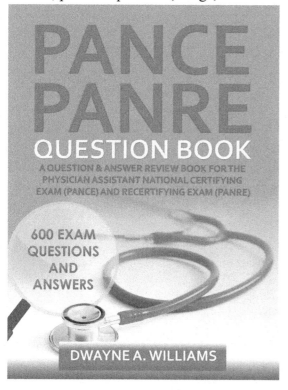

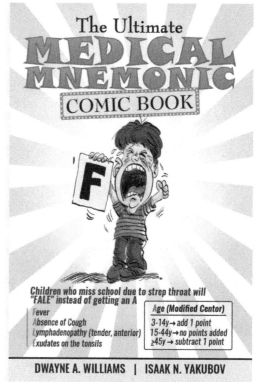

Earn 20 AAPA-approved Category 1 Self-assessment CME with the QUESTION BOOK!

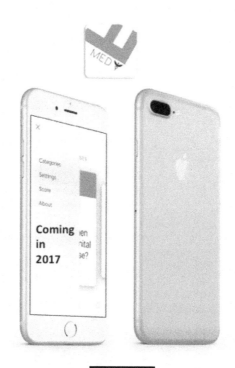

Made in the USA
Columbia, SC
02 February 2018